AF834641

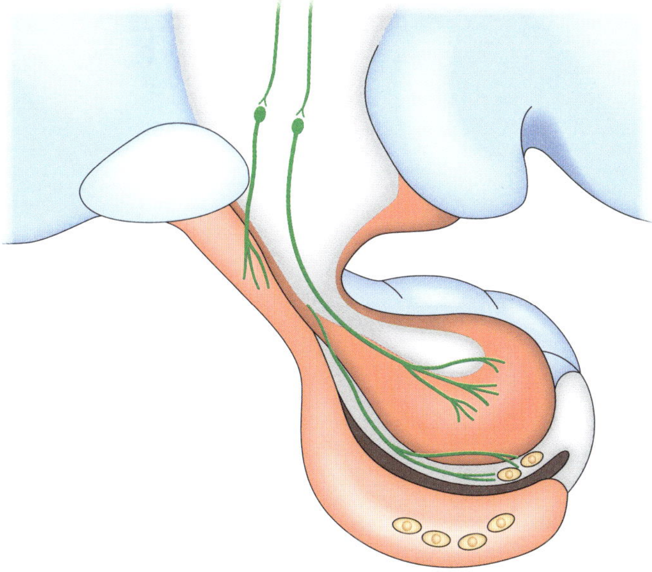

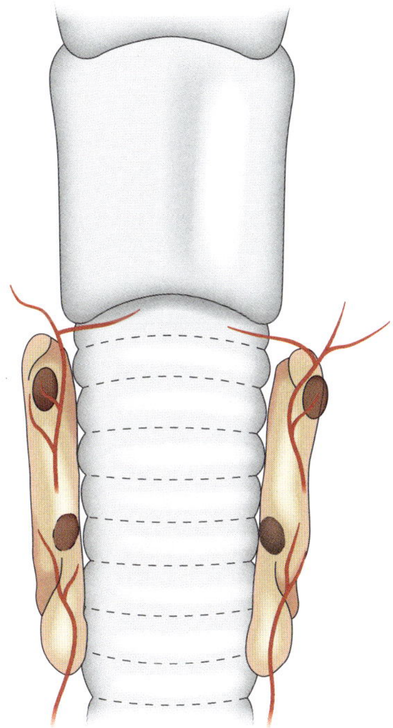

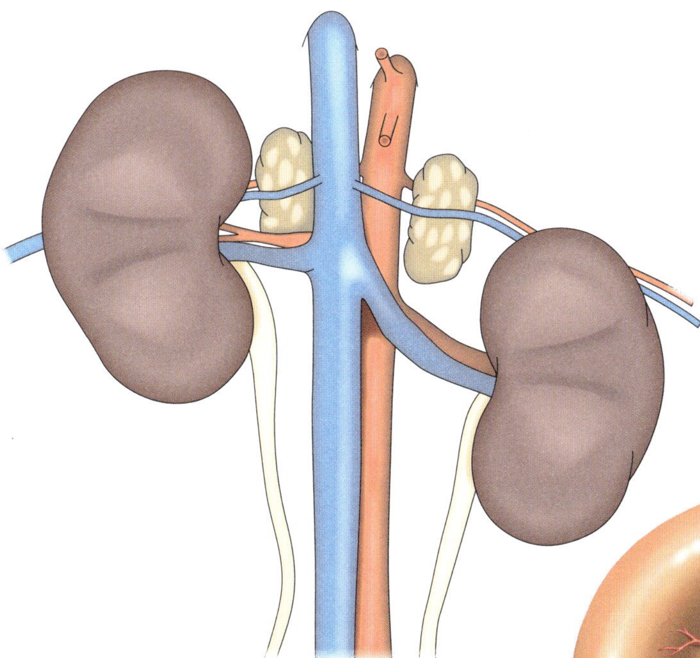

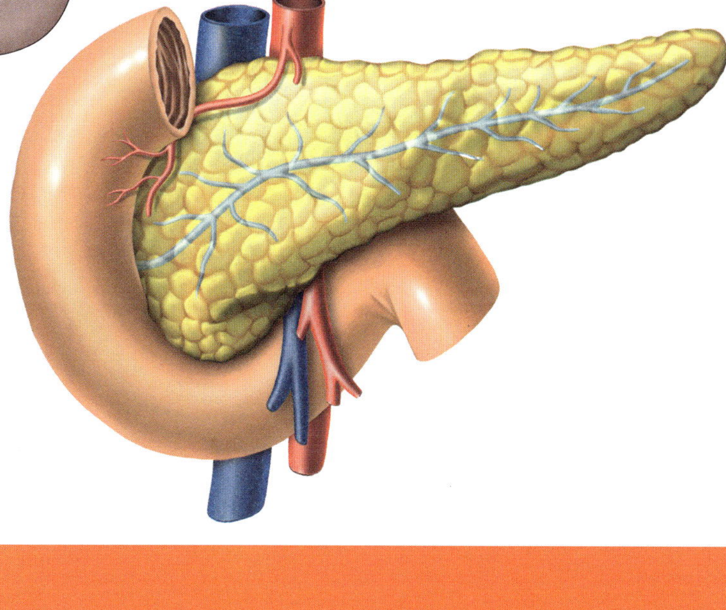

VETERINARY
INTERNAL
MEDICINE

EDITORS-IN-CHIEF
EDWARD FELDMAN
FEDERICO FRACASSI

CANINE ENDOCRINOLOGY

EDITORS

Sara Galac
Federico Fracassi

edra
PUBLISHING

VETERINARY INTERNAL MEDICINE SERIES - Edward Feldman, Federico Fracassi. Editors-in-chief.
Sara Galac, Federico Fracassi - Canine endocrinology

ISBN: 978-1-957260-45-7
eISBN: 978-1-957260-64-8

Book Publishing Manager: Costanza Smeraldi

Paper, printing and Binding Manager: Paolo Ficicchia

Cover: Laura Barzacca

Layout: T&T studio s.a.s, Milano

Copyediting: Mercedes González Fernández de Castro – Science & Health Publications

edra
PUBLISHING

Edra Publishing US LLC
3309 Northlake Boulevard
Suite 203, Palm Beach Gardens
FL, 33403
EIN: 844113980
info@edrapublishing.com
www.edrapublishing.com

Printed in Italy by "Erregiemme printing" S.r.l., August 2024

Series editors

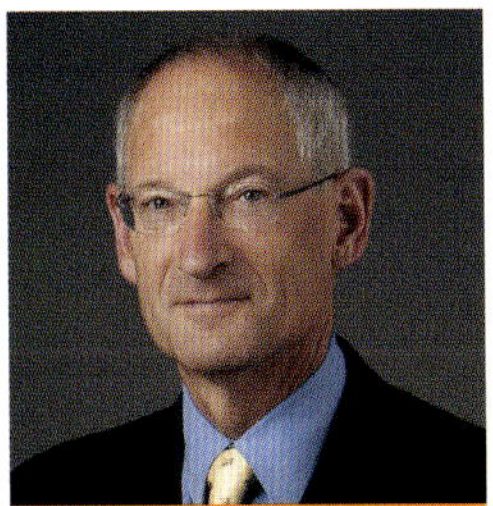

Edward C. Feldman
DVM, ACVIM Diplomate (SAIM), Emeritus Professor of Small Animal Internal Medicine,
University of California, Davis, USA

Dr. Feldman earned his DVM from the University of California in 1973. He joined the Davis faculty in 1979 after an internship at the Animal Medical Center in New York City, a Residency with Dr. Stephen Ettinger in the world's first referral only private veterinary practice in Berkeley California, a year in general practice and another on faculty at the University of Saskatchewan, in Canada. He has authored more than 160 peer-reviewed scientific publications, 110 scientific abstracts, and 75 book chapters.

Dr. Feldman has coedited the last six editions of The Textbook of Veterinary Internal Medicine with Dr. Stephen Ettinger and the last two also with Dr. Etienne Côté. He coauthored the four editions of Canine and Feline Endocrinology with Dr. Richard Nelson and the 4th edition also with Drs. Claudia Reusch, Catharine Scott-Moncrieff, and Ellen Behrend. He coedited Feline Endocrinology with Dr. Fracassi and Dr. Peterson.

Dr. Feldman has lectured in more than 45 of the 50 United States and 43 countries.

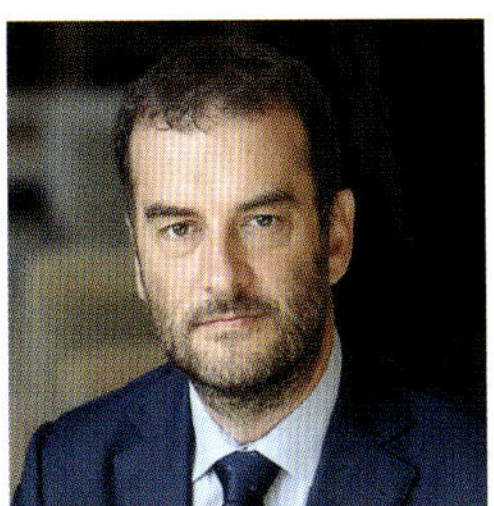

Federico Fracassi
DVM, ECVIM Diplomate (SAIM)
Professor of Small Animal Internal Medicine
University of Bologna, Italy

Dr. Fracassi graduated in Veterinary Medicine (DVM) at the University of Bologna, Italy. In 2005 he defended his PhD thesis and then completed a Residency in Internal Medicine at the University of Zurich, Switzerland.

He is now an Associate Professor of Veterinary Internal Medicine at the University of Bologna. His publication list consists of more than 100 journal articles.

He is the editor of "Veterinaria", a peer-reviewed journal and associate editor of JSAP. He coedited Feline Endocrinology with Dr. Feldman and Dr. Peterson. He has edited the book "Diagnostic and therapeutic algorithms in internal medicine for dogs and cats".

Dr. Fracassi has lectured in 22 countries.

Book editor

Sara Galac

DVM, PhD
Department of Clinical Sciences
Faculty of Veterinary Medicine
Utrecht University
The Netherlands

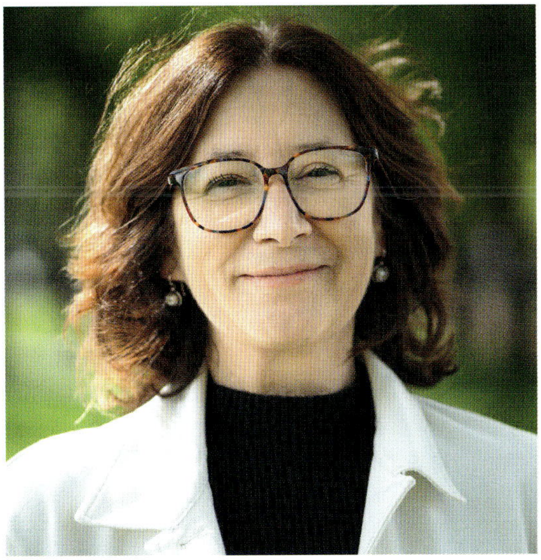

Sara Galac graduated from the Veterinary Faculty in Ljubljana, Slovenia. After graduation, she moved to the Netherlands and completed an internship and residency at the Department of Clinical Sciences, Faculty of Veterinary Medicine in Utrecht, the Netherlands. She completed her first PhD thesis on the use of a progesterone receptor antagonist in dogs at the University of Ljubljana in 2001. Her second PhD, about Cushing's syndrome in dogs, she successfully defended at Utrecht University in 2010.

Nowadays, she is a staff member of the Department of Clinical Sciences, Faculty of Veterinary Medicine in Utrecht. She holds the position of associate professor and leads the veterinary oncology research group. Her main interest is endocrinology. She is involved in clinical work and teaching, and in her research, she focuses on pituitary and adrenal tumors.

Her publication list includes journal articles, research abstracts, case reports, and book chapters. She is a frequent speaker at veterinary conferences and is involved in continuing education. She also served as president of the European Society of Veterinary Endocrinology (ESVE).

Federico Fracassi

DVM, ECVIM Diplomate (SAIM)
Professor of Small Animal Internal Medicine
University of Bologna, Italy

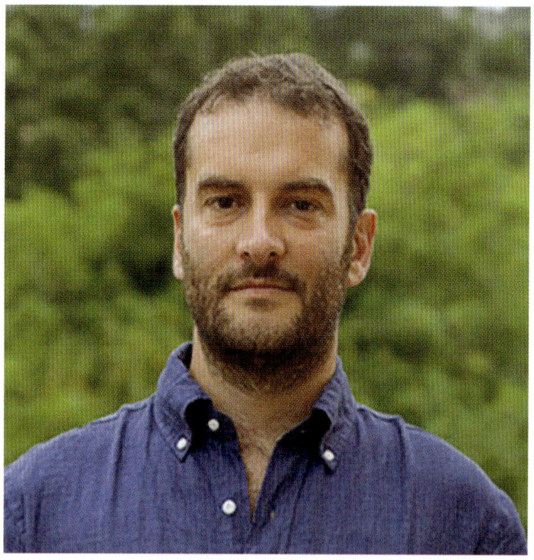

Federico Fracassi graduated in Veterinary Medicine (DVM) "cum laude" at the University of Bologna, Italy. He did an internship and started a Ph.D. at the same veterinary school, and defended his Ph.D. thesis in 2005. After the Ph.D., he became a permanent staff member at the Department of Veterinary Medical Sciences – University of Bologna (Italy) where at present he is Associate Professor of Internal Medicine. He completed a Residency in Internal Medicine at the Clinic for Small Animal Internal Medicine, University of Zurich, Switzerland, and gained his status of European Specialist in Internal Medicine in 2012 (Diplomate ECVIM-CA-internal medicine). Dr. Fracassi's duties include patient care, education (to students, postgraduate training, and training of interns and residents), and research in internal medicine of companion animals, with special emphasis on endocrinology. He is the past-president of the European Society of Veterinary Endocrinology (ESVE), past-president of the Italian Society of Veterinary Internal Medicine (SIMIV), and board member of the executive committee of the ECVIM-CA congress. He is editor of "Veterinaria", a peer-review journal, and associate editor of the Journal of Small Animal Practice. His publication list consists of more than 100 journal articles, research abstracts, case reports, and book chapters. He coedited Feline Endocrinology with Dr. Feldman and Dr. Peterson. He has edited the book "Diagnostic and therapeutic algorithms in internal medicine for dogs and cats".
Dr. Fracassi has lectured in 22 countries.

Contributors

Francesco Albanese, DVM
Centro Dermatologico Veterinario Toscano
Arezzo, Italy
CDVet - Laboratorio Analisi Veterinarie
Roma, Italy

Carolina Arenas, DVM, PhD, DECVIM-CA (Internal Medicine)
AniCura Valencia Sur Veterinary Hospital
Valencia, Spain
VetCT, Cambridge, UK

Ghita Benchekroun, DVM, DECVIM-CA (Internal medicine), PhD
École Nationale Vétérinaire d'Alfort
Maisons-Alfort, France

Jérôme Benoit, DVM, MRCVS, DACVR-Radiation Oncology, DECVDI-Radiation Oncology
Clinique Vétérinaire Oncovet
Villeneuve d'Ascq, France
IVC Evidensia France
Courbevoie, France

Felicitas S. Boretti, Prof., Dr. med. vet., FVH, DACVIM, DECVIM-CA (Internal Medicine)
Clinic for Small Animal Internal Medicine, Vetsuisse Faculty
University of Zurich
Zurich, Switzerland

Charlotte Bjørnvad, DVM, PhD, DECVCN
Department of Veterinary Clinical Sciences
University of Copenhagen
Copenhagen, Denmark

Miguel Campos, DVM, PhD, DECVIM-CA (Internal Medicine)
AniCura Medisch Centrum voor Dieren
Amsterdam, The Netherlands

Roberto Chiocchetti, DVM, PhD
Department of Veterinary Medical Sciences
Alma Mater Studiorum - University of Bologna
Ozzano Emilia (BO), Italy

Andrea Corsini, DVM, PhD, DECVIM-CA (Internal Medicine)
Department of Veterinary Medical Sciences
University of Parma
Parma, Italy

Sylvie Daminet, DVM, PhD, DACVIM, DECVIM-CA (Internal Medicine)
Small Animal Department, Faculty of Veterinary Medicine
University of Ghent
Ghent, Belgium

Lucy Davison, MA, VetMB, PhD, DSAM, DECVIM-CA (Internal Medicine), MRVCS
Department of Clinical Science and Services
Royal Veterinary College
Hawkshead, United Kingdom

Viviani De Marco, DVM PhD
VetUnity Specialties, Endocrinology Service
Sao Paulo, Brazil

Francesca Del Baldo, DVM, MRCVS, PhD, DECVIM-CA (Internal Medicine)
Department of Veterinary Medical Sciences
Alma Mater Studiorum - University of Bologna
Ozzano Emilia (BO), Italy

Sara Del Magno, DVM, PhD, DECVS
Department of Veterinary Medical Sciences
Alma Mater Studiorum - University of Bologna
Ozzano Emilia (BO), Italy

M.M. Diaz Espineira, DVM, PhD, DECVIM-CA (Internal Medicine)
Department of Clinical Sciences, Faculty of Veterinary Medicine
Utrecht University
Utrecht, The Netherlands

Edward C. Feldman, DVM, DACVIM (SAIM)
Emeritus Professor of Small Animal Internal Medicine
University of California
Davis, USA

Linda Fleeman, BVSc, PhD, MANZCVS
Animal Diabetes Australia
Mulgrave, Australia

Paula García San José, DVM, PhD
Department of Medicine and Animal Surgery
Complutense University of Madrid
Madrid, Spain

Alexander German, BVSc(Hons), PhD, CertSAM, DECVIM-CA (Internal Medicine), SFHEA, FRCVS
Institute of Life Course and Medical Sciences
University of Liverpool
Neston, UK

Chen Gilor, DVM, PhD, DACVIM (SAIM)
Department of Small Animal Clinical Sciences, College of Veterinary Medicine
University of Florida
Gainesville, FL (USA)

Stefania Golinelli, DVM, PhD
Department of Veterinary Medical Sciences
Alma Mater Studiorum - University of Bologna
Ozzano Emilia (BO), Italy

Peter A Graham, BVMS, PhD, CertVR, DECVCP, SFHEA, MRCVS
School of Veterinary Medicine and Science
University of Nottingham
Sutton Bonington, Loughborough, UK

Sean Hulsebosch, DVM, DACVIM (SAIM)
School of Veterinary Medicine
University of California - Davis
Davis, CA (USA)

Rosanne E. Jepson, BVSc, MVetMed, PhD, DACVIM (SAIM), DECVIM-CA (Internal Medicine)
Department of Clinical Science and Services
Royal Veterinary College
Hawkshead, UK

Hans S. Kooistra, DVM, PhD, DECVIM-CA (Internal Medicine)
Department of Clinical Sciences, Faculty of Veterinary Medicine
Utrecht University
Utrecht, The Netherlands

Daniel K. Langlois, DVM, DACVIM (SAIM)
College of Veterinary Medicine
Michigan State University
East Lansing, MI (USA)

Thomas A. Lutz, DVM, PhD
Institute of Veterinary Physiology, Vetsuisse Faculty
University of Zurich
Zurich, Switzerland

Eleonora Malerba, DVM, PhD
Department of Veterinary Medical Sciences
Alma Mater Studiorum - University of Bologna
Ozzano Emilia (BO), Italy

Björn Meij, DVM, PhD, DECVS
Department of Clinical Sciences, Faculty of Veterinary Medicine
Utrecht University
Utrecht, The Netherlands

Carlos Melian, DVM, PhD
Department of Animal Pathology, Animal Production, and Food Science and Technology
Universidad de Las Palmas de Gran Canaria
Las Palmas, Spain

Diego Miceli, DVM, PhD
National Council of Scientific and Technical Research (CONICET)
Buenos Aires, Argentina

Stijn J.M. Niessen, DVM, PhD, DECVIM, PGCertVetEd, FHEA MRCVS
Royal Veterinary College
University of London
London, UK

Rodolfo Oliveira Leal, DVM, PhD, DECVIM-CA (Internal Medicine)
Centre for Interdisciplinary Research in Animal Health, University of Lisbon, Portugal
Associate Laboratory for Animal and Veterinary Sciences (AL4AnimalS), Portugal

Darja Pavlin, DVM, PhD
Veterinary Faculty, Small animal clinic
University of Ljubljana
Ljubljana, Slovenija

Maria Dolores Pérez-Alenza, DVM, PhD
Department of Medicine and Animal Surgery
Complutense University of Madrid
Madrid, Spain

Tera Pijnacker, DVM, DECVIM-CA (Internal Medicine)
Department of Clinical Sciences, Faculty of Veterinary Medicine
Utrecht University
Utrecht, The Netherlands

Álan Gomes Pöppl, DVM, MSc, DSc
Departamento de Medicina Animal, Faculdade de Veterinária
Universidade Federal do Rio Grande do Sul - UFRGS
Porto Alegre, RS, Brasil

Dan Rosenberg, DVM, PhD
MICEN VET Referal Center
Créteil, France

Johan P. Schoeman, BVSc, MMedVet, PhD, DSAM, DECVIM -CA (Internal Medicine), FRCVS
Department of Companion Animal Clinical Studies, Faculty of Veterinary Science
University of Pretoria
Onderstepoort, South Africa

Robert Shiel, MVB, ProfCertBiostatistics ProfDipUTL, PhD, DECVIM-CA (Internal Medicine)
School of Veterinary Medicine
Murdoch University
Murdoch, West Australia

Nadja S. Sieber-Ruckstuhl, Prof., Dr. med. vet., DACVIM, DECVIM-CA (Internal Medicine)
Clinic for Small Animal Internal Medicine, Vetsuisse Faculty
University of Zurich
Zurich, Switzerland

Barbara J. Skelly, MA, VetMB, PhD, CertSAM, DACVIM (SAIM), DECVIM-CA (Internal Medicine), MRCVS
Queen's Veterinary School Hospital, Department of Veterinary Medicine
University of Cambridge
Cambridge, UK

Lisa Stammeleer, DVM, DECVIM (Internal Medicine)
Small Animal Department, Faculty of Veterinary Medicine
University of Ghent
Ghent, Belgium

Antonio Maria Tardo, DVM
Department of Veterinary Medical Sciences
Alma Mater Studiorum - University of Bologna
Ozzano Emilia (BO), Italy

Santiago Teyssandier, DVM
University Hospital and Private practice
Universidad del Salvador
Buenos Aires, Argentina

Chiara Valtolina, DVM, PhD, DECVECC, DACVECC
Department of Clinical Sciences, Faculty of Veterinary Medicine
Utrecht University
Utrecht, The Netherlands

Marit F. van den Berg, DVM, DECVIM-CA (Internal Medicine)
Department of Clinical Sciences, Faculty of Veterinary Medicine
Utrecht University
Utrecht, The Netherlands

Henk van den Broek, DVM, PhD, DECVDI
Department of Clinical Sciences, Faculty of Veterinary Medicine
Utrecht University
Utrecht, The Netherlands

Sebastiaan A. van Nimwegen, DVM, PhD, DECVS
Department of Clinical Sciences, Faculty of Veterinary Medicine
Utrecht University
Utrecht, The Netherlands

Stefanie Veraa, DVM, PhD, DECVDI
Department of Clinical Sciences, Faculty of Veterinary Medicine
Utrecht University
Utrecht, The Netherlands

Annemarie M.W.Y. Voorbij DVM, PhD, DECVIM-CA (Internal Medicine)
Department of Clinical Sciences, Faculty of Veterinary Medicine
Utrecht University
Utrecht, The Netherlands

Tim Williams MA, VetMB, PhD, AFHEA, FRCPath, DECVCP, MRCVS
Department of Veterinary Medicine
University of Cambridge
Cambridge, UK

Panagiotis G. Xenoulis, DVM, PhD
Faculty of Veterinary Science
University of Thessaly, Karditsa, Greece
School of Veterinary Medicine & Biomedical Sciences
Texas A&M University, College Station, TX, USA

Maurice Zandvliet, DVM, MVR, PhD, DECVIM-CA (Internal Medicine and Oncology)
Department of Clinical Sciences, Faculty of Veterinary Medicine, Faculty of Veterinary Medicine
Utrecht University
Utrecht, The Netherlands

Florian Zeugswetter, Priv. Doz., DVM
Clinical Department for Small Animals and Horses
University of Veterinary Medicine Vienna
Vienna, Austria

Series preface

"Oh! You are a veterinarian? I (or my brother, my sister, my son, my daughter…) always wanted to be a veterinarian." All of us, as veterinary students and later as veterinarians, have often heard comments like this. Becoming a veterinarian seems to be such a wonderful career to nonveterinarians: helping helpless dogs and cats. Veterinarians should be happy and satisfied in their *chosen* profession because they are able to earn a living by caring for loved pets. The journey to satisfaction and happiness for veterinarians, however, never seems to follow an obvious, straight, or level path.

The 1950s witnessed a dramatic growth in the popularity of pet dogs and in the number of veterinarians who cared exclusively for pets. The popularity of cats soon followed. Today, more dogs and cats are considered "members of the family" than ever before in human history, and their owners want to protect their family members from illness or to resolve any illness. There are more veterinarians who care for dogs and cats currently than ever before in human history. Veterinary medicine has evolved remarkably to meet the ever-growing medical care expectations and demands of dog and cat owners.

When learning of a diagnosis, prognosis, treatment, and/or the cost of care for their ill pet, some owners become distressed. These emotions are often directed at the "messenger" of the bad news: the veterinarian. The veterinarian, in turn, may not respect their own knowledge and feel inadequate. One reason that a veterinarian may feel inadequate is the realization that it is impossible for anyone in general practice to be expert and current on all the canine and feline conditions encountered in a day, week, or month: everything from orthopedics to oncology, from vaccinology to dermatology, from ophthalmology to cardiology. Nor is it possible for an internal medicine specialist to be expert and current in each condition they encounter, from endocrinology to gastroenterology or from respiratory conditions to chronic kidney disease. Further, it is clear that cats are not small dogs. Perceived "knowledge deficiencies" can cause veterinarians to feel they are failing to meet their clients' expectations.

The internal medicine textbooks in this new series offer one approach for enjoying veterinary practice. We encourage colleagues to embrace developing expertise in one area. By focusing on and studying one organ system in either the dog or cat, one can achieve greater knowledge and skills and, in turn, greater confidence. Each book in this series offers a clear path to learning current opinions on pathophysiology, diagnosis, treatment, prognosis, and costs associated with illnesses involving one system in one species. Confidence gained in a focused area can be sensed by devoted owners. Further, confidence in one area of internal medicine also creates confidence in sharing limitations: "I am extremely confident in diagnosing and managing some conditions but I lack that level of expertise in all other conditions".

The books in this series have been constructed to help build expertise in one organ system in either the dog or the cat. Each book is edited by one or two specialists with outstanding international credentials. Each editor was tasked with building a text that contains all the information found in general internal medicine textbooks, but with much more in-depth discussions on each condition. Each book has early chapters focusing on differential diagnoses of owner concerns, physical examination findings, and laboratory and/or imaging results. These are excellent for students as they begin to apply their basic knowledge to clinical cases. These chapters also provide a quick review for experienced general practitioners and specialists. Each chapter provides at least one algorithm designed to take the reader from a vague owner concern, physical examination finding, or laboratory abnormality to a specific diagnosis with step-by-step instructions. The "techniques section" in each text teaches currently employed procedures, most with videos. In-depth chapters on known illnesses comprise 70 to 80% of each book's content. The editors have provided a larger number of chapters, a larger number of expert contributors, and greater depth on each organ system than any general textbook can supply. The material has a level of credibility that no internet site can claim. Each book can guide the reader through a more complete journey of understanding than is available in any other veterinary resource.

Edward Feldman
Federico Fracassi

Preface

In the fascinating world of endocrinology, scientific knowledge and technology have advanced greatly in recent years. Alongside, our ability to diagnose, treat, and manage various endocrine disorders has progressed too. The goal of this textbook is to provide an up-to-date, comprehensive, yet accessible resource for understanding and managing endocrine disorders in dogs.

The book is divided into two parts. The first part adopts a problem-oriented approach to the most common clinical and laboratory abnormalities in dogs with endocrine diseases. We provide algorithms that guide veterinarians step by step in diagnostic evaluation and setting up the treatment. This section serves as a quick reference guide in clinical situations. Additionally, part one covers practical topics such as blood pressure measurement and glucose monitoring. The chapters are supplemented by video material, enhancing comprehension of handling and procedures. These videos do not only facilitate learning for the professionals but can also be shared with owners.

Part two focuses on endocrine diseases. Each chapter starts with the basic anatomy and physiology of the specific endocrine glands, followed by detailed discussions on clinical signs, diagnostic methodologies, and management strategies. Chapters are richly supplemented with boxes, tables, algorithms, charts, imaging studies, and illustrations. Each chapter features a key fact box summarizing the most crucial information. The chapters on diabetes mellitus and Cushing's syndrome are broken down into multiple subchapters. This allows for the inclusion of additional experts offering insights on specific subject matter, such as nutrition, radiation therapy, and diagnostic imaging.

In writing this book, we have had the privilege of collaborating with phenomenal veterinary experts from around the globe. While you will encounter well-known authors, you will also discover some new names. One of our key missions was to pair emerging talents with their professional mentors. The expertise and critical attitude of the authors were indispensable throughout the writing process, making editorial tasks both enjoyable and rewarding. Additionally, special thanks to Edra, and particularly Constanza Smeraldi, for providing state-of-the-art visuals in the book. They significantly ensure that the reading material is easy to understand. Finally, whenever we had doubts, we had the privilege of receiving immediate advice from a friend who is one of the "fathers" of veterinary endocrinology. Thank you, Ed Feldman, for the constant positive and professional support you have provided us.

The recommendations provided in our book are based on research, clinical experience, and expertise, but also practicality and cost-effectiveness. Nonetheless, what may be effective today may be improved upon tomorrow. Science encourages curiosity and urges us to challenge existing beliefs. Therefore, while providing a go-to reference book for veterinarians, veterinary students, residents, and enthusiasts of endocrinology, we also aspire for our book to serve as an inspiration, reminding readers to maintain an open-minded attitude.

Sara Galac
Federico Fracassi

Abbreviations

131I radioactive iodine-131
17OHP 17-alpha-hydroxyprogesterone
3MT 3-methoxytyramine
3D-CRT 3D-conformal radiotherapy
α-MSH alpha-melanocyte-stimulating hormone
β-OHB β-hydroxybutyrate
AA abiraterone acetate
AC adenylate cyclase
AcAc acetoacetate
ACEi angiotensin-converting enzyme inhibitors
AChR acetylcholine receptor
ACTH adrenocorticotropic hormone
ACTHst ACTH stimulation test
ACVIM American College of Veterinary Internal Medicine
AD adrenal-dependent
ADH antidiuretic hormone
ADHC adrenal dependent hypercortisolism
AIA autoinsulin antibody
AKI acute kidney injury
ALIVE Agreeing Language in Veterinary Endocrinology
ALP alkaline phosphatase
ALT alanine aminotransferase
Ang II angiotensin II
ANS aniline naphthalene sulphonic acid
APS autoimmune polyendocrine syndrome
AQP aquaporin
ARB angiotensin receptor blockers
AST aspartate aminotransferase
AT adrenal/adrenocortical tumor
ATP adenosine triphosphate
AVP arginine vasopressin
BAL bronchoalveolar lavage
BARF biologically appropriate raw food
BCS body condition score
BGc blood glucose concentration
BGC blood glucose curve
BHB beta-hydroxybutyrate
BHD black hair follicular dysplasia
bid bis in die
BP blood pressure
cAMP cyclic adenosine monophosphate
CaSR calcium-sensing receptor
CAR cortisol-to-ACTH ratio
CBC complete blood count
CCD canine cognitive dysfunction
CCK cholecystokinin
CDA color dilution alopecia
CDI central diabetes insipidus
CECT contrast-enhanced computed tomography
CEN concurrent endocrine neoplasia
CEUS contrast-enhanced ultrasound
CMG congenital myasthenia gravis
CGM continuous glucose monitoring
CGMS continuous glucose monitoring system
CGRP calcitonin gene-related peptide
CHG congenital hypothyroidism with goiter
CK creatine kinase
CKD chronic kidney disease
CLIA chemiluminescent immunoassay
CLIP corticotropin-like intermediate-lobe peptide
CNS central nervous system
CO cardiac output
COMT catechol-O-methyltransferase
CPB canine pattern baldness
CPD central pontine demyelination
cPL canine pancreatic lipase
cPLI canine pancreatic lipase immunoreactivity
cRECIST canine response evaluation criteria for solid tumors
CRF corticotropin-releasing factor
CRI continuous rate infusion
CRT capillary refill time
CRH corticotropin-releasing hormone
CRP C reactive protein
CSF cerebrospinal fluid
CSF-1R colony stimulating factor-1 receptor
CT computed tomography
cTnI cardiac troponin I
cTSH canine thyroid-stimulating hormone
CTV clinical target volume
CVA coefficient of variation
CVC caudal vena cava
DA dopamine
DDAVP desmopressin acetate
DEXA dual-energy X-ray absorptiometry
DHA docosahexaenoic acid
DHEAS dehydroepiandrostenedione
DI diabetes insipidus
DIC disseminated intravascular coagulation
DIT diiodotyrosine
DK diabetic ketosis
DKA diabetic ketoacidosis
DLA dog leucocyte antigen
DM diabetes mellitus
DOCP desoxycorticosterone pivalate
DRD2 dopamine receptor D2
DTM dermatophyte test médium
eACTH endogenous ACTH
ECF extracellular fluid
ECG electrocardiogram
EDTA ethylenediaminetetraacetic acid

EGA Error Grid Analysis
EI exercise intolerance
EIC exercise-induce collapse
ELISA enzyme-linked immunosorbent assay
EMG electromyography
EPA eicosapentanoic acid
ESVE European Society of Veterinary Endocrinology
FEK fractional urinary excretion of potassium
FFA free fatty acid
FGMS flash glucose monitoring system
FSH follicle-stimulating hormone
fT4 free tetraiodothyronine, free thyroxine
FTC follicular cell thyroid carcinoma
FTS follicular thyroid carcinoma
GFR glomerular filtration rate
GH growth hormone
GHRH growth hormone-releasing hormone
GIP gastric inhibitory polypeptide
GIP glucose-dependent insulinotropic peptide
GLP-1 glucagon-like peptide-1
GlyHb glycated hemoglobin
GnRH gonadotropin-releasing hormone
GTV gross tumor volume
GV glycemic variability
HC hypercortisolism
HCT hematocrit
HHM humoral hypercalcemia of malignancy
HHS hyperosmolar hyperglycemic state
HR heart rate
HSS hyperosmolar hyperglycemic syndrome
IAPP islet amyloid polypeptide
IBD inflammatory bowel disease
IBW ideal body weight
iCa ionized calcium
ICF intracellular fluid
IDDM insulin-deficient diabetes mellitus
IG interstitial glucose
IGc interstitial glucose concentration
IGF-1 insulin-like growth factor 1
IGF-2 insulin-like growth factor 2
IHC immunohistochemistry
IM intramuscular
IMRT intensity-modulated radiotherapy
IR insulin resistance
IRDM insulin-resistant diabetes mellitus
IRMA immunoradiometric assay
ISF interstitial fluid
KB ketone body
KCS keratoconjunctivitis sicca
LC-MS/MS liquid chromatography-tandem mass spectrometry
L-DOPA L-dihydroxyphenylalanine
LDDST low-dose dexamethasone suppression test
LH lipohypertrophy
LH luteinizing hormone
LMN lower motor neuron
LoD limit of detection
LoQ limit of quantification
L-T4 levothyroxine
MACS mild autonomous cortisol syndrome
MC2R melanocortin 2 receptor
MCS muscle condition score
MDWT modified water deprivation test
MEN multiple endocrine neoplasia
MER maintenance energy requirements
MG myasthenia gravis
MHC major histocompatibility complex
MIBG metaiodobenzylguanidine
MIT monoiodotyrosine
MLC multileaf collimator
MODS multiorgan dysfunction
MPA medroxyprogesterone acetate
MPR multiplanar reconstruction
MR mineralocorticoid receptors
MRI magnetic resonance imaging
MST median survival time
MTC medullary thyroid carcinoma
MV megavoltage
NDI nephrogenic diabetes insipidus
NFA non-hormonally functional adenomas
NIS sodium/iodide symporter
NMJ neuromuscular junction
NO nitric oxide
NPH neutral protamine Hagedorn
NPY neuropeptide Y
NSP nutritional secondary hyperparathyroidism
NT-proBNP N-terminal pro B-type natriuretic peptide
NTI non-thyroidal illness
oHDDST oral high-dose dexamethasone suppression test
P/B pituitary-to-brain value
PASS Pheochromocytoma of the Adrenal gland Scaled Score
PAV phrenicoabdominal vein
PBGM portable blood glucose meter
PCC pheochromocytoma
PD polydipsia
PD pituitary-dependent
PDH pituitary dependent hypercortisolism
PDGFR platelet-derived growth factor receptor
PDH pituitary-dependent hypercortisolism
PET-CT positron emission computed tomography CT
PFS progression-free survival
PHPTH primary hyperparathyroidism
PK pharmacokinetics
PLI pancreatic lipase immunoreactivity
PNMT phenylethanolamine-N-methyltransferase
PNS peripheral nervous system
POMC pro-opiomelanocortin
Posm plasma osmolality
PRH prolactin-releasing hormone
PRL prolactin
PT prothrombin time
PTE pulmonary thromboembolism
PTH parathyroid hormone
PTHrp PTH-related protein
PTV planning target volume
PU polyuria
PU/PD polyuria/polydipsia
PZI protamine zinc insulin
RAAS renin-angiotensin-aldosterone system
RER resting energy requirements
rhTSH human recombinant thyroid-stimulating hormone
SAA serum amyloid A
SBP systolic blood pressure
SBW start body weight
SC subcutaneous
SDMA symmetric dimethylarginine
SF surviving fraction
SF-1 steroidogenic factor-1
SGLT2 sodium-glucose cotransporter 2

SH systemic hypertension
SIAD syndrome of inappropriate ADH release
SNS sympathetic nervous system
SOAT1 sterol-o-acyltransferase 1
SP substance P
SPECT single-photon emission computed tomography
SRS stereotactic radiosurgery
SRT stereotactic radiotherapy
SST somatostatin
SSTR2 somatostatin receptor subtype 2
SSTR5 somatostatin receptor subtype 5
SV stroke volume
SVR systemic vascular resistance
T3 tri-iodothyronine
T3AA T3 autoantibodies
T4 tetraiodothyronine, thyroxine
T4AA T4 autoantibodies
TBG thyroglobulin
tCa total calcium
TgAAs antithyroglobulin antibodies
TEG thromboelastography
THRT thyroid hormone replacement treatment
tid ter in die
TKI tyrosine kinase inhibitor
TLI trypsin-like immunoreactivity
TOD target organ damage
TPO thyroid peroxidase
TPR total peripheral resistance
TRH thyrotrophin-releasing hormone
TSH thyroid-stimulating hormone
UA urinalysis
UCCR urine cortisol-to-creatinine ratio
UMN upper motor neuron
Uosm urine osmolality
UPCR urine protein to creatinine ratio
US ultrasound
USG urine specific gravity
UTI urinary tract infection
VEGFR vascular endothelial growth factor receptor
VLDL very-low-density lipoprotein
VMA vanillylmandelic acid
VMAT volumetric modulated arc therapy
VP vasopressin
VR venous return
WAT white adipose tissue
WBC white blood cell
WHO World Health Organization
WSAVA World Small Animal Veterinary Association

Table of contents

SECTION I Differential diagnoses for owner chief concerns and physical examination findings

SECTION II Differential diagnoses for clinicopathologic abnormalities

Growth retardation

Federico Fracassi
DVM, PhD, DECVIM (SAIM)

Dolores Pérez Alenza
DVM, PhD

Hans S. Kooistra
DVM, PhD, DECVIM-CA (Internal Medicine)

Pathophysiology

Growth is a complex yet tightly regulated process. Genetic factors play a major role in linear growth, with numerous genes involved in its regulation. After the domestication of the dog, the selection of such genes by humans has resulted in breeds with a wide variety of body sizes and growth rates. For example, selection by people for the genes that give rise to angular limb formation and short legs has resulted in chondrodystrophic dog breeds. As these breeds have been created intentionally, they are generally not considered to have growth retardation.
Dogs must consume sufficient calories and nutrients to meet the full (genetic) potential for growth. After food intake, food must be digested and absorbed adequately. Next, nutrients must be transported to the tissues for metabolic maintenance and growth. Based on these processes, the causes of growth retardation can be subdivided into three major groups: inadequate intake of calories and nutrients, increased use of energy, and increased loss of energy.
Several hormones are known to be important determinants of linear growth. Consequently, hormonal disturbances at a young age may be associated with growth retardation (Table 1.1).
The intake of insufficient calories and nutrients at a young age is, next to genetic factors, the most important reason for growth retardation, i.e., nutritional deprivation severely impairs growth. Selective deficiencies in vitamins or minerals may also cause growth retardation. In addition to the quantity, food quality and palatability should also be considered.
A poor appetite, e.g., due to a systemic disease, may result in less food intake. Oropharyngeal disorders, including swallowing problems, may cause hyporexia. Regurgitation or vomiting could cause insufficient nutrients to reach the intestines. A vascular ring anomaly due to a persistent right aortic arch should be considered in puppies with stunted growth and chronic regurgitation, especially after weaning. Maldigestion, e.g., due to exocrine pancreatic insufficiency or biliary obstruction, and malabsorption, e.g., due to an intestinal wall disorder in case of an enteropathy, can result in decreased uptake of nutrients. Intestinal parasites may cause inadequate uptake of nutrients, mainly in puppies.
Catabolic processes, such as those associated with inflammatory processes and fever, will increase energy use. Congenital heart anomalies and endocarditis may result in tachycardia, which, in turn, means extra loss of energy, leaving fewer calories for growth. Disorders involving organs that play a central role in metabolism, i.e., the liver and the kidneys, may also result in growth retardation. Both congenital renal disorders and acquired kidney disease, e.g., pyelonephritis, can result in stunted growth. Portosystemic shunting resulting in hepatic encephalopathy is the most common liver disorder associated with growth retardation. Hepatitis and glycogen storage disease have also been associated with stunted growth. Growth retardation in young dogs with chronic anemia may be associated with impaired oxygen delivery to tissues as well as increased cardiovascular effort. Failure to grow normally cannot only be associated with glucosuria due to (juvenile) diabetes mellitus but may also result from glucosuria due to defects in the proximal tubules of the kidneys. Persistent proteinuria and protein-losing enteropathies decrease growth potential.

Diagnostic approach

Algorithm 1.1 shows the approach to the dog with failure to grow.

Algorithm 1.1 Note 1 A detailed nutritional history should be obtained to get information regarding the amount, quality, and palatability of the food offered to the dog.

Algorithm 1.1 Note 2 A poor appetite, despite the feeding of sufficient palatable, high-quality food, suggests a disorder of the gastrointestinal tract or the presence of systemic disease. Growth retardation in dogs with very good or ravenous appetite may point to maldigestion, malabsorption or loss of energy. History-taking may also reveal treatment with steroids for an unrelated problem. Concurrent clinical signs may help identify an underlying cause for the growth retardation. Diarrhea or voluminous stools may be due to maldigestion and/or malabsorption.

TABLE 1.1 Endocrine causes of growth retardation.

Growth hormone and insulin-like growth factor-1 deficiency. (For more information, see chapter 24)	
Physiology	■ Growth hormone (GH), produced and secreted from the anterior lobe of the pituitary gland, plays a central role in the modulation of growth. ■ Although GH directly affects many tissues, most of its growth-promoting actions are mediated by insulin-like growth factor-1 (IGF-1). ■ Circulating IGF-1 is mainly produced in the liver. In other tissues, IGF-1 stimulates anabolic processes in a paracrine or autocrine manner. For example, linear growth largely depends on the local production of IGF-1 in growth plates. ■ In adult dogs, there is a strong linear correlation between the plasma IGF-1 concentration and body size, while basal plasma GH concentrations are quite similar among various breeds. This implies that breed-specific reference ranges must be used to determine whether growth retardation is due to insufficient circulating IGF-1 concentrations.[1-3]
Etiology	■ Congenital GH deficiency or pituitary dwarfism is the best-known example of such a deficiency. ■ In German Shepherd dogs and Czechoslovakian Wolfdogs, congenital GH deficiency is due to a mutation in the gene encoding for the transcription factor LHX3.
Pathophysiology	■ In the case of complete GH deficiency, linear growth occurs at about a third to a quarter of the normal rate. ■ Growth hormone deficiency in a young animal affects the growth of almost all tissues, resulting in "proportionate dwarfism", meaning that all body components are equally small.
Main clinical signs	■ During the first weeks after birth, pituitary dwarfs may be of similar size as their litter mates. ■ Proportionate growth retardation. ■ Retention of puppy hair coat. ■ Bilateral symmetrical alopecia. ■ Skin hyperpigmented and scaly. ■ Pointed muzzle and relatively long pointy ears, resembling the face of a fox.
Hypothyroidism. (For more information, see chapter 27)	
Physiology	■ Thyroid hormones are essential for central nervous system (CNS) maturation, bone growth, and chondrogenesis. ■ Adequate circulating thyroid hormone concentrations appear to be a prerequisite for normal growth. ■ The effect of IGF-1 on cartilage cells is dependent on thyroid hormones. ■ Thyroid hormones exert direct effects on cell metabolism.
Etiology	■ Congenital dyshormonogenesis or thyroid dysgenesis (congenital primary hypothyroidism). ■ Congenital central hypothyroidism due to isolated TSH deficiency.
Pathophysiology	■ Because skeletal growth strongly depends on thyroid hormones that promote chondrogenesis, in synergy with GH and IGF-1, juvenile hypothyroidism is associated with delayed epiphyseal closure, retarded epiphyseal growth, reduced long bone growth and, consequently, "disproportionate dwarfism".[4]
Main clinical signs	■ Growth retardation with disproportionate dwarfism (short and broad skull, shortened mandible and ears, enlarged or protruding tongue, short thick neck, wide/square trunk, shortened limbs). ■ Impaired mental development (cretinism).
Insulin deficiency	
Physiology	■ Insulin is the most important anabolic hormone in the body. ■ The anabolic actions of insulin include stimulation of protein synthesis and cell division.
Etiology/ pathophysiology	■ Insulin deficiency at a young age, i.e., juvenile diabetes mellitus, is associated with growth retardation. ■ The failure of normal growth, typical of dogs with juvenile diabetes mellitus, is also due to a decrease in insulin-dependent transportation of glucose and fatty acids into muscle and fat cells. ■ Juvenile diabetes mellitus results in glucosuria, i.e., loss of energy in the urine.
Glucocorticoid excess	
Physiology/ pathophysiology	■ The catabolic effects of glucocorticoids are increased gluconeogenesis, decreased glucose uptake by muscle and fat cells, increased protein breakdown, and lipolysis. ■ Glucocorticoid excess suppresses pituitary GH secretion, mainly due to stimulation of hypothalamic somatostatin release. ■ Long-term administration of glucocorticoids to young, growing animals may result in growth retardation.
Gonadal steroids excess	
Physiology/ pathophysiology	■ Gonadal androgens and estrogens affect linear growth. ■ Prepubertal gonadectomy may result in taller individuals.[5] ■ Administration of androgens or estrogens at an early age may result in growth retardation due to premature closure of the growth plates.
Other endocrine hypofunctions	
Physiology/ pathophysiology	■ Hypoadrenocorticism may occur at any age. When hypoadrenocorticism develops in a young growing dog, it may result in growth retardation. ■ Hypoadrenocorticism is often associated with a decrease in appetite, vomiting, and diarrhea, resulting in reduced nutrient intake and, consequently, may result in growth retardation. ■ Hypoparathyroidism may also occur at a young age. ■ Parathyroid hormone has an important role in bone metabolism, and therefore, parathyroid hormone deficiency may result in growth retardation. ■ Disorders associated with severe polydipsia, such as central diabetes insipidus, may result in impaired appetite and failure to adequate growth.

Polyuria may point to renal disease, hepatic disease, diabetes mellitus, diabetes insipidus, or other conditions. Mental dullness may point to hypothyroidism or (hepatic or renal) encephalopathy. Symmetrical truncal alopecia can be seen in dogs with growth hormone deficiency or hypothyroidism. Regurgitation since weaning may point to vascular ring anomaly or megaesophagus. A thorough physical examination is essential in dogs with growth retardation, as specific physical findings may point to a specific disorder. For example, dogs with hypothyroidism usually will have a weak pulse. A heart murmur associated with tachycardia may disclose a cardiac abnormality as a cause of growth retardation.

Algorithm 1.1 Note 3 Body proportions must be carefully evaluated in dogs with growth retardation. Relatively short limbs compared to

ALGORITHM 1.1

Diagnostic approach to growth retardation.

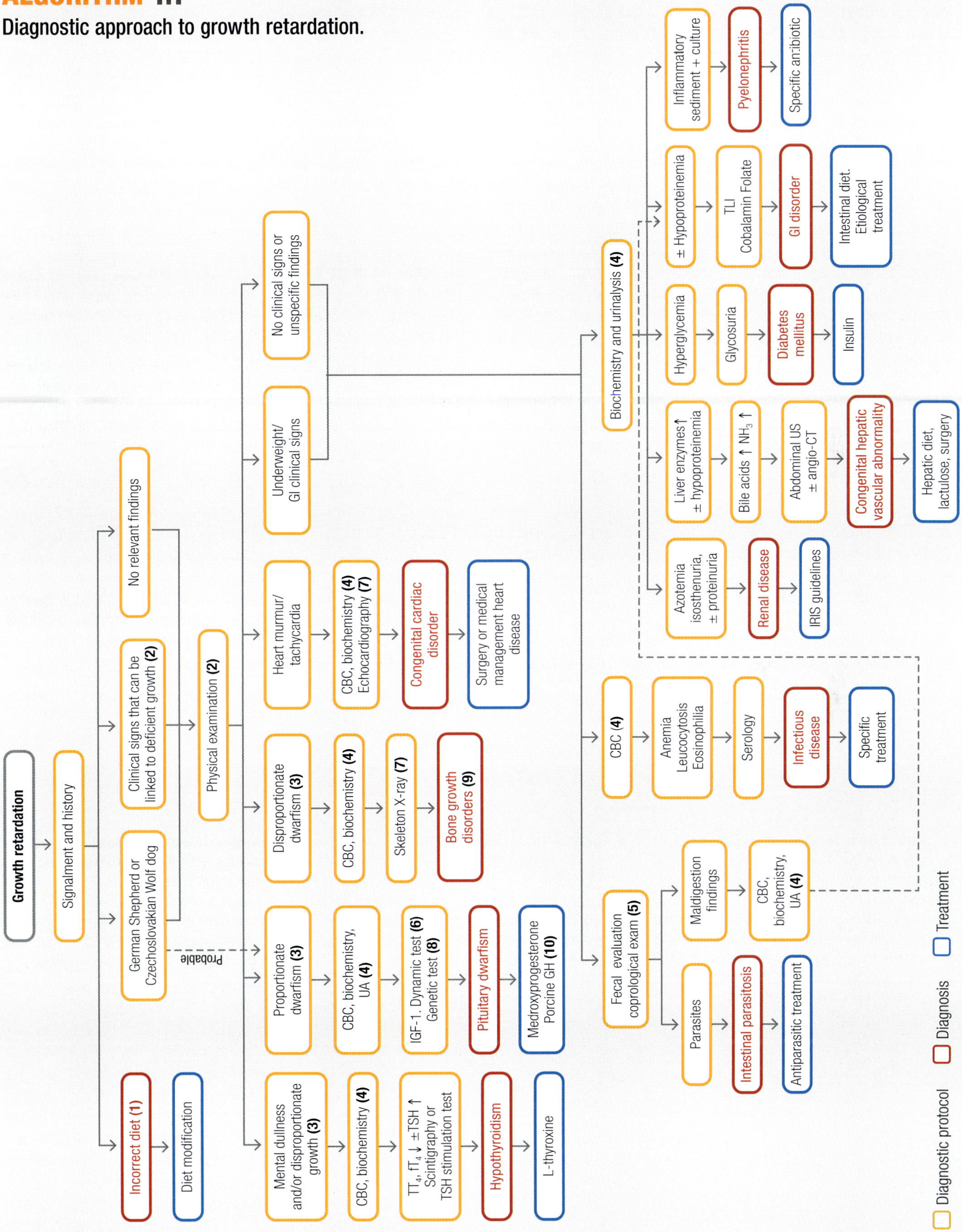

the trunk may point to juvenile hypothyroidism or chondrodystrophy. In contrast, growth hormone deficiency causes proportionate dwarfism. It is also important to note the ratio of height to weight. An animal with stunted growth that is overweight for its height is more likely to have an endocrine disorder such as growth hormone deficiency or hypothyroidism. Malnutrition or systemic disorders are more likely to result in underweight dogs.

Algorithm 1.1 Note 4 Urinalysis may reveal proteinuria, glucosuria, or hyposthenuria. Indications for pyelonephritis may be found in the urine sediment. A complete blood count should be performed to detect anemia, inflammation, or eosinophilia. It has to be taken into account that puppies normally have lower red blood cell counts than adults. Eosinophilia may point to parasitism or hypoadrenocorticism. The results of a routine serum biochemistry profile can help identify renal disease, hepatic disease, diabetes mellitus, or hypoadrenocorticism. Decreased serum protein concentrations may indicate hepatic disease, protein-losing enteropathy, or nephropathy.

Algorithm 1.1 Note 5 Laboratory evaluations should include multiple fecal examinations for intestinal parasites, such as *Giardia* spp. A fecal examination may also provide information regarding (mal)digestion and (mal)absorption.

Algorithm 1.1 Note 6 A low serum IGF-1 concentration may point to growth hormone deficiency. The absence of a significant increase in circulating growth hormone concentration after intravenous administration of GH-releasing hormone can be used to demonstrate growth hormone deficiency (see chapter 24).

Algorithm 1.1 Note 7 Radiological evaluation of the thorax and skeleton and abdominal ultrasound or echocardiography are useful in congenital cardiac diseases, respiratory disorders, liver diseases, renal diseases, and bone growth abnormalities.

Algorithm 1.1 Note 8 Pituitary dwarfism in German Shepherd Dogs is quite often caused by a mutation in a gene that encodes for the transcription factor LHX3.[6] The availability of a diagnostic DNA test not only allows for proper diagnosis of dogs with pituitary dwarfism due to this mutation but also enables breeders to prevent dwarfs from being born to identifying carriers of the LHX3 mutation. If all breeding animals were genetically tested for the presence of the LHX3 mutation and a correct breeding policy were implemented, this disease could be eradicated completely.

Algorithm 1.1 Note 9 Several musculoskeletal disorders may cause failure to grow in young animals. Most of them are congenital and inherited, such as dyschondroplasia (especially in Poodles, Scottish Terriers, and Alaskan Malamutes), dystrophy-like myopathies, osteochondrosis, osteochondromatosis, osteogenesis imperfecta, osteopetrosis, angular limb deformities (abnormal development of the radius and ulna), and hypertrophic osteodystrophy and glycogen storage disease. In addition, nutritional imbalances, such as secondary hyperparathyroidism, a deficiency of vitamin D, and/or excessive vitamin A, may cause failure to grow.

Algorithm 1.1 Note 10 Treating canine hyposomatotropism involves administering synthetic progestins: either medroxyprogesterone acetate at a dosage of 5 mg/kg SC initially every 3 weeks and subsequently at 6-week intervals or proligestone at a dosage of 10 mg/kg SC every 3 weeks, both until 12 months of age. There are, however, some adverse effects, including recurrent periods of pruritic pyoderma and, occasionally, the development of mammary tumors. Porcine GH (pGH) is another potential option. Treatment with either progestagens or pGH should be accompanied by thyroid hormone replacement.

References

1. Favier RP, Mol JA, Kooistra HS, et al. Large body size in the dog is associated with transient GH excess at a young age. *J Endocrinol* 170:479-484, 2001.
2. Nap RC, Mol JA, Hazewinkel HAW. Age related plasma concentrations of growth hormone (GH) and insulin-like growth factor I (IGF-I) in Great Dane pups fed different dietary levels of protein. *Domest Anim Endocrinol* 10:237-247, 1993.
3. Nap RC, Mol JA, Hazewinkel HAW. Growth and growth hormone in the dog. *Vet Quart Suppl* 1:31S-32S, 1994.
4. Saunders HM, Jezyk PK. The radiographic appearance of canine congenital hypothyroidism: skeletal changes with delayed treatment. *Vet Radiol Ultrasound* 32:171-177, 1991.
5. Salmeri KR, Bloomberg MS, Scruggs SL, et al. Gonadectomy in immature dogs: effects on skeletal, physical, and behavioral development. *J Am Vet Med Assoc* 198:1193-1203, 1991.
6. Voorbij AMWY, Van Steenbeek FG, Vos-Loohuis M, et al. A contracted DNA repeat in LHX3 intron 5 is associated with aberrant splicing and pituitary dwarfism in German shepherd dogs. *PLoS One* 6:2011. doi:10.1371/journal.pone.0027940

CHAPTER 2

Alopecia

Francesco Albanese
DVM

Alopecia refers to hair loss in areas of the body where it is usually present. Other terms, such as hypotrichosis, are also used to define a partial lack of hair. However, some dermatologists prefer to reserve it for congenital alopecia. To additionally confuse the nomenclature, the term alopecia is also incorrectly used to define a hair disorder known as postclipping alopecia in which hairs, numerically normal but shorter as shaved, give a "false" aspect of hair loss.

Pathophysiology

The causes of alopecia are numerous and include pruritic diseases (e.g., allergies), infectious diseases (e.g., dermatophytosis, and bacterial folliculitis), parasitic diseases of the hair follicle (e.g., demodicosis), physiological or functional abnormalities of the hair follicle (e.g., endocrinopathies, alopecia X, metabolic diseases), anatomical abnormalities (e.g., congenital alopecia, follicular dysplasia), immune mediated-autoimmune diseases (e.g., alopecia areata, pseudopelade, mural folliculitis, sterile periadnexal granulomatous/pyogranulomatous syndrome), vasculitis (ischemic dermatopathy linked to low-grade vasculitis), and neoplastic diseases (e.g., cutaneous epitheliotropic lymphoma).

Classification and clinical signs

Alopecia can be clinically classified based on the number of skin lesions, their localization and extension, and the simultaneous presence or absence of other lesions on the skin. Regarding the number of areas without hairs, alopecia is classified as focal, multifocal, symmetrical, and diffuse while looking at the presence or absence of associated skin lesions such as erythema, papules, scales, pustules, etc. Alopecia is commonly differentiated as inflammatory and noninflammatory.

A clear clinical differentiation between inflammatory and noninflammatory alopecia is not free from interpretative problems. Indeed, in some hypothyroid dogs or dogs with hypercortisolism, multifocal inflammatory alopecia due to a secondary pyoderma could be the unique dermatological sign in the early stage of the disease in which a clear symmetrical/diffuse alopecia is not yet present.

Endocrine-based alopecias are classically noninflammatory and have a symmetrical and diffuse distribution that usually spares the hairs of the head and extremities. Other dermatological or systemic signs can be observed in animals affected by endocrinopathies and can help the clinician guide the diagnosis. Nevertheless, the clinician must remember that several nonendocrine disorders can present symmetrical and/or diffuse alopecia, mimicking an endocrinopathy; therefore, a meticulous workup is necessary to obtain a definitive diagnosis (Table 2.1).

This chapter focuses on providing the diagnostic workup in a patient with symmetrical and diffuse noninflammatory alopecia.

Diagnostic approach

Algorithm 2.1 Note 1 Although it is uncommon that diffuse noninflammatory alopecia is caused by an infectious agent or a parasite, a complete dermatological workup including Wood's lamp test, trichoscopy, adhesive acetate tape test, cytology, skin scrapings, and fungal culture on dermatophyte test medium (DTM) should always be carried out in any case of alopecia.

Algorithm 2.1 Note 2 Pyoderma, dermatophytosis, and demodicosis are the most common causes of focal and multifocal inflammatory alopecia. Less frequently, the above-mentioned infectious agents can complicate any noninflammatory alopecia, transforming them into inflammatory alopecia.

Algorithm 2.1 Note 3 Apart from alopecic breeds, hair loss from birth is typical of congenital alopecia or X-linked ectodermal dysplasia. In the latter, defects of dentition and tearing are constantly associated with alopecia. Some breeds, such as Chesapeake Bay Retrievers, Irish Water Spaniels, and Portuguese Water Dogs, are predisposed to genetic follicular dysplasia. Dogs have normal coats at birth and, at a young age, develop noninflammatory symmetrical and diffuse alopecia that can mimic an endocrinopathy. The diagnosis is confirmed by skin biopsy.

TABLE 2.1 Differential diagnoses for noninflammatory symmetrical and diffuse alopecia.

Alopecia due to endocrinopathy	Alopecia due to genetic disorders	Alopecia due to temporary hair cycle arrest
■ Hypothyroidism ■ Hypercortisolism ■ Hyperestrogenism ■ Hyposomatotropism	■ Alopecic breeds ■ Congenital alopecia ■ X-linked ectodermal dysplasia ■ Follicular dysplasia not linked to hair color ■ Follicular dysplasia linked to hair color	■ Alopecia X ■ Seasonal flank/ recurrent alopecia ■ Postclipping alopecia ■ Telogen effluvium ■ Anagen effluvium

Algorithm 2.1 Note 4 When noninflammatory alopecia is associated with systemic signs, endocrinopathies must be considered. Polyuria, polydipsia, polyphagia, panting, and weight gain are frequent systemic signs associated with hypercortisolism. Other skin lesions such as thinning of the skin with lost of elasticity, comedones, and skin mineralization (calcinosis cutis) can be observed in this endocrinopathy. Lethargy, exercise intolerance, and weight gain are suggestive of hypothyroidism. In this endocrinopathy, adjunctive and suggestive skin changes are alopecia with shiny and hyperpigmented skin on the bridge of the nose along with an alopecia of the tail that, when complete, shows a so-named "rat tail" appearance. The latter aspect is erroneously thought to be linked only to hypothyroidism since in other endocrinopathies (hyperestrogenism and hypercortisolism). In temporary or permanent alopecic follicular diseases such as alopecia X or follicular dysplasia, partial to complete hair loss on the tail can also be observed.

Hyperestrogenism is caused by endogenous estrogen sources such as an ovarian cyst, granulosa cell tumor, Sertoli cell tumor, or exogenous estrogens used for therapeutic purposes. It is characterized by vulvar enlargement, prolonged estrus and pyometra in females, testicle mass, gynecomastia, and linear preputial erythema/hyperpigmentation in males. In some affected males, behavioral changes, such as urination without lifting the leg and loss of interest in bitches in heat, are also reported. Although not pathognomonic, hyperpigmented spots are commonly observed on the alopecic skin, especially on the rear thighs. Treatment involves the withdrawal of the estrogen source by surgical castration or ceasing estrogen treatment.

Algorithm 2.1 Note 5 In diffuse noninflammatory alopecia with no systemic signs and negative testing on endocrinopathies, several differential diagnoses are possible, and in all, the diagnosis can only be reached by skin biopsy.[5,6,7]

In dogs born with a dilute haircoat, a so-called color dilution alopecia (CDA) can occur; large clumps of melanin are irregularly distributed into the hair's cortex, deforming the cuticula and causing the fracture of the hair shafts. These microscopic findings are often minimal and not so clearly evident at trichoscopic examination.[4] Similar clinicopathological aspects are observed in black hair follicular dysplasia (BHD).

Alopecia X (hair cycle arrest) is a common skin disorder of unknown origin mainly observed in Pomeranians. In this breed, hormonal dysregulation has been demonstrated, specifically of estrogen metabolism at the skin level.[2] Since the clinical presentation can be identical to many endocrine disorders, the diagnosis of alopecia X is made when endocrinopathies are ruled out via endocrine tests, and a compatible histomorphological pattern is observed on skin biopsies.[1]

Seasonal flank/recurrent alopecia usually starts and remains localized at the flank region in most affected dogs. It must highlighted that in some breeds, such as Lagotto Romagnolo, hair loss starts as more diffuse alopecia, involving large skin areas of the back and trunk, mimicking an endocrinopathy or another noninflammatory alopecia. So, recurrent alopecia must not be ruled out if lesions are not only on the flanks.

A history of clipping is diagnostic of "postclipping alopecia" in dogs with shortened haircoat. At the same time, the anamnesis of a stressful event (pregnancy, lactation, severe illness) or a chemotherapy treatment (e.g., with doxorubicin) suggests telogen and anagen effluvium, respectively.

Finally, canine pattern baldness (CPB) is typical of many short-haired breeds, such as Pinschers, Whippets, Dachshunds, etc. Miniaturized hairs on the ventral neck, temporal and retroauricular areas, and posterior thighs are the hallmarks of this localized skin disorder. The posterior profile of the rear legs is the only affected skin area in Greyhounds with the so-called "bald thigh syndrome", a localized variant of CPB. Although lesions are more localized and not spread to the trunk in CPB, as it happens in endocrinopathies, in rare cases, alopecia can be so widespread that it also involves the lower and middle part of the trunk. This extension makes the disease less characteristic and can be confused with other noninflammatory alopecic diseases.

Algorithm 2.1 Note 6 The therapy of endocrinopathies will be discussed in dedicated sections of the book.

Algorithm 2.1 Note 7 For follicular dysplasia (CDA, BHD, non-color linked dysplasia, breed-linked dysplasia, pattern baldness), pharmacological therapy is not available.

Algorithm 2.1 Note 8 Treatment of alopecia X involves various approaches and variable success rates. Treatment with melatonin and trilostane, as well as chemical castration with suprelorin, are reported to be the most successful.[1,3] Treatment with trilostane led to complete hair regrowth in 85% of Pomeranians with alopecia X within 4 to 8 months.[1] When trilostane is used, the protocol for treating hypercortisolism is applied (see chapter 35). In 60-75% of non-neutered male dogs, hair regrowth was observed within three months after suprelorin treatment.[1]

Algorithm 2.1 Note 9 A spontaneous recovery is observed in seasonal flank/recurrent alopecia. Both telogen and anagen effluvium spontaneously resolve when the causative underlying cause is eliminated.

Algorithm 2.1 Note 10 In some breeds affected by canine pattern baldness, including Dachshunds, Boston Terriers, and Miniature Pinschers, partial benefit has been anecdotally reported with melatonin at the dosage of 3 mg/dog tid. Since some dogs show spontaneous improvement of alopecia, the efficacy of the melatonin remains questionable.

ALGORITHM 2.1

Diagnostic approach to alopecia.

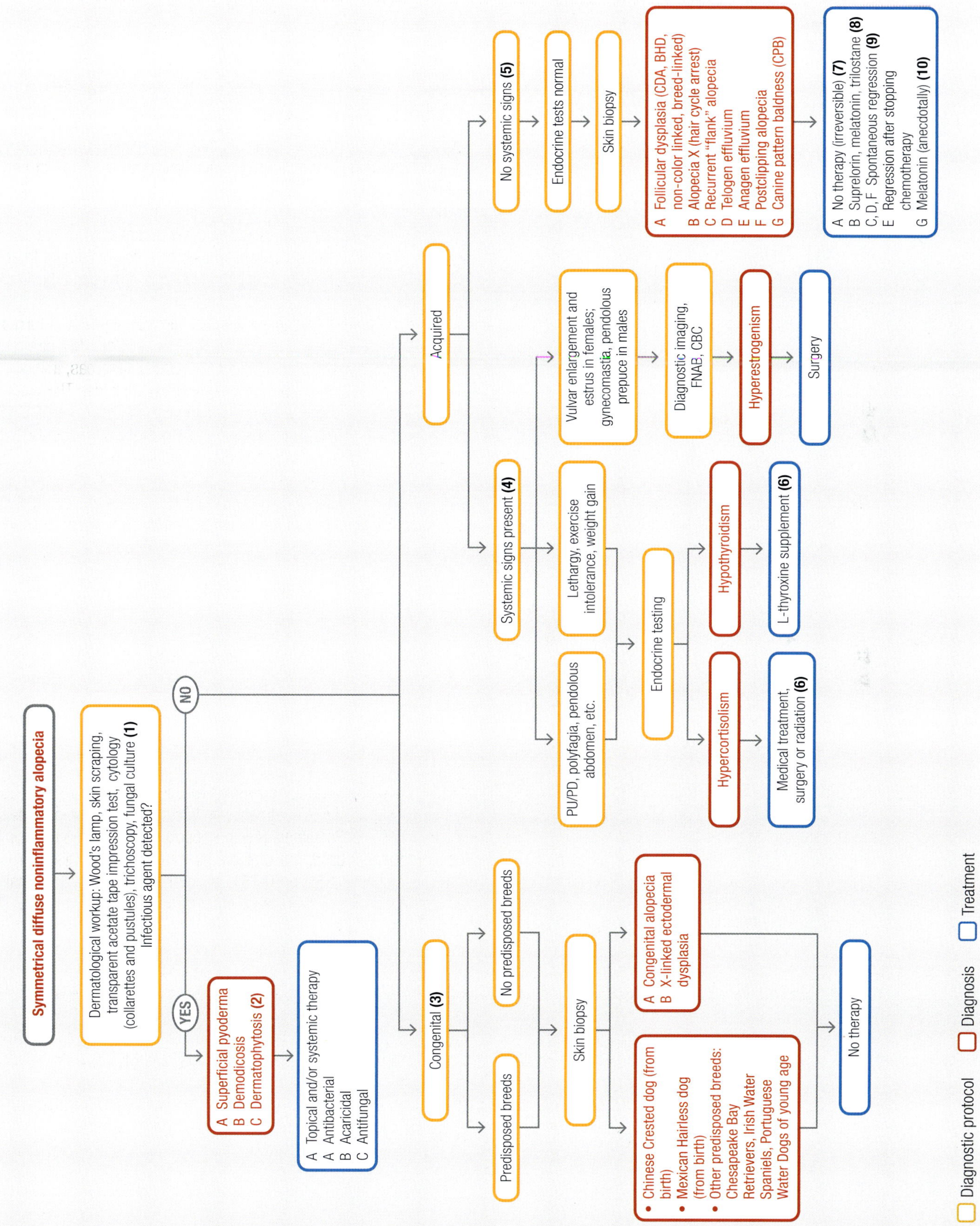

References

1. Albanese F, Malerba E, Abramo F, Miragliotta V, Fracassi F. Deslorelin for the treatment of hair cycle arrest in intact male dogs. *Vet Dermatol* 25(6):519-522, e87-e88, 2014. doi:10.1111/vde.12148.
2. Brunner MAT, Jagannathan V, Waluk DP, Roosje P, Linek M, Panakova L, Leeb T, Wiener DJ, Welle MM. Novel insights into the pathways regulating the canine hair cycle and their deregulation in alopecia X. *PLoS One* 12(10):e0186469, 2017. doi:10.1371/journal.pone.0186469.
3. Cerundolo R, Lloyd DH, Persechino A, Evans H, Cauvin A. Treatment of canine Alopecia X with trilostane. *Vet Dermatol* 15(5):285-293, 2004. doi:10.1111/j.1365-3164.2004.00403.x.
4. Drögemüller C, Philipp U, Haase B, Günzel-Apel AR, Leeb T. A noncoding melanophilin gene (MLPH) SNP at the splice donor of exon 1 represents a candidate causal mutation for coat color dilution in dogs. *J Hered* 98(5):468-473, 2007. doi:10.1093/jhered/esm021.
5. Müntener T, Doherr MG, Guscetti F, Suter MM, Welle MM. The canine hair cycle –A guide for the assessment of morphological and immunohistochemical criteria. *Vet Dermatol* 22(5):383-395, 2011. doi:10.1111/j.1365-3164.2011.00963.x.
6. Müntener T, Schuepbach-Regula G, Frank L, Rüfenacht S, Welle MM. Canine noninflammatory alopecia: a comprehensive evaluation of common and distinguishing histological characteristics. *Vet Dermatol* 23(3):206-e44, 2012. doi:10.1111/j.1365-3164.2012.01049.x.
7. Welle MM. Canine noninflammatory alopecia: An approach to its classification and a diagnostic aid. *Vet Pathol* 60(6):748-769, 2023. doi:10.1177/03009858231170295.

CHAPTER 3

Weight loss

Sean E. Hulsebosch
DVM, DACVIM (SAIM)

Pathophysiology

Weight loss is a common presenting complaint in small animal practice with an extensive list of causes. Therefore, the clinician must obtain a detailed history and perform a thorough physical exam in order to reach a diagnosis efficiently. Noting the dog's appetite is of paramount importance, as this helps to narrow the list of differential diagnoses.

Weight loss can be intentional or unintentional; this chapter will focus on unintentional weight loss, which is defined in human and veterinary medicine as >5% loss of usual body weight over the prior 6-12 months.[1] When approaching a problem with so many underlying causes, it is helpful to remember the various pathophysiological mechanisms of unintentional weight loss, which include insufficient caloric intake, maldigestion, malabsorption, increased utilization of calories, loss of calories, or due to multifactorial reasons.

Insufficient caloric intake can be due to inadvertent underfeeding by the client, decreased food intake secondary to dysphagia, or hyporexia to anorexia secondary to either gastrointestinal (GI) or various systemic diseases. Maldigestion and malabsorption result from either GI disease or exocrine pancreatic disease. Increased utilization of calories generally occurs due to an increased metabolic rate from an endocrinopathy, neoplasia, systemic infection, or other systemic inflammatory illness. Loss of calories in dogs can occur due to GI or renal disease. Some diseases lead to weight loss via multiple mechanisms (e.g., neoplasia via inappetence and increased utilization).[2] See Table 3.1.

Inflammatory cytokines such as tumor necrosis factor, interleukin-1, and interleukin-6 promote anorexia and catabolism of fat and muscle in neoplasia and certain inflammatory diseases.[3] These diseases can also lead to a hypermetabolic state, which in turn upregulates gluconeogenesis, lipolysis, protein catabolism, and recycling of lactate.[2,3,4] Weight loss with low body fat and consequent low leptin levels should, under physiologic conditions, increase appetite. However, despite low leptin concentrations in illness, the above inflammatory mediators are thought to interfere with appetite signaling. There can also be dysregulation in the hormones involved in decreasing appetite (e.g., leptin, insulin, GLP-1, peptide YY, cholecystokinin, and the above inflammatory cytokines) and those hormones involved in increasing appetite (e.g., ghrelin, neuropeptide Y).[2,3,4]

In order to assess whether a dog is being inadvertently underfed, the dog's resting energy requirements (RER) can be calculated using the exponential formula: $70 \times (\text{body weight in Kg})^{0.75}$. Maintenance energy requirements (MER) can then be estimated using the following conversion factors: $1.2\text{-}1.4 \times \text{RER}$ for an inactive or

TABLE 3.1 Causes of unintentional weight loss in the dog, according to pathophysiology.

Insufficient caloric intake	Maldigestion or malabsorption	Increased utilization/ metabolic rate	Loss of calories	Multifactorial/ miscellaneous
■ Inadvertent underfeeding ■ Oral pain (e.g., severe dental disease) ■ Dysphagia (e.g., megaesophagus) ■ Inappetence from systemic disease (e.g., uremia, advanced liver disease, moderate-severe anemia, neoplasia, etc.) ■ Hypothalamic disease affecting appetite center ■ Cognitive dysfunction ■ Iatrogenic (medication-induced)	■ Exocrine pancreatic insufficiency (EPI) ■ Inflammatory bowel disease (IBD) ■ Food-responsive enteropathy ■ Gastrointestinal (GI) neoplasia (e.g., small cell lymphoma) ■ Primary lymphangiectasia ■ Severe endoparasitism ■ Chronic-partial foreign body obstruction	■ Neoplasia ■ Pregnancy ■ Hyperthyroidism ■ Hypercortisolism (when muscle atrophy exceeds fat deposition) ■ Systemic infection ■ Systemic inflammation ■ Cardiac disease/failure	■ GI disease (protein-losing enteropathy) ■ Renal disease (protein-losing nephropathy) ■ Cutaneous (uncommon in dogs)	■ Neoplasia ■ Hypoadrenocorticism ■ Diabetes mellitus ■ Age-related sarcopenia ■ Cardiac cachexia

ALGORITHM 3.1

Diagnostic approach to weight loss.

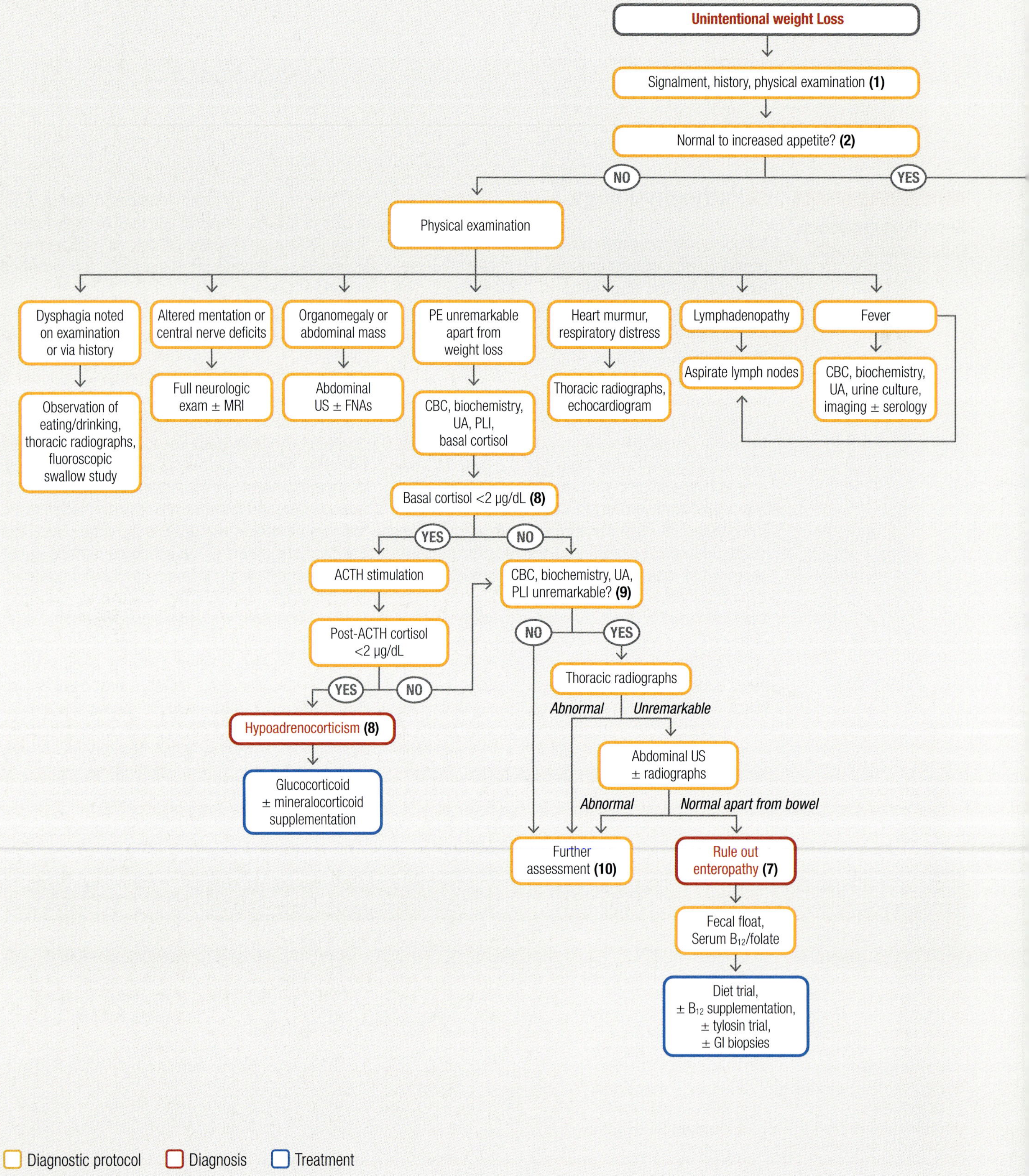

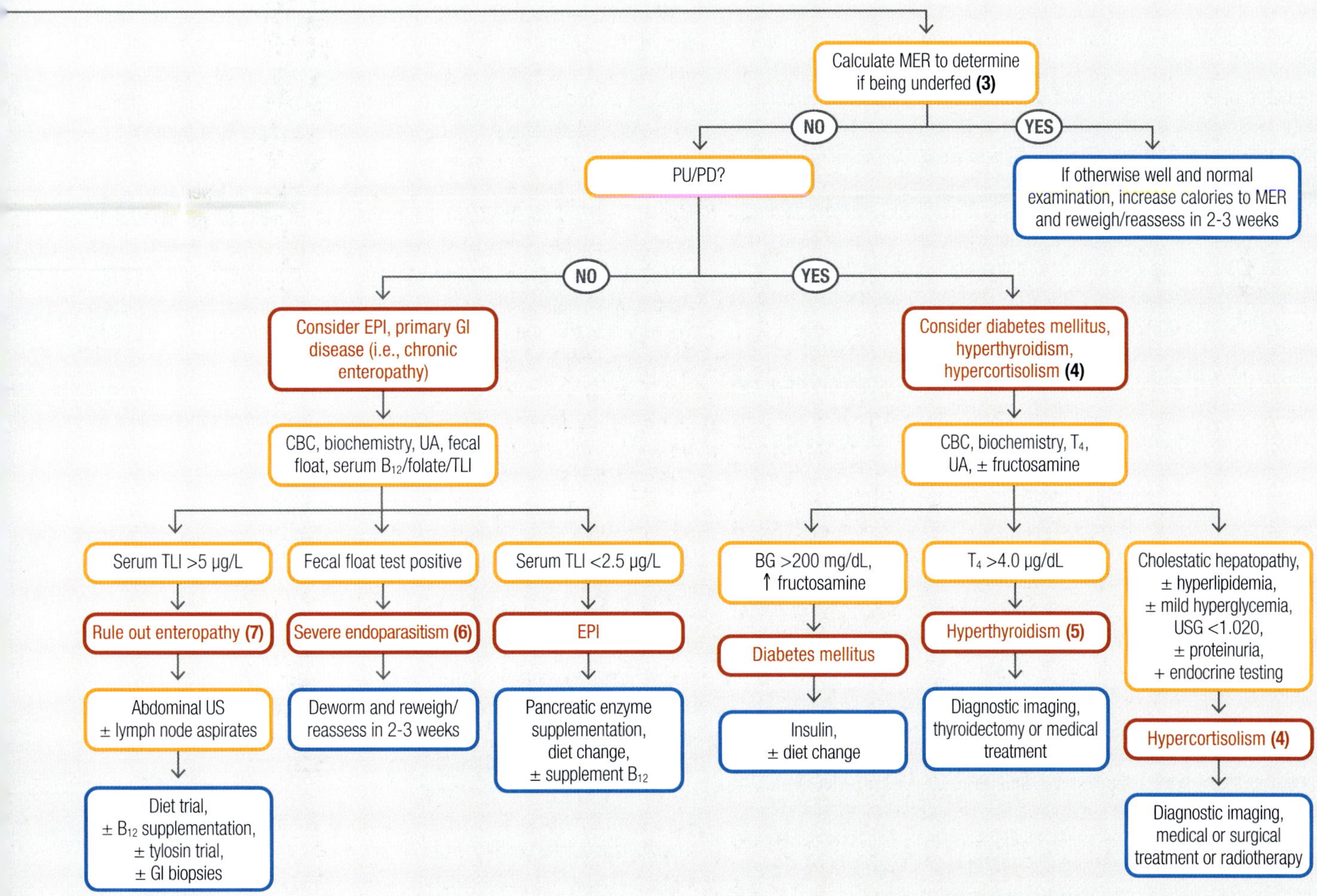
Calculate MER to determine if being underfed (3)
NO
YES
PU/PD?
If otherwise well and normal examination, increase calories to MER and reweigh/reassess in 2-3 weeks
NO
YES
Consider EPI, primary GI disease (i.e., chronic enteropathy)
Consider diabetes mellitus, hyperthyroidism, hypercortisolism (4)
CBC, biochemistry, UA, fecal float, serum B12/folate/TLI
CBC, biochemistry, T4, UA, ± fructosamine
Serum TLI >5 μg/L
Fecal float test positive
Serum TLI <2.5 μg/L
BG >200 mg/dL, ↑ fructosamine
T4 >4.0 μg/dL
Cholestatic hepatopathy, ± hyperlipidemia, ± mild hyperglycemia, USG <1.020, ± proteinuria, + endocrine testing
Rule out enteropathy (7)
Severe endoparasitism (6)
EPI
Diabetes mellitus
Hyperthyroidism (5)
Hypercortisolism (4)
Abdominal US ± lymph node aspirates
Deworm and reweigh/reassess in 2-3 weeks
Pancreatic enzyme supplementation, diet change, ± supplement B12
Insulin, ± diet change
Diagnostic imaging, thyroidectomy or medical treatment
Diagnostic imaging, medical or surgical treatment or radiotherapy
Diet trial, ± B12 supplementation, ± tylosin trial, ± GI biopsies

obesity-prone dog, 1.4-1.6 × RER for a neutered dog, 1.8 × RER for an intact dog, 2-3 × RER for a puppy (depending on age), and 3 × RER for a late-term pregnant bitch.[4,5,6] The clinician should recognize that some dogs being fed their MER can still lose weight in the absence of disease due to individual dog variation.

Clinical signs

In addition to the weight loss observed by the owner or veterinarian, other additional clinical signs that might be present include lethargy, changes in appetite, vomiting, diarrhea, polyuria (PU), polydipsia (PU), coughing, sneezing, pruritus, and changes in skin or hair coat (Video 3.1). Occasionally, clinical signs are less obvious, such as taking longer to finish meals, eating only high-value foods, or lip licking in the absence of vomiting. Appetite is often diminished, and there are a myriad of differentials for weight loss with a decreased appetite in dogs. Conversely, there are limited differentials for weight loss with polyphagia, including exocrine pancreatic insufficiency (EPI), some chronic enteropathies, severe endoparasitism, diabetes mellitus, hyperthyroidism, and occasionally hypercortisolism (if the peripheral muscle atrophy exceeds central fat deposition). When the client reports a "normal" appetite despite weight loss, further questioning and history are needed to determine if there is truly no change in appetite.

Noting which of the aforementioned clinical signs are present can help discern if there is a primary GI or extra-GI cause of the weight loss. For example, PU/PD more likely suggests metabolic or endocrine disease as opposed to primary GI disease. Fever might suggest systemic infectious or inflammatory disease. Changes in stool quality are more consistent with primary GI or exocrine pancreatic disease but also occur with extra-GI disease (e.g., hyperthyroidism). Importantly, the absence of vomiting, diarrhea, and inappetence does not exclude the possibility of primary GI disease.[6,7]

Primary GI disease is one of the more common reasons for weight loss in dogs. As mentioned, this differential is often, but not always, accompanied by the clinical signs of vomiting, diarrhea, and variable appetite. Of the many GI differentials for weight loss, chronic enteropathies are the most abundant, including food-responsive enteropathy, antibiotic-responsive enteropathy, and immune-responsive enteropathy or inflammatory bowel disease.[8] Other primary GI considerations for weight loss include severe endoparasitism, infectious enteropathy (e.g., histoplasmosis), lymphangiectasia, and GI neoplasia. Exocrine pancreatic diseases, including chronic pancreatitis and exocrine pancreatic insufficiency, present with similar clinical signs as GI disease.

Extra-GI disorders can be ruled in or out with blood and urine testing and/or imaging diagnostics. There are myriad metabolic disorders that can lead to weight loss, including uremia, advanced hepatic disease, and endocrinopathies, and there are typically additional clinical signs, such as PU/PD, panting, nausea, etc., that accompany these metabolic diseases. For example, hyperthyroidism, hyperparathyroidism, diabetes mellitus, hypoadrenocorticism, and hypercortisolism are examples of endocrinopathies that can cause weight loss, and all of these also typically cause PU/PD. While hypercortisolism (and exogenous glucocorticoids) cause appendicular muscle atrophy and truncal weight gain, which classically leads to "weight redistribution", this can lead to weight loss in certain dogs (Video 3.1).

Video 3.1

A 12-year-old male intact mixed breed dog with severe polyphagia, weight loss, muscle atrophy, and muscle stiffness from uncontrolled ACTH-dependent hypercortisolism and a suspected enteropathy.

Diagnostic approach

Algorithm 3.1 shows the approach to weight loss in dogs. Weight loss >5% of body weight in 6-12 months warrants investigation.[1] Serial weight measurements can easily confirm weight loss. Dogs of any age are at risk for weight loss, although in a puppy, weight loss can be masked by physiological growth. Therefore, comparing body condition score (BCS) estimations can be more helpful in a growing puppy.

Algorithm 3.1 Note 1 A thorough history is critical when addressing a problem with as many differential diagnoses as weight loss. Special attention should be given to diet, medications, environment, travel history, and systems review, including vomiting, diarrhea, thirst, and appetite. Evaluation of whether the dog is generally unwell or well helps to dictate the urgency and the number of diagnostics performed. A meticulous physical examination is also paramount.

Algorithm 3.1 Note 2 There are a limited number of differentials for weight loss with a normal to increased appetite, highlighting the importance of this history information.

Algorithm 3.1 Note 3 Reminder that some dogs being fed MER can lose weight due to variations in a given dog's inherent metabolism and activity level.

Algorithm 3.1 Note 4 There are a limited number of differentials for weight loss, polyphagia, and PU/PD. While dogs with hypercortisolism classically have "weight redistribution" (i.e., peripheral muscle atrophy and truncal fat deposition), in some dogs, the muscle atrophy exceeds fat deposition, leading to weight loss (Video 3.1).

Algorithm 3.1 Note 5 Hyperthyroidism is uncommon in dogs and is typically associated with thyroid carcinoma. Confirm that hyperthyroidism is not caused by diet, such as a raw food diet that includes animal thyroid glands.

Algorithm 3.1 Note 6 In order to cause significant weight loss, endoparasitism must be severe.

Algorithm 3.1 Note 7 While often associated with vomiting, diarrhea, and changes in appetite, chronic enteropathies can lead to weight loss as the sole clinical sign. Additionally, while appetite is typically decreased, some dogs with chronic enteropathy can present with polyphagia due to malabsorption. Abdominal ultrasonography can imply GI disease (e.g., thickened bowel loops, abnormal bowel wall layering, functional ileus). Serum markers of intestinal absorption, including albumin, globulin, cholesterol, magnesium, calcium, cobalamin, and folate, may be decreased, suggesting GI disease is the source of weight loss.

Algorithm 3.1 Note 8 A basal serum cortisol >55 nmol/L (2 μg/dL) excludes hypoadrenocorticism. If basal cortisol is <55 nmol/L (2 μg/dL), an ACTH stimulation test should be performed; hypoadrenocorticism is confirmed when serum cortisol post-ACTH is <55 nmol/L (2 μg/dL) in a dog that has not received consistent glucocorticoids in the previous 2 months. A urinary cortisol/creatinine ratio below the reference range is suggestive of hypoadrenocorticism and should be confirmed with post-ACTH cortisol measurement.[9]

Algorithm 3.1 Note 9 If the animal presents significantly unwell or debilitated, then CBC, serum biochemistry panel, and urinalysis should be performed earlier in the diagnostic process after physical examination.

Algorithm 3.1 Note 10 At this step, further assessment of abnormal thoracic radiographs might include a CT scan, bronchoscopy, tracheal wash, and/or ultrasound-guided percutaneous fine-needle aspiration cytology. Further assessment of abnormal abdominal radiographs or ultrasonography might include ultrasound-guided percutaneous fine-needle aspiration cytology and/or biopsy, laparoscopic biopsies, and/or laparotomy. Further assessment of abnormal CBC might include a workup of anemia, polycythemia, leukocytosis, leukopenia, or thrombocytopenia. Further assessment of abnormal biochemistry panel might include a workup of azotemia, hepatopathy, electrolyte derangements, dyslipidemias, hypoalbuminemia, hyperglobulinemia, or hypoglycemia. Further assessment of abnormal urinalysis might include further workup of inappropriate urine specific gravity, bacteriuria, pyuria, or findings consistent with Fanconi's syndrome.

References

1. Bosch X, Monclús E, Escoda O, et al. Unintentional weight loss: clinical characteristics and outcomes in a prospective cohort of 2677 patients. *PloS One* 12(4):e0175125, 2017. doi.org/10.1371/journal.pone.0175125.
2. Johannes CM, Musser ML. Anorexia and the cancer patient. *Vet Clin North Am Small Anim Pract* 49(5):837-854, 2019. doi:10.1016/j.cvsm.2019.04.008.
3. Perera LAM, Chopra A, Shaw AL. Approach to patients with unintentional weight loss. *Med Clin North Am* 105(1):175-186, 2021. doi:10.1016/j.mcna.2020.08.019.
4. Johnson LN, Freeman LM. Recognizing, describing, and managing reduced food intake in dogs and cats. *J Am Vet Med Assoc* 2017 251(11): 1260-1266. doi.org/10.2460/javma.251.11.1260.
5. Hand MS, Thatcher CD, Remillard RL, Roudebush P, Novtony BJ (editors). Small Animal Clinical Nutrition 5th edition. Topeka, Kansas, Mark Morris Institute, 2010.
6. Tolbert MK, Murphy M, Gaylord L, et al. Dietary management of chronic enteropathy in dogs. *J Small Anim Pract* 63(6):425-434, 2022. https://doi.org/10.1111/jsap.13471.
7. Craven MD, Washabau RJ. Comparative pathophysiology and management of protein-losing enteropathy. *J Vet Intern Med* 33(2):383-402, 2019. doi:10.1111/jvim.15406.
8. Dandrieux JR, Mansfield CS. Chronic enteropathy in canines: prevalence, impact and management strategies. *Vet Med Res Rep* 6:203-214, 2019. doi.org/10.2147/VMRR.S162774.
9. Del Baldo F, Gerou Ferriani M, Bertazzolo W, et al. Urinary cortisol-creatinine ratio in dogs with hypoadrenocorticism. *J Vet Inter Med* 36(2): 482-487, 2022. doi:10.1111/jvim.16358

CHAPTER 4

Polyuria and polydipsia

Stijn J.M. Niessen
DVM, PhD, DECVIM, PGCertVetEd, FHEA, MRCVS

Federico Fracassi
DVM, PhD, DECVIM (SAIM)

Sara Galac
DVM, PhD

Edward C. Feldman
DVM, DACVIM (SAIM)

Physiology and pathophysiology

In health, 85-90% of the fluid filtered by glomeruli is reabsorbed iso-osmotically with sodium and glucose in the proximal nephron. Sodium is selectively reabsorbed from the proximal nephron, creating the hypotonic fluid that flows into distal nephrons. Water balance is maintained primarily via interactions between the distal nephrons/collecting ducts and the pituitary hormone vasopressin (antidiuretic hormone; ADH). As much as 90% of distal nephron fluid can be absorbed when ADH opens water channels within kidney distal tubular cells, causing water resorption by osmotic gradient (kidney interstitial fluid is hypertonic).

ADH is synthesized in hypothalamic supraoptic and paraventricular nuclei before being transported along axons to the posterior pituitary, from which it is released into the circulation with appropriate stimulation. In the presence of water overload, increased blood volume, and/or decreased blood osmolarity, ADH secretion is suppressed, large volumes of dilute urine (as low as 1.001) can be produced because the water channels are closed, "drowning" is prevented, and water balance maintained. In the presence of water deficiency, decreased blood volume, and/or increased blood osmolarity, ADH secretion is stimulated, water channels are opened, small volumes of concentrated urine (as high as 1.060) are produced, dehydration is prevented, and water balance is maintained. Blood osmolarity/sodium is mainly monitored by specific and sensitive cells in the hypothalamus. Blood volume/pressure is monitored primarily by specific cells located in the cardiac atria and the aortic arch.

Water intake and urine output in healthy dogs vary. On random sampling, most healthy dogs produce urine with a specific gravity >1.018 and <1.045. Warm environmental temperatures, exercise, dry food diets, diarrhea, and vomiting are among the factors that should mildly increase water intake and are not usually of concern to owners.

Definitions and initial considerations

A dog with polyuria/polydipsia (PU/PD) consumes abnormally large volumes of water (>100 mL/kg/day) and produces abnormally large volumes of urine. The first task for the veterinary clinician is to discriminate the dog with pollakiuria/dysuria from one with polyuria (PU) since either can cause an owner to observe increased frequency and/or what appears to be prolonged periods of urination. Urinalysis results are always valuable, especially if collected by the owner within 12-24 hours before consultancy. Dogs with PU/PD can have solute diuresis, an insensitivity to ADH, or an ADH deficiency, each of which can be medically induced. In all these conditions, water lost due to PU stimulates polydipsia (PD). It is rare for a dog to have "primary PD", which leads to PU.

Solute diuresis

When there is an excess solute in the glomerular filtrate, water absorption from the proximal nephrons is impaired, and increased volumes of water flow into the distal nephrons, where their ability to absorb water is overwhelmed, and PU develops. To compensate for this water loss, affected dogs increase their water intake (PD). In chronic renal failure, there are an ever-decreasing number of functioning nephrons. There is a compensatory increase in glomerular filtration rate per surviving nephron, and the amount of fluid presented to the distal tubules is increased. Increased tubular flow rate causes less urea, sodium, and other substances to be reabsorbed. The result is an osmotic diuresis further complicated by a reduced medullary concentration gradient. All these factors contribute to the development of PU.

Another common and classic solute diuresis in dogs occurs secondary to excess glucose in the glomerular filtrate due to diabetes mellitus (DM). Primary renal glucosuria is quite uncommon. Owners are usually aware if their dog is given a solute diuretic, e.g., mannitol.

Primary and secondary ADH deficiency

Central diabetes insipidus (CDI) can be caused by hypothalamic/pituitary pathology that decreases or completely eliminates ADH synthesis/secretion. It is an extremely uncommon congenital condition. CDI is uncommonly caused by an expanding pituitary mass or even less commonly due to trauma. Primary ADH deficiency should only be considered after all common causes for PU/PD have been ruled out. It is unclear whether or not the remarkable PU/PD observed in dogs with iatrogenic or naturally occurring hypercortisolism is due, in part, to suppressed ADH synthesis/secretion (secondary CDI) due to secondary NDI (see below) or both.

Primary ADH resistance

Primary nephrogenic diabetes insipidus (NDI) is an extremely rare congenital condition in which nephrons are insensitive to ADH, causing profound PU, which stimulates PD.

Secondary ADH resistance

Secondary NDI is among the most common causes of PU/PD in dogs. PU/PD associated with many of these conditions is reversible. The most common causes of secondary NDI are pyometra, cortisol excess (iatrogenic cortisol administration or any form of naturally occurring Cushing's syndrome), and hypercalcemia. Uncommon-to-rare causes of secondary NDI include (in decreasing order of frequency) severe liver disease/failure, pyelonephritis, hypokalemia, hyperthyroidism (naturally occurring and iatrogenic caused by improperly prepared raw meat diets), and acromegaly.

Signalment, history, physical examination

Each PU/PD patient evaluation component can be extremely valuable. Non-spayed females may have pyometra. The Norwegian Elkhound and Basenji are predisposed to primary renal glycosuria. Dogs with enlarged lymph nodes or an anal sac mass could have hypercalcemia of malignancy. Dogs with progressive weight loss and poor appetites may have CKD. Dogs with progressive weight loss and an excellent appetite may have DM. Dogs with apparent weight gain and excellent appetites may have hypercortisolism.

Diagnostic approach

Algorithm 4.1 shows a practical approach to the patient presenting with PU/PD. Given the many possible diseases underlying PU/PD, the workup requires a systematic medical approach.

Diagnosis

In case of any doubt over whether there is PU/PD, a water diary (water consumption in 24 hours) could be conducted by owners at home or in-clinic. The latter can be interesting since dogs with (predominantly) primary polydipsia often show a sudden decrease in volumes drunk when the environment is changed.

The volume urinated is often difficult to establish by direct measurement. A useful substitute is simple urine specific gravity (USG) measurement, ideally on an early morning sample; early morning increases the chance maximum concentrating ability is shown. The obtained value can be used to guide the location of the problem. Hyposthenuria (USG <1.008), for instance, would be associated with conditions where active dilution of urine occurs (e.g., problems connected with lack of ADH production, secretion, or action). A structural kidney disease commonly causes isosthenuria (USG 1.008-1.015).

Algorithm 4.1 Note 1 Urinary specific gravity is a parameter commonly used by veterinarians in routine practice. Ideally, in association with the USG, urinary osmolality could be assessed. Urinary osmolality provides more precise information, but its correlation with USG is good.[2] Although there are many different causes for PU/PD, many hints about its etiology can be obtained by considering the signalment, a thorough history, physical examination as well as basic blood biochemistry.

Algorithm 4.1 Note 2 Routine biochemistry is essential in the workup of cases with PU/PD. As examples, blood sodium concentration can provide subtle hints over whether PU/PD is induced by polydipsia (sodium more likely low normal or low) or induced by polyuria (sodium more likely high normal or high); the presence of ALP and cholesterol elevations could fit with hypercortisolism; azotemia, despite inappropriate dilute urine, suggests renal dysfunction. Abdominal ultrasound can highlight adrenal masses or other alterations potentially connected to PU/PD (e.g., liver disease, nephropathy, masses).

Algorithm 4.1 Note 3 Measure USG or Uosm in serial urine samples collected by the owner at home over the day or perform a modified water deprivation test (MDWT) (see chapter 25). Both tests are combined with the administration of DDAVP: intraocular or oral in the urine test and parenteral in the MDWT. If USG increases to >1.020 or UOsm >1.000 mOsm/kg, central diabetes insipidus is very likely.

Algorithm 4.1 Note 4 Equivocal results, with a trend towards USG concentration but slightly less than 50%, may indicate partial central diabetes insipidus.

Algorithm 4.1 Note 5 When central diabetes insipidus is diagnosed, supplementation with DDAVP (ADH analog) conjunctival drops, injections, or oral tablets is indicated.

DDAVP is a synthetic analog of ADH. Initial therapy includes doses of 0.05 mg PO q12h for dogs <5 kg, 0.1 mg PO q12h for dogs between 5 to 20 kg, 0.2 mg PO q12h for dogs >20 kg, up to a maximum of 0.4 mg q8h. If these doses are not enough to control PU/PD, it is possible to try the administration q8h. If necessary, the conjunctival or subcutaneous route can also be used.[4]

ALGORITHM 4.1

Diagnostic approach to polyuria/polydipsia.

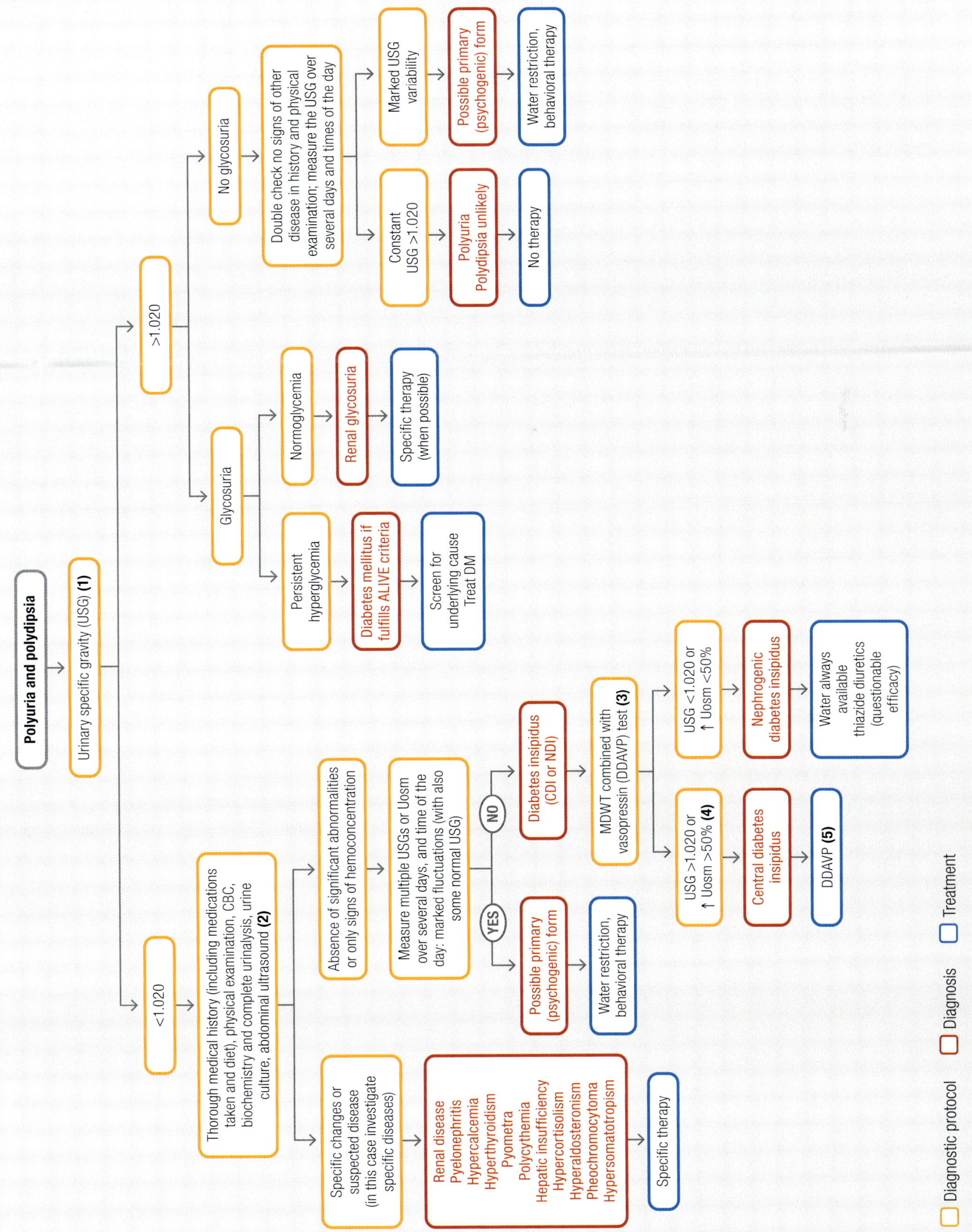

References

1. Ayoub JA, Beaufrere H, Acierno MJ Association between urine osmolality and specific gravity in dogs and effect of commonly measured urine solutes on that association. *Am J Vet Res* 74;1542-1545, 2013.
2. Rijnberk A, Kooistra HS. Protocols and function tests. In Rijnberk A, Kooistra HS (editors). Clinical Endocrinology of Dogs and Cats. Hannover, Schlütersche, 2010, pp. 305-314.
3. Niessen SJM, Bjornvad C, Church DB, Davison L, Esteban-Saltiveri D, Fleeman LM, Forcada Y, Fracassi F, Gilor C, Hanson J, Herrtage M, Lathan P, Leal RO, Loste A, Reusch C, Schermerhorn T, Stengel C, Thoresen S, Thuroczy J; ESVE/SCE membership. Agreeing Language in Veterinary Endocrinology (ALIVE): Diabetes mellitus –A modified Delphi-method-based system to create consensus disease definitions. *Vet J* 289:105910, 2022. doi: 10.1016/j.tvjl.2022.105910. Epub ahead of print.
4. Feldman EC, Nelson RW, Reusch CE, Scott-Moncrieff JCR, Behrend E (editors). Canine and Feline Endocrinology 4th edition. St. Louis, Elsevier, 2015.

CHAPTER 5

Polyphagia

Dan Rosenberg
DVM, PhD

Polyphagia (or hyperphagia) refers to excessive food consumption or appetite.[1-3]

In many aspects, the term "excessive" is subjective, and this subjectivity may explain why, to date, no study investigating underlying causes of polyphagia has ever been published in dogs.

Hyperphagia may be preferred over the term polyphagia when the increase in food consumption results from a compensatory mechanism toward physiological or pathological increases in energy demand (Table 5.1). Inappropriate polyphagia refers in this chapter to predominantly pathological situations in which overeating is not, or not solely, triggered by an increase in energy demand.

TABLE 5.1 Causes of polyphagia in the dog.

Compensatory polyphagia (hyperphagia)	Inappropriate polyphagia
■ Low food intake	■ Encephalic related
■ Contextual	– Diencephalic mass
– Insufficient feeding rations	– Palatable diet
– Hypocaloric diet	– Postictal
■ Pathological	– Psychogenic
– Megaesophagus	– Stress-induced
– Esophagus compression secondary to aortic arch anomalies	■ Endocrine (non compensatory) related
– Parasitic spoliation	– Acromegaly
■ Maldigestion/malabsorption	– Hyperadrenocorticism
– Exocrine pancreatic insufficiency	– Insulinoma
– Inflammatory or neoplastic bowel disease	– Neutering
– Intestinal lymphangiectasia	■ Drug-induced
■ Decreased cell energy supply	– Bromides
– Diabetes mellitus	– Glucocorticoids
– Hypoglycemia	– Imepitoin
■ High metabolic consumption	– Orexigenic (and ghrelin receptor agonist) agents
■ Physiological	– Phenobarbital
– Growth	– Primidone
– Lactation	– Theophylline
– Pregnancy	– Thyroxine overdosage (infrequent)
– Cold environment	■ Miscellaneous
– Increased exercise	– Breed-associated (e.g., Labrador Retriever)
■ Pathological	– Sudden acquired retinopathy
– Inflammation and neoplastic process (at early stages)	– Presumed cancer-associated retinopathy
– Hyperthyroidism	– Portosystemic shunt
	– Liver encephalopathy

Pathophysiology

Appetite regulation has not been studied in depth in dogs. Most concepts discussed in this section are extrapolated from rodent and primate data. The regulation of appetite involves central and peripheral mechanisms. The historical distinction of satiety and hunger center,[4,5] located in the ventromedial area and the lateral area of the hypothalamus, respectively, has been replaced by a more subtle description of different regions, cell types, and even more specific axonal projections involved in the stimulation or suppression of food consumption.[6] Both ventromedial (refined as the arcuated nucleus) and lateral areas comprise highly differentiated neurons that activate or inhibit appetite under regulation from multiple hypothalamic, brainstem, and cortical (mainly limbic) areas, allowing response to behavioral, sensorial (e.g., olfaction, taste, vision), endocrine, and autonomic stimuli. Most peripheral stimuli regulating appetite belong to the so-called "gut-brain axis" and "adipose tissue-brain axis".[7] In the gut, chemoreceptors and mechanoreceptors activate a response to meals through nervous (vagal) and endocrine signals, including different anorexigenic peptides secreted by digestive cells such as glucagon-like peptide-1 (GLP-1), peptide YY, and cholecystokinin, whereas fasting stimulates gastric secretion of the orexigenic hormone ghrelin. Neurons involved in appetite stimulation express the ghrelin receptor and depolarize after binding with this hormone. Most of them also express the leptin receptor with opposite downstream signaling (physiologic hyperpolarization in case of energy storage in adipose tissue resulting in leptin secretion and satiety).

The main causes of canine polyphagia are listed in Table 5.1. The frequency of occurrence of polyphagia varies significantly from one entity to another in this list, ranging, for example, from approximately 50% of cases observed in hypercortisolism to less than 5% of patients with insulinoma.[8-9]

The concept of compensatory polyphagia, in which an unmet energy need leads to the activation of the "gut-brain" and "adipose tissue-brain" axes, seems logical and allows for a mnemonic appropriation of the table. However, the implication of these pathogenic mechanisms

ALGORITHM 5.1

Diagnosis approach of a dog with polyphagia.

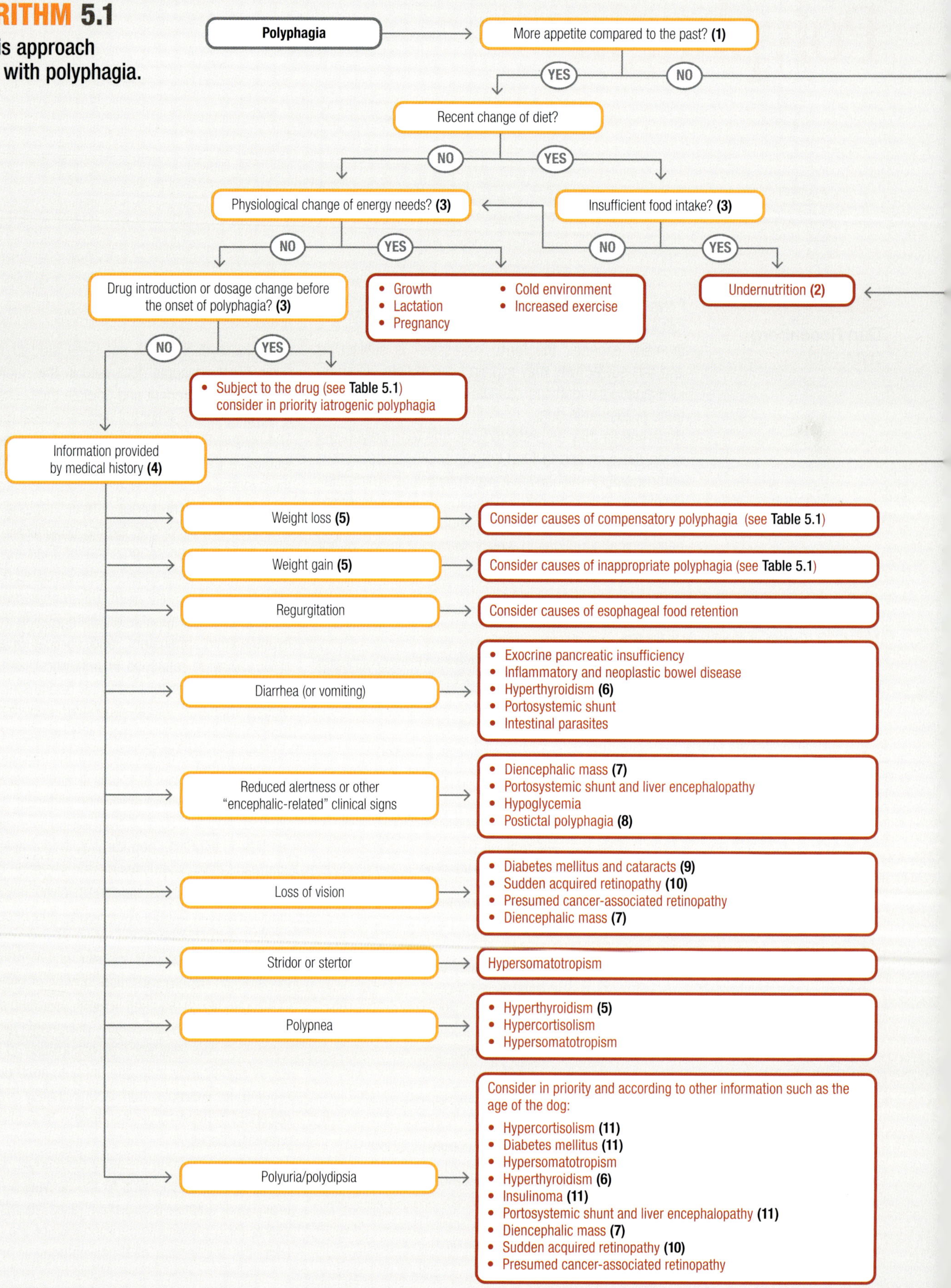

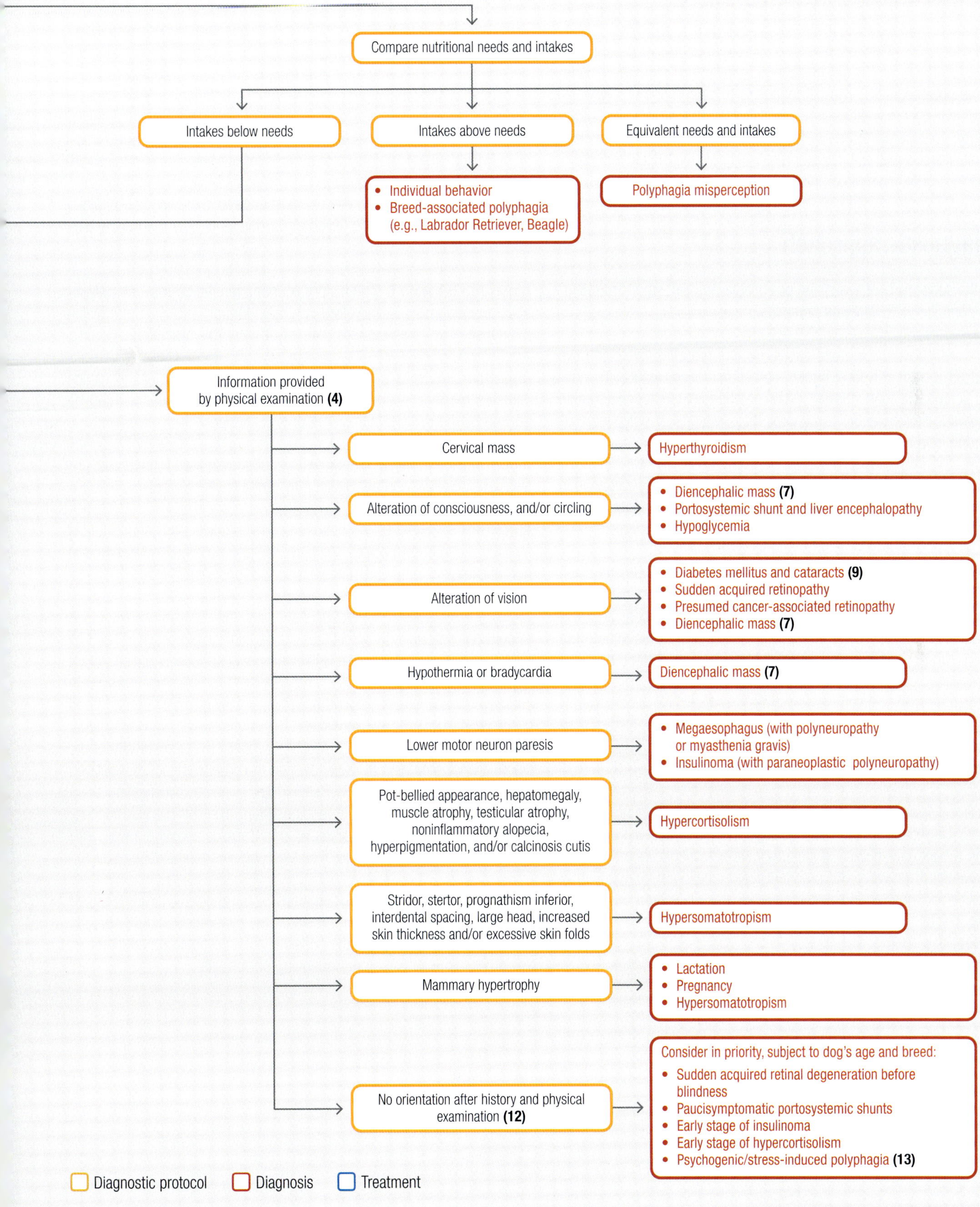
Compare nutritional needs and intakes
Intakes below needs
Intakes above needs
Equivalent needs and intakes
• Individual behavior
• Breed-associated polyphagia (e.g., Labrador Retriever, Beagle)
Polyphagia misperception
Information provided by physical examination (4)
Cervical mass
Hyperthyroidism
Alteration of consciousness, and/or circling
• Diencephalic mass (7)
• Portosystemic shunt and liver encephalopathy
• Hypoglycemia
Alteration of vision
• Diabetes mellitus and cataracts (9)
• Sudden acquired retinopathy
• Presumed cancer-associated retinopathy
• Diencephalic mass (7)
Hypothermia or bradycardia
Diencephalic mass (7)
Lower motor neuron paresis
• Megaesophagus (with polyneuropathy or myasthenia gravis)
• Insulinoma (with paraneoplastic polyneuropathy)
Pot-bellied appearance, hepatomegaly, muscle atrophy, testicular atrophy, noninflammatory alopecia, hyperpigmentation, and/or calcinosis cutis
Hypercortisolism
Stridor, stertor, prognathism inferior, interdental spacing, large head, increased skin thickness and/or excessive skin folds
Hypersomatotropism
Mammary hypertrophy
• Lactation
• Pregnancy
• Hypersomatotropism
No orientation after history and physical examination (12)
Consider in priority, subject to dog's age and breed:
• Sudden acquired retinal degeneration before blindness
• Paucisymptomatic portosystemic shunts
• Early stage of insulinoma
• Early stage of hypercortisolism
• Psychogenic/stress-induced polyphagia (13)
Diagnostic protocol
Diagnosis
Treatment

has not been thoroughly studied, even for seemingly straightforward scenarios such as exocrine pancreatic insufficiency.

Although polyphagia associated with hyperthyroidism is commonly presented as a compensatory mechanism for the increased metabolic activity in affected patients, this pathophysiological mechanism remains speculative and is likely accompanied by direct central and peripheral orexigenic effects of thyroid hormones, resulting in concurrent inappropriate polyphagia.[10-11] The pathogenesis of inappropriate polyphagia associated with the entities listed in the right column of Table 5.1 is also often considered to be multifactorial and poorly understood, with polyphagia associated with hypercortisolism or glucocorticoid treatment, serving as a good example of this lack of comprehension.[12]

Diagnostic approach

Given the subjectivity of assessing polyphagia, the first step in the diagnostic approach is to verify its presence (Algorithm 5.1).

Algorithm 5.1 Note 1 In most cases, owners reporting this sign have noticed an increase in food intake, sometimes associated with scavenging behavior or food stealing. When no change in food consumption is observed, it is essential to confirm the existence of polyphagia by comparing food needs and intakes.

Algorithm 5.1 Note 2 Undernutrition with no perception of a change in appetite is unlikely, as it typically refers to a prolonged period of insufficient feeding, which would have led to a highly cachectic state.

Algorithm 5.1 Note 3 Many causes of compensatory polyphagia, such as a physiological increase in metabolic needs or insufficient food intake, and inappropriate polyphagia, such as neutering, the recent adoption of a palatable diet, or the introduction or adjustment of the dose of an orexigenic drug, can be easily screened through questioning the owner.

Algorithm 5.1 Note 4 In other cases, mostly pathological, since polyphagia is almost never the sole clinical sign of the disease, history, and physical examination often provide significant information, allowing the prioritizing of a low number, if not one, of hypotheses.

Algorithm 5.1 Note 5 Changes in body weight may play a pivotal role in further diagnostic steps.[1-3] An increase in food intake will generally result in weight gain in case of inappropriate polyphagia, whereas, with the exception of growing and pregnant dogs, dogs with compensatory polyphagia will most often experience a decrease in weight or, at best, a stable weight.

Algorithm 5.1 Note 6 Most dogs with hyperthyroidism present with an easily palpable cervical mass, with the exception of cases with nutritional hyperthyroidism.

Algorithm 5.1 Note 7 Polyphagia is mostly observed in dogs with hypercortisolism secondary to small to mid-sized corticotroph or somatotroph adenomas. In larger tumors, polyphagia is generally gradually replaced by hyporexia and other signs resulting from hypothalamus, third ventricle and thalamus compression, such as hypothermia, bradycardia, lethargy or reduced alertness (chapter 35). In contrast to these vague clinical signs, vision alterations may also be present but are scarce in dogs with difficulties distinguishing between real troubles of vision and disorientation in these cases. In other diencephalic masses, including non-pituitary tumors and non-neoplastic lesions, polyphagia is only theoretical (i.e., undescribed in dogs yet).

Algorithm 5.1 Note 8 The history is characteristic of postictal polyphagia, and diagnosis is, therefore, a straightforward event if determining the cause of seizures remains unresolved after this first step.

Algorithm 5.1 Note 9 Rapid onset cataracts are frequent in canine diabetes mellitus (chapter 39); depending on the cases, they can be noticed by the owners themselves or practitioners.

Algorithm 5.1 Note 10 In dogs with sudden acquired retinopathy, polyphagia, polyuria, and polydipsia may precede vision loss.

Algorithm 5.1 Note 11 As opposed to hypercortisolism and diabetes mellitus, concurrent polyphagia, polyuria, and polydipsia are scarce in portosystemic shunts, liver encephalopathy, and insulinomas.

Algorithm 5.1 Note 12 In exceptional cases, the clinician is encouraged to consider entities with sometimes subtle clinical expressions, such as portosystemic shunts, early-onset insulinoma, sudden acquired retinal degeneration (before vision loss), and paucisymptomatic hypercortisolism and psychogenic/stress-induced polyphagia. These should be prioritized according to the dog's age and breed. This subtle nature exposes a higher risk of overdiagnosing these entities, regardless of the specificity of the diagnostic tools employed. Depending on the clinical impact of a delayed diagnosis, careful consideration should be given to investigating them through sensitive tests (e.g., pre- and postprandial serum bile acid concentrations to screen for a portosystemic shunt) versus adopting a wait-and-see approach (e.g., in the case of sudden acquired retinal degeneration).

Algorithm 5.1 Note 13 The diagnosis of psychogenic/stress-induced polyphagia is a diagnosis of exclusion. This hypothesis should not lead to overlooking, for instance, the possibility of a corticotroph adenoma or any other metabolic disorder underlying polyphagia.

References

1. Laflamme D. Polyphagia and hyperphagia. In Washabau RJ, Day MJ (editors). Canine and Feline Gastroenterology. St. Louis, Missouri, Elsevier, 2013, pp. 148-150.
2. Daminet S. Polyphagia. In Ettinger SP, Feldman EC, Côté E (editors). Textbook of Veterinary Internal Medicine 8th edition. St. Louis, Missouri, Elsevier, 2017, pp. 490-495.
3. Batchelor DJ, German AJ. Polyphagia. In Hall EJ, Williams DA, Kathrani A (editor). BSAVA Manual of Canine and Feline Gastroenterology. Gloucester, BSAVA Library, 2019, pp. 46-48.
4. Hetherington AW, Ranson SW. Hypothalamic lesions and adiposity in the rat. *Anat Rec* 78:149-172, 1940.
5. Anand BK, Brobeck JR. Hypothalamic control of food intake. *Yale J Biol Med* 24(2):123-140, 1951.
6. Heisler LK, Lam DD. An appetite for life: brain regulation of hunger and satiety. *Curr Opin Pharmacol* 37:100-106, 2017.
7. Haspula D, Cui Z. Neurochemical basis of inter-organ crosstalk in health and obesity: focus on the hypothalamus and the brainstem. *Cells* 12(13):1801, 2023. doi: 10.3390/cells12131801.
8. Bennaim M, Shiel RE, Mooney CT. Diagnosis of spontaneous hyperadrenocorticism in dogs. Part 1: Pathophysiology, aetiology, clinical and clinicopathological features. *Vet J* 62(7):531-539, 2021. doi:10.1016/j.tvjl.2019.105342.
9. Ryan D, Pérez-Accino J, Gonçalves R, et al. Clinical findings, neurological manifestations and survival of dogs with insulinoma: 116 cases (2009-2020). *J Small Anim Pract* 62(7):531-539, 2021.
10. Miller ML, Randolph JF, Peterson ME. Hyperthyroidism: clinical signs and physical examination findings. In Feldman EC, Fracassi F, Peterson ME (editors). Handbook of Feline Endocrinology. Milan, Edra Publishing, 2019, pp. 130-140.
11. Mullur R, Liu YY, Brent GA. Thyroid hormone regulation of metabolism. *Physiol Rev* 94(2):355-382, 2014.
12. Kuckuck S, van der Valk ES, Scheurink AJW, et al. Glucocorticoids, stress and eating: The mediating role of appetite-regulating hormones. *Obes Rev* 24:e13539, 2023. doi:10.1111/obr.13539.

CHAPTER 6

Exercise intolerance

M. Montserrat Diaz Espineira
DVM, PhD, DECVIM-CA (Internal Medicine)

Exercise intolerance (EI) is the inability or decreased ability to perform physical activity considered normal concerning the dog's age, breed, and physical condition.

Pathophysiology

Several organ systems and disorders may be involved in the development of EI (Table 6.1):

- Cardiovascular system: animals with heart failure and/or severe arrhythmias are unable to maintain an appropriate cardiac output to deal with adequate levels of physical activity. Impaired muscular perfusion, decreased oxygen delivery to organs, pulmonary hypertension, and edema contribute to poor exercise tolerance. Arrhythmias can cause sudden declines in cardiac output and provoke EI, collapse, or syncope.[1]
- Respiratory disorders: impairment of blood oxygenation due to decreased lung function causes EI with more or less visible signs of respiratory distress, which worsens with exercise.
- Endocrine diseases are associated with EI due to different mechanisms. Some endocrinopathies cause electrolyte imbalances (hypoadrenocorticism, diabetes mellitus, hyperparathyroidism, hyperaldosteronism). Others are associated with myopathies and/or neuropathies (hypothyroidism, diabetes mellitus, hypoglycemia, hypercortisolism). Hyperglycemia (diabetes mellitus) or hypoglycemia (insulinoma) directly affects physical exercise tolerance and mental status. Secretion of excessive amounts of catecholamines in pheochromocytomas provokes hypertension and episodic, potentially life-threatening tachycardia, tachyarrhythmias, and collapse. Hypothyroidism decreases the metabolic rate and oxygen consumption of most tissues and causes lethargy, weight gain, and unwillingness to exercise. Myopathy could also play a role.
- Anemia decreases the oxygen supply to tissues, which provokes intolerance to expected levels of physical activity. The severity of the EI and other clinical signs depends on the gravity, onset, and underlying cause of the anemia.
- Polycythemia provokes changes in cerebral blood flow due to an increased red blood cell mass which raises blood viscosity. This has a direct impairing effect on brain function.
- Neurological diseases: brain disorders, spinal cord diseases, and neuropathies are associated with variable severity of EI. Based on the localization of the lesion, certain clinical manifestations and specific neurological deficits on neurologic exam are present. Inflammatory disorders, infections, neoplasia, traumas, hemorrhages, infarcts, toxins, metabolic and endocrine diseases, and congenital, hereditary, or degenerative disorders are possible etiologies.
- Neuromuscular disorders: myasthenia gravis (MG) is the most common neuromuscular junction (NMJ) disorder in dogs. Dogs with MG show generalized and/or focal weakness and exhaustion of skeletal muscle. This muscle fatigability typically worsens with exercise and improves after rest. Impaired neuromuscular transmission can be congenital, but it is mainly an acquired autoimmune disease with antibodies against the acetylcholine receptor (AChR) in the skeletal muscle NMJ. Even though the EI in these patients may be severe, their neurological examination is usually normal.[2] The congenital form of MG (CMG) is rare and includes a heterogeneous group of genetic disorders that cause impairment of the neuromuscular transmission. CMG results from one or more deficiencies of the presynaptic, synaptic, or postsynaptic components of the NMJ. In CMG, there are no antibodies targeted against the AChR. This heterogeneous group is now referred to as "congenital myasthenic disorders" (CMSs). The onset of clinical signs in CMSs is observed in the first weeks to months of the dog's life.[2]
- Blood pressure: both hyper- and hypotension can provoke episodical weakness and EI. Severe systemic

TABLE 6.1 Causes of exercise intolerance in dogs.

Cardiovascular diseases	Electrolyte disturbances	Immune-mediated disease
Respiratory diseases	Hypoglycemia	Neoplasia
Endocrine diseases	Metabolic diseases	Obesity
Neurological diseases	Blood pressure abnormalities	Aging
Neuromuscular disorders	Orthopedic disorders	Pain and discomfort
Muscular disorders	Inflammation, infection	Drugs and therapies
Hematologic abnormalities		

hypertension is commonly associated with endocrinopathies (e.g., pheochromocytoma, hypercortisolism, hyperaldosteronism) and can lead to target organ damage (see chapter 9).

- Obesity and aging are obvious reasons for exercise intolerance and predisposition to other diseases.[3,4] Neoplasia and their different paraneoplastic syndromes cause fatigue and impaired tolerance to physical activity in oncologic patients.
- Pain, discomfort, and drugs associated with many disorders diminish exercise tolerance. Dogs with orthopedic problems (e.g., arthroses, arthritis), congenital conditions (e.g., Chiari-like malformation, syringomyelia, hydrocephalus, atlantoaxial subluxation, Wobbler syndrome), nausea and abdominal pain (e.g., gastrointestinal disease) can be reluctant to walk and have less capacity to resist high demands on physical activity. Certain therapies and drugs (e.g., corticosteroids, antiepileptics, diuretics) play a role in the reduction of physical activity and endurance in these animals.

Clinical signs

The problem of EI is easily noted, as dogs share physical activities with their owners. These seek veterinary help if their pets cannot deal with a certain expected level of endurance. Achieving a diagnosis in a patient with EI can be a challenge, especially when there are no specific clinical signs and/or abnormal physical findings identified.[5] Therefore, a systematic approach is essential. Patient's signalment (breed, age, sex, neutered status) and a thorough problem-oriented clinical history are the first information sources. A detailed problem-oriented anamnesis with questions about the exact descriptions of the complaints and the specific moments when the problems are evident (e.g., after fasting, after meals, during activity/excitement, after laying down), is mandatory. All the patient's clinical signs have to be specified: e.g., dyspnea, coughing, cyanosis, pale mucous membranes, paresis, ataxia, lameness, reluctance to walk, collapse, pain, polyuria/polydipsia, vomiting, diarrhea. The onset of clinical signs (acute, subacute, chronic) and their course (progressive, intermittent, stationary) support certain more likely differential diagnoses. Nowadays, the availability of videos showing the animal's problems provides clinicians a valuable aid. Even healthy dogs can have trouble dealing with high environmental temperatures, and not every owner is aware of this.

Diagnostic approach

Algorithm 6.1 shows the approach to the dog with EI.

Algorithm 6.1 Note 1 Thorough general physical and organ systems exams: neurologic, respiratory, cardiovascular, digestive, and orthopedic examinations are required in exercise-intolerant patients. Specific abnormal findings are crucial for further targeted workup and allow the veterinarian to reach the diagnosis easily. Nevertheless, the physical examination can be inconclusive, and an additional general diagnostic workup is needed (Video 6.1).

Algorithm 6.1 Note 2 Respiratory tract disorders can be caused by pneumonia, bronchitis, lung fibrosis, neoplasia, pleural effusion, pneumothorax, lung edema showing dyspnea, coughing, cyanosis, abnormal thoracic auscultation and reluctance or impossibility to exercise. Upper respiratory disorders explain EI with stridor, cyanosis, and/or inspiratory dyspnea. EI is the most frequent clinical sign in dogs with pulmonary hypertension, which can be caused by many respiratory diseases.[6]

Algorithm 6.1 Note 3 Brain disorders can cause abnormal consciousness, seizures, abnormal or compulsive behavior, circling, hemineglect, and abnormal postural reactions in contralateral limbs. Brainstem lesions involve abnormal mentation (sopor, stupor, coma), cranial nerve deficits, upper motor neuron (UMN) hemiparesis (ipsilateral), and/or abnormalities in breathing and cardiac parameters. Dogs with cerebellar disorders have normal mentation, intention tremor, and ataxia of the head, trunk, and/or limbs (hypermetric). There is no paresis, and the postural reactions are present but may be hypermetric, and the spinal reflexes are normal. Neurological examination characterizes upper (UMN) or lower (LMN) motor neuron signs in spinal cord disease.

Spinal cord disease is localized in four spinal cord segments: C1-C6 (UMN in all limbs), C6-T2 (LMN in forelimbs and UMN in hindlimbs), T2-L3 (normal forelimbs and UMN hindlimbs) and L3-S3 (normal forelimbs and LMN hindlimbs).

Peripheral nerve system (PNS) disorders (12 pairs of cranial nerves, peripheral nerves that innervate the muscle of the limbs and originate from cervical and lumbar intumescences) cause LMN signs in the affected limbs. Sensory components are mostly not involved.

Polyneuropathies affect different peripheral nerve groups, causing generalized LMN signs. Acute polyradiculoneuritis is commonly diagnosed in dogs, and hindlimb paresis can quickly progress in a few days to tetraparesis/paralysis.

Algorithm 6.1 Note 4 Myopathies (immune-mediated inflammation, infectious, hereditary, metabolic, degenerative) explain EI and muscle weakness because of muscle damage (inflammation, atrophy, swelling, degenerative changes, pain). Gait abnormalities, muscle contractures, muscle atrophy, swelling, or pain with a normal neurological examination may indicate muscle disease.[7] In idiopathic polymyositis, diffuse inflammation of the skeletal muscle is caused by a primary autoimmune process. Glucocorticoid therapy is administered and tapered for weeks or months.

Algorithm 6.1 Note 5 Dogs with myasthenia gravis show generalized skeletal muscle weakness and fatigability which worsens with activity and improves after rest. Impaired NM transmission can be congenital, but it is mainly an acquired autoimmune disease with antibodies against the skeletal muscle NMJ.

Algorithm 6.1 Note 6 Exercise-induced collapse (EIC) has been reported in young Labrador Retrievers and other breeds. EIC is an autosomal recessive neuromuscular disorder caused by a mutation in the dynamin 1 (DNM1) gene. The clinical signs of EI, hyperthermia, and even collapse arise during different levels of physical activity.[8] A DNA test is available for diagnosis.

ALGORITHM 6.1

Diagnostic approach to the dog with exercise intolerance.

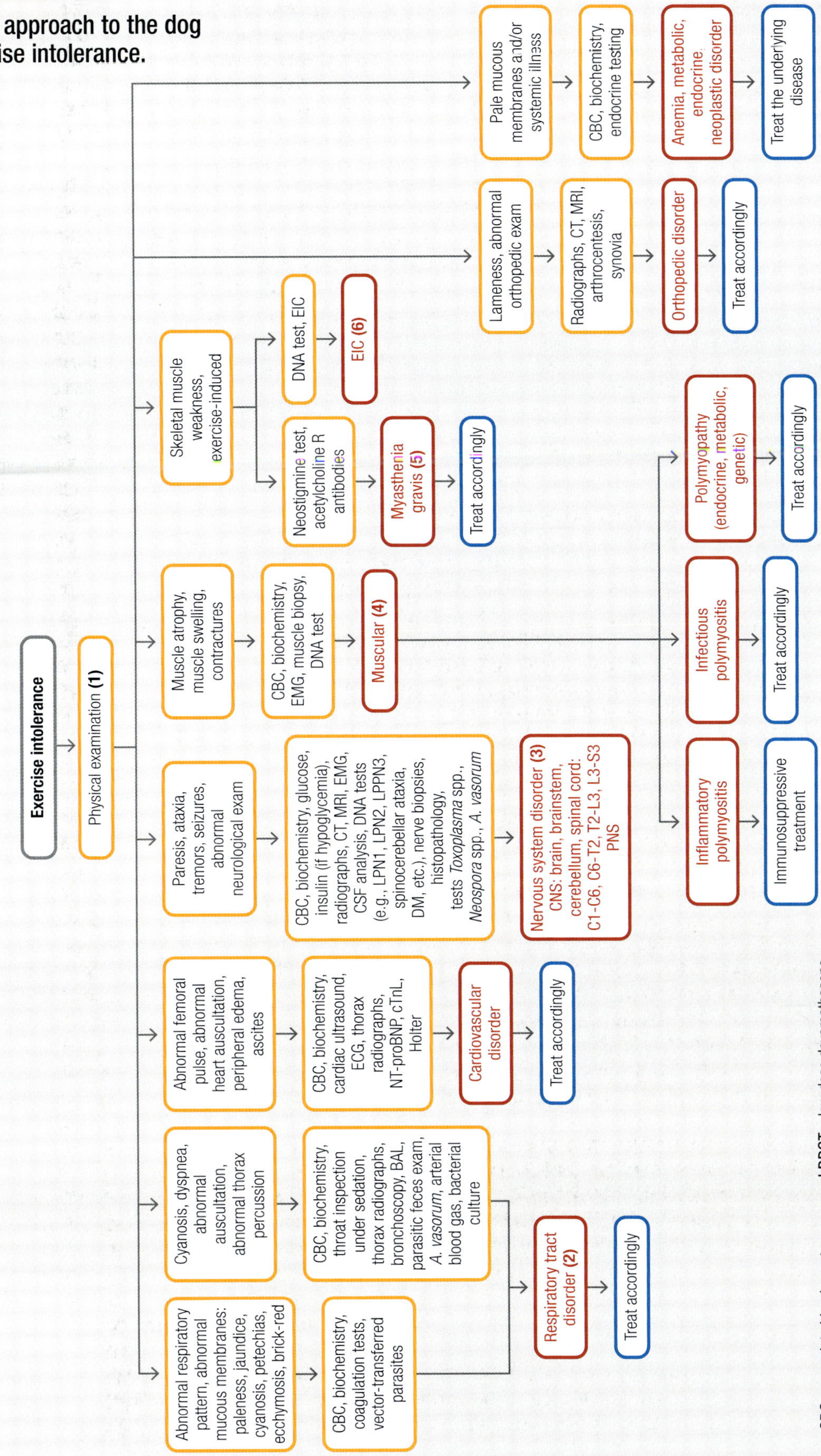

Diagnostic protocol | Diagnosis | Treatment

CBC: complete blood count
CK: Creatine kinase
CSF: cerebrospinal fluid
cTnI: cardiac troponin I
DM: degenerative myelopathy
eACTH: basal ACTH
ECG: electrocardiogram
EIC: Exercise induced collapse
EMG: electromyogram
fT4: free T4
LDDST: low dose dexamethasone suppression test
LPN1: Leonberger polyneuropathy 1
LPN2: Leonberger polyneuropathy 2
LPPN3: Leonberger laryngeal paralysis and polyneuropathy
NT-proBNP: N-terminal pro b-type natriuretic peptide
T4: thyroxine
UCCR: urinary cortisol creatinine ratio
US: ultrasound

Video 6.1

11-year-old male English Springer Spaniel diagnosed with insulinoma. The dog presented mainly with exercise intolerance, muscle contractures, and ataxia when going with the owners for long walks (at least one hour) in the forest without receiving a recent meal. Eventually, the dog got seizures when exercising further. Physical examination (general, cardiovascular, and neurologic) was unremarkable. Blood exam showed very low glucose with a normal serum insulin concentration. Abdominal ultrasound revealed a nodule in the tip of the right pancreatic lobe. The final diagnosis was exercise intolerance caused by hypoglycemia as a result of insulinoma.

References

1. Little WC, Kitzman DW, Cheng CP. Diastolic dysfunction as a cause of exercise intolerance. *Heart Fail Rev* 5(4):301-306, 2000. doi:10.1023/a:1026503028065.
2. Mignam T, Targett M, Lowrie M. Classification of myasthenia gravis and congenital myasthenic syndromes in dogs and cats. *J Vet Intern Med* 34(5):1707-1717, 2020. doi:10.1111/jvim.15855.
3. German AJ. The growing problem of obesity in dogs and cats. *J Nutr* 136(7 Suppl):1940S-1946S, 2006. doi:10.1093/jn/136.7.1940S.
4. McKenzie BA, Chen FL. Assessment and management of declining physical function in aging dogs. *Top Comp Anim Med* 51:100732, 2022. doi:10.1016/j.tcam.2022.100732.
5. Barnett L, Martin MWS, Todd J, Smith S, Cobb M. A retrospective study of 153 cases of undiagnosed collapse, syncope or exercise intolerance: the outcomes. *J Small Anim Pract* 52(1):26-31, 2011. doi:10.1111/j.1748-5827.2010.01013.x.
6. Campbell FE. Cardiac effects of pulmonary disease. *Vet Clin North Am Small Animal Pract* 37(5): 949-962, 2007. doi:10.1016/j.cvsm.2007.05.006.
7. Shelton GD, Engvall E. Muscular dystrophies and other inherited myopathies. *Vet Clin North Am Small Anim Pract* 32(1):103-124, 2002. doi:10.1016/s0195-5616(03)00081-0.
8. Furrow A, et al. Relationship between dynamin 1 mutation status and characteristics of recurrent episodes of exercise-induced collapse in Labrador Retrievers. *J Am Vet Med Assoc* 242(6):786-791, 2013. doi:10.2460/javma.242.6.786.

CHAPTER 7

Obesity

Alexander German
BVSc(Hons), PhD, CertSAM, DECVIM-CA (Internal Medicine), FRCVS

Etiology and pathophysiology

Obesity results from disordered energy homeostasis, resulting from an imbalance between energy intake and energy use. Many risk factors have been suggested (Table 7.1), including genetic, "biological", behavioral, owner, and environmental (food environment, living space) categories. Further, some comorbidities can predispose to weight gain, including hypercortisolism, hypothyroidism, and insulinoma. Hypothyroidism disrupts energy homeostasis as a result of decreased metabolism, whilst weight gain associated with hypercortisolism results from increased food intake (due to polyphagia), fat redistribution (increased visceral fat), and organomegaly. Weight gain can also occur as a result of drug therapy (e.g., corticosteroids and anticonvulsants).

For energy homeostasis, energy intake from dietary macronutrients (e.g., protein, fat, and carbohydrates) must be balanced by energy expenditure, comprising essential metabolic processes, thermoregulation, and physical activity. Surplus energy is predominantly stored in white adipose tissue, leading to its expansion through adipocyte hypertrophy and hyperplasia. Risk factors can influence energy homeostasis by determining the relative ease with which energy is gained or lost.

Expansion of white adipose tissue (WAT) is initially a physiological process to enable energy storage but, when excessive, can become pathological as a result of adipose tissue hypoxia, macrophage recruitment, and release of proinflammatory adipokines. Both the expanded adipose tissue mass and its altered chemical environment are linked to the pathological consequences downstream[1] and are also associated with the functional impairments that occur as a result of two mechanisms. The adverse health effects of obesity (Table 7.2) include associations with comorbidities, functional impairment, shortening of the lifespan, and poorer quality of life.[7,13]

Clinical signs

Signs of obesity include subcutaneous (neck, thorax, pelvic region, and tail base) and visceral fat deposition (abdominal distension); lethargy; altered respiratory effort, rate, and sounds (e.g., stetor); exercise intolerance; reduced mobility; and poor skin and coat condition. There might also be signs related to comorbidity, including lameness (orthopedic disease), vomiting and abdominal pain (pancreatitis); polydipsia and polyuria (hypercortisolism), incontinence (urethral sphincter mechanism incompetence) or dermatological signs associated with an endocrine disorder (e.g., mental dullness, lethargy, exercise intolerance, alopecia, dryness, hyperpigmentation). Owners' reports about their dog's appetite are often inconsistent, with some reporting increased appetite (and sometimes coprophagia, stealing, and scavenging) but others suggesting a picky appetite. The latter is usually due to owners offering excessive and varied amounts of food, meaning they can pick and choose, leading to excessive intake despite not eating everything offered.

Diagnostic approach

Obesity should be differentiated from other causes of weight gain (Algorithm 7.1 Note 1), including fluid accumulation or diseases that lead to increased tissue mass (e.g., abdominal neoplasia), as explained in Algorithm 7.1. Once obesity is known to be the cause, the degree of obesity then needs to be quantified, risk factors associated with its development should be identified and possible comorbidities diagnosed. Pertinent investigations will vary from case to case since this will depend upon the exact clinical signs, likely possible causes, and also comorbidities that are present. Investigations that can be used for the diagnosis and characterization of obesity include:

- History and physical examination. In addition to a standard medical history, a full nutritional assessment should be performed (for details, see the WSAVA nutrition guide).[3] Information about current physical activity, environment, the family unit (pets and people), lifestyle, and neuter status should also be recorded. Finally, signs related to possible comorbidities should be reported.
- Body weight measurement. Body weight will be a key metric for monitoring throughout weight management. Ideally, the same set of electronic scales should be used to ensure consistency.

TABLE 7.1 Risk factors for canine obesity.

Category	Risk factor
Genetic	■ Deletion (14 base pairs) in the pro-opiomelanocortin (POMC) gene in retrievers (Labrador and Flat Coated) associated with appetite and weight gain ■ Breed associations suggest genetic effects. Obesity-prone breeds include Beagles, Cocker Spaniels, French Bulldogs, Golden Retrievers, Labrador Retrievers, Pugs, and Rottweilers
Age and early-life factors	■ Rapid growth rate associated with future risk of obesity
Sex and neutering	■ No consistent effect of sex on obesity risk ■ Neutering associated with increased obesity risk
Other diseases	Positive associations between canine obesity and: ■ Hypercortisolism ■ Hypothyroidism ■ Insulinoma ■ Other diseases affecting energy balance (e.g., orthopedic disease affecting mobility ■ Drug therapy (e.g., corticosteroids, anticonvulsants)
Environment and activity	Positive associations between canine obesity and: ■ Indoor living ■ Low physical activity (frequency and/or duration)
Dietary factors	*Food type* ■ Positive association with "grocery store" dog foods ■ Dogs fed a mix of commercial and home-made food are at greater risk of obesity than dogs fed either home-prepared food or commercial food alone *Feeding method.* Positive associations between canine obesity and: ■ Offering food *ad libitum* ■ Once-daily feeding ■ Feeding of additional snacks ■ Dog being present during food preparation ■ Using a scoop to measure food portions ■ Dog stealing food from another pet in the household ■ Owner sharing food with dog at meal times
Owner factors and behavior	■ Negative associations with owner income or gross-domestic product of the country (some, but not all, studies) ■ Positive association between overweight status in dog and owner ■ Positive association in dogs whose owners smoke ■ Positive associations where a close owner-dog bond exists (e.g., tendency to "over-humanize" dog, allowing dog to sleep on bed, seeing dog as "a baby") ■ Positive association with owners using food as a reward ■ Negative association with interest in preventive health care for pet ■ Negative association with the acceptance of obesity as a disease

TABLE 7.2 Associations between obesity and other conditions in dogs.

Disease category	Condition
Cardiorespiratory	■ Altered cardiovascular function ■ Brachycephalic airway obstruction syndrome ■ Decreased ventilation and oxygenation ■ (Mild) hypertension ■ Myocardial hypoxia ■ Tracheal collapse
Endocrine and metabolic	■ Diabetes mellitus, insulin resistance, and obesity-related metabolic dysfunction ■ Hypercortisolism ■ Hypothyroidism ■ Insulinoma
Gastrointestinal	■ Oral cavity disease (epidemiological studies) ■ Pancreatitis
Musculoskeletal	■ Cruciate ligament disease ■ Hip dysplasia ■ Humeral condylar fractures ■ Intervertebral disc disease ■ Osteoarthritis
Neoplastic	■ Increased neoplasia risk (in epidemiological studies) ■ Mammary carcinoma (some but not all studies) ■ Transitional cell carcinoma
Urogenital	■ Abnormal urinary functional markers ■ Calcium oxalate urolithiasis ■ Glomerular disease (experimental) ■ Lower urinary tract disease (epidemiological studies) ■ Transitional cell carcinoma ■ Urethral sphincter mechanism incompetence
Other	■ Anesthesia risk ■ Oxidative stress ■ Undesirable behaviors (aggression, nervousness, food seeking and stealing, food guarding)

- Body condition scoring (**Algorithm 7.1 Note 2**). Body condition scoring (BCS) is a validated, semiquantitative, non-invasive method for assessing body composition, with different systems reported, including a 9-unit scale, a 5-unit scale, a 7-unit algorithm-based system, and a 6-unit "body fat index" scale. The 9-unit scale is most widely accepted[11] and has been recommended by the WSAVA. With this system, scores of 6-7 and 8-9 represent overweight (10-20% above the ideal body weight, IBW) and obese (>20% above IBW) conditions, respectively. The BCS can also be used to determine the degree of obesity (Box 7.1). Recently, the author has identified many dogs with a greater degree of obesity than is accommodated by the chart, suggesting that refinements to the original BCS system (extending the categories) are required.
- Muscle condition scoring. In addition to BCS, muscle mass should be indirectly quantified using a 4-unit muscle condition score,[12] not least because BCS scales do not adequately reveal changes in muscle mass, not least in dogs with excessive body fat.
- Zoometry. Zoometry involves using a tape measure to take dimensional measurements, including those that correlate with stature (e.g., head, thorax, and limb length) and those with fat mass (e.g., thorax, abdominal and neck circumference), which, when combined, can indicate estimate adiposity. However, such systems are complicated and time-consuming, making them impractical for regular use.
- Advanced imaging for body composition analysis. Dual-energy X-ray absorptiometry (DEXA) is a precise and reliable non-invasive method of assessing body composition and has been used in research studies, but the requirement for sedation limits and limited availability means that this

ALGORITHM 7.1

Approach to the investigation of weight gain in the dog.

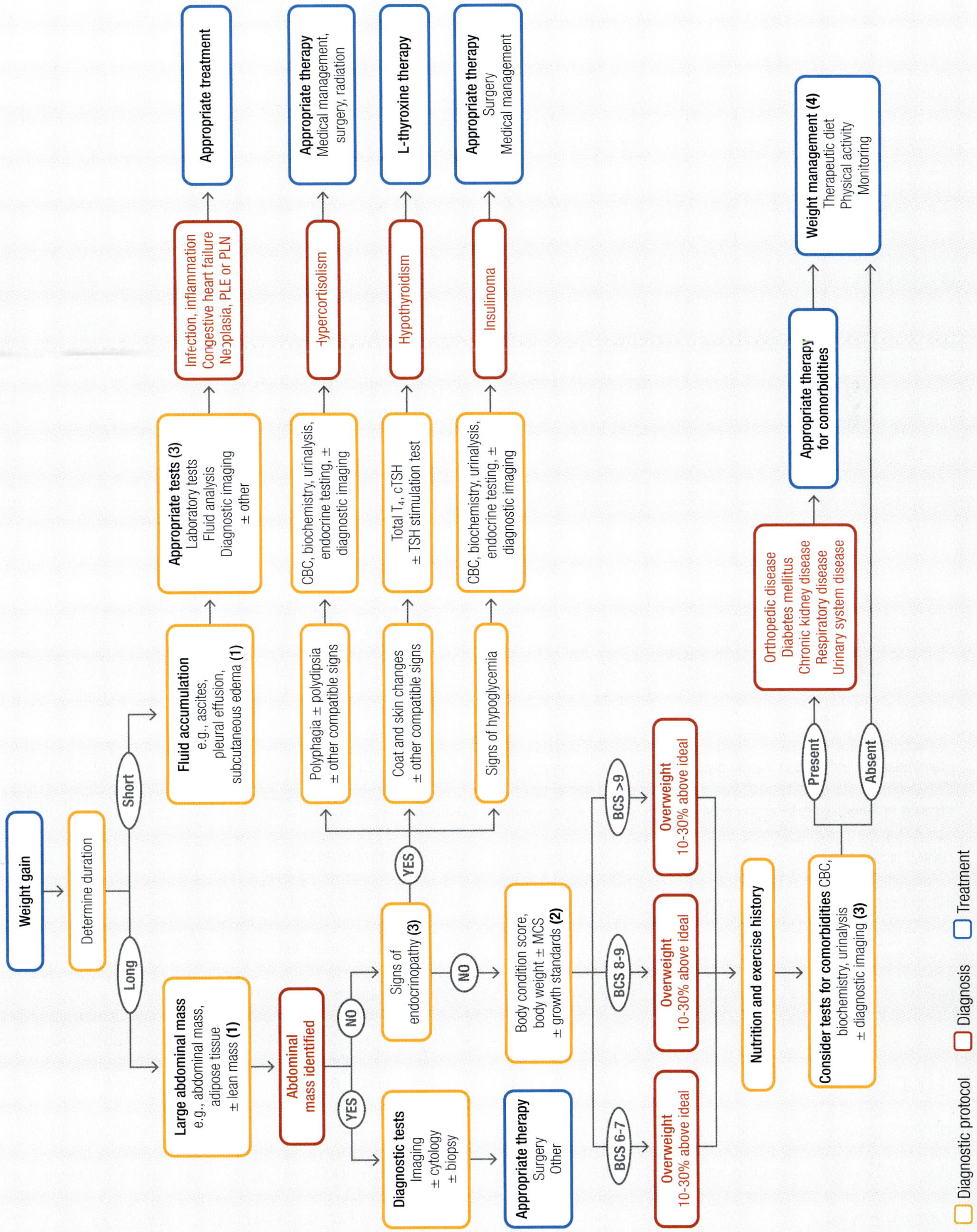

Box 7.1 Estimating ideal body weight (IBW) in a dog with obesity.[1,2]

Research studies have indicated that each unit on the 9-point BCS system, between 5/9 and 9/9, is associated with approximately 10% of additional weight. Therefore, the IBW can be calculated from current body weight and current body condition scoring using one of the following equations:

- **BCS 6/9:** IBW = current weight ÷ 1.1
- **BCS 7/9:** IBW = current weight ÷ 1.2
- **BCS 8/9:** IBW = current weight ÷ 1.3
- **BCS 9/9:** IBW = current weight ÷ 1.4

For example, the IBW of a dog weighing 48.0 kg and with a BCS of 9/9 would be:

48.0 kg ÷ 1.4 = 34.3 kg

[1] *This method only provides an estimate of ideal weight because there can be marked variability either side of this estimate amongst dogs. If possible, other information should be used to confirm the estimnate (e.g., revising historical medical records for a weight before the onset of obesity.*

[2] *Note also that some dogs might have a greater degree of obesity than tht represented by BCS 9/9 (~40% above ideal weight). Unless historical weight records are available, It can be difficult to determine the ideal accurately.*

is only available at specialist referral centers.[5]. Methods for assessing body fat mass using either CT or MRI have also been reported.[10,15]

- Photography. Periodic photography (before, during, and after the weight management protocol) is useful for demonstrating body shape changes to owners, provided that positioning is standardized (Fig. 7.1).
- Growth charts. Given that BCS or other methods have not been properly validated in puppies, regular weight measurements are recommended for monitoring weight gain during growth, with reference to evidence-based growth standards. Such standards confirm whether the rate of weight gain is appropriate and can identify rapid growth, enabling corrective measures to be implemented.[14]
- Further investigations (**Algorithm 7.1 Note 3**). Clinicopathological investigations such as complete blood count (CBC), clinical chemistry, and urinalysis are recommended to ascertain health status and identify possible comorbidities. Additional investigations might also be required, including blood pressure measurement, thyroid and adrenal gland function assessment, insulin and glucose measurements for possible insulinoma, and diagnostic imaging (ultrasonography and advanced imaging, as required).

Therapy

Algorithm 7.1 Note 4 The above investigations should enable the dog to be comprehensively assessed in terms of the degree of obesity and the presence of comorbidities, enabling a tailored weight-reduction plan to be developed. In preparing for the weight reduction phase, the following should be determined:

1. Goals of obesity care, namely the expected improvements that weight loss will bring, for example, improved mobility, improved insulin sensitivity, or improved quality of life. Success will, ultimately, be determined by how well these goals are met.
2. Ideal weight, defined as a weight at which the dog's body fat mass would be optimal, which can either be determined from historical medical records (e.g., an early-adult weight when body condition was reported to be optimal) or from current weight and BCS (Box 7.1). It should be emphasized that IBW (and NOT target weight is used to set the initial dietary energy intake for weight reduction).
3. Target weight, defined as the goal weight set for the period of controlled weight reduction. Variables used to set the target weight include age, comorbidities, and expected benefits of weight reduction. Sometimes, the target weight is the same as IBW (e.g., young dog, no comorbidities), but often (e.g., older animals, comorbidities present), the target weight is deliberately set to be greater than IBW. Such a target weight is more modest and can be easier to achieve whilst still facilitating enough weight loss to significantly improve health and well-being.
4. Therapeutic plan for comorbidities, including drug therapies or surgery and their relative timing, as well as whether adjustments to the weight management plan may be required.

There are two phases to an obesity care plan: weight reduction and weight maintenance. The aim of weight reduction is controlled weight loss until, hopefully, the predetermined target weight is reached; the aims of weight maintenance are first to stabilize weight and prevent weight regain.

Weight reduction

Although, historically, a rate of loss of 1-2% start body weight (SBW) per week is recommended, this rate is based on research colony studies and is unrealistic in pet dogs with obesity. A more realistic goal is an average rate of weight loss of 0.5-1.0% per week, which seems to be safe.[5] However, given marked variability amongst dogs, the actual rate of weight loss can be highly variable, such that slower-than-expected rates of weight loss (<0.5% per week) are acceptable if the owner remains compliant. The two main components of a weight management plan are dietary management and lifestyle alterations, including increasing physical activity.

Dietary management

It is recommended that a purpose-formulated wet or dry therapeutic diet be used. Such diets have a reduced energy density and increased protein (amino acid) and micronutrients relative to energy, meaning that essential nutrient intake is usually maintained despite moderate-to-severe energy restriction.[9] Supplementing protein and L-carnitine helps to maintain lean mass, whilst supplementing protein and dietary fiber improves satiety.[17] The starting food allocation for weight reduction can be calculated in various ways, including methods based on resting energy requirement. However, the author's preferred approach involves tailoring initial intake to IBW, sex, and neuter status:

1. Calculate IBW (Box 7.1).
2. Calculate starting energy intake using the following equations:
   - Sexually intact males: 80 kcal per $kg^{0.75}$ IBW per day.
   - Neutered males and sexually intact females: 70 kcal per $kg^{0.75}$ IBW per day.
   - Neutered females: 60 kcal per $kg^{0.75}$ IBW per day.

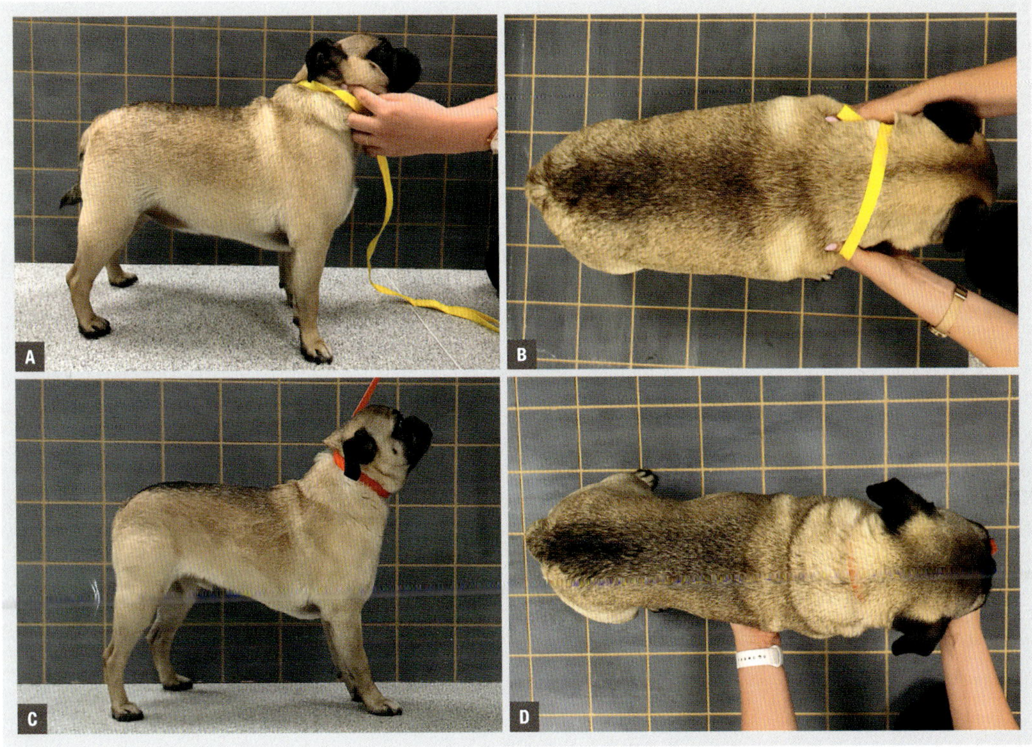

FIG. 7.1 (**A, B**) Photographs of a 3-year-old neutered female Pug with obesity, weighing 14.8 kg and a body condition score of 9/9. (**C, D**) Photographs of the same dog, after successful weight loss on a high protein and high fiber diet, when body weight was 8.7 kg and body condition score was 5/9. Total weight lost was 41% of the starting body weight over 461 days, at a rate of 0.63% per week. Images courtesy of the Royal Canin Weight Management Clinic, University of Liverpool, UK.

Further adjustments can be required in some cases, such as if a comorbidity, like an orthopedic disease, is present. In these circumstances, the author reduces the above amounts by ~10% (e.g., 5 kcal per $kg^{0.75}$ IBW). This initial allocation might promote weight loss at the start of the program, but not uncommonly, the rate slows, and adjustments to the feeding amount are needed, typically in small adjustments (~5% decrease) each time.

Owners should be instructed to measure food portions accurately, if possible (e.g., using electronic gram scales), since alternative methods, such as measuring cups, are imprecise and can lead to overfeeding.[6] Usually, the daily food allocation is fed over at least two meals per day, and if dry food is used, some can also be reserved for use in training or as treats. Interactive feeding devices (e.g., puzzle feeder toys or modified feeding bowls) can also be used. Not only do they provide mental stimulation and enjoyment, but slowing food intake might also improve satiety.

Beyond the main meal, additional sources of food (e.g., treats, table scraps, etc.) should be minimized. One option, as mentioned above, would be to use a portion of the main meal, though many owners do not favor such a strategy. An alternative would be to use low-energy treats, including cucumber or cooked zucchini. Such treats are often readily consumed without adding too many calories to the daily total.

Physical activity

Daily (or more frequent) exercise should be included in the weight loss plan, with options including lead walking, hydrotherapy, swimming, and play. The exact recommendation for physical activity must be tailored to the individual, considering comorbidities. The main benefits include minimizing lean tissue mass[16] and improving owner and dog well-being. However, the impact on weight loss during weight management is limited: in one randomized controlled trial, physical activity was less effective than the use of a therapeutic weight reduction diet, and the amount of weight lost was insignificant.[2]

Monitoring weight reduction

The weight reduction process should be monitored by regular reassessments, ideally every 2-4 weeks. The primary outcome measure is change in body weight, although other metrics can also be monitored, including BCS and zoometric measurements. Ideally, owners should be encouraged to keep a diary, which can be reviewed when weight loss is not progressing as expected. If a cause for the poor progress is not identified (e.g., feeding additional food, illness leading to reduced activity), an adjustment to the daily food allocation should be considered (see above).

Weight maintenance

Once the target weight is reached, dogs can be transitioned to the maintenance phase, usually by increasing (e.g., by ~5%) the food intake and rechecking weight 2 weeks later. This process continues until body weight remains stable; no further adjustments are made at this point, but weight continues to be checked (at gradually increasing intervals 2 weeks, 4 weeks, 3 months, etc.). Long-term monitoring in maintenance is strongly recommended because many will suffer rebound.[8] One variable strongly associated with weight regain is the diet chosen for maintenance; in one study, the odds of rebounding was twenty times less when the therapeutic diet used during weight reduction is continued, albeit being fed for maintenance requirements.[8] Thus, the author usually recommends against switching to a different food at this point unless necessitated by other factors (e.g., a comorbidity requiring a different food, such as chronic kidney disease).

Prevention of obesity

Prevention of obesity is arguably more critical than managing it once developed but, until recently, has received little attention. Given that weight gain, during the development of obesity, occurs gradually and is then resistant to change, strategies for prevention can be challenging. Any strategy needs to be proactive, commence early in life, and be lifelong. The key stage for obesity prevention is the early-life phase, during which individuals at risk should be identified based on risk factors, enabling interventions to be started as soon as possible. The risk factors that can be used include breed, whether and when the dog is neutered, growth pattern, and a known history within the family (e.g., having other family pets with obesity). Growth patterns are associated with future obesity risk in humans and dogs.[14] Therefore, the author recommends taking regular weight measurements throughout development and using these to monitor the growth pattern using validated growth standards (https://www.waltham.com/resources/puppy-growth-charts). Starting at 8-12 weeks, at least monthly weight measurements are commended until 6 months, and then measurements at least every 3 months after until skeletal maturity. Additional weight measurements are also needed after neutering (e.g., 2 weeks, 4 weeks, 8 weeks) so that any impact on weight gain can rapidly be spotted and addressed. Compliance with such a weight monitoring strategy can be improved if they coincide with other preventive medicine visits (e.g., vaccination, deworming, microchipping, etc.). When a growth pattern that deviates from the standards is seen (e.g., crossing centile lines up or down), the feeding plan should be adjusted (i.e., by increasing or decreasing the amount fed as relevant), and further weight checks should be used to ensure that the issue has been addressed.

Once the dog reaches early adult life, their body condition can be verified using BCS, and this "early adult" weight is recorded in the medical records. From then on, regular weight assessments should be continued at least every 12 months (e.g., at annual vaccination), but more frequently if possible, including at non-routine visits. The "early adult weight" should be used as a reference for any future checks to maintain the dog's weight to within ±5% of this reference. This weight could also be used as an IBW (see above) should a formal weight-reduction plan be required in the future.

References

3. Bray GA, Kim KK, Wilding JPH. Obesity: a chronic relapsing progressive disease process. A position statement of the World Obesity Federation. *Obes Rev* 18:715-723, 2017. doi: 10.1111/obr.12551
4. Chapman M, Woods GRT, Ladha C, Westgarth C, German AJ. An open-label randomised clinical trial to compare the efficacy of dietary caloric restriction and physical activity for weight loss in overweight pet dogs. *Vet J* 243:65-73, 2019. doi: 10.1016/j.tvjl.2018.11.013
5. Freeman L, Becvarova I, Cave N, et al. WSAVA Nutritional Assessment Guidelines. *J Small Anim Pract* 52:385-396, 2011. doi: 10.1111/j.1748-5827.2011.01079.x
6. German AJ. Weight management in obese pets: the tailoring concept and how it can improve results. *Acta Vet Scand* 20;58(Suppl 1):57, 2016. doi: 10.1186/s13028-016-0238-z
7. German AJ, Holden SL, Bissot T, et al. Dietary energy restriction and successful weight loss in obese client-owned dogs. *J Vet Intern Med* 21:1174-1180, 2007. doi: 10.1892/06-280.1.
8. German AJ, Holden SL, Mason SL, et al. Imprecision when using measuring cups to weigh out extruded dry kibbled food. *J Anim Physiol Anim Nutr (Berl)* 95:368-373, 2011. doi: 10.1111/j.1439-0396.2010.01063.x
9. German AJ, Holden SL, Wiseman-Orr ML, et al. Quality of life is reduced in obese dogs but improves after successful weight loss. *Vet J* 192:428-434, 2012a. doi: 10.1016/j.tvjl.2011.09.015
10. German AJ, Holden SL, Morris PJ, Biourge V. Long-term follow-up after weight management in obese dogs: the role of diet in preventing regain. *Vet J* 192:65-70, 2012b. doi: 10.1016/j.tvjl.2011.04.001
11. German AJ, Holden SL, Serisier S, et al. Assessing the adequacy of essential nutrient intake in obese dogs undergoing energy restriction for weight loss: a cohort study. *BMC Vet Res* 11:253, 2015b. doi:10.1186/s12917-015-0570-y
12. Gifford A, Kullberg J, Berglund J, Malmberg F, Coate KC, Williams PE, Cherrington AD, Avison MJ, Welch EB. Canine body composition quantification using 3 tesla fat-water MRI. *J Magn Reson Imaging* 39(2):485-491, 2014. doi: 10.1002/jmri.24156
13. Laflamme D. Development and validation of a body condition score system for dogs. *Canine Pract* 22:10-15, 1997.
14. Michel KE, Anderson W, Cupp C, Laflamme DP. Correlation of a feline muscle mass score with body composition determined by dual-energy X-ray absorptiometry. *Br J Nutr* 106 Suppl 1:S57-559, 2011. doi: 10.1017/S000711451100050X.
15. Salt C, Morris PJ, Wilson D, et al. Association between life span and body condition in neutered client-owned dogs. *J Vet Intern Med* 33:89-99, 2019. doi: 10.1111/jvim.15367
16. Salt C, Morris PJ, Butterwick RF, et al. Comparison of growth patterns in healthy dogs and dogs in abnormal body condition using growth standards. *PLoS One* 23;15(9):e0238521, 2020. doi: 10.1371/journal.pone.0238521.
17. Turner RBS, Hepworth G, Wilson K, Tyrrell D, Dunshea FR, Mansfield CS. Abdominal volume computed tomography assessment of body composition in dogs. *BMC Vet Res* 15(1):21, 2019. doi: 10.1186/s12917-018-1768-6
18. Vitger AD, Stallknecht BM, Nielsen DH, Bjornvad CR. Integration of a physical training program in a weight loss plan for overweight pet dogs. *J Am Vet Med Assoc* 248:174-182, 2016. doi: 10.2460/javma.248.2.174
19. Weber M, Bissot T, Servet E, et al. A high protein, high fiber diet designed for weight loss improves satiety in dogs. *J Vet Intern Med* 21:1203-1208, 2007.

CHAPTER 8

Hypertension

Rosanne E. Jepson
BVSc, MVetMed, PhD, DACVIM (SAIM) DECVIM-CA (Internal Medicine), PGCertVetEd, FHEA, MRCVS

Video 8.1

Hypertension target organ damage associated with endocrine disease.

Pathophysiology

Systemic hypertension (SH) is defined as an increase in systolic blood pressure (SBP) >160 mmHg that can cause target organ damage (TOD), including the eye, kidneys, cardiovascular and central nervous system (CNS). Where underlying disease conditions contribute to the development of hypertension, e.g., endocrine disease, SH is considered secondary[1] (Video 8.1).

In dogs, a number of endocrine disease conditions can be associated with SH, including hypercortisolism (pituitary- and adrenal-dependent), hyperaldosteronism, pheochromocytoma, diabetes mellitus, hypothyroidism, and hyperthyroidism.[2] Some of these endocrine conditions are rare in their own right, and specific data on the prevalence of hypertension can be limited. Pathophysiological mechanisms for the development of hypertension associated with endocrine disease in dogs are poorly explored, and suggested mechanisms are extrapolated mainly from human and experimental studies. However, the pathophysiology of hypertension is dependent on common key regulatory pathways.

SBP is the product of cardiac output (CO) and total peripheral resistance (TPR), which resides mainly in the systemic arterioles with CO dependent on both heart rate (HR) and stroke volume (SV). Circulating blood volume relative to venous capacitance vessels determines the venous return. Regulation of SBP involves integrated interaction between the kidney, the heart, and the vasculature, which are regulated by the sympathetic nervous system (SNS), endocrine mediators, particularly those from the adrenal and other glands, and paracrine mediators. In health, complex feedback loops maintain normotension by regulating circulating fluid volume via sodium homeostasis, vascular resistance, vascular capacitance, HR, and force of contraction.

Changes in SBP are sensed, and modifications are triggered by the following mechanisms: baroreceptors (arterial stretch receptors) adapting rapidly to minute-by-minute changes in SBP, atrial stretch receptors which determine circulatory filling, renal afferent arteriolar stretch receptors determining renal perfusion, and macula densa in the kidney sensing delivery of chloride and adjusting renal hemodynamics to maintain stable tubular flow and volume status (tubuloglomerular feedback). Therefore, it is apparent that many endocrine disease conditions identified in the dog have the capacity to impact the regulation of SBP.[2] Potential mechanisms involved in different endocrine disorders are described in Table 8.1.

Clinical signs

It is uncommon for dogs with endocrine disease to present with clinical signs directly related to SH. More commonly, the clinical history and physical examination findings will reflect the underlying endocrine disorder, and SH will only be recognized when SBP is measured and/or more in-depth examinations are performed, e.g., fundic examination.

TOD that can be recognized as part of clinical presentation includes hypertensive ocular injury (e.g., hyphema, retinal detachment) leading to advanced ocular abnormalities and/or sudden onset blindness, which may be apparent to the owner, hypertensive encephalopathy (e.g., altered mentation, behavioral change, seizures) or potentially hypertension contributing to cardiovascular manifestations (e.g., arrhythmias, syncope, collapse). These clinical signs may be more likely with sudden and severe SH (i.e., hypertensive crisis) and/or SH that is paroxysmal, for example, in patients with pheochromocytoma. Epistaxis has also been reported as a presenting sign for SH. For other endocrine disease conditions, where an increase in SBP may be more gradual, clinical manifestations of hypertension are less common, e.g., diabetes mellitus, hypercortisolism, and hypothyroidism.

In dogs with endocrine disease, SH diagnosis will depend on the measurement of SBP and evaluation for TOD. This should include fundic examination for evaluation of hypertensive retinopathy/choroidopathy, including narrowing of retinal arterioles, vascular tortuosity, retinal hemorrhages, retinal and subretinal edema, retinal detachment, and optic disc edema. Whilst studies exploring hypertensive ocular injury include dogs with endocrine disease, the risk of ocular TOD in specific endocrine diseases frequently cannot be extrapolated from available

TABLE 8.1 Proposed pathophysiological mechanisms associated with endocrine hypertension in the dog and reported hypertension prevalence.

Endocrine condition	Prevalence of systemic hypertension	Proposed pathophysiological mechanisms involved in development of systemic hypertension
Hypercortisolism	20-80%*** May be higher in dogs with AD-HC than PD-HC. SH may develop during management and treatment of HC	■ Activation of RAAS ■ Mineralocorticoid activity of cortisol ■ Enhanced pressor response to catecholamines, vasopressin, and Ang II ■ Increased beta-adrenergic sensitivity ■ Inhibition of vasodilatory mechanisms (e.g., NO, prostacyclin and kinin-kallikrein system) ■ Increased vascular resistance
Hyperaldosteronism	Very rare disease; no data on prevalence**	■ Renal: aldosterone-associated contribution to inflammation, fibrosis, and proteinuria leading to development and progression of CKD ■ Aldosterone-mediated sodium and volume retention ■ Aldosterone-mediated effects on vascular remodeling and endothelial dysfunction ■ CNS effects on SNS and altered baroreceptor reflex
Pheochromocytoma	43-86%*** Limited data on whether SH is persistent or paroxysmal	■ Peripheral vascular smooth muscle stimulation for alpha-1 adrenoceptors leading to vasoconstriction and increased SVR ■ Activation of beta-1 adrenoceptors on cardiomyocytes leading to positive inotropic and chronotropic effects increasing HR, SV, and CO ■ Stimulation of beta-1 adrenoceptors in juxtamedullary apparatus of kidney stimulating renin production and RAAS activation resulting in vasoconstriction (Ang II) and sodium/volume retention
Diabetes mellitus	24-67%*	■ Obesity and chronic low-grade inflammation ■ RAAS activation ■ Adipokine stimulation of aldosterone ■ Endothelial dysfunction (impaired vascular relaxation) ■ SNS activation ■ Altered renal handling of sodium
Hypothyroidism	No data on prevalence*	■ Decreased cardiac output and decreased availability of NO as a potent vasodilator results in increased SVR ■ In humans, it leads to increased diastolic blood pressure and narrow pulse pressure ■ In humans, links with hypercholesterolemia and atherosclerosis
Hyperthyroidism	Rare condition; no data on prevalence**	■ Relative situational effect ■ Stimulation of SNS ■ Direct action of T_3 on gene regulation of cardiac proteins (e.g., myosin chains, sarcoplasmic reticulum proteins, Ca^{2+}ATPase, phospholamban) and extranuclear action on cardiac myocytes leading to increase in HR and SV with net increase in CO ■ Dilation of resistance arterioles, decreasing SVR, effective arteriolar filling, and stimulating RAAS leading to sodium and water retention, increase blood volume and VR with net increase in CO ■ Increased erythropoietin production leading to increased red cell mass and increased blood volume contributing to net increase in CO
Acromegaly	Very rare condition; no data on prevalence*	■ Poorly understood mechanism in human medicine ■ Possible increase in volume status and CO ■ Possible increased catecholamines ■ Association with diabetes mellitus ■ Alteration in SVR due to increased wall thickness in resistance arterioles ■ Endothelial dysfunction

*Low risk of SH; **mild risk of SH; ***moderate risk of SH.

data. However, it should be noted that punctate retinal hemorrhages have been reported in dogs with hypercortisolism without SH.[3]

Cardiovascular TOD can include left ventricular hypertrophy and arteriosclerosis, with the former identified on echocardiography.[4] Aortic undulation and dilation have been reported on thoracic radiographs of dogs with SH.[5] Systolic heart murmurs, arrhythmias, and gallop sounds may be audible on examination. However, while some dogs included in studies evaluating cardiovascular manifestations of SH have underlying endocrine disease, the prevalence of these findings associated with specific endocrine conditions is again poorly reported and must be differentiated from other primary or secondary cardiovascular diseases. For example, left ventricular hypertrophy has been reported in 67% of dogs with hypercortisolism, but of these, only 27% were reported to be hypertensive,[6] and left ventricular hypertrophy has been identified in dogs that have been diabetic for >1 year without SH.[7]

Neurological manifestations of SH are rarely reported in association with most canine endocrine diseases. Where neurological signs are reported in dogs with hypercortisolism, they must be differentiated from signs attributable to a pituitary macroadenoma,[8] and in dogs with neurological signs associated with pheochromocytoma, consideration should be given to whether such signs are the consequence of SH or could be attributed to hemorrhage or metastatic disease.[9]

SH may also lead to hypertensive renal injury and contribute to the development of proteinuria. In hypertensive patients, assessment of proteinuria with urine protein to creatinine ratio (UPCR) may be informative, particularly when considering the choice of antihypertensive medication. However, given that many endocrine diseases are identified in the older canine population, consideration must also be given to concurrent renal disease and that certain endocrine disease conditions, e.g., hypercortisolism, may contribute to proteinuria.

Diagnostic approach

Algorithm 8.1 shows the approach to the patient with systemic hypertension.

Diagnosis

Algorithm 8.1 Note 1 The diagnosis of SH must consider individual patient factors. The behavior of the patient should be used to consider the risk of situational (white coat) hypertension. SBP is recognized to increase with age. Therefore, the relative risk of SH will increase in an older dog. Measurements of SBP should be considered in light of the breed, given that higher SBP measurements in health are identified in Sighthounds and brachycephalic breeds. Concurrent disease conditions that could influence SBP, e.g., chronic kidney disease (CKD), must be considered. The relative risk of SH in the specific endocrine disease must be considered; for example, this may be deemed high for pheochromocytoma, moderate-high for hyperaldosteronism, moderate for hyperthyroidism and hypercortisolism, and moderate to low for diabetes mellitus and hypothyroidism.

Algorithm 8.1 Note 2 Measurement of SBP (see chapter 21) must be performed in a quiet and calm environment to reduce the risk of situational hypertension. Serial assessment of SBP may be required for conditions such as pheochromocytoma, where SH may be paroxysmal. 8.1 Note that hypotension has also been reported with pheochromocytoma.

Algorithm 8.1 Note 3 Criteria used for SBP diagnosis of SH should be based on the American College of Veterinary Internal Medicine (ACVIM) hypertension guidelines,[1] where SBP >160 mmHg is considered hypertensive and SBP >180 mmHg severe hypertension.

Algorithm 8.1 Note 4 All dogs with suspected SH should be evaluated for ocular and neurological TOD, including a fundic examination. For many patients with endocrine disease, e.g., hypercortisolism, hyperaldosteronism, and diabetes mellitus, it is prudent also to assess renal function and proteinuria. Antiproteinuric therapy may be indicated for dogs that are identified to be persistently proteinuric. The presence of concurrent proteinuria and SH may have an impact on the choice of drug for the treatment of these conditions. Echocardiographic assessment is least frequently performed but may be considered if there is a clinical concern based on auscultatory findings.

Algorithm 8.1 Note 5 A diagnosis of SH can be made based on a single SBP >160 mmHg when in conjunction with evidence of ocular or neurological TOD.

Algorithm 8.1 Note 6 The presence of severe ocular and/or neurological manifestations of SH should prompt emergency hospitalized management for hypertension. The risk of ocular and neurological TOD is of particular concern in patients with pheochromocytoma where severe hypertension >180-300 mmHg and hypertensive crisis can be recognized. For all patients simultaneously diagnosed with an endocrine disorder, concurrent management of that disease process and SH is required.

Algorithm 8.1 Note 7 For patients where no TOD is identified, repeat assessment of SBP within 1-2 weeks is recommended in order to establish where there is persistence of SH. For dogs with SBP persistently >160 mmHg and an underlying endocrine disease associated with SH and/or other predisposing risk factors present, antihypertensive treatment should be started alongside management of the underlying endocrine disease.

Algorithm 8.1 Note 8 For dogs with SBP <160 mmHg, SH can be excluded, and treatment and management should focus on the endocrine disease. However, there is evidence that SH may develop in certain conditions with time, e.g., hypercortisolism,[10] and therefore, repeat assessment of SBP is prudent as part of the standard monitoring of endocrine disease where hypertension is recognized.

Considerations for treatment

Treatment of SH in endocrine disease will depend not only on the rate of onset and severity of hypertension (i.e., identification of hypertensive crisis) but also on the specific endocrine disease condition and any comorbid disease conditions that may also be present. It will be important to manage the primary disease for all endocrine disease conditions as this treatment may impact SBP. For example, a significant reduction in SBP may be seen with trilostane treatment of hypercortisolism[10] (see chapter 35). Similarly, for dogs with hyperaldosteronism, specific treatment with aldosterone inhibitors, e.g., spironolactone, may result in small improvements in SBP (see chapter 36). For dogs with pheochromocytoma, specific antiadrenergic therapy is recommended for ~2 weeks in the preoperative period or long-term if surgical treatment is not a viable option, e.g., phenoxybenzamine[11,12] (Table 8.2; chapter 37). However, for all these endocrine disorders, it is common that the management of the underlying endocrine disease alone is insufficient to achieve normotension.

The target for treatment of SH should be SBP <160 mmHg or ideally <140 mmHg in line with the ACVIM guidelines.[1] In general, the principle of antihypertensive therapy is a gradual reduction in SBP. In dogs, where proteinuria is identified, there is potential for RAAS activation, and/or there is evidence of concurrent renal disease, angiotensin receptor blockers (ARB), e.g., telmisartan are widely considered first-choice antihypertensive agents (Table 8.2). Alternatively, angiotensin-converting enzyme inhibitors (ACEi), e.g., benazepril, can be used. When starting these drugs, careful monitoring of renal parameters (urea, creatinine, symmetric dimethylarginine) and electrolytes (potassium) should be performed. The calcium channel blocker, amlodipine besylate, is a common second-line treatment. In dogs with SH, it is common for multimodal antihypertensive therapy to be required. After every drug addition or dose adjustment, careful monitoring of SBP should be performed within 7-14 days, and hypotension (SBP <120 mmHg) should be avoided.

ALGORITHM 8.1

Approach to the patient with systemic hypertension.

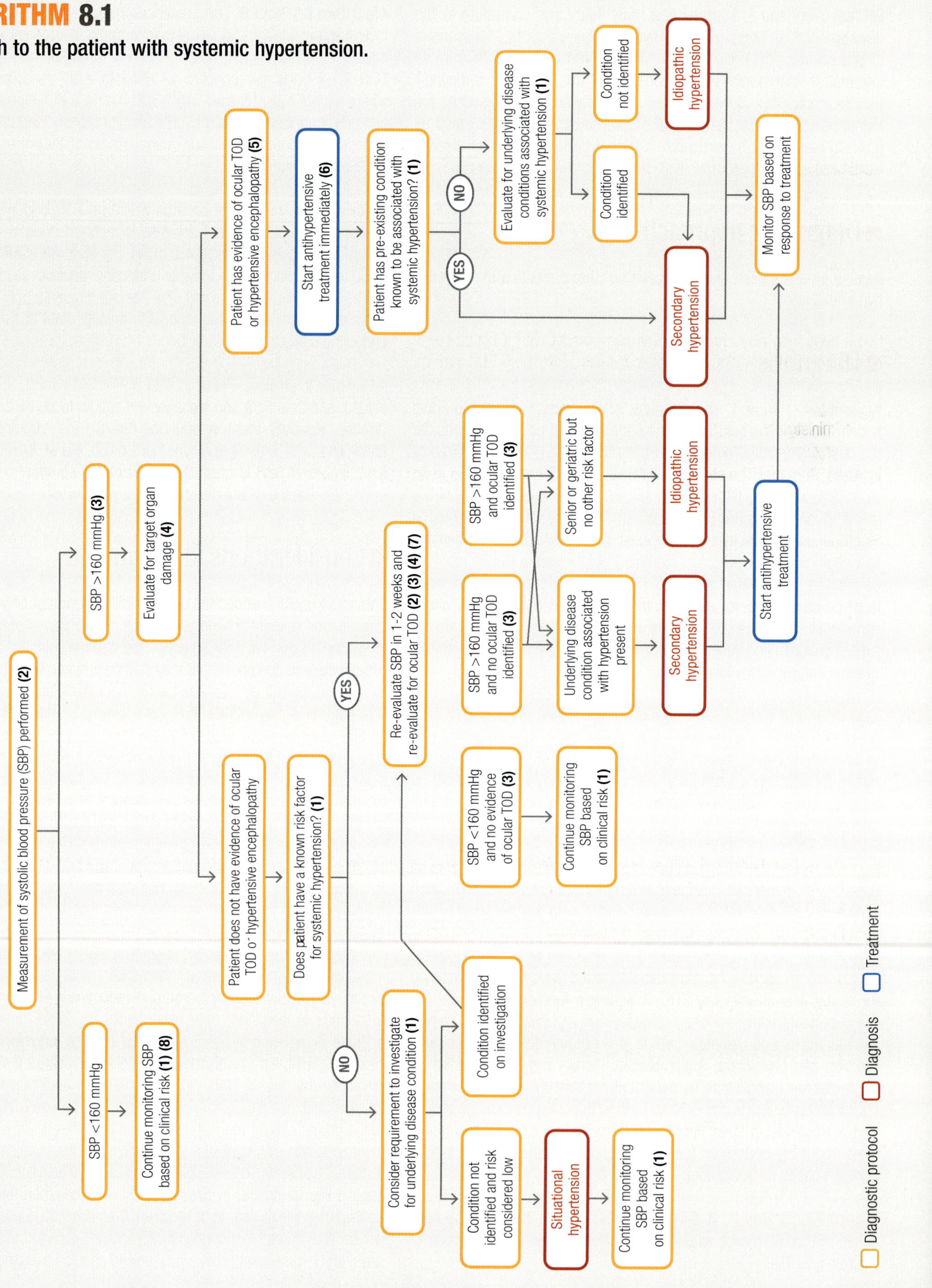

TABLE 8.2 Commonly used oral antihypertensive agents in dogs with endocrine hypertension.

Drug group	Drug name	Commonly used starting dose for oral antihypertensives
Angiotensin receptor blocker	Telmisartan	1 mg/kg q24h up to 2 mg/kg q24h
Angiotensin-converting enzyme inhibitor	Benazepril	0.5 mg/kg q12-24h
	Enalapril	0.5 mg/kg q12-24h
Calcium channel blocker	Amlodipine	0.1-0.25 mg/kg q24h up to 0.5 mg/kg q24h
Direct vasodilator	Hydralazine	0.5-2 mg/kg q12h (start at low end of range)
Alpha-adrenergic blocker	Phenoxybenzamine	0.2-1.5 mg/kg q12h (for preoperative management of pheochromocytoma, start at lower end of dose range and titrate upwards q2-3 days to ~1 mg/kg q12h over ~2 weeks prior to surgery)

Some dogs with pheochromocytoma can present with a hypertensive emergency: SBP elevation that is rapid in onset, extreme (>200 mmHg), and associated with hypertensive encephalopathy. In this situation, hospitalization for urgent and rapid reduction in SBP is required. Where oral administration is possible, phenoxybenzamine can be initiated.[11,12] However, parenteral antihypertensive agents may be required. Here, the preferred drug is phentolamine, a short-acting competitive alpha-adrenergic blocking drug (loading dose 0.1 mg/kg IV followed by continuous rate infusion (CRI): 1-2 μg/kg/min. For further information on parenteral antihypertensive agents, see the ACVIM hypertension guidelines.[1]

For those endocrine disease conditions where definitive treatments are available, e.g., adrenalectomy for hypercortisolism, pheochromocytoma, hyperaldosteronism, SBP should be controlled in advance of surgical procedures. The evidence base for ongoing antihypertensive therapy after definitive treatment is limited. SBP should be carefully monitored in the postoperative period, and antihypertensive therapy can, in some situations, be gradually titrated and discontinued. However, for those dogs where multiple disease conditions may contribute to the hypertensive state, ongoing antihypertensive treatment may be required, while disease-specific drugs may be discontinued.

KEY POINTS

- Endocrine diseases, including hypercortisolism, pheochromocytoma, hyperaldosteronism, diabetes mellitus, hypo- and hyperthyroidism, have been associated with systemic hypertension in dogs.
- Diagnosis of SH should be based on knowledge of predisposing risk factors, measurement of SBP, and evaluation for target organ damage.
- For some endocrine diseases, specific therapies targeting the endocrine disease process may result in a reduction in systolic blood pressure, but where SH is present, they are frequently insufficient for the return of normotension. Additional antihypertensive therapies are therefore required.
- First-line antihypertensive drugs in dogs with SH usually include inhibition of the renin-angiotensin-aldosterone system, e.g., angiotensin receptor blockers or angiotensin enzyme inhibitors with calcium channel blockers used as second-line agents. In dogs, it is common to need a multimodal antihypertensive treatment.
- Certain endocrine conditions, e.g., pheochromocytoma, can be associated with severe hypertension and hypertensive emergency requiring hospitalization and emergency parenteral antihypertensive therapy.
- Where SH is diagnosed, management will be long-term, together with ongoing management of the endocrine disease.
- For dogs where a definitive surgical procedure is available for the management of the endocrine disease, SBP should be carefully monitored in the postoperative period to determine the requirement for ongoing antihypertensive treatment. Requirement may be dependent on the presence of other contributing risk factors.

References

1. Acierno M, Brown S, Coleman A, et al. Guidelines for the identification, evaluation and management of systemic hypertension in dogs and cats. *J Vet Intern Med* 32:1803-1822, 2018.
2. Elliott J, Syme HM, Jepson RE, editors. Hypertension in the dog and cat. Cham: Springer Nature, 2020.
3. Violette NP, Ledbetter EC. Punctate retinal hemorrhage and its relation to ocular and systemic disease in dogs: 83 cases. *Vet Ophthalmol* 21(3):233-239, 2018.
4. Holland M, Hofmeister E, Hudson J. Echocardiographic changes in the shape and size of the aortic cusps in dogs with confirmed systemic hypertension. *Vet Radiol Ultrasound* 62(6):697-704, 2021.
5. Holland M, Hudson J, Hofmeister E. An observational thoracic radiographic study of aortic remodeling in dogs with confirmed systemic hypertension. *Vet Radiol Ultrasound* 63(3):254-263, 2022.
6. Takano H, Kokubu A, Sugimoto K, et al. Left ventricular structural and functional abnormalities in dogs with hyperadrenocorticism. *J Vet Cardiol* 17(3):173-181, 2015. Available from: http://dx.doi.org/10.1016/j.jvc.2015.07.002
7. Vichit P, Rungsipipat A, Surachetpong SD. Changes of cardiac function in diabetic dogs. *J Vet Cardiol* 20(6):438-450, 2018. Available from: https://doi.org/10.1016/j.jvc.2018.08.001
8. O'Neill DG, Scudder C, Faire JM, et al. Epidemiology of hyperadrenocorticism among 210,824 dogs attending primary-care veterinary practices in the UK from 2009 to 2014. *J Small Anim Pract* 57(7):365-373, 2016.
9. Barthez PY, Marks SL, Woo J, et al. Pheochromocytoma in dogs: 61 cases (1984-1995). *J Vet Intern Med* 1(5):272-278, 1997.
10. García San José P, Arenas Bermejo C, et al. Changes in systolic blood pressure in dogs with pituitary-dependent hyperadrenocorticism during the first year of trilostane treatment. *J Vet Intern Med* 35(1):130-141, 2021.
11. Herrera MA, Mehl ML, Kass PH, et al. Predictive factors and the effect of phenoxybenzamine on outcome in dogs undergoing adrenalectomy for pheochromocytoma. *J Vet Intern Med* 22:1333-1339, 2008.
12. Reusch CE. Pheochromocytoma and multiple endocrine neoplasia. In Feldman EC, Nelson RW, Reusch CE, Scott-Moncrieff JCR, Behrend EN (editors). Canine and Feline Endocrinology 4th edition. St. Louis, 2015, Elsevier Saunders, pp. 521-554.

Hyperglycemia

Florian Z. Zeugswetter
Priv. Doz., DVM

Pathophysiology

Hyperglycemia is defined as an increase in blood glucose concentrations above the upper reference limit for a given species.

Under physiologic conditions, glucose homeostasis, i.e., normoglycemia, is ensured by a complex interplay of neuroendocrine and cellular mechanisms, balancing glucose uptake, production, utilization, and excretion. Insulin, a peptide hormone produced by pancreatic ß-cells exerts potent hypoglycemic actions and is the key player in opposing the hyperglycemic effects of hormones including cortisol, catecholamines, glucagon, thyroid hormones, growth hormone (GH), resistin, and proinflammatory cytokines (e.g., tumor necrosis factor, interleukin 6). Endogenous insulin sensitizers such as adiponectin, secreted by adipose tissue, and gastrointestinal incretins, including glucagon-like peptide-1 (GLP-1) and glucose-dependent insulinotropic peptide (GIP), augment its effects. The dynamic equilibrium may be tilted towards a hyperglycemic state by diseases or drugs reducing insulin secretion and/or pathological processes causing insulin resistance (Table 9.1). Although obesity causes insulin resistance and insulin hypersecretion, and the fact that some obese dogs may have persistent hyperglycemia and pronounced postprandial glucose peaks, additional factors are necessary to trigger overt diabetes mellitus (DM).

Under normal conditions, about 90% of freely filtered glucose is reabsorbed by insulin-independent sodium-glucose cotransporters 2 (SGLT 2) located at the renal proximal tubular cells. In dogs, tubular reabsorptive capacities are exceeded at blood glucose concentrations above 10-11.1 mmol/L (180-200 mg/dL), leading to osmotic diuresis and associated energy, electrolyte, and water losses. Clinical signs are usually not observed at blood glucose concentrations below this so-called "renal threshold".

Clinical signs

In clinical DM, signs usually develop rapidly and progress over time. When renal reabsorptive capacities are exceeded, osmotic diuresis leads to polyuria with subsequent dehydration and the activation of the renin-angiotensin-aldosterone system (RAAS). Water, glucose, and electrolyte losses lead to polydipsia, polyphagia, weight loss, and lethargy/depression, whereby polydipsia is by far the most prevalent first sign.

Insulin deficiency and increased counter-regulatory hormones trigger glycogenolysis, gluconeogenesis, lipolysis, and muscle proteolysis.

Weight loss and skeletal muscle wasting may thus be dramatic and rapid. In contrast to cats, gait abnormalities (e.g., plantigrade stance) are rarely reported.

Accumulation of polyols, glycosylation of lens proteins, and oxidative injury lead to bilateral cataract formation and may be associated with blindness. Cataract development is common and documented in 50% of diabetic dogs within the first 5 to 6 months after diagnosis.

In advanced cases, a sweet odor on the dog's breath, indicative of exhaled acetone, may be appreciated. Left untreated, the accumulation of ketoacids and associated acidemia may result in anorexia, nausea, vomiting, abdominal pain, or a deep labored breathing pattern (Kussmaul breathing).

In subclinical DM, hyperglycemia is identified by chance during routine laboratory evaluations, and the diagnosis has to be confirmed by repeated blood glucose measurements or alternative glycemic parameters.

Diagnostic approach

Glucose concentrations in healthy dogs are surprisingly stable and rarely exceed 6.7 mmol/L (120 mg/dL) in adults and 8.0 mmol/L (144 mg/dL) in puppy dogs aged up to 2 months. Algorithm 9.1 shows the approach to the hyperglycemic patient.

Algorithm 9.1 Note 1 As very mild glucose surges are observed in healthy dogs fed a high-starch diet, the need for a 12-hour fasting time has been questioned. Nevertheless, as glucose peaks up to 7 mmol/L (126 mg/dL) and lasting up to 90 minutes were observed in healthy dogs consuming a glucose-enriched diet (2 g/kg D-glucose added to a high protein meal), withholding food for a minimum of 8 hours is recommended.

TABLE 9.1 Drugs that inhibit insulin secretion and/or cause insulin resistance.

	Hormones, drugs and diseases causing an insulin-deficient state	Hormones, drugs and diseases causing an insulin-resistant state
Hormones (endogenous or exogenous causes)	■ Glucocorticoids (stress, hypercortisolism) ■ Mineralocorticoids (hyperaldosteronism) ■ Gestagens (luteal phase: pregnancy/diestrus, adrenocortical neoplasia, medication) ■ Catecholamines (pheochromocytoma)	■ Glucocorticoids (stress, hypercortisolism) ■ Gestagens (pregnancy, diestrus, adrenocortical neoplasia, medication) ■ Catecholamines (stress, pheochromocytoma, paraganglioma) ■ Growth hormone (pituitary tumor, mammary origin, hypothyroidism) ■ Thyroid hormones (thyroid tumors, food, medication) ■ Glucagon (stress, pancreatic neuroendocrine tumors)
Drugs (other than hormones)	■ Alpha 2-agonists (e.g., dexmedetomidine, medetomidine, xylazine, amitraz) ■ Atypical antipsychotics (e.g., clozapine, olanzapine) ■ Benzothiadiazine derivatives (diazoxide) ■ Beta-blockers (e.g., propranolol, atenolol, metoprolol) ■ Calcineurin inhibitors (ciclosporine A, tacrolimus) ■ Cyproheptadine ■ Fluoroquinolones (ciprofloxacine, ofloxacine) ■ L-asparaginase ■ Loop diuretic (furosemide) ■ Phenytoin ■ Somatostatin analogs (octreotide, lanreotide, pasireotide) ■ Streptozotocin and alloxane ■ Theophylline ■ Thiazide diuretics (e.g., hydrochlorothiazid)	■ Atypical antipsychotics (e.g., clozapine, olanzapine) ■ Beta-blockers (e.g., propranolol, atenolol, metoprolol) ■ Loop diuretic (furosemide) ■ Niacin ■ Thiazide diuretics (e.g. hydrochlorothiazide)
Diseases/conditions	■ Exocrine pancreatic disease (pancreatitis, neoplasia, pancreatectomy, idiopathic) ■ Inborn endocrine pancreatic disease (aplasia, abiotrophy, hypoplasia) ■ Acquired endocrine pancreatic disease (immune-mediated, infection, toxicity, idiopathic) ■ Hyperglycemia (glucotoxicity) ■ Hyperlipidemia (lipotoxicity)	■ Obesity (low adiponectin, high resistin, cytokines TNF-α, IL-6) ■ Inflammation (cytokines TNF-α, IL-6, and MCP-1 (monocyte chemotactic protein 1) ■ Hyperglycemia (glucotoxicity) ■ Hyperlipidemia (lipotoxicity)

Algorithm 9.1 Note 2 The pivotal ALIVE criteria for diagnosing DM in dogs include a random (fasted or unfasted) blood glucose ≥11.1 mmol/L (≥200 mg/dL) in combination with classical clinical signs. DM can be differentiated from stress-induced hyperglycemia in dogs with fasting glucose concentrations ≥7 mmol/L (≥126 mg/dL) but <11.1 mmol/L (<200 mg/dL) by the documentation of persistent hyperglycemia for more than 24 hours or increased glycated blood proteins. Persistently increased fasting blood glucose concentrations >8 mmol/L (>144 mg/dL) have also been suggested to define overt canine DM by others. All cutoffs currently used to define DM are arbitrary and primarily intended to facilitate the classification and comparison of studies.

Algorithm 9.1 Note 3 For the correct interpretation of glucose concentrations, knowledge of pretreatment is important. Very high glucose concentrations are possible in dogs sedated with α2 receptor agonists (e.g., medetomidine and xylazine) or after ample glucose administration. For drugs inhibiting insulin secretion and/or causing insulin resistance, see Table 9.1.

Algorithm 9.1 Note 4 As glucose concentration in random spot canine urine samples rarely exceeds 1.3 mmol/L (23.4 mg/dL), any quantitative glucose measurement above this limit or any positive urine dipstick result using traditional dipstick tests should encourage a detailed diagnostic workup. Documented causes of glucosuria include DM, renal glucosuria, Fanconi syndrome, acute and chronic renal failure, leptospirosis, lead toxicity, and the application of α2 receptor agonists or sodium-glucose cotransporter 2 inhibitors. False-positive dip test results are possible in dogs receiving cephalosporines, when testing contaminated urine (oxidizing agents, e.g., hydrogen peroxide), or after prolonged exposure of the reagent strips to air.

Algorithm 9.1 Note 5 Although the measurement of glycated proteins is not required *per se* to diagnose DM, it is recommended in ambiguous cases. Fructosamines are glycated proteins, primarily albumin, and are considered to reflect the median glucose concentration over the preceding 1-2 weeks. With a sensitivity and specificity of 0.93 and 0.95 in diagnosing canine DM, plasma/serum fructosamine measurement is considered a test with high accuracy. Nevertheless, diseases influencing protein concentrations (e.g., protein-losing enteropathy or nephropathy [reduced concentrations] and paraproteinemia [increased concentrations]), protein metabolism (e.g., hypothyroidism [increased concentrations]), metabolic situations modifying glycation, and finally interindividual variations of deglycation, hamper its diagnostic value. Furthermore, false high or low fructosamine measurements are possible in case of severe hemolysis and marked hypertriglyceridemia, respectively. An alternative indicator of glycemic status is glycated hemoglobin, which, for technical reasons, is rarely used in veterinary medicine.

ALGORITHM 9.1
Approach to the hyperglycemic patient.

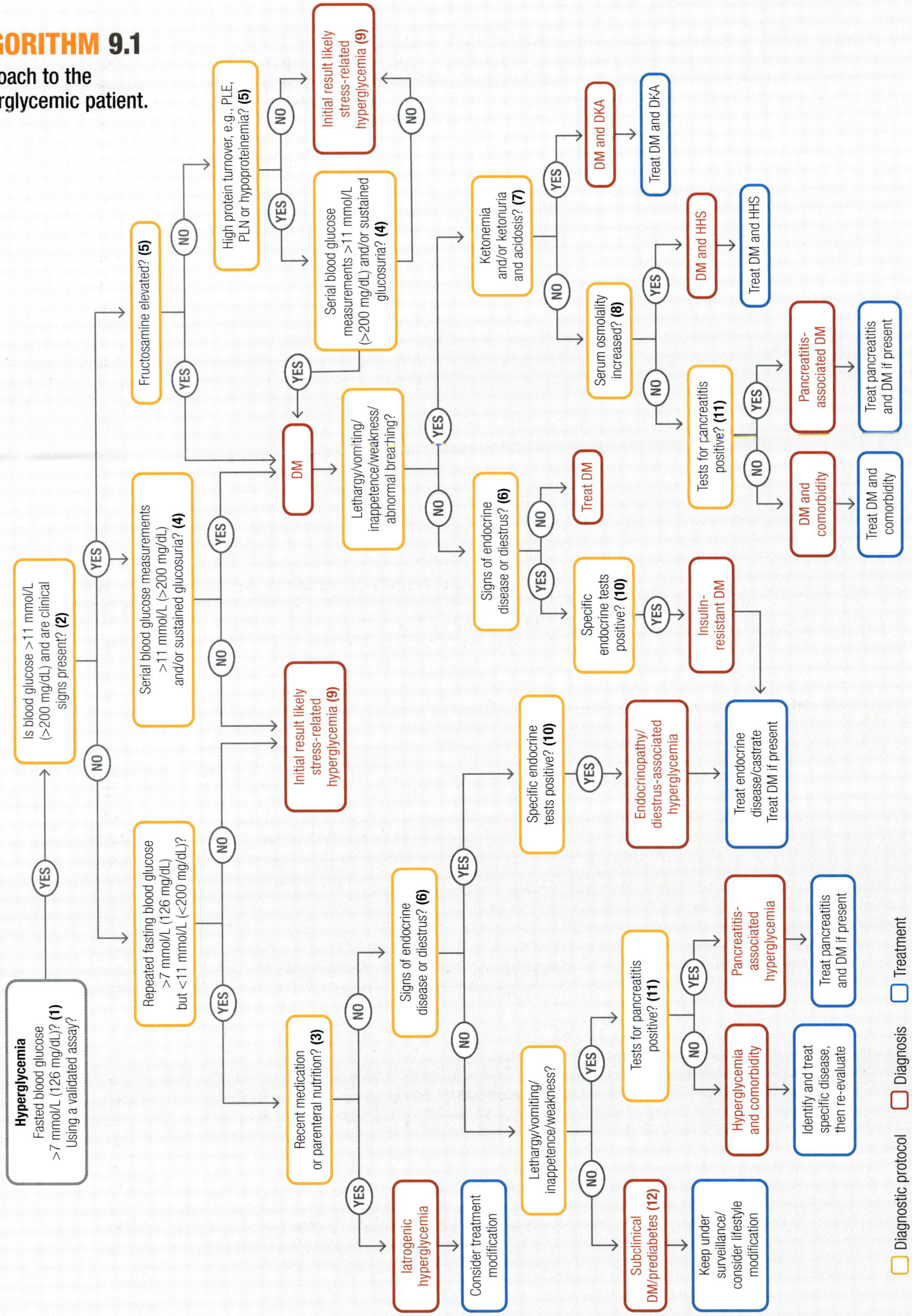

Algorithm 9.1 Note 6 Endocrine diseases/conditions associated with canine DM are primarily hypercortisolism, GH excess in the luteal phase, and hypersomatotropism. There is considerable overlap of clinical signs between dogs with DM and hypercortisolism, such as polyuria, polydipsia and polyphagia, but thin skin, comedones, a potbellied appearance, bilateral symmetrical alopecia, and calcinosis cutis should draw the attention to the latter. Hypersecretion of GH may be observed during diestrus, pregnancy and hypothyroidism, and clinical signs may include a large tongue, widened interdental spaces, an altered facial appearance, and organomegaly. Superficial necrolytic dermatitis may be diagnosed in dogs with glucagonoma. Although obesity causes insulin resistance in dogs, as in other species, progression to overt DM is not recognized in dogs.

Algorithm 9.1 Note 7 Life-threatening diabetic ketoacidosis (DKA) is easily ruled out by measuring capillary or venous β-hydroxybutyrate (β-OHB) using hand-held ketone meters. At concentrations below 1.9 mmol/L, DKA is unlikely to be present, whereas β-OHB exceeding 3.8 mmol/L is highly specific (>90%) for diagnosing DKA. If blood gas analysis is unavailable, any unwell diabetic patient with a β-OHB-concentration above 1.9 mmol/L should be suspected of suffering from DKA and must be treated accordingly. Although semiquantitative urinary acetoacetate measurement using reagent strips is a simple alternative method to test for ketonemia, its sensitivity of 80% precludes its use as a reliable test.

Algorithm 9.1 Note 8 Hyperosmolar hyperglycemic syndrome (HSS) is defined by the combination of glucose concentrations exceeding 33.3 mmol/L (600 mg/dL) and an effective osmolarity above 320 mOsm/kg [effective osmolarity is calculated 2 × Na (mmol/L) × glucose (mg/dL)/18] in the absence of DKA. In HSS, insulin secretion and sensitivity are enough to prevent lipolysis and ketogenesis but not hyperglycemia. Further, additional factors that cause reduced water intake and/or increased water losses (e.g., renal failure) lead to hemoconcentration and aggravate hyperglycemia. The resultant effects of hyperosmolarity on the central nervous system initiate a vicious circle. Changes in mentation, circling, seizures, ataxia, or abnormal pupillary light reflexes may be observed.

Algorithm 9.1 Note 9 Stress-induced hyperglycemia is considered part of a graded adaptive immune-neurohormonal response during acute illness. In a recent study, the incidence of hyperglycemia in non-diabetic hospitalized dogs in the intensive care unit of a veterinary clinic was 16%. In 11% of these dogs, glucose exceeded 11.1 mmol/L (200 mg/dL), and non-survivors had higher concentrations. Whereas data suggest that transient surges during stress or illness are protective and part of graded adaptive responses conferring a survival advantage, the proinflammatory, prothrombotic, and pro-oxidant effects of prolonged hyperglycemia are detrimental (i.e., glucose toxicity) and associated with a myriad of harmful complications including β-cells desensitization and decreases of downstream action of insulin in target tissues (i.e., insulin resistance).

Algorithm 9.1 Note 10 In dogs with poorly regulated DM, the influence on the results of adrenocortical function tests has to be considered. As a result of hepatic lipidosis, alkaline phosphatase activity can be markedly elevated in diabetic dogs without concurrent hypercortisolism. As false-positive test results are possible, the diagnosis of hypercortisolism should ideally be confirmed by diagnostic imaging of the pituitary and adrenal glands. The suspicion of diestrus and acromegaly could be evidenced by elevated progesterone and IGF-1 levels, respectively.

Algorithm 9.1 Note 11 The relationship between DM and pancreatitis is bidirectional. Thus, pancreatitis can be causal or consequential to DM. Pancreatitis has been estimated to be present in 28 to 40% of canine DM patients, but it is rarely possible to differentiate between cause and effect. Unfortunately, there is no single gold-standard test to diagnose pancreatitis, including pancreatic lipase assays and diagnostic imaging. Accordingly, although this may be selected for severe cases, the diagnosis should be based on the combination of clinical history, physical examination findings, pancreatic lipase concentration, and ultrasonographic or advanced imaging findings.

Algorithm 9.1 Note 12 DM is considered subclinical in dogs with persistent fasting hyperglycemia without the presence of classic clinical signs. The term prediabetes may be applicable to dogs with intermediate hyperglycemia and glycemic variables higher than normal, but there is currently no consensus on its definition or clinical relevance.

References

1. Ambrisko TD, Hikasa Y. Neurohormonal and metabolic effects of medetomidine compared with xylazine in beagle dogs. *Can J Vet Res* 66(1):42-9, 2002. PMID:11858648; PMCID: PMC226981.
2. Duarte R, Simoes DM, Franchini ML, et al. Accuracy of serum beta-hydroxybutyrate measurements for the diagnosis of diabetic ketoacidosis in 116 dogs. *J Vet Intern Med* 16(4):411-417, 2002. doi: 10.1892/0891-6640(2002)016<0411:aosmft>2.3.co;2.
3. Gal A, Odunayo A. Diabetes ketoacidosis and hyperosmolar hyperglycemic syndrome in companion animals. *Vet Clin North Am Small Anim Pract* 53(3):531-550, 2023. doi: 10.1016/j.cvsm.2023.01.005
4. Gomez-Fernandez-Blanco C, Peeters D, Moyse E, et al. Interbreed variation of biomarkers of lipid and glucose metabolism in dogs. *Vet Clin Pathol* 47(4):582-588, 2018. doi: 10.1111/vcp.12673
5. Hagley SP, Hopper K, Epstein SE. Etiology and prognosis for dogs with abnormal blood glucose concentrations evaluated in an emergency room. *J et Emerg Crit Care (San Antonio)* 30(5):567-573, 2020. doi: 10.1111/vec.12996
6. Hewson-Hughes AK, Gilham MS, Upton S, et al. Postprandial glucose and insulin profiles following a glucose-loaded meal in cats and dogs. *Br J Nutr* 106 Suppl 1:S101-104, 2011. doi: 10.1017/S0007114511000857
7. Niessen SJM, Bjornvad C, Church DB, et al. ESVE/SCE membership. Agreeing Language in Veterinary Endocrinology (ALIVE): Diabetes mellitus – A modified Delphi-method-based system to create consensus disease definitions. *Vet J* 289:105910, 2022. doi: 10.1016/j.tvjl.2022.105910
8. Silva NLT, Bonatto NCM, Oliveira PL, et al. Post-prandial lipemia and glycemia in dogs fed with industrialized pet food. *Comp Clin Pathol* 28:253-258, 2019. https://doi.org/10.1007/s00580-018-2824-0.
9. Syring RS, Otto CM, Drobatz KJ. Hyperglycemia in dogs and cats with head trauma: 122 cases (1997-1999). *J Am Vet Med Assoc* 218(7):1124-1129, 2001. doi: 10.2460/javma.2001.218.1124.
10. Zeugswetter FK, Schwendenwein I. Basal glucose excretion in dogs: the impact of feeding, obesity, sex, and age. *Vet Clin Pathol* 49(3):428-435, 2020. doi: 10.1111/vcp.12899

CHAPTER 10

Hypoglycemia

Federico Fracassi
DVM, PhD,
DECVIM (SAIM)

Pathophysiology

Hypoglycemia is defined as a blood glucose concentration below 60 mg/dL (3.5 mmol/L).[1] In healthy dogs, the blood glucose concentrations are kept within the normal range thanks to complex neuroendocrine and cellular mechanisms linked together. Carbohydrate homeostasis is maintained by the interaction between food absorption, liver deposits and their release, and the effects of the main hormones that control blood glucose (insulin and glucagon). The liver acts as a storage organ for glucose, which is stored as glycogen and can be released following glycogenolysis or through the mobilization of fatty acids or amino acids (gluconeogenesis). Other hormones, in addition to insulin and glucagon, are also involved in glycemic control; these include glucocorticoids, catecholamines, and growth hormone.

Insulin stimulates glucose uptake by cells and inhibits gluconeogenesis, glycogenolysis, and glucagon secretion. Glucagon stimulates hepatic glycogenolysis and gluconeogenesis; the latter process converts amino acids to glucose. Glucagon also decreases peripheral glucose utilization. Cortisol stimulates hepatic gluconeogenesis and decreases peripheral tissue utilization of glucose. Epinephrine increases glucagon secretion, decreases insulin secretion, and promotes lipolysis. Growth hormone increases lipolysis and reduces peripheral glucose utilization.[2]

The hypoglycemic condition can be the result of several mechanisms, such as the excessive consumption of glucose by the cells (e.g., insulinoma and insulin growth factor II [IGF-II]-secreting neoplasms, insulin overdose), abnormalities of hepatic gluconeogenesis, and/or glycogenolysis (e.g., hepatic insufficiency), a deficiency of counterregulatory hormones (e.g., hypoadrenocorticism), an insufficient dietary intake of glucose (especially in young animals), or a combination of one or more of these mechanisms.[3] Furthermore, it can derive from the administration or ingestion of drugs or toxins such as insulin, sulphonylurea, and xylitol[4] (Table 10.1).

TABLE 10.1 Causes of hypoglycemia in the dog, according to pathophysiological classification.

Hypoglycemia due to reduced glucose production	Hypoglycemia due to increased removal of glucose	Other causes: combination of factors/unknown

■ Hepatic vascular abnormalities
■ Acute liver failure
■ Chronic end-stage hepatopathy (fibrosis/cirrhosis)
■ Hypoadrenocorticism
■ Toxins: ethylene glycol/ethanol
■ Medications/toxins: propranolol
■ Growth hormone deficiency
■ Neonatal and juvenile hypoglycemia
■ Toy breed hypoglycemia
■ Glycogen storage disease:
  ■ Type I: von Gierke's disease
  ■ Type III: Cori's disease
	■ Insulin overdose
	■ Oral hypoglycemic agents
	■ Insulinoma
	■ Insulin-like-substance-producing tumors: hepatoma, leiomyoma, leiomyosarcomas, carcinomas, melanomas, plasma cell tumors, etc.
	■ Nesidioblastosis
	■ Polycythemias: primary erythrocytosis, leukemias
	■ Toxins: xylitol, oleander
	■ Renal glycosuria
		■ Sepsis
		■ *Babesia* spp. infection
		■ Toxins: alpha-lipoic acid
		■ Hunting dog

Modified from Nelson, 2015.[5]

Clinical signs

Glucose is the primary energy source for the body; in particular, the central nervous system cannot synthesize or store glucose and is totally dependent on plasma glucose concentrations. Therefore, a condition of neuroglycopenia produces neurological clinical signs of central origin. The clinical manifestations depend on the duration and intensity of the hypoglycemic episode, the length of time with which the dog has lived with hypoglycemia, and the counter-regulatory response. Patients with mild hypoglycemia (45-60 mg/dL; 2.5-3.3 mmol/L) may have subtle clinical signs or be clinically normal. The clinical signs are usually evident when blood glucose concentrations are below 45 mg/dL (2.5 mmol/L). Dogs may remain asymptomatic at blood glucose as low as 45 mg/dL (2.5 mmo/L), but the more rapid the fall in glucose levels concentration, the more likely clinical signs are to be present. The clinical manifestations of hypoglycemia are believed to result from both lack of glucose supply to the brain (neuroglycopenia) and stimulation of the sympathoadrenal system.[4] The neuroglycopenic clinical signs include weakness, lethargy, ataxia, disorientation, behavioral abnormalities, blindness, and seizures. The stimulation of the sympathoadrenal system produces tremors, nervousness, shaking, and restlessness (Video 10.1). Prolonged, severe hypoglycemia can cause irreversible brain damage and potentially death. The clinical signs can be acute or progress over time.

Diagnostic approach

Algorithm 10.1 shows the approach to the hypoglycemic patient.
Dogs of any age, sex, or breed can develop hypoglycemia. Normal canine blood glucose concentrations range from 70-120 mg/dL (3.9-6.7 mmol/L). Hypoglycemia is defined as a blood glucose concentration below 60 mg/dL (3.3 mmol/L).[1]

Algorithm 10.1 Note 1 Laboratory error and sample handling must be considered when a concentration is low but the dog has no clinical signs. Failure to separate erythrocytes and leukocytes from serum within 30 minutes results in artifactual hypoglycemia due to cellular consumption of glucose. Glucose levels can also decrease by 10% every 30-60 minutes at room temperature.[6] Many portable human glucose meters tend to underestimate the real blood glucose concentration of dogs. If clinical signs are not consistent with hypoglycemia before embarking on an extensive work-up, re-remeasuring glucose concentration on a properly handled and processed fresh sample is appropriate. Hexokinase is the gold standard method for measuring blood glucose and should be used to confirm suspected cases of hypoglycemia.

Video 10.1

A 10-year-old male Poodle with insulinoma and worsening neurological clinical signs during the day. In the first part of the day, during the walk performed shortly after the morning meal, almost no anomalies are detectable. Later in the day, when the dog is filmed at home, restlessness, ataxia, and tremors are increasingly noticeable. Finally, the dog is no longer able to get up 10 hours after the last meal.

Algorithm 10.1 Note 2 A careful evaluation of the history can provide essential indications for reaching the diagnosis. Specific attention must be given to the diet (especially in a young puppy or a toy breed dog), to the administration of medications (e.g., insulin), or potential exposure to toxic drugs (e.g., xylitol).

Algorithm 10.1 Note 3 A diabetic patient receiving insulin injections is at risk of hypoglycemia in three scenarios. Firstly an accidental insulin overdose, secondly the provision of insulin when a patient has not consumed sufficient calories (e.g., inappetence, vomiting) and thirdly, when endogenous insulin concentration or sensitivity begins to recover (resolution of insulin resistance or diabetes remission) and exogenous insulin is less or no longer required. Diabetic remission is an uncommon event in dogs. Still, it can be observed after cessation of corticosteroid therapy or after ovariectomy/ovariohysterectomy of a bitch in the progesterone-dominated phase of diestrus or pregnancy. In case of a massive overdose, hypoglycemia can last several days and requires intensive care treatment with constant rate infusion with glucose, with careful electrolyte management.

Algorithm 10.1 Note 4 The artificial sweetener xylitol, commonly found in "sugar-free" products such as chewing gum or toothpaste for human use, can cause signs of hypoglycemia by stimulating the release of insulin from beta cells.

Algorithm 10.1 Note 5 Limited hepatic glycogen stores, small muscle mass, lack of adipose tissue, and decreased use of free fatty acids as an alternative source place the neonate/young animal at risk of developing hypoglycemia within hours of fasting. A similar condition can be observed in toy breed dogs.

Algorithm 10.1 Note 6 A complete blood count, serum chemistry, and urinalysis should be evaluated for all hypoglycemic patients to help determine the underlying cause. Depending on a patient's history and clinical signs, further testing may be indicated.

Algorithm 10.1 Note 7 Fructosamine is glycosylated albumin and reflects the average blood glucose during the preceding 1-2 weeks. Persistent hypoglycemia may produce low fructosamine concentration.

Algorithm 10.1 Note 8 If no causes of hypoglycemia are found, it may be useful to carry out an ACTH stimulation test also in normokalemic and normonatremic dogs. Serum basal cortisol assessment can also be useful. A basal serum cortisol >2 μg/dL excludes hypoadrenocorticism. If basal cortisol <2 μg/dL is found, the ACTH stimulation test should always be performed to confirm or exclude the disease. Detection of a urinary cortisol/creatinine ratio in the normal range is another method that can be used to rule out hypoadrenocorticism. Hypoadrenocorticism is confirmed when serum cortisol post-ACTH is <2 μg/dL, in a dog that has not received corticosteroid in the previous 2 months.

Algorithm 10.1 Note 9 Functional tumors arising from the beta cells of the pancreatic islets are usually malignant tumors that secrete insulin. The detection of metastasis at the time of diagnosis is common. The most common sites of tumor spread are the regional lymphatics and lymph nodes (duodenal, mesenteric, hepatic, splenic), the liver, and the peripancreatic omentum. Pulmonary metastases are uncommon.

ALGORITHM 10.1

Approach to the hypoglycemic patient

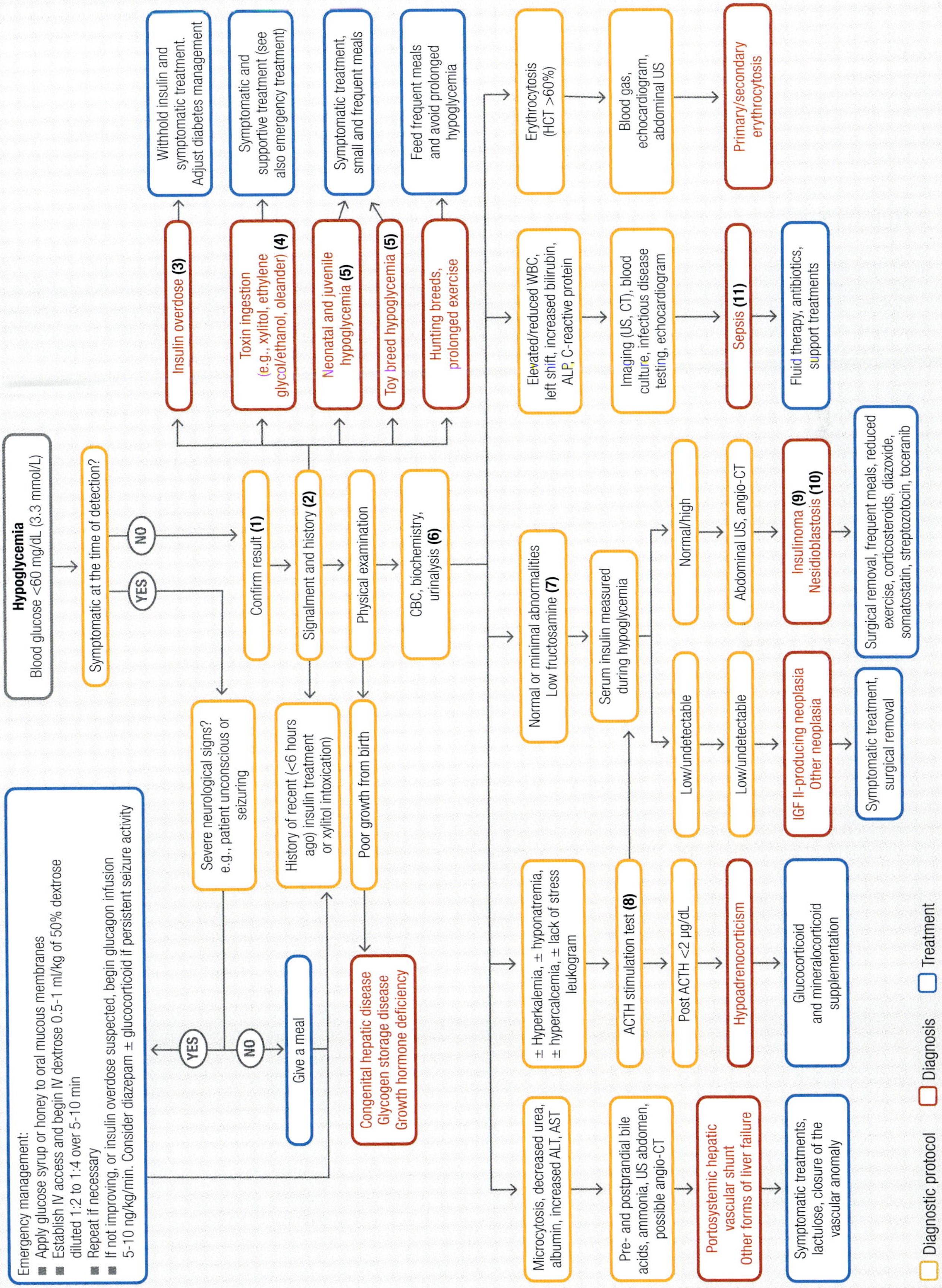

Algorithm 10.1 Note 10 Nesidioblastosis (non-insulinoma pancreatic hypoglycemia syndrome) is an increasingly recognized syndrome in people that can be congenital or acquired. It is secondary to focal or diffuse, non-neoplastic beta cell hypertrophy and/or hyperplasia within the pancreas. This condition has also been described in dogs, and the diagnosis is reached based on the histopathology of the pancreas. Partial pancreatectomy is the treatment of choice.[7]

Algorithm 10.1 Note 11 The mechanism(s) for hypoglycemia with sepsis is not well defined. Depleted glycogen stores, impaired gluconeogenesis, and increased peripheral glucose utilization may all be contributing factors. In one study, sepsis was the reason for hypoglycemia in about one-fourth of non-diabetic dogs presented to a veterinary emergency room.[8]

References

1. Niessen SJM, Bjornvad C, Church DB, et al. Agreeing Language in Veterinary Endocrinology (ALIVE): Diabetes mellitus –A modified Delphi-method-based system to create consensus disease definitions. *Vet J* 289:105910, 2022.
2. Rucinsky R. Hypoglycemia. In: Byers CG, Giunti M, eds. Feline Emergency and Critical Care Medicine. Milan, 2021, Edra, pp. 434-437.
3. Fracassi F, Davison L. In: Fracassi F, ed. Diagnostic and therapeutic algorithms in internal medicine for dogs and cats. Milan, 2022, Edra, pp. 173-176.
4. Murphy LA, Dunayer EK. Xylitol toxicosis in dogs: an update. *Vet Clin North Am Small Anim Pract* 48(6):985-990, 2018.
5. Nelson RW. Beta-cell neoplasia: insulinoma. In: Feldman EC, Nelson RW, Reusch C, Scott-Moncrieff JC (eds.). Canine and Feline Endocrinology 4th edition. St. Louis, 2015, Elsevier Saunders, pp. 355.
6. Willard MD. Small animal clinical diagnosis by laboratory methods 5th edition. St. Louis, 2012, Elsevier Saunders, p. 165.
7. Polansky BJ, Martinez SA, Chalkley MD. Resolution of hyperinsulinemic hypoglycemia following partial pancreatectomy in a dog with nesidioblastosis. *J Am Vet Med Assoc* 253(7):893-896, 2018.
8. Hagley SP, Hopper K, Epstein SE. Etiology and prognosis for dogs with abnormal blood glucose concentrations evaluated in an emergency room. *J Vet Emerg Crit Care (San Antonio)* 30(5):567-573, 2020.

CHAPTER 11

Low thyroxine

Robert E. Shiel
MVB, PhD, DECVIM-CA
(Internal Medicine)

Pathophysiology

Serum total thyroxine (T_4) concentrations are routinely measured as part of the investigation of hypothyroidism and are sometimes included on extended biochemical screening profiles. A low total T_4 concentration is supportive of hypothyroidism; however, several other factors influence circulating T_4 concentrations. These include nonthyroidal illness (NTI) syndrome, exercise and use of certain medications. Finally, some breeds have physiologically low T_4 concentrations.

Breed

Thyroid hormone concentrations in euthyroid dogs can vary between individual breeds. Often, these differences are statistically significant but do not result in values outside of non-breed-specific reference intervals.[1] However, in some breeds, total T_4 values are decreased in a large proportion of healthy dogs (Table 11.1). This is best characterized in Greyhounds, where approximately 90% of total T_4 values are below non-breed-specific reference intervals and often below the limit of quantification of commonly used assays.[2] Decreased total T_4 may be associated with thyroid hormone-binding protein variants,[3] altered T_4:triiodothyronine (T_3) secretion ratio, or altered thyroid hormone receptor sensitivity or metabolism.[4] Regardless of the mechanism, the presence of low T_4 concentrations in health suggests physiological variation rather than a pathological cause.

TABLE 11.1 Factors most commonly associated with decreased total T_4 concentrations in euthyroid dogs.

Breed	Drugs	Other factor
Greyhound[a]	Glucocorticoids[c]	Nonthyroidal illness syndrome
Whippet	Barbiturates[c]	Exercise
Saluki[a]	Potentiated sulfonamides[d]	Age
Basenji	Carprofen	
Sloughi	Clomipramine	
Scottish Deerhound		
Sled dogs[a,b]		
Dogue de Bordeaux		

[a]Decreased free T_4 values also reported in the breed. [b]Not a defined breed, but related to Siberian Huskies and Alaskan Malamutes. [c]Most common medications to cause marked suppression of total T_4. [d]May induce clinical primary hypothyroidism.

Nonthyroidal illness syndrome

Nonthyroidal illnesses can have a profound suppressive effect on thyroid hormone concentrations, with the magnitude of the effect dependent upon the type, severity, and duration of the disease.[6] These effects may be mediated through modification of the hypothalamic-pituitary-thyroid axis, altered thyroid hormone metabolism or binding to plasma proteins, or altered thyroid hormone receptor expression or function.[5]

Several illnesses have been shown to cause NTI syndrome, including hypercortisolism, a variety of infectious diseases, neoplasia (especially when associated with cachexia), and kidney disease. However, any concurrent disease may suppress thyroid hormone concentrations, particularly if severe.

Medication

Several drugs affect thyroid hormone concentrations through a variety of mechanisms, including alteration of thyroid hormone secretion, protein binding in plasma, cellular uptake, and metabolism of thyroid hormones.[7] The magnitude of the effect is dependent on the dose, route of administration, and duration of therapy. Clearly, the administration of antithyroid medications (thiamazole or carbimazole) will decrease circulating thyroid hormone concentrations due to their suppressive effects on thyroid peroxidase function, a key enzyme involved in thyroid hormone synthesis. In dogs, glucocorticoids and barbiturates have the most suppressive effects. Immunosuppressive (2 mg/kg/day) dosages of glucocorticoids consistently decrease total and free T_4 concentrations. Most studies have shown a suppressive effect of phenobarbitone on total and free T_4 concentrations, as well as a mild increase in TSH concentrations. Potentiated sulfonamides also inhibit thyroid peroxidase function, and administration can be associated with decreased thyroid hormone concentrations, increased TSH concentrations, and the development of reversible clinical goitrous primary hypothyroidism. Clomipramine can decrease total and free T_4 concentrations by approximately one-third, potentially below the lower limit of the reference interval. Toceranib phosphate does not decrease total T_4 concentrations but may decrease free T_4 and increase TSH concentrations.

By contrast, the effects of most other drugs, including carprofen, are relatively mild and unlikely to affect thyroid function testing.

Other factors influencing total thyroxine concentrations

Training and exercise have a suppressive effect on total T_4 concentrations, with lower values reported in competing sled dogs and Greyhounds. Similarly, experimental treadmill exercise significantly decreases total T_4 concentrations by approximately 10-15% in dogs. Potential suppression of total T_4 concentrations should be considered in dogs engaged in rigorous activity and training.

The effect of age on thyroid hormones is most prominent in young dogs. Total T_4 values increase from approximately twice the mean adult value at birth, peak at approximately five times the adult value at 3-4 weeks, and decrease to approximately twice the adult value by 12 weeks. Total T_4 values decline with advancing age but typically remain with reference interval.

Effects of sex, neutering status, body condition, and body weight on total T_4 concentrations have been described, but values typically remain within the reference interval.

Finally, the effect of the thyroid hormone assay should be considered. As outlined in the European Veterinary Endocrine Quality Assurance Scheme, total T_4 concentrations can vary between different laboratories and different methods.[8] Therefore, repeat measurement should be considered, particularly if results and clinical presentation are discordant or if a result is generated in a laboratory without rigorous quality assurance and control. The presence of T_4 autoantibodies in dogs can also impact the measurement of total T_4, resulting in an erroneous increase in concentration with most commonly used assays.

Clinical signs

Total T_4 concentrations are most commonly measured in dogs as part of the diagnosis of hypothyroidism. Given the poor specificity of total T_4, in clinical cases, it is essential that concentrations are only measured in dogs in which there is a suspicion of hypothyroidism, based on findings such as nonpruritic, truncal alopecia, weight gain, hypercholesterolemia or the presence of a gallbladder mucocele, as detailed in chapter 27.

Dogs with significant nonthyroidal illness usually have signs relating to that disease process, which may not be consistent with hypothyroidism. The identification of such signs should prompt investigation of the nonthyroidal illness prior to investigation of thyroid function, if possible.

Diagnostic approach

Before measuring total T_4 concentrations in any dog, potential effects of breed, NTI syndrome, and thyroid-suppressive medications should be considered to reduce the likelihood that a decreased T_4 concentration is due to a factor other than the presence of hypothyroidism.

Algorithm 11.1 shows the diagnostic and treatment path for low thyroxine findings.

Algorithm 11.1 Note 1 Clinical signs raising the suspicion of hypothyroidism are based on consistent history, physical examination, and clinicopathological or diagnostic imaging findings.

Algorithm 11.1 Note 2 Total T_4 concentrations may also be measured in young, healthy dogs to identify animals with early thyroid disease prior to use for breeding. In such cases, concurrent measurement of thyroglobulin autoantibody and TSH concentrations is usually recommended to identify dogs with lymphocytic thyroiditis and subclinical hypothyroidism, respectively, which can be identified months or years prior to the development of clinical hypothyroidism.

Algorithm 11.1 Note 3 In breeds that frequently display physiologically low T_4 concentrations, such as Greyhounds, a decreased T_4 value is not supportive of hypothyroidism, especially in the absence of clinical signs. However, maintenance of reference interval values may markedly decrease the likelihood of this diagnosis.

Algorithm 11.1 Note 4 In dogs with significant nonthyroidal illness or in those receiving thyroid-suppressive medications, thyroid function testing should be postponed, if possible, until at least 4-6 weeks after resolution of disease and/or discontinuation of medication. In some cases, this may not be possible. For example, a cure may not be attainable in dogs with severe immune-mediated, metabolic, or neoplastic diseases, and discontinuation of prednisolone or phenobarbitone may not be possible in dogs with immune-mediated disease or seizures, respectively.

Algorithm 11.1 Note 5 Plasma TSH concentrations should be measured in the same sample in which low T_4 was detected. If TSH was not measured initially (or following treatment of illness or removal of thyroid suppressive medications), both total T_4 and TSH should be measured concurrently before proceeding further. Low total T_4 concentration should not be interpreted in the absence of TSH concentration.

Algorithm 11.1 Note 6 Approximately 75-80% of hypothyroid dogs have increased TSH concentrations. Increased TSH concentrations are not observed in any of the breeds with physiologically decreased total T_4 concentrations. Likewise, most nonthyroidal illnesses and drugs are not associated with increased TSH concentrations. However, TSH concentrations may increase transiently during the recovery phase of nonthyroidal illness or following discontinuation of thyroid suppressive medication. Increased TSH concentrations have also been described in euthyroid dogs with primary hypoadrenocorticism.

Algorithm 11.1 Note 7 Concurrent measurement of free T_4 and TSH may increase confidence in the diagnosis of hypothyroidism, although free T_4 concentrations (by analogue or equilibrium dialysis methods) may also be decreased in dogs with severe nonthyroidal illness and those receiving glucocorticoid or barbiturate therapy, and TSH concentrations are not increased in all hypothyroid dogs. Additional tests, including thyroid scintigraphy or TSH response testing, could be considered if the diagnosis remains uncertain.[9,10] Measurement of thyroglobulin autoantibody (TgAA) concentrations does not provide any information on thyroid function, but positivity at least confirms the presence of thyroid disease (lymphocytic thyroiditis).

Algorithm 11.1 Note 8 Measurement of TgAA does not provide any information on thyroid function, but the presence of TgAA positivity confirms the presence of thyroid pathology.

ALGORITHM 11.1

Diagnostic approach to low thyroxine concentration.

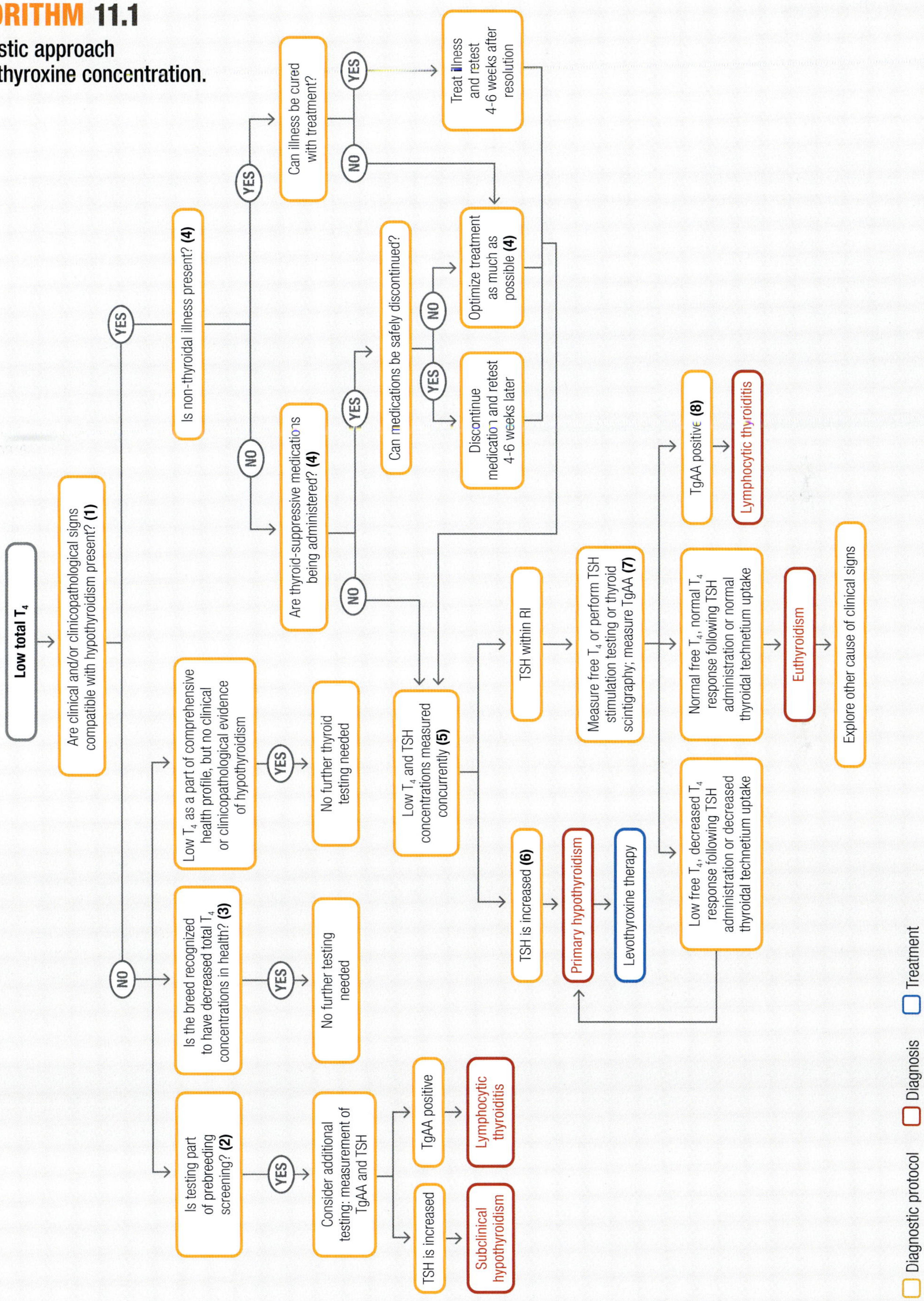

References

1. Hegstad-Davies RL, Torres SM, Sharkey LC, et al. Breed-specific reference intervals for assessing thyroid function in seven dog breeds. *J Vet Diagn Invest* 27(6):716-727, 2015.
2. Shiel RE, Brennan SF, Omodo-Eluk AJ, et al. Thyroid hormone concentrations in young, healthy, pretraining greyhounds. *Vet Rec* 161(18):616-619, 2007.
3. Mimoto MS, Refetoff S. Clinical recognition and evaluation of patients with inherited serum thyroid hormone-binding protein mutations. *J Endocrinol Invest* 43:31-41, 2020.
4. Shiel RE, Nolan CM, Nally JE, et al. Qualitative and semiquantitative assessment of thyroid hormone binding proteins in greyhounds and other dog breeds. *Dom Anim Endocrinol* 76:106623, 2021.
5. Warner MH, Beckett GJ. Mechanisms behind the non-thyroidal illness syndrome: an update. *J Endocrinol* 205(1):1-3, 2009.
6. Mooney CT, Shiel RE, Dixon RM. Thyroid hormone abnormalities and outcome in dogs with non-thyroidal illness. *J Small Anim Pract* 49(1):11-16, 2008.
7. Daminet S, Ferguson DC. Influence of drugs on thyroid function in dogs. *J Vet Intern Med* 17(4):463-472, 2003.
8. European Veterinary Endocrine Quality Assurance Scheme [Internet]. Cited 24 July 2023. https://www.esve.org/esve/eve-qas/default.aspx
9. Shiel RE, Pinilla M, McAllister H, et al. Assessment of the value of quantitative thyroid scintigraphy for determination of thyroid function in dogs. *J Small Anim Pract* 53(5):278-285, 2012.
10. Corsini A, Faroni E, Lunetta F, et al. Recombinant human thyrotropin stimulation test in 114 dogs with suspected hypothyroidism: a cross-sectional study. *J Small Anim Pract* 62(4):257-264, 2021.

CHAPTER 12

Hyperlipidemia

Panagiotis G. Xenoulis
DVM, PhD, cECVCN

Hyperlipidemia is a common condition in dogs. In the last decade, several studies in both humans and dogs have associated specific forms of hyperlipidemia with a much wider range of diseases than previously thought. Postprandial hyperlipidemia is physiologic and typically resolves within 7-12 hours after a meal. Therefore, determination of serum lipid concentrations should always follow a fast of at least 12 hours.

Pathophysiology

Persistent fasting hyperlipidemia can be either primary (typically due to an inborn inherited error in lipid metabolism) or secondary to other diseases or drug administration. Secondary hyperlipidemia is the most common form of hyperlipidemia in dogs. Most commonly, secondary hyperlipidemia (hypertriglyceridemia and/or hypercholesterolemia) is the result of an endocrine disorder such as hypothyroidism, diabetes mellitus, or hypercortisolism. Hyperlipidemia (hypertriglyceridemia and/or hypercholesterolemia) has also been associated with naturally-occurring pancreatitis in dogs, but in most cases, this is relatively mild unless another cause of hyperlipidemia is also present. Another important cause of secondary hyperlipidemia in dogs is obesity. Other possible causes of hyperlipidemia include protein-losing nephropathy (nephrotic syndrome), cholestasis, high-fat diets, and possibly other conditions (e.g., infections, inflammation, neoplasia, congestive heart failure). Administration of certain drugs, mainly glucocorticoids and estrogens (such as megestrol acetate), can induce marked hyperlipidemia. Other drugs reported to cause hyperlipidemia in dogs include phenobarbital, potassium bromide, and progestagens.

Primary lipid abnormalities in dogs are usually, but not always, associated with certain breeds. Depending on the breed, the prevalence of a primary lipid abnormality can vary widely. Also, the geographic region of the canine population tested seems to play an important role due to genetic differences. Primary hyperlipidemia is very common in Miniature Schnauzers in the United States (>30% of Miniature Schnauzers are affected based on one study).[1,2] There are no published studies regarding the European population. Primary hyperlipidemia in the Miniature Schnauzer is typically characterized by hypertriglyceridemia. Although hypercholesterolemia may also be present, it is not found in all affected dogs and is always present in association with hypertriglyceridemia. Other breeds, such as Shetland Sheepdogs, Beagles, Briards, Doberman Pinschers, and Rottweilers, may also have different forms of primary hyperlipidemias.

Clinical signs

Hyperlipidemia *per se* does not appear to lead to any clinical signs. However, dogs with secondary hyperlipidemia often display clinical signs of the primary disease (e.g., polyuria and polydipsia in dogs with diabetes mellitus). In addition, many animals with hyperlipidemia develop diseases or conditions as a result of hyperlipidemia, and clinical signs develop as a result of those diseases. Therefore, canine hyperlipidemia is now considered an important clinical condition that requires a systematic diagnostic approach and appropriate treatment. Such diseases include pancreatitis, hepatobiliary disease (increased liver enzyme activity, vacuolar hepatopathy, and gallbladder mucocele), insulin resistance, atherosclerosis, ocular disease, xanthomatosis (benign granulomatous lesions on the skin or internal organs), proteinuria and glomerular lipidosis, and neurologic disease (e.g., seizures, ischemic strokes).

Diagnostic approach

Algorithm 12.1 shows the diagnostic approach to dogs with hyperlipidemia.

Diagnosis

Algorithm 12.1 Note 1 Hyperlipidemia is typically diagnosed by measurement of fasting serum triglyceride and/or cholesterol concentrations or suspected when a lipemic serum sample is visually identified (Fig. 2.1). In some cases, fasting serum triglyceride concentrations

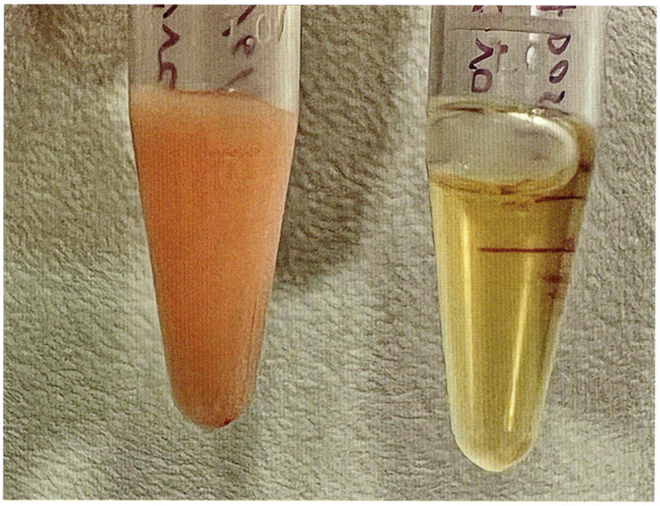

FIG. 12.1 Serum with high (left) and normal (right) triglyceride concentrations. The sample on the right is "lipemic" as indicated by the "cloudy" or "milky" appearance.

may be normal, while abnormal hypertriglyceridemia might be evident postprandially.

Algorithm 12.1 Note 2 After hyperlipidemia has been diagnosed, the next step is to determine whether the patient has a primary or a secondary lipid disorder, based initially on clinical presentation and results from routine testing. This is crucial because animals with secondary hyperlipidemia typically show clinical signs of the primary disease (e.g., obesity, polyuria, and polydipsia in dogs with hypercortisolism) and/or laboratory abnormalities (e.g., hyperglycemia and glucosuria in diabetes mellitus), which can help prioritize the selection of diagnostic tests and lead the way towards an appropriate diagnostic plan. Dogs with primary hyperlipidemia commonly do not have clinical signs unless hyperlipidemia has led to a secondary disease (such as pancreatitis or biliary mucocele).

Algorithm 12.1 Note 3 Specific diagnostic investigations should be performed to diagnose or rule out specific diseases that can cause secondary hyperlipidemia. The selection of tests to be performed is based on information from the history and physical examination and is tailored to each individual case. A more general and wide selection of tests might be necessary for patients with vague or no clinical signs.

Algorithm 12.1 Note 4 One possible exception is the Miniature Schnauzer, in which primary hyperlipidemia is common. A detailed diagnostic investigation of hyperlipidemia might not be necessary for this breed in the absence of clinical signs, and routine clinicopathologic testing suggests an underlying cause because primary hyperlipidemia is very common and well-characterized in this breed. The main clinicopathological finding in these dogs is hypertriglyceridemia. Hypercholesterolemia might also be present, but isolated hypercholesterolemia is not a feature of primary hyperlipidemia in this breed.

Algorithm 12.1 Note 6 If secondary hyperlipidemia is excluded, a tentative diagnosis of a primary lipid disorder can be made.

Algorithm 12.1 Note 8 In some cases, additional specialized testing might be implemented to determine the nature of hyperlipidemia (e.g., ultracentrifugation to determine the lipoprotein fractions that are responsible for the hyperlipidemia). For example, hypertriglyceridemia, which is a result of increased chylomicrons, is more likely to respond to dietary treatment as opposed to increased very-low-density-lipoproteins (VLDLs).

Treatment

Algorithm 12.1 Note 5 If hyperlipidemia is secondary, the condition causing hyperlipidemia should be treated. This typically resolves or at least improves hyperlipidemia. Resolution of secondary hyperlipidemia after treatment of the cause should always be confirmed by laboratory testing (typically 4-6 weeks after initiation of treatment of the primary disease and periodically thereafter). If severe hyperlipidemia persists after treatment of the primary disease, treatment for primary hyperlipidemia should be implemented.

Algorithm 12.1 Note 7 Treatment of primary or persistent secondary hypertriglyceridemia is clinically important. Management of hypercholesterolemia seems to be of less clinical importance. In most cases, treatment should initially be pursued with dietary management, while drug therapy can be initiated later if deemed necessary. It has been traditionally recommended that hypertriglyceridemia should be treated only when exceeding 500 mg/dL (27.7 mmol/L). However, recent studies have shown that insulin resistance, hepatobiliary disease, and possibly other complications of hypertriglyceridemia can exist even with serum triglyceride concentrations below 500 mg/dL (27.7 mmol/L). Therefore, treatment should be considered even in patients with less severe hypertriglyceridemia to keep serum triglyceride concentrations as low as possible and lower the risk for complications.

Dietary management

Typically, the first step in the management of primary or persistent secondary hyperlipidemia is dietary modification. The most commonly used and likely most effective dietary option for hyperlipidemia in dogs is feeding a low-fat diet. Dogs with persistent primary hyperlipidemia should be offered a low-fat diet throughout their lives, while animals with transient primary or persistent secondary hyperlipidemia should be offered low-fat diets on the basis of repeated testing and effectiveness of control of the primary disease. Many commercially available diets are labeled as low-fat, but their fat content can vary widely. It needs to be pointed out that the percentage of fat content in the diet (commonly listed on food labels) does not reliably reflect the amount of fat the animal is consuming. Therefore, fat content should be assessed on a metabolizable energy basis. The author generally recommends diets that contain less than 25 g of total fat per 1,000 Kcal (metabolizable energy).[3,4] Home-made low-fat diets have not been systematically evaluated for the management of hyperlipidemia in dogs. If such diets are used, care should be taken to make sure that these diets are balanced, especially when intended for long-term feeding, and that the minimum nutrient requirements are met for all nutrients, including essential fatty acids. In some dogs, additional dietary modifications may be used if low-fat diets are not effective.

Other options in the dietary management of dogs with abnormal serum lipid concentrations include the addition of dietary fiber. Complex carbohydrates seem to have a positive effect on clinical disorders of lipid

ALGORITHM 12.1

Diagnostic approach to hyperlipidemia.

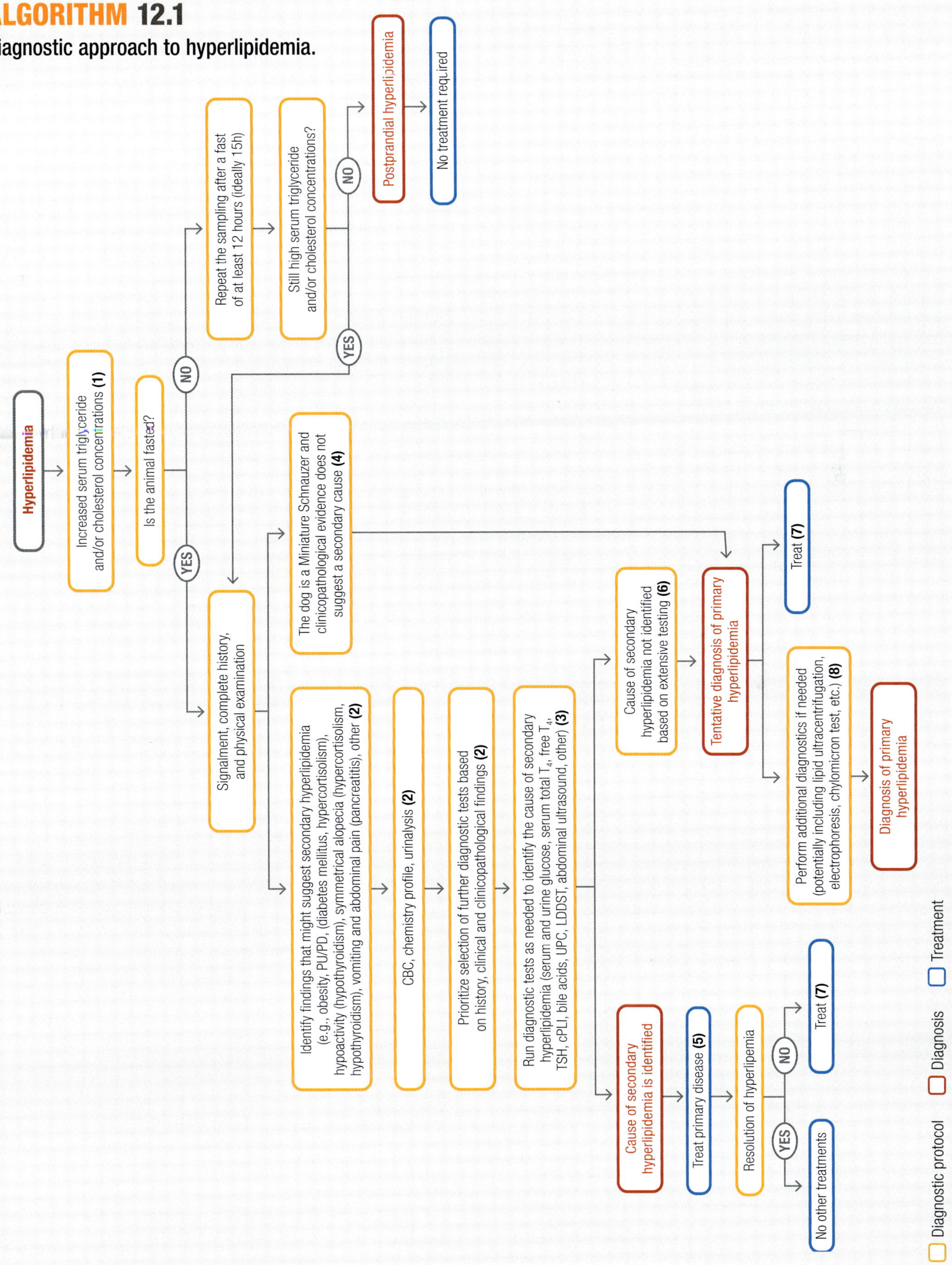

metabolism. Although explicit studies in dogs are lacking, it might be useful, based on experience in humans and other animals, to achieve a reduction in blood lipid levels via the inclusion of dietary fiber. Sources of fiber can be soluble and insoluble. While insoluble fibers, for example, cellulose, have a typical bulk effect, soluble fibers can, depending on their character, lead to a change in the viscosity of the digest. Furthermore, they can influence the composition and metabolic activity of the intestinal microbiota.

Polyunsaturated fatty acids of the n-3 series (omega-3 fatty acids, eicosapentaenoic acid [EPA], and docosahexaenoic acid [DHA]) are abundant in marine fish. Omega-3 fatty acid supplementation has been shown to lower serum triglyceride concentrations in experimental animals and humans, including cases of primary hypertriglyceridemia. However, studies evaluating the efficacy and safety of omega-3 fatty acid supplementation in dogs with hyperlipidemia are lacking. A "fishy" odor is often noted in dogs receiving high doses of omega-3 fatty acids, and it might be unacceptable for some owners. Omega-3 fatty acids may be used in dogs at doses ranging from 200 mg/kg to 300 mg/kg, PO, once a day, and their effect on serum triglyceride concentrations is dose-dependent.

Niacin is a form of vitamin B_3 that has been used successfully to treat hyperlipidemia in humans for many years. When used in pharmacological doses, niacin is a broad-spectrum lipid-modifying drug. Clinical trials regarding the efficacy and safety of niacin in dogs with primary hypertriglyceridemia are lacking, and clinical experience is limited. In some dogs, niacin reduced serum triglyceride concentrations for several months without causing side effects. As is often the case in humans, niacin administration in dogs may be associated with side effects such as erythema and pruritus, which may require discontinuation of therapy. Long-term risks for myotoxicity and hepatotoxicity may also exist. Niacin may be administered to dogs at a dose of 50 to 100 mg/day.

Medical management

Some animals with primary hyperlipidemia may not sufficiently respond to dietary modification, or faster and more predictive lowering of serum lipid concentrations may be required. In these cases, medical treatment may be required. Drugs that are more commonly used in the management of hyperlipidemia are shown in Table 12.1.

Fibrates (fabric acid derivatives)

Fibrates are weak agonists of peroxisome proliferator-activated receptor-α (PPARα), a nuclear transcription factor that regulates lipid and lipoprotein synthesis and catabolism. Gemfibrozil is one of the most commonly used fibrates in humans, and it has also been used anecdotally in dogs with hypertriglyceridemia. It can be administered at 10 mg/kg q12h, PO, in dogs. No side effects have been observed in dogs, although no studies have evaluated its safety in this species. In the author's experience, many canine patients with primary hyperlipidemia do not respond well to treatment with gemfibrozil. Bezafibrate, another fibric acid derivative, may be both more effective and associated with fewer adverse effects in the treatment of humans and

TABLE 12.1 Dietary and medical options for the management of hyperlipidemia in dogs.

		Dosage regimen	Side effects	Comments
Dietary modification	Low-fat diets	Fat <25 g/1000 Kcal	None known	■ Cornerstone of treatment. ■ Effective in many cases. ■ Percentage of fat in diet not accurate. ■ Diet fat content should be expressed in metabolizable energy.
	Dietary fiber	Unkown	None known	■ Unknown effectiveness.
	Omega-3 fatty acids	200-300 mg/kg, q24h, PO	Fishy odor, gastrointestinal signs	■ Questionable effectiveness in severe cases.
	Niacin	50-200 mg/day (total dose)	Erythema, pruritus, myotoxicity, hepatotoxicity	■ Questionable effectiveness. ■ Possibly modest effect.
	Chitosan	3 g/cat, q24h, PO	None known	■ Limited experience. ■ Possibly modest effect.
	5-aminolevulinic acid	1 mg/kg, q24h, PO	None known	■ Exact effectiveness unkown.
Drug *Fibrates*	Bezafibrate	4-10 mg/kg, q24h, PO	Potentially myotoxicity and hepatotoxicity	■ Highly effective in both primary and secondary hypertriglyceridemia. ■ Long-term safety unknown.
	Fenofibrate	10 mg/kg, q24h, PO	Potentially myotoxicity and hepatotoxicity	■ Highly effective in both primary and secondary hypertriglyceridemia. ■ Long-term safety unknown.
	Gemfibrozil	10 mg/kg, q12h, PO	Potentially myotoxicity and hepatotoxicity	■ Questionable effectiveness.
Drug *Statins*		Depends on specific drug. Not established for dogs and cats.	Unknown; possible hepatotoxicity	■ Very limited experience. ■ May be used for hypercholesterolemia.

dogs with hyperlipidemia. Bezafibrate has been evaluated for treating hyperlipidemia of various causes (both primary and secondary) in dogs and was found to be highly effective in reducing serum triglyceride and cholesterol concentrations. In one study, bezafibrate was used at a dose ranging from 4 mg/kg to 10 mg/kg, q24h, for 30 days. Normalization of serum triglyceride and cholesterol concentrations was achieved in 91% and 68% of cases, respectively.[3,5] No side effects were observed. In a more recent study, fenofibrate (10 mg/kg, q24h) was also evaluated in the treatment of severe hypertriglyceridemia in dogs (both primary and secondary) and was found to be highly effective, leading to the normalization of serum triglyceride concentrations in 86% of dogs.[3,6] In that study, normalization of serum cholesterol concentrations occurred in only about 50% of dogs. No significant adverse effects were reported. Periodic testing of serum triglyceride concentration and liver enzyme activities is recommended.

Statins

Statins (HMG-CoA reductase inhibitors) are among the most potent and commonly used lipid-lowering drugs and constitute first-line therapy for treating hypercholesterolemia in humans. They are reversible inhibitors of the enzyme HMG-CoA reductase, which is the rate-limiting step for cholesterol biosynthesis. Therefore, statins are mainly cholesterol-lowering drugs (in humans, they specifically lower LDL-cholesterol) with less potent effects on triglyceride metabolism. This makes them less than ideal for cases with hypertriglyceridemia as the main lipid abnormality. Statins have been associated with myopathy, rhabdomyolysis, and hepatotoxicity in humans. In humans, concurrent administration of statins and fibrates (especially gemfibrozil) is not recommended because the latter has been shown to affect the pharmacokinetics of statins, leading to increased risk for toxicity. However, other fibrates (e.g., bezafibrate) appear to be safer and better tolerated than gemfibrozil when combined with statins.

References

1. Xenoulis PG, Steiner JM. Canine hyperlipidaemia. *J Small Anim Pract* 56(10):595-605, 2015.
2. Xenoulis PG, Suchodolski JS, Levinski MD, et al. Investigation of hypertriglyceridemia in healthy miniature schnauzers. *J Vet Intern Med* 21:1224-1230, 2007.
3. Xenoulis PG, Zentek J. Nutritional and medical considerations in hyperlipidemia. In Ettinger SJ, Feldman EC, Côté E (editors). Textbook of Veterinary Internal Medicine 9th edition. In press.
4. Xenoulis PG, Cammarata PJ, Walzem RL, et al. Effect of a low-fat diet on serum triglyceride and cholesterol concentrations and lipoprotein profiles in Miniature Schnauzers with hypertriglyceridemia. *J Vet Intern Med* 34:2605-2616, 2020.
5. De Marco V, Noronha KSM, Casado TC, et al. Therapy of canine hyperlipidemia with bezafibrate. *J Vet Intern Med* 31:717-722, 2017.
6. Miceli DD, Vidal VP, Blatter MFC, et al. Fenofibrate treatment for severe hypertriglyceridemia in dogs. *Dom Anim Endocrinol* 74:106578, 2021.

CHAPTER 13

Hyperkalemia

Daniel K. Langlois
DVM, DACVIM (SAIM)

Pathophysiology

Potassium is one of the most abundant cations in the body and is vital for numerous physiologic processes. The most critical functions of potassium are often considered to be its roles in membrane voltage and the generation of action potentials in cells of the nervous, muscular, and endocrine systems.[1,2] There are approximately 50 mEq of potassium per kg of body weight in dogs, and nearly 98% of these potassium stores are within the intracellular compartment.[3] The large concentration gradient from the intracellular compartment (approximately 130-140 mEq/L) to the extracellular compartment (approximately 4-5 mEq/L) is essential for maintaining the normal membrane resting potential and cell excitability.[1] As such, extracellular potassium is tightly controlled. The kidneys are the major regulator of total body potassium balance (i.e., external potassium balance) through the processes of filtration, reabsorption, and excretion.[1,2,4] Aldosterone is the primary modifier of this renal potassium regulation, where it acts in the distal tubules and collecting ducts to promote the excretion of potassium and the reabsorption of sodium and water. Some aldosterone-mediated excretion of potassium also occurs within the intestinal tract. The major regulators of internal potassium balance are insulin and catecholamines, both of which promote the intracellular sequestration of potassium.[1,2]

Non-artifactual hyperkalemia is generally caused by either decreased elimination, transcellular or trans-compartmental shifts, or increased intake.[1] Disruptions in the normal renal-urinary elimination of potassium are the most common cause of hyperkalemia in dogs. Hypoaldosteronism, kidney injury/disease, and urinary outflow obstruction (urethral or ureteral) are the main diseases resulting in decreased urinary potassium elimination and subsequent hyperkalemia.[2,5,6] A variety of drugs targeting the renin-angiotensin-aldosterone system also have the potential to cause hyperkalemia. Abnormal or inappropriate transcellular shifts can result in hyperkalemia; examples include severe metabolic acidosis and massive tissue breakdown.[5,6] Increased dietary potassium intake seldom causes hyperkalemia unless other homeostatic mechanisms are disrupted, but aggressive intravenous administration of potassium salts can result in hyperkalemia. Finally, some gastrointestinal diseases sporadically cause hyperkalemia, but the mechanisms are not fully characterized (Table 13.1).[5,7]

TABLE 13.1 Differentials for non-artifactual hyperkalemia in dogs.[1-6]

Decreased renal excretion	Trans-compartmental shifts	Miscellaneous causes

■ Hypoaldosteronism
  ■ Primary hypoadrenocorticism
  ■ Hyporeninemic hypoaldosteronism (rare)
  ■ Isolated primary hypoaldosteronism (rare)
  ■ Drug-induced hypoaldosteronism (e.g., heparin; rare)
■ Kidney disease
  ■ Acute kidney injury
  ■ Chronic kidney disease (usually end-stage)
■ Urinary obstruction
■ Bladder rupture
■ Drugs targeting RAAS
  ■ ACE inhibitors
  ■ Aldosterone-receptor antagonists
  ■ Angiotensin receptor blockers
	■ Insulin deficiency and concurrent diabetic ketoacidosis
	■ Pleural and peritoneal effusions
	■ Massive tissue breakdown
	  ■ Rhabdomyolysis
	  ■ Aortic thromboembolism
	  ■ Tumor lysis syndrome
	■ Severe metabolic acidosis (rare)
	■ Severe hypertonicity (rare)
		■ Certain gastrointestinal diseases
		  ■ Intestinal parasitism (trichuriasis)
		  ■ Salmonellosis (rare)
		  ■ Other severe enteropathies (rare)
		■ Excess administration of IV potassium
		■ Increased dietary intake (rare, unless complicated by concurrent decreased excretion)
		■ Liver failure (rare)
		■ Late gestation Greyhounds (rare)

Clinical signs

As described above, hyperkalemia increases the resting membrane potential of cells, resulting in a weakened action potential. The subsequent clinical consequences are a result of these effects on cardiac and skeletal muscle cells.[1,2,4] Mild to moderate hyperkalemia (serum potassium <6.5 mmol/L) seldom results in overt abnormalities. Clinical abnormalities in dogs with mildly increased potassium concentrations can usually be attributed to the underlying disease process (e.g., uremia associated with severe kidney disease) rather than hyperkalemia itself. Clinical signs of hyperkalemia are more likely to occur when increases in potassium concentrations become more severe (e.g., serum potassium >6.5-7.5 mmol/L).[2-4] However, there is not a reliable cutpoint at which clinical signs predictably occur, and some dogs with seemingly severe hyperkalemia experience minimal consequences.[2] Both the severity and acuity in which hyperkalemia develops, in conjunction with myriad other physiologic factors, are thought to influence the occurrence of clinical signs.

Moderate to severe hyperkalemia is a potentially life-threatening problem. Hyperkalemia-induced cardiotoxicity and associated rhythm disturbances are well-described in dogs. ECG abnormalities associated with hyperkalemia include tall and tented T waves, prolonged PR intervals, blunted to absent P waves, widened QRS complexes, sine wave complexes, and finally, ventricular fibrillation.[2,3,6] Bradycardia is also common and should prompt consideration of hyperkalemia in any hypovolemic dog. Clinicians should also be mindful that other electrolyte and acid-base disturbances, such as hypocalcemia, hyponatremia, and acidemia, can exacerbate the cardiotoxic effects of hyperkalemia.[2] The most notable non-cardiac consequence of hyperkalemia is muscle weakness.[1-4] This might be most apparent in the pelvic limbs, although any muscles can be affected, and generalized weakness is common.

Diagnostic approach

Hyperkalemia is generally considered to be a serum potassium concentration >5.0-5.5 mmol/L. It should be noted that serum potassium concentrations are slightly higher than plasma potassium concentrations because a small amount of potassium is released from platelets during clotting. If a plasma sample is utilized for analysis, heparin is preferred over K_3EDTA as an anticoagulant in order to avoid spurious hyperkalemia.[2] Algorithm 13.1 shows the diagnostic approach to hyperkalemia.[1-8]

Algorithm 13.1 Note 1 Artifactual causes of hyperkalemia should be considered and excluded, especially in clinically healthy dogs with minimal biochemical abnormalities. Severe thrombocytosis can cause hyperkalemia in serum specimens because platelets release a small amount of potassium during clotting.[2] This artifact can be avoided in dogs with severe thrombocytosis by measuring potassium in a plasma sample instead of serum. Hemolysis in certain dog breeds with high intraerythrocyte potassium stores (Akitas, Shiba Inus) can also cause hyperkalemia, as can severe leukocytosis in any breed, although the latter is exceedingly rare. Samples obtained from IV catheters in dogs being administered IV potassium supplementation could be contaminated. Finally, severe hyperlipidemia or hyperproteinemia could interfere with some methods of potassium measurement, but assays using ion-specific electrode measurements should not be affected.[2,4]

Algorithm 13.1 Note 2 A thorough history is essential in recognizing potential iatrogenic or drug-induced causes of hyperkalemia. The signalment and history might also heighten suspicion for certain disease processes such as hypoadrenocorticism or even trichuriasis. The history may also point the clinician toward a tumor lysis syndrome.

Algorithm 13.1 Note 3 There are many medications that can alter potassium homeostasis, most of which target the renin-angiotensin-aldosterone system (RAAS). This includes angiotensin-converting enzyme inhibitors (ACEi), aldosterone receptor antagonists, and angiotensin receptor blockers.[1,2] Severe hyperkalemia is uncommon with these drugs, and dose modifications are usually all that is needed to resolve any drug-associated hyperkalemia. Various other medications have sporadically been shown to alter potassium concentrations, and these include heparin, beta-blockers, and cardiac glycosides.

Algorithm 13.1 Note 4 A detailed physical exam can aid in identifying pleural or peritoneal effusions, which are known causes of hyperkalemia. Furthermore, the identification of bradycardia in sick or hypovolemic animals should heighten concern for the possibility of hyperkalemia and similarly should prompt ECG evaluation.

Algorithm 13.1 Note 5 A minimum database consisting of a CBC, chemistry profile, and urinalysis is indicated in all dogs with suspected or confirmed hyperkalemia. In fact, the results of these routine tests often provide strong clinical support for a tentative diagnosis. A fecal flotation should also be considered a part of the initial testing to further evaluate for parasitism in a dog with diarrhea.

Algorithm 13.1 Note 6 Primary glucocorticoid- and mineralocorticoid-deficient hypoadrenocorticism is a differential diagnosis for almost all hyperkalemic dogs, especially those with concurrent hyponatremia or even low-normal sodium. Distinguishing between hypoadrenocorticism and kidney disease can be challenging in dogs with electrolyte disturbances and azotemia, but most dogs with hypoadrenocorticism will have other hematologic and biochemical indicators of cortisol deficiency. Fortunately, initial stabilization measures are similar for both conditions, pending the results of ACTH stimulation testing.

Algorithm 13.1 Note 7 Most dogs with mild to moderate hyperkalemia require no treatment beyond intravenous fluid therapy and management of the underlying disease process. More targeted treatment of hyperkalemia is typically reserved for those dogs with severe hyperkalemia and concurrent ECG abnormalities.

Calcium gluconate alters the resting cell membrane potential but does not affect plasma potassium concentrations. These cardioprotective effects only last for 20-30 minutes, and calcium administration is not without possible adverse arrhythmogenic effects. As such, this therapy should be reserved for those dogs with truly life-threatening hyperkalemia, and ECG monitoring is essential.

Dextrose, as well as the coadministration of dextrose and insulin, are reasonable choices for severe hyperkalemia that requires treatment beyond initial IV fluid therapy. However, it is essential that blood glucose concentrations are carefully monitored when insulin is used, especially in those dogs with suspected hypoadrenocorticism.[2,4,6] Beta-agonists, such as albuterol, have not been studied in detail, but they are likely a benign one-time treatment option. Sodium bicarbonate should be used with extreme caution due to concerns with hyperosmolarity or paradoxical cerebrospinal fluid acidosis.[6] The author considers this a last resort.

ALGORITHM 13.1

Approach to the patient with hyperkalemia.

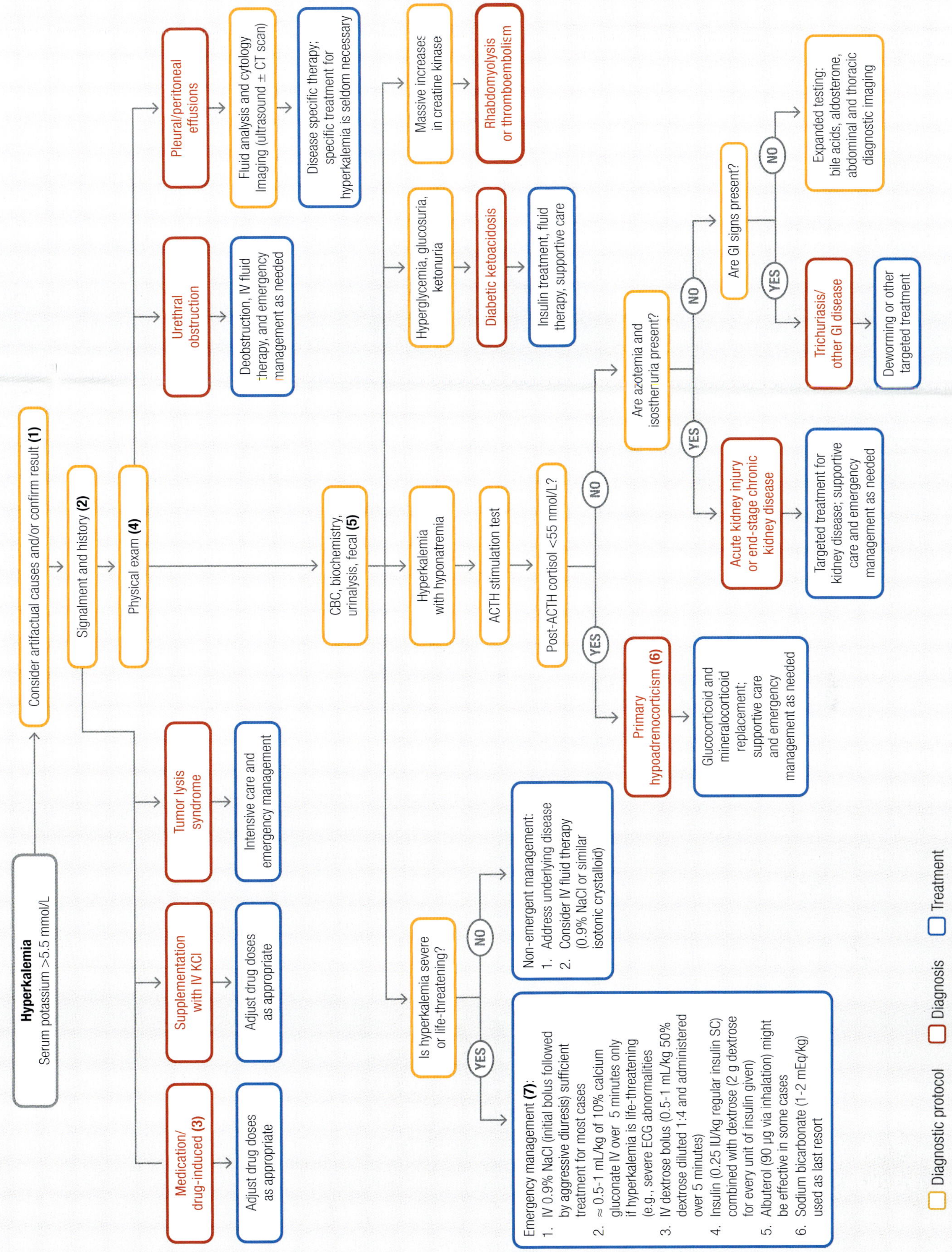

References

1. Kettritz R, Loffing J. Potassium homeostasis: physiology and pharmacology in a clinical context. *Pharmacol Ther* 249:108489, 2023.
2. Willard MD. Disorders of potassium homeostasis. *Vet Clin North Am Small Anim Pract* 19:241-263, 1989.
3. Feldman EC, Church DB. Electrolyte disorders: potassium (hyper/hypokalemia). In Ettinger SJ, Feldman EC (editors). Textbook of Veterinary Internal Medicine 7th edition. St. Louis, Saunders Elsevier, 2010, pp. 303-307.
4. DiBartola SP, de Morais HA. Disorders of potassium: hypokalemia and hyperkalemia. In DiBartola SP (editor). Fluid, Electrolyte, and Acid-Base Disorders in Small Animal Practice 3rd edition. St. Louis, Saunders Elsevier, 2006, pp. 91-121.
5. Kogika MM, de Morais HA. A quick reference on hyperkalemia. *Vet Clin North Am Small Anim Pract* 47:229-234, 2017.
6. Schaer M. Therapeutic approach to electrolyte emergencies. *Vet Clin North Am Small Anim Pract* 38:513-533, 2008.
7. Graves TK, Schall WD, Refsal K, Nachreiner RF. Basal and ACTH-stimulated plasma aldosterone concentrations are normal or increased in dogs with trichuriasis-associated pseudohypoadrenocorticism. *J Vet Intern Med* 8:287-289, 1994.
8. Ogrodny A, Jaffey JA, Kreisler R, et al. Effect of inhaled albuterol on whole blood potassium concentration in dogs. *J Vet Intern Med* 36:2002-2008, 2022.
9. Manual of Canine and Feline Endocrinology 5th edition. British Small Animal Veterinary Association, 2023, pp. 97-107.
10. Feldman EC, Hoar B, Pollard R, et al. Pretreatment clinical and laboratory findings in dogs with primary hyperparathyroidism: 210 cases (1987-2004). *J Am Vet Med Assoc* 227(5):756-761, 2005.
11. Arenas C. Hypercalcemia. In Fracassi F (editor). Diagnostic and Therapeutic Algorithms in Internal Medicine for Dogs and Cats. Milan, Edra, 2022, pp. 137-140.
12. Bailey DB. Paraneoplastic syndromes. In Vail DM, H.Thamm D, Liptak JM (editors). Withrow & MacEwen's Small Animal Clinical Oncology. Missouri, Elsevier, 2020, pp. 98-112.
13. Lee JA. Chemical toxicoses. In Ettinger SJ, Feldman EC, Côté E (editors). Textbook of Veterinary Internal Medicine. Missouri, Elsevier, 2017, pp. 1660-1670.
14. Galvao JB, Schenck P, Chew D. A quick reference on hypercalcemia. *Vet Clin North Am Small Anim Pract* 47:241-248, 2017.
15. Coady M, Fletcher DJ, Goggs R. Severity of ionized hypercalcemia and hypocalcemia is associated with etiology in dogs and cats. *Front Vet Sci* 6:276, 2019.

CHAPTER 14

Hypokalemia

Ghita Benchekroun
DVM, DECVIM-CA
(Internal medicine), PhD

Pathophysiology

Potassium is the major intracellular cation: intracellular stores account for 90 to 95% of the entire bodily potassium reservoir. Potassium plays a pivotal role in preserving cell volume and growth within the cellular milieu, whereas extracellular potassium undergoes tight regulation. Any fluctuation in potassium concentration, whether an increase or decrease, can potentially lead to life-threatening repercussions. Hypokalemia is defined by serum potassium below 3.5 mmol/L, but this threshold may vary depending on the sample used and the analyzer. Potassium concentration in plasma is lower than in serum because potassium is released from platelets during the clotting process. Ion-selective electrode methods are recommended to avoid artifactual hypokalemia.

Sodium, potassium-adenosine triphosphatase (Na^+, K^+-ATPase) has a central role in maintaining a normal balance between intracellular and extracellular fluid: this enzyme pumps sodium out and potassium into the cell. The most important function of intracellular potassium is to maintain a normal resting cell membrane potential. Thus, hypokalemia hyperpolarizes the cell, increasing the resting potential and decreasing membrane excitability. These effects are mostly noticed in skeletal and cardiac muscles, leading to cardiovascular and neuromuscular signs.[1]

Oral intake of potassium is essential to maintain total potassium status. Potassium is absorbed from the gastrointestinal tract and excreted mainly by the kidneys and the colon to a lesser extent. Aldosterone plays a pivotal role in potassium regulation as it is necessary for efficient potassium excretion, and it can enhance this process in the renal distal convoluted tubule and collecting ducts. Insulin and catecholamines increase potassium uptake by muscle and liver cells. Finally, acute changes in pH will shift K^+ between fluid compartments: alkalemia may result in hypokalemia, while acidemia may cause hyperkalemia.[2]

A recent study has identified that in dogs presented in an emergency department, hypokalemia, even mild, was associated with a higher mortality rate compared to dogs with normokalemia.[10] Further studies are required to know if hypokalemia has a direct effect on mortality and if prompt control of hypokalemia improves the outcome.

Hypokalemia can result from several mechanisms (Table 14.1), including gastrointestinal losses, renal losses, and transcellular shifting. Unlike cats, dogs' decreased oral intake does not typically lead to profound hypokalemia. However, prolonged anorexia may contribute to electrolyte imbalances.

TABLE 14.1 Etiology of hypokalemia in dogs.

Hypokalemia	
Increased loss	**Renal** ■ Chronic kidney disease ■ Distal renal tubular acidosis ■ Hyperaldosteronism (rare in dogs) ■ Drug-induced: iatrogenic (furosemide, thiazide diuretics, amphotericin B, mineralocorticoids) ■ Postobstructive diuresis (rare in dogs) ■ Diabetic ketoacidosis ■ Hyperadrenocorticism ■ Renal acidifying diet **Intestinal** ■ Vomiting ■ Diarrhea
Decreased intake	■ Anorexia ■ Inadequate fluid therapy (fluid free potassium)
Intracellular shift	■ Metabolic alkalosis ■ Treatement of proximal renal tubular acidosis with bicarbonate ■ Perfusion fluids containing glucose ■ Total parenteral nutrition ■ Pheochromocytoma ■ Iatrogenic (salbutamol, insulin)

Renal losses

Kidney losses can occur in intrinsic renal disease, leading to direct impairment of potassium tubular reabsorption. Kaliuresis can also increase with severe polyuria/polydipsia or as a result of iatrogenic factors.

Hypokalemia can be significant in dogs with renal tubular acidosis (potassium reabsorption impairment). Renal tubular acidosis can be congenital or acquired following many diseases such as leptospirosis, copper storage disease, jerky treats administration, ethylene glycol toxicosis, gentamicin treatment, or acute pancreatitis.[3,4]

Another cause of potassium loss in urine is primary hyperaldosteronism, where aldosterone is secreted autonomously. This disease seems very rare in dogs, with less than five dogs reported in the veterinary literature.[5] Finally, hypokalemia may occur in dogs with severe hypercortisolism due to the mineralocorticoid effect of glucocorticoids.[6]

Gastrointestinal losses

Gastrointestinal disease may cause potassium loss. Therefore, it is advisable to check for hypokalemia in any dog that presents with symptoms such as diarrhea or vomiting. Hypokalemia may occur with chronic or acute gastrointestinal disease.

Transcellular shifts

Another mechanism that can potentially lead to hypokalemia is potassium translocation from extracellular fluid to intracellular fluid. In patients with ketoacidosis, hypokalemia is usually multifactorial, with digestive and urinary loss, decreased intake, and potassium translocation in response to insulin administration or sodium bicarbonate. In these cases, it is critical to monitor potassium concentration closely.

Iatrogenic causes

Hypokalemia can also be iatrogenic and should be rechecked in dogs receiving aggressive, potassium-depleted fluid therapy. Diuretic treatment can also lead to hypokalemia by inhibition of the renal tubular electrolyte pumps. Dogs with hypoadrenocorticism that receive mineralocorticoid supplementation may develop hypokalemia, but it is usually mild and subclinical.

Clinical signs

The severity of clinical signs is directly correlated with potassium concentration and varies depending on the acuteness of potassium depletion. It is important to bear in mind that kalemia does not represent the total body store of potassium, and a dog may show only slight hypokalemia despite being severely depleted at the whole-body level.

Common clinical signs of hypokalemia include anorexia, muscle weakness (focal or generalized), polyuria, and impaired urinary concentrating capacity. In cases of severe hypokalemia, flaccid ventroflexion of the neck can be present (although it is more characteristic of hypokalemia in cats). Low potassium concentration may also cause ventricular or supraventricular tachyarrhythmias. Hypokalemia should be suspected in any dogs presenting cardiovascular (arrhythmia) or neuromuscular signs (weakness). Severe hypokalemia has been associated with rhabdomyolysis and respiratory muscle paralysis.[7]

Diagnostic approach

The diagnostic approach to hypokalemia is displayed in Algorithm 14.1.

Algorithm 14.1 Note 1 When hypokalemia is identified, it may be useful to store urine and blood samples for further investigation as needed before K^+ supplementation.

Algorithm 14.1 Note 2 In the presence of severe hypokalemia, it is advisable to perform an electrocardiogram (ECG) to assess arrhythmias linked to low potassium levels and to monitor their improvement following potassium supplementation.

Algorithm 14.1 Note 3 History of previous fluid therapy, parenteral nutrition, peritoneal dialysis, and drug administration such as loop diuretics, thiazide diuretics, amphotericin B, penicillin, insulin, or catecholamine should be reviewed because they all cause hypokalemia. Salbutamol toxicosis by oral ingestion of a salbutamol inhaler may cause profound hypokalemia with associated clinical signs.[8]

Algorithm 14.1 Note 4 If no drug administration or toxicosis is reported in the history, CBC, biochemistry, blood gas analysis, systolic blood pressure measurement, and urinalysis are required.

The fractional urinary excretion of potassium (FE_K) can be calculated and is used to help localize the source of potassium loss, whether renal or not. It is calculated as:

$$FE_K\ (\%) = UK \times SCr\ /\ SK \times UCr \times 100,\ \text{where:}$$

UK = urine concentration of potassium; UCr = urine concentration of creatinine; SK = serum concentration of potassium; SCr = serum concentration of creatinine.[1]

Algorithm 14.1 Note 5 The clinical history and initial workup often indicate the likely cause of hypokalemia: vomiting and diarrhea are evocative of gastrointestinal loss; azotemia with glucosuria is evocative of renal tubular acidosis and urinary loss, or insulin treatment in a dog with ketoacidosis is evocative of potassium translocation.

Algorithm 14.1 Note 6 If FE_K is less than 4 to 6%, gastrointestinal loss is likely in dogs with gastrointestinal signs such as vomiting or diarrhea. Hypokalemia is reported in dogs with gastric foreign bodies in addition to metabolic alkalosis, hyponatremia, and hypochloremia, but also dogs with acute gastroenteritis (enteric parvovirosis or acute hemorrhagic diarrhea syndrome).

Algorithm 14.1 Note 7 If FE_K is above 4 to 6%, a renal source of loss is suspected. Differentials include endocrine diseases, tubular acidosis, or diabetic ketoacidosis.

Algorithm 14.1 Note 8 Hyperchloremic metabolic acidosis is suggestive of renal tubular acidosis. In distal renal tubular acidosis, hypokalemia is reported at diagnosis, while in proximal renal tubular acidosis, hypokalemia tends to appear after sodium bicarbonate therapy. Several causes of renal tubular acidosis are reported, and they may be congenital or acquired. Metabolic acidosis with a high anion gap and hyperglycemia is suggestive of ketoacidosis. Hypokalemia may worsen after treatment initiation, and close monitoring is required in these cases.[9] In chronic kidney disease, hypokalemia is uncommon.

Algorithm 14.1 Note 9 In cases with systemic hypertension, and eventually with an adrenal mass, primary hyperaldosteronism should be suspected (Video 14.1). The final diagnosis requires measuring serum aldosterone concentration. Another possibility is hyperadrenocorticism or any disease-causing polyuria.

ALGORITHM 14.1

Diagnostic algorithm for hypokalemia.

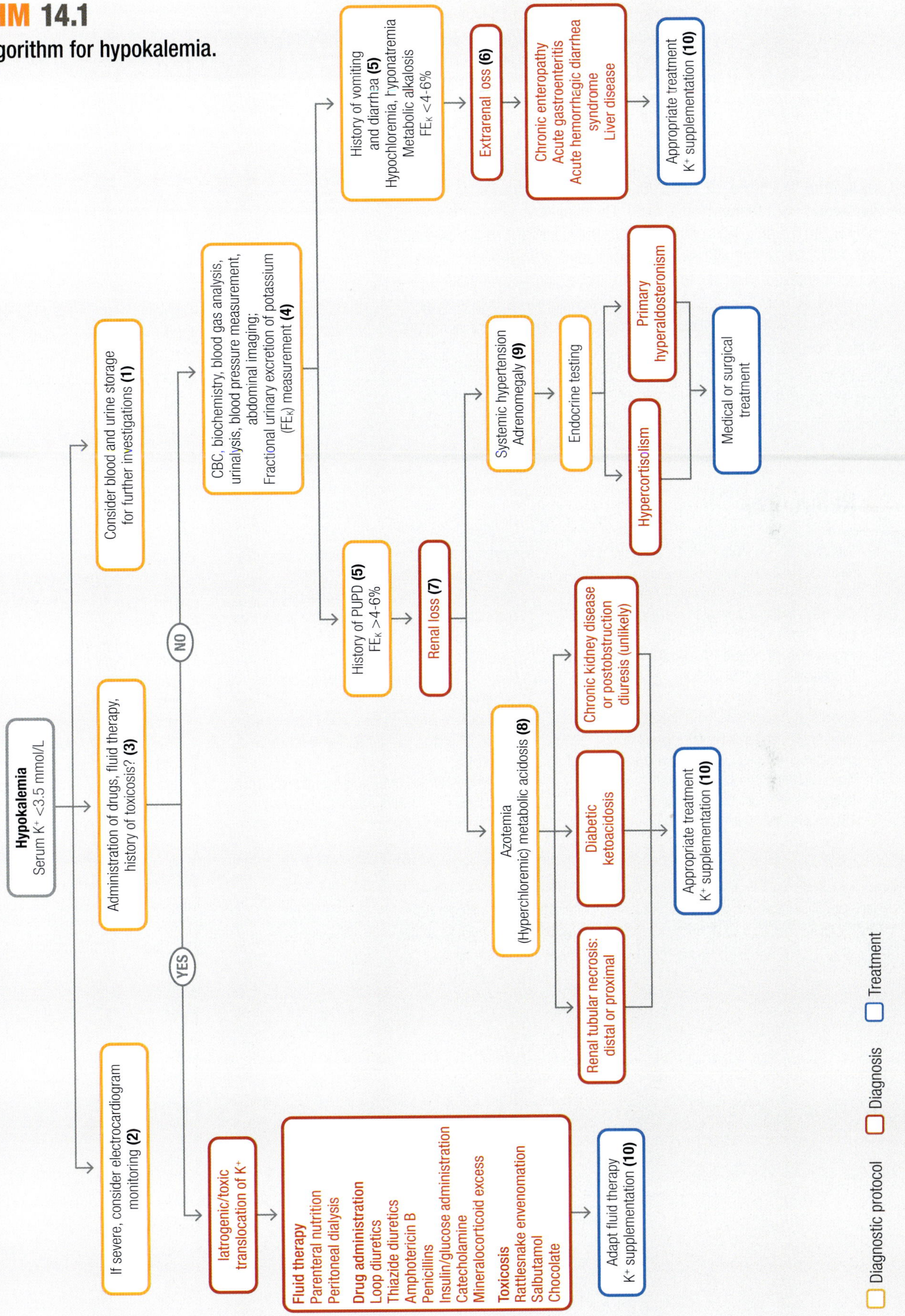

Video 14.1

Cervical ventroflexion caused by a hypokalemic polymyopathy in a dog with primary hyperaldosteronism. Cervical ventroflexion is a specific sign of hypokalemia. Its recognition in the clinical examination can direct the diagnostic approach. (Courtesy of Dr. Lorenzo Golini from the University of Zurich).

Algorithm 14.1 Note 10 Potassium is usually supplemented through intravenous fluid therapy (Table 14.2). The supplementation rate should not exceed 0.5 mEq/kg/h, which dictates the maximal fluid rate depending on the amount of potassium chloride added to the fluid. Sometimes, supplementation may fail to normalize potassium concentration, but it should resolve the clinical signs of hypokalemia. If hypokalemia is refractory to supplementation, hypomagnesemia should be investigated and, if needed, corrected.

TABLE 14.2 Degree of hypokalemia and fluid correction required.

Serum K^+ (mmol/L)	Potassium chloride (mEq) in 1L of 0.9% saline	Maximal fluid rate (ml/kg/h)
<2	80	7
2-2.4	60	9
2.5-2.9	40	12
3-3.4	28	18
3.5-5	20	25

References

1. DiBartola SB, De Morais HA. Disorders of potassium: hypokalemia and hyperkalemia. In DiBartola SB (editor). Fluid, Electrolyte, and Acid-Base Disorders in Small Animal Practice 4th edition. St Louis, Elsevier, 2021, pp. 92-119.
2. Kogika MM, de Morais HA. A quick reference on hypokalemia. *Vet Clin North Am Small Anim Pract* 47(2):229-234, 2017.
3. Knöpfler S, Mayer-Scholl A, Luge E, et al. Evaluation of clinical, laboratory, imaging findings and outcome in 99 dogs with leptospirosis. *J Small Anim Pract* 58(10):582-588, 2017.
4. Nybroe S, Bjørnvad CR, Hansen CFH, Andersen TSL, Kieler IN. Outcome of acquired Fanconi syndrome associated with ingestion of jerky treats in 30 dogs. *Animals* 12(22):1-11, 2022.
5. Rijnberk A, Kooistra HS, Van Vonderen IK, et al. Aldosteronoma in a dog with polyuria as the leading symptom. *Domest Anim Endocrinol* 20(3):227-240, 2001.
6. Behrend EN. Canine hyperadrenocorticism. In Feldman EC, Nelson RW, Reusch CE, Scott-Moncrieff JCR (editors). Canine and Feline Endocrinology 4th edition. St. Louis, Elsevier, 2015, pp. 377-451.
7. Granfone M, Walker JM. Acute nontraumatic rhabdomyolysis in a Greyhound after albuterol toxicosis. *J Vet Emerg Crit Care* 31(6):818-822, 2021.
8. Crouchley J, Bates N. Retrospective evaluation of acute salbutamol (albuterol) exposure in dogs: 501 cases. *J Vet Emerg Crit Care* 32(4):500-506, 2022.
9. Gal A, Odunayo A. Diabetes ketoacidosis and hyperosmolar hyperglycemic syndrome in companion animals. *Vet Clin North Am Small Anim Pract* 53(3):531-550, 2023.
10. Hoehne SN, Hopper K, Epstein SE. Retrospective evaluation of the severity of and prognosis associated with potassium abnormalities in dogs and cats presenting to an emergency room (January 2014–August 2015): 2441 cases. *J Vet Emerg Crit Care* 29(6):653-661, 2019.

CHAPTER 15

Hypernatremia

Chiara Valtolina
DVM, PhD, DECVECC, DACVECC

Pathophysiology

Hypernatremia is defined as a serum sodium concentration ([Na^+]) above 150 mmol/L.

Sodium is the most abundant extracellular fluid (ECF) electrolyte and the primary determinant of ECF osmolality and volume. Serum [Na^+] reflects the amount of Na^+ relative to the volume of water in the body and is not an estimation of total body Na^+ content. In fact, abnormalities in water balance are the most common cause of changes in serum [Na^+] in dogs.[1,2,3]

Serum [Na^+] and plasma osmolality are maintained within a strict range by the interplay of different mechanisms: the effect of antidiuretic hormone (ADH or vasopressin) released by the posterior pituitary, able to increase or decrease water excretion via the kidney and the thirst mechanism. Another important factor that stimulates the release of ADH and the thirst mechanism, independently from plasma osmolarity, is the decrease in the effective circulating volume in shock situations. The alteration of the effective circulating volume can also affect the sodium excretion rate via the kidney via the effect of the hormones aldosterone, angiotensin II, and natriuretic peptides.[1,2,3]

Hypernatremia is a common electrolyte disorder in critical care and develops more commonly secondary to hypotonic fluid losses (water loss in excess of Na^+) or excessive Na^+ gain. Intense thirst protects against hypernatremia unless animals cannot replace their water loss with intake for different reasons (i.e., altered mental state, water deprivation).[1,2] In dogs presented to a university hospital, the development of hypernatremia was associated with gastrointestinal fluid loss (39.3%), followed by central diabetes insipidus (CDI, 23.2%) and fever or hyperthermia (23.2%). Almost half of the patients developed hypernatremia when hospitalized, and the magnitude of hypernatremia was linearly associated with a higher case fatality rate.[4]

Numerous classifications of hypernatremia exist; the one that reflects mostly the pathophysiological changes is the classification based on volume status[2,3] (Table 15.1). Hypernatremic patients can be normovolemic when hypernatremia is secondary to free water losses in the case of central or nephrogenic diabetes insipidus, free water loss via the expirium due to excessive panting (stress, fever/hyperthermia, and pain), or it can be seen in patients suffering from hypodipsia. Hypernatremic dogs can present with signs of hypovolemia if the fluid lost is hypotonic, secondary to vomiting and diarrhea, inability of the kidneys to concentrate urine (chronic kidney disease [CKD], non-oliguric acute kidney disease and postobstructive diuresis). Hypotonic fluid losses can be seen with other polyuric conditions like diabetes mellitus and diabetes ketoacidosis and the administration of chemical or osmotic diuretics. Signs of hypervolemia (although not common) can be seen in dogs with salt intoxication, bicarbonate, and hypertonic saline administration.

TABLE 15.1 Causes of hypernatremia in dogs classified based on volume status.

Fluid loss		Solute gain
Normovolemia (free water loss)	**Hypovolemia (hypotonic fluid loss)**	**Hypervolemia**
■ Diabetes insipidus ▪ Central (neurogenic) ▪ Congenital/acquired nephrogenic ■ Fever ■ Decreased access to water ■ Hyperventilation ■ Hypodipsia (uncommon)	■ Renal losses ▪ Chronic kidney disease ▪ Non-oliguric acute renal failure ■ Gastrointestinal losses ■ Third space losses ■ Burns ■ Diuresis (osmotic or chemical) ▪ Diabetes mellitus ▪ Diabetic ketoacidosis ▪ Hyperosmolar nonketotic syndrome ▪ Mannitol infusion ▪ Furosemide ▪ Postobstructive diuresis	■ Salt intoxication ▪ Iatrogenic ▪ Sea water ingestion ■ Hypertonic saline infusion ■ Sodium bicarbonate infusion ■ Primary hyperaldosteronism ■ Hypercortisolism

Modified from Guillaumin J, and DiBartola.[5]

Clinical signs

In dogs, clinical signs of hypernatremia are often observed when the serum [Na^+] concentration exceeds 170 mmol/L, although their severity depends more on the rapidity of the Na^+ changes and development of hypernatremia than on the value of $[Na^+]$ itself.[1,2,3] Clinical signs of hypernatremia are often nonspecific: lethargy, altered mental state, vomiting, and weakness are commonly reported findings. If hypernatremia develops acutely, these signs can quickly progress to tremors, altered mental state, seizure, coma, and death due to the movement of water out of the brain cells, which might result in focal intracerebral and subarachnoid hemorrhages.

In chronic hypernatremia, patients can be fairly asymptomatic due to the brain's osmotic adaptation to the increase in $[Na^+]$. Within hours from the development of hypernatremia, the brain will begin to adapt to the new hyperosmolar state with an increased uptake of Na^+ and potassium in the brain cells and the production of intracellular osmolytes that facilitate the increase in brain cell osmolality. The increased brain osmolarity will result in water movement back into the brain and normalization of brain volume.[1,2,3]

It is also important to remember that severe neurological clinical signs might develop if chronic hypernatremia is corrected too rapidly, causing the development of brain edema (Video 15.1).

Diagnostic approach

Algorithm 15.1 shows the approach to the hypernatremic patient. Normal $[Na^+]$ ranges from 140 mEq/L to 150 mEq/L for dogs.

The approach to a patient with hypernatremia involves taking a detailed anamnesis from the caretakers and performing an in-depth physical examination. The anamnesis should focus on current medical therapy, water intake over the last days and urinary production, gastrointestinal fluid losses (vomiting and diarrhea), and possible exposure to salt or play dough. Physical examination should detect changes in the cardiovascular status of the patient and evaluate the patient's hydration state. A complete electrolytes panel, urea and creatinine, total protein and albumin, and urine sample collection should be performed in every patient with hypernatremia. Other blood work depends on the patient's suspected underlying condition and clinical condition. Besides correcting the hypernatremia, addressing the underlying condition is paramount.

Algorithm 15.1 Note 1 Hypoproteinemia and/or hypolipidemia can cause spurious hypernatremia if serum $[Na^+]$ is measured using an indirect ion-selective electrode methodology.

Algorithm 15.1 Note 2 Hypoperfusion is recognized in dogs with tachycardia, weak peripheral pulse, pale mucous membranes, and prolonged capillary refill time (CRT).

Video 15.1

Salt intoxication in a dog. Dog with acute iatrogenic salt intoxication after the owners administered too much salt at home to induce emesis. At presentation, $[Na^+]$ was 199.7 mmol/L and the dog had severe metabolic acidosis. The dog was showing whole body and head tremors and decreased mental state signs of hypoperfusion hemorrhagic diarrhea. Video courtesy of Dr. Marco Bertoli.

Algorithm 15.1 Note 3 If signs of hypoperfusion are present, administer (based on the severity of the hypoperfusion) smaller boluses of crystalloid fluid (10-20 mL/kg in 10-20 minutes). The fluid used should have a sodium concentration similar to that of the patient (within 10 mmol/L of the patient's $[Na^+]$). Often, hypertonic saline added to an isotonic fluid needs to be used to prepare such solution. Repeat bolus until the patient is cardiovascular stable.[2,3] Monitor serum $[Na^+]$ every 20 minutes after the bolus, then follow algorithm notes 4 or 5.

Algorithm 15.1 Note 4 If the onset of the hypernatremia is acute and there are neurological signs present, it is recommended to decrease the patients' $[Na^+]$ rapidly at the rate of 2 mEq/L/h for 2-3 hours until the clinical signs subdue.[2,3] Then follow algorithm note 5.

To calculate how much water to administer to the patient to decrease serum $[Na^+]$, numerous (more or less complicated) formulas exist to calculate free water deficit. The one mostly used is:

$$\text{Free water deficit (L)} = ([\text{current } [Na^+] / [\text{normal } [Na^+]] - 1) \times 0.6 \times \text{BW (body weight in kg)}.$$

Where current $[Na^+]$ is the patient's actual $[Na^+]$ and normal $[Na^+]$ is 145 mmol/L.

The author and other clinicians use the rule of thumb that 3.7 mL/kg/h of free water (i.e., dextrose 5%) will decrease the serum $[Na^+]$ by 1 mEq/L/h.[2,3]

Following the above-mentioned rule, in acute situations and severe clinical signs, a dextrose 5% solution is used at a rate of 7 mL/kg/h for 2-3 hours until the clinical signs subdue.[2,3]

$[Na^+]$ should be checked initially every hour, then every 2-4 hours.

Algorithm 15.1 Note 5 If the onset of hypernatremia is chronic (>48h) but clinical signs are present, it is recommended to decrease the patients' sodium rapidly at the rate of 2 mEq/L for the first 2-3 hours the decrease in $[Na^+]$ should not exceed 1 mEq/L/h. As in practice, the decrease in $[Na^+]$ is less predictable, limiting the decrease in $[Na^+]$ to a total of 10 mEq/L during the first 24h and 18 mEq/L for the first 48h.[2,3]

Algorithm 15.1 Note 6 If the onset of hypernatremia is chronic (>48h) and no clinical signs are present, the decrease in $[Na^+]$ should not exceed 0.5 mEq/L/h to avoid any rapid decrease in plasma osmolarity compared to the ICF and the development of brain edema. As in practice, the decrease in $[Na^+]$ is less predictable; limit the decrease in $[Na^+]$ to a total of 10 mEq/L during the first 24h and 18 mEq/L for the first 48h.[2,3]

Algorithm 15.1 Note 7 Hypodipsia is uncommon and has been reported to be congenital in Miniature Schnauzers. In other dog breeds, hypodipsic hypernatremia has been associated with central nervous system disease or malformation.

Algorithm 15.1 Note 8 In CDI, the lack of production or release of the ADH by the hypothalamus and posterior pituitary, respectively, causes the loss of free water via the urine, which becomes hyposthenuric. Nephrogenic diabetes insipidus (NDI) refers to the inability of the kidney to concentrate the urine secondary to structural or functional renal abnormalities.

Algorithm 15.1 Note 9 The treatment of CDI is the administration of the synthetic hormone desmopressin acetate (DDAVP); the intranasal solution can be administered in the conjunctival sac alternating left and

ALGORITHM 15.1

Diagnostic approach to hypernatremia.

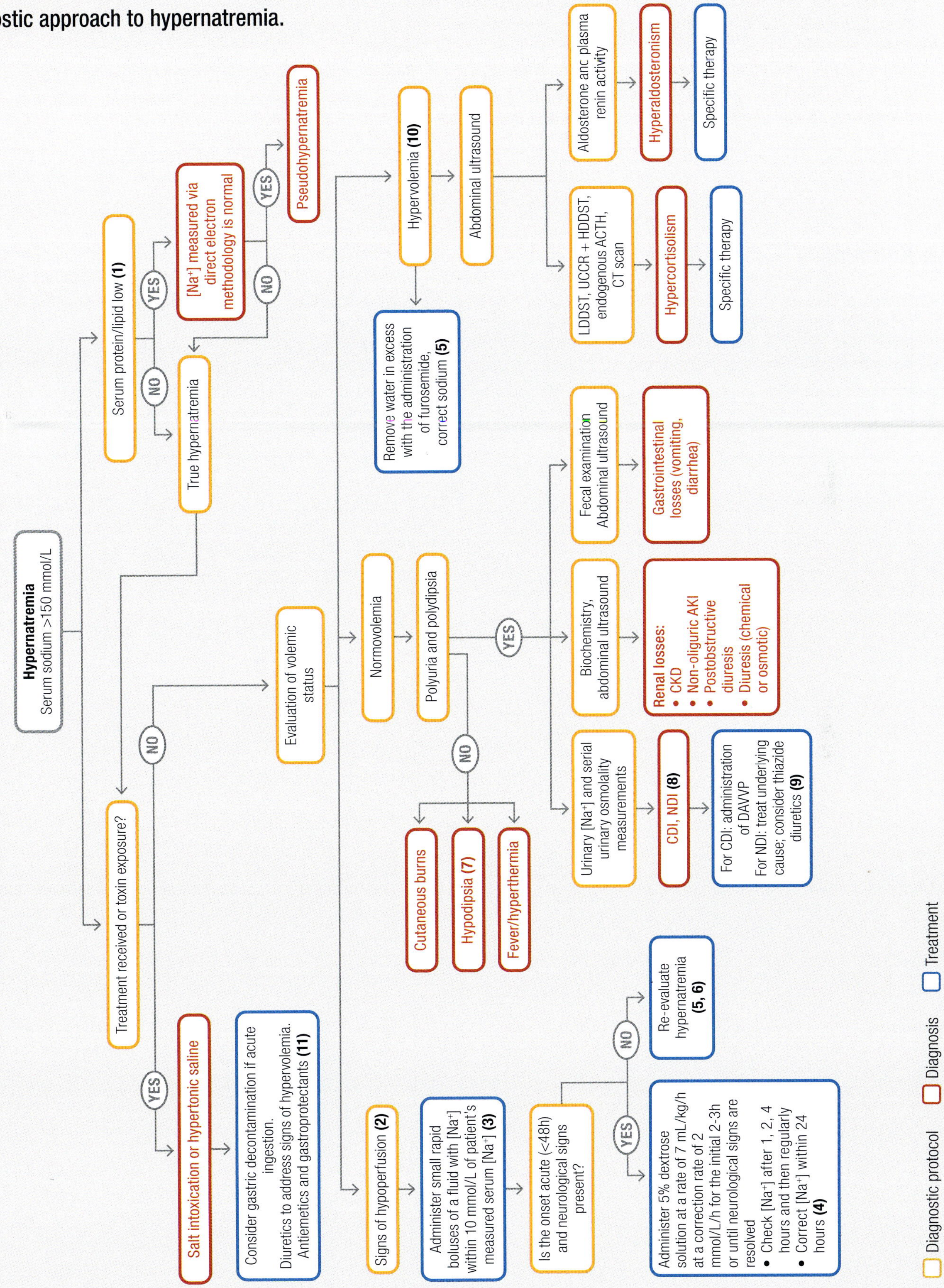

right eye (1 drop bid or tid), or desmopressin tablets can be given orally (0.1 mg bid or tid). Patients with NDI do not often respond to DDAVP. Thiazide diuretics or a sodium-restricted diet have been advocated for the treatment of NDI.

Algorithm 15.1 Note 10 Signs of hypervolemia can often be subtle: pleural effusion, peripheral and organ edema, and lung edema.

Algorithm 15.1 Note 11 If hypernatremia is secondary to excessive isotonic fluid administration in a patient that is not drinking, consider the use of a hypotonic solution (0.45% NaCl + 2.5% glucose) as maintenance fluid.

References

1. DiBartola S. Disorders of sodium and water: hypernatremia and hyponatremia. In DiBartola SP (editor). Fluid, Electrolyte, and Acid-base Disorders in Small Animal Practice. St Louis, Saunders Elsevier, 2012, pp. 45-79.
2. Ueda and Hopper K. Sodium and water balance. In Drobatz K.J., Hopper K. Rozanski E, Silverstein D (editors). Textbook of Small Animal Emergency. John Wiley & Sons, 2019, pp. 690-699.
3. Guillaumin J, DiBartola S. Disorders of sodium and water homeostasis. *Vet Clin North Am Small Anim Pract* 47:293-312, 2017.
4. Ueda Y, Hopper K, Epstein SE. Incidence, severity and prognosis associated with hypernatremia in dogs and cats. *J Vet Intern Med* 29:794-800, 2015.
5. Guillaumin J, DiBartola S. A quick reference to hypernatremia. *Vet Clin North Am Small Anim Pract* 47:209-212, 2017.

CHAPTER 16

Hyponatremia

Chiara Valtolina
DVM, PhD, DACVECC, DECVECC

Pathophysiology

Hyponatremia is defined as a serum sodium concentration ([Na+]) below 135 mmol/L.

Sodium is the most abundant extracellular fluid (ECF) electrolyte and the primary determinant of the ECF osmolality and volume. Serum [Na+] reflects the amount of sodium relative to the volume of water in the body and is not an estimation of total body sodium content. In fact, abnormalities in water balance are the most common causes in dogs for changes in serum [Na+].[1,2,3]

Serum [Na+] and plasma osmolality are maintained within a strict range by the interplay of different mechanisms: the effect of antidiuretic hormone (ADH or vasopressin) released by the posterior pituitary, able to increase water retention via the kidney and the thirst mechanism. Another important factor that stimulates the release of ADH and the thirst mechanism independently from plasma osmolarity is the decrease in the effective circulating volume (ECV) in shock situations. In the latter condition, adequate ECF volume maintenance is prioritized over normal osmolality maintenance, causing the release of ADH and free water retention. The alteration of the EVC can also affect the sodium excretion rate via the kidney via the effect of the hormones aldosterone, angiotensin II, and natriuretic peptides.[1,2,3]

Hyponatremia is a very common disturbance in small animal patients. In dogs presented to a university hospital, the most common cause of hyponatremia was gastrointestinal fluid loss (55.8%), followed by third-space fluid loss (21.7%) and fluid shift from intracellular fluid (ICF) to ECF because of moderate to severe hyperglycemia (13.4%).[4] This study also demonstrated a significant association of hyponatremia with non-survival and that the severity of hyponatremia was linearly associated with higher case fatality rates.[4]

Hyponatremic patients may have decreased, increased, or normal total body sodium content. The cause of hyponatremia can be further divided into three categories based on plasma osmolality and volume status. Most patients are in the hypovolemic and hypo-osmolar categories (Table 17.1).[1,2,3,5]

Clinical signs

Clinical signs of hyponatremia range from asymptomatic to severe neurological signs. The severity of hyponatremia (usually [Na+] <120 mmol/L) and, even more critical, the rapidity in which the hyponatremia develops or is corrected determine the severity of clinical signs.[1,2,3,5]

The majority of clinical signs associated with hyponatremia are nonspecific, like nausea, vomiting, lethargy, and disorientation. If hyponatremia develops acutely, neurological signs will be present. They may involve focal and diffuse neurological deficits and seizures and become more severe, like coma and death. The severity of clinical signs depends on the ability of the brain to adapt to the changes of [Na+] and the new plasma osmolarity; with acute and rapid changes, the brain has no time to adapt, and it will suffer from cell swelling and brain edema causing increase intracranial pressure, brain herniation, and

TABLE 16.1 Causes of hyponatremia in dogs according to the pathophysiological classification based on plasma osmolarity and volume status.

Hypo-osmolar			Normo-osmolar	Hyperosmolar
Normovolemic	**Hypovolemic**	**Hypervolemic**		
■ Primary/psychogenic polydipsia ■ Syndrome of inappropriate ADH release (SIAD) ■ Antidiuretic drugs ■ Myxedema coma ■ Hypotonic fluid infusion	■ Shock ■ Gastrointestinal losses ■ Third space losses ■ Cutaneous losses ■ Hypoadrenocorticism ■ Diuretic administration	■ Severe liver disease ■ Congestive heart failure ■ Nephrotic syndrome ■ Acute or chronic renal failure ■ Water intoxication	■ Hyperlipemia ■ Hyperproteinemia	■ Hyperglycemia ■ Mannitol infusion ■ Severe azotemia

death. When hyponatremia develops over several days, the brain adapts by removing intracellular electrolytes and idiogenic osmoles, creating a gradient that will shift some of the water out of the brain cell, restoring partly normal brain volume.[1,2,3,5]

During the correction of hyponatremia, a too-rapid increase in serum [Na$^+$] causes osmotic water movement out of the cells, and brain cell shrinkage occurs. Brain shrinkage will cause vascular rupture and cerebral bleeding and is responsible for acute neurologic signs, such as seizures, decreased mental state, and even death. In addition to the immediate changes, rapid correction of hyponatremia may cause a delayed syndrome called osmotic demyelination syndrome or central pontine demyelination (CPD). This syndrome is characterized by severe neurologic damage, often not reversible, like ataxia, paresis, or coma.[1,2,3,5]

Diagnosis

Algorithm 16.1 shows the approach to the hyponatremic patient.

The normal reference range might change slightly among laboratories. Normal [Na$^+$] for dogs ranges from 140 mmol/L to 150 mmol/L.

The approach to a patient with hyponatremia involves taking a detailed anamnesis from the caretakers and performing an in-depth physical examination. Physical examination should detect changes in the cardiovascular status of the patient and evaluate the patient's hydration state. A complete serum/plasma electrolytes panel, urea and creatinine, total protein and albumin, and urine sample collection should be performed in every patient with hyponatremia. The measurement of urine and serum [Na$^+$] can also be very helpful in differentiating between appropriate and inappropriate ADH secretion. The urinary [Na$^+$] of a normovolemic patient should be >30 mmol/L; a lower urinary [Na$^+$] is suggestive of the effect of aldosterone and urinary sodium reabsorption, typical of a decreased extracellular volume. Besides correcting the hypernatremia, addressing the underlying condition is paramount.

Algorithm 16.1 Note 1 In animals with hyperproteinemia or hyperlipidemia, when flame photometry methodology is used to determine [Na$^+$], a low [Na$^+$] can be a measurement artifact.

Algorithm 16.1 Note 2 Hyperglycemia (or administration of a hypertonic agent such as mannitol) by increasing plasma osmolarity and attracting water to the intravascular space, will cause a dilution in plasma [Na$^+$] called pseudohyponatremia. The relationship between glucose ([Glu]) and [Na$^+$] is not linear. With [Glu] up to 400 mg/dL (22.2 mmol/L), [Na$^+$] decreases by 1.6 mEq/L for every 100 mg/dL (5.6 mmol/L) rise in [Glu] and for [Glu] above 400 mg/dL (22.2 mmol/L), [Na$^+$] decreases by 2.4 mEq/L for every 100 mg/dL (5.6 mmol/L) rise in [Glu].

Algorithm 16.1 Note 3 Hypoperfusion is recognized in dogs with tachycardia, weak peripheral pulse, pale mucous membrane, and prolonged capillary refill time (CRT).

Algorithm 16.1 Note 4 If signs of hypoperfusion are present, based on the severity of the hypoperfusion, administer small boluses of crystalloid fluid (10-20 mL/kg in 10-20 minutes) with a [Na$^+$] within 10 mmol/L of the patient's [Na$^+$]. Ringer's solution or Ringer's lactate contains 130 mmol/L [Na$^+$] and can be a good isotonic balanced solution to use. A suitable fluid can eventually be created by adding an appropriate volume of dextrose 5% to a standard replacement fluid. Monitor serum [Na$^+$] 20 minutes after the fluid has been administered and then follow algorithm notes 6 or 7. Often, the resolution of hypoperfusion is enough to correct the hyponatremia.

Algorithm 16.1 Note 5 In dogs with acute clinical hyponatremia, [Na$^+$] should be rapidly increased at the rate of 1-2 mEq/L/h by increasing serum [Na$^+$] by 3 to 7 mEq/L until [Na$^+$] reaches a value >125 mmol/L and severe neurological signs disappear. Protocols using 2 mL/kg of hypertonic 3% NaCl over 30-60 minutes have been reported in the literature. This is expected to increase [Na$^+$] by 2 mmol/L. The dose of hypertonic saline can be repeated until [Na$^+$] >125 mmol/L and clinical signs disappear. However, for an inexperienced clinician, it is safer to use a solution like NaCl 0.9%. The total sodium increase over the first 24 hours should not exceed 10 to 12 mmol/L.

Algorithm 16.1 Note 6 If the onset of hyponatremia is chronic (>48h of duration), and no neurological signs are present, sodium supplement should be slowly increased with a rate of 0.5 mEq/L/h. Limit the increase in [Na$^+$] to a total of 10 mEq/L during the first 24h and 18 mEq/L for the first 48h. If the administration of isotonic crystalloids is inadequate in increasing [Na$^+$], then the amount of [Na$^+$] deficit in mmol/L can be calculated using the formula below and administered at a rate <0.5mEq/L/h:

$$\text{Na deficit} = \text{BW (kg)} \times 0.6 \times (\text{normal } [Na^+] - \text{patient } [Na^+])$$

Algorithm 16.1 Note 7 If the onset of hyponatremia is chronic (<48h) but neurological signs are present, follow Algorithm 16.1 Note 5 for the first 1-2h. Then, slowly increase of [Na$^+$] with a rate of 0.5-1 mEq/L/h. The above formula can be used to calculate the [Na$^+$] deficit.

Algorithm 16.1 Note 8 Hypervolemic patients may have ascites, jugular distention, peripheral edema, or pulmonary edema.

Algorithm 16.1 Note 9 The syndrome of inappropriate ADH release (SIAD) (see chapter 25) is characterized by normovolemia, low serum [Na$^+$], high urine [Na$^+$], increased urine osmolarity and decreased urinary output.

Algorithm 16.1 Note 10 In hypoadrenocorticism, hyponatremia is secondary to hypoaldosteronism and decreased ECV. Low cortisol also stimulates ADH release, contributing to hyponatremia.

ALGORITHM 16.1

Diagnostic approach to the hyponatremic patient.

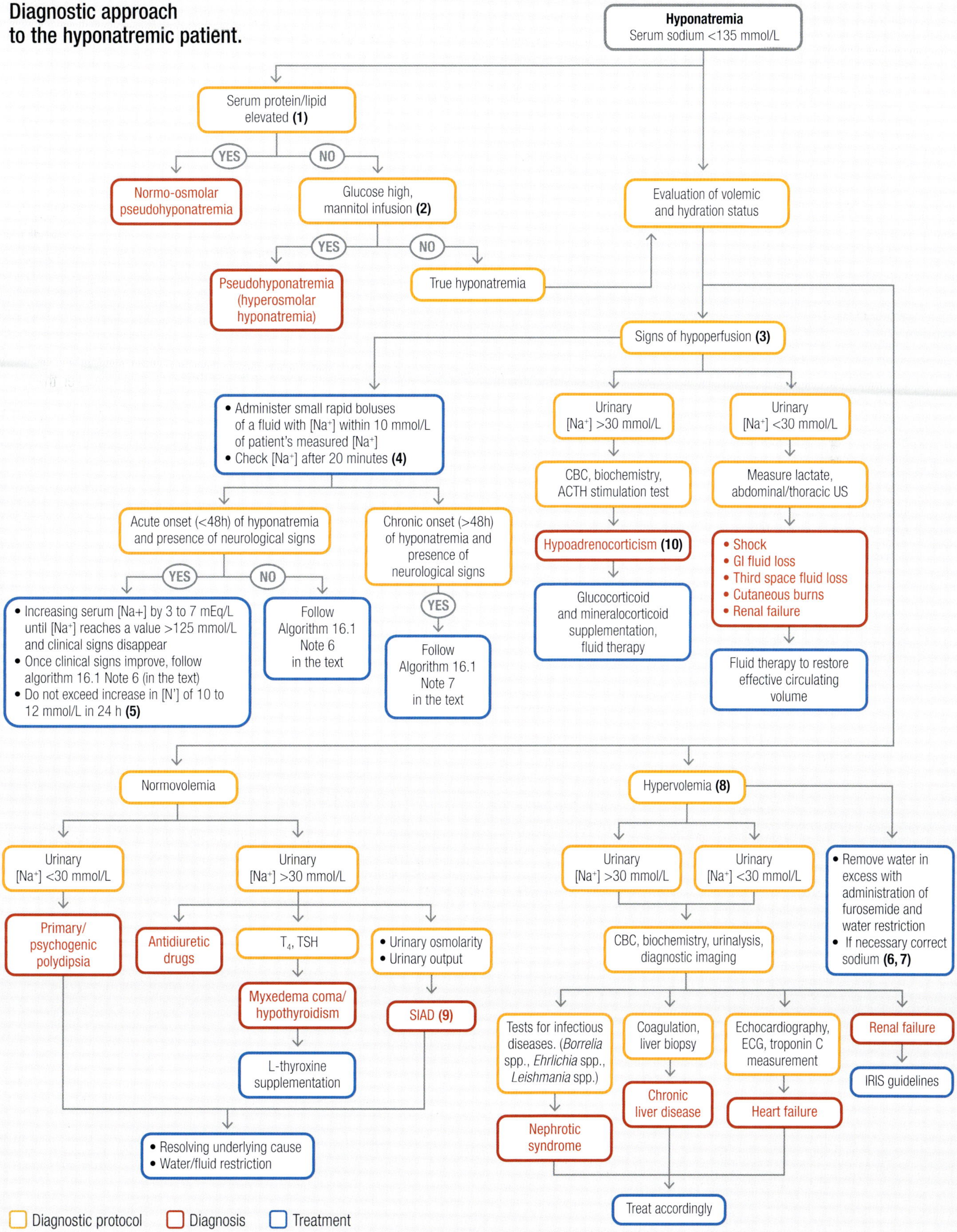

References

1. DiBartola S. Disorders of sodium and water: hypernatremia and hyponatremia. In DiBartola SP (editor). Fluid, Electrolyte, and Acid-base Disorders in Small Animal Practice. St Louis, Saunders/Elsevier, 2012, pp. 45-79.
2. Ueda and Hopper K. Sodium and Water Balance. In Textbook of Small Animal Emergency. In Drobatz KJ, Hopper K, Rozanski E, Silverstein D (editors). Textbook of Small Animal Emergency. John Wiley & Sons, 2019, pp. 690-699.
3. Guillaumin J, DiBartola S. Disorders of sodium and water homeostasis. *Vet Clin North Am Small Anim Pract* 47:293-312, 2017.
4. Ueda Y, Hopper K, Epstein SE. Incidence, severity and prognosis associated with hyponatremia in dogs and cats. *J Vet Intern Med* 29:801-807, 2015.
5. Burton A, Hopper K. Hyponatremia in dogs and cats. *J Vet Emerg Crit Care* 29:461-471, 2019.

CHAPTER 17

Hypocalcemia

Santiago Teyssandier
DVM

Pathophysiology

Hypocalcemia is a clinical and biochemical condition associated with multiple endocrine and nonendocrine disorders. Calcium acts on many vital intracellular and extracellular processes. Enzymatic reactions, membrane transport and stability, blood coagulation, nerve conduction, neuromuscular transmission, muscle contraction, vascular smooth muscle tone, hormone secretion, bone formation and resorption are only a part of the many actions where calcium is required.

Calcium exists in the blood in three fractions: 55% ionized (iCa or Ca^{2+}), 10% complexed (bound to phosphate, bicarbonate, sulfate, citrate, and lactate), and 35% bound to proteins.[1] The regulation depends on the relationship between absorption, excretion, and storage. The gut, kidneys, and bones play an important role in calcium homeostasis along with the parathyroid hormone (PTH), calcitriol (1,25-dihydroxyvitamin D_3), and calcitonin.

TABLE 17.1 Conditions associated with hypocalcemia from an electronic database of electrolyte analyses in 1467 dogs with hypocalcemia conducted at the Cornell University Hospital from 2007 to 2017.

Cause	N (%)
Nonpathologic, transient, or inconsequential	646 (44)
Critical illness	255 (17.4)
Kidney injury	152 (10.4)
Toxicity	110 (7.5)
Nutritional or gastrointestinal	93 (6.3)
Diabetes mellitus	64 (4.4)
Acute pancreatitis	51 (3.5)
Eclampsia	38 (2.6)
Undetermined	32 (2.2)
Parathyroid-related	11 (0.7)
Soft tissue trauma	14 (1.0)

Extracted from Coady M, Fletcher DJ, Goggs R. Severity of ionized hypercalcemia and hypocalcemia is associated with etiology in dogs and cats. *Front Vet Sci* 6:276, 2019. doi:10.3389/fvets.2019.00276.

The main effect of PTH is to increase extracellular fluid calcium concentrations by mobilizing calcium from bones, increasing tubular reabsorption of calcium from the kidneys, and indirectly increasing calcitriol synthesis in the intestine. Calcitriol increases the reabsorption of calcium and phosphorus from the intestine and kidneys and plays an essential role in the formation of osteoclasts. The effects of calcitonin on calcium homeostasis are considered mild, with the main action during hypercalcemia being the inhibition of bone resorption the main effect.

Ionized calcium (iCa) is the physiologically active form of calcium, although the initial evaluation of calcium disorders usually begins with the measurement of total calcium (tCa) concentration being more widely available. Interferences and discrepancies between iCa concentration and tCa concentration occur.[2] Hemolysis and lipemia increase calcium concentration. Anticoagulants (oxalate, citrate, ethylenediaminetetraacetic acid) and hyperbilirubinemia decrease it. Dogs younger than 3 months have slightly higher calcium concentrations. Acidic pH increases iCa concentration, and alkaline pH decreases it. Therefore, for an accurate assessment of iCa concentration, samples must be taken and processed anaerobically not to alter the pH.

Hypocalcemia is defined as total calcium (tCa) concentrations lower than 9.0 mg/dL (2.2 mmol/L) and iCa concentrations lower than 1.25 mmol/L (5 mg/dL). Conditions associated with hypocalcemia in the dog are summarized in Table 17.1.[3] Other causes not cited in the table are tumor lysis syndrome, secondary nutritional hyperparathyroidism, and medullary thyroid carcinoma due to low incidence in large populations or described as undetermined.

Clinical signs

Clinical signs depend on the duration, severity, and sensitivity of the individual patient to hypocalcemia. tCa concentrations less than 7 mg/dL (1.75 mmol/L) or iCa concentrations of approximately 0.7 mmol/L (2.8 mg/dL) are considered concentrations at which clinical signs are usually observed.[4] Despite all the functions in which calcium is involved, neurological signs are the most

recognized. When iCa concentration decreases, the threshold potential required to trigger an action potential in the neurons decreases, causing excitability in the peripheral and central nervous system (CNS).
Mild to moderate neurological clinical signs observed include:

- Behavioral changes: anxiety, panting, hypersensitivity, irritability, facial rubbing.
- Neuromuscular: stiff gait (Video 17.1), tremors (Video 17.2), tetany (Video 17.3 and Video 17.4).
- CNS: seizures.

Severe cases will manifest as:

- Tachyarrhythmia.
- Bradycardia and negative inotropism.
- Respiratory failure.

Uncommon signs:

- Vomiting.
- Diarrhea.
- Cataracts.
- Weakness.

Signs of chronic hypocalcemia

Nutritional secondary hyperparathyroidism (NSP) can cause hypocalcemia. Diets containing an excessive amount of phosphorus (e.g., meat-based diet) with normal/low calcium levels induce a compensatory response with increased plasma concentrations of PTH. This can lead to bone resorption, causing severe bone pain and reluctance to move (Video 17.5), especially in growing animals. Spontaneous fractures and long bone deformities are also signs of NSP.

Video 17.1

Stiff gait in a patient with hypocalcemia secondary to primary hypoparathyroidism. Primary hypothyroidism was also present in this case.

Video 17.2

Tremors and panting in a patient with hypocalcemia secondary to eclampsia.

Video 17.3

Tetany in a patient with hypocalcemia secondary to eclampsia.

Video 17.4

Tetany in a patient with hypocalcemia secondary to eclampsia.

Diagnostic approach

Algorithm 17.1 shows the approach to the hypocalcemic patient.
Normal tCa and iCa concentrations for most laboratories range from 9.0-11.5 mg/dL (2.2-3.8 mmol/L) and 1.2-1.5 mmol/L (5.0-6.0 mg/dL), respectively. Hypocalcemia is defined as tCa concentrations lower than 9.0 mg/dL (2.2 mmol/L) and iCa concentrations lower than 1.25 mmol/L (5 mg/dL). However, clinical signs usually manifest at tCa concentrations below 7 mg/dL (1.75 mmol/L) or iCa concentrations below 0.7 mmol/L (2.8 mg/d/L).

Algorithm 17.1 Note 1 Tetany is defined as a random stiffening or tightening of various muscle groups. Status epilepticus is defined as an ictal event >5 minutes or three or more generalized seizures. Generally, these symptomatic events of hypocalcemia are secondary to eclampsia or primary hypoparathyroidism.

Algorithm 17.1 Note 2 Hypocalcemic crisis should be treated with intravenous administration of calcium salts.[4] A solution of 10% calcium gluconate is recommended. A 0.15-1.5 mL/kg bolus should be administered slowly over 10-30 minutes or until effect (Video 17.6). If required, a constant rate infusion of calcium gluconate can be continued at 2.3-3.75 mg/kg/h (calculated with elemental calcium). Suspending the infusion is indicated in the event of bradycardia or an increase in the Q-T interval.

Algorithm 17.1 Note 3 tCa concentration is affected by lipemia, albumin concentration, hyperbilirubinemia, hemolysis and anticoagulants such as EDTA, oxalate, and citrate.[1] iCa concentration is mainly affected by acidosis and alkalosis, so the sample must be obtained under anaerobic conditions. Check for all analytical interferences and confirm hypocalcemia.[3]

Algorithm 17.1 Note 4 Administration of furosemide, phosphate enemas, or blood transfusion bags containing excessive citrate could cause hypocalcemia. Ethylene glycol intoxication has also been implicated.[5]

Algorithm 17.1 Note 5 Rapid destruction of tumor cells (mainly lymphoid or bone marrow tumors) after chemotherapy could cause hypocalcemia due to the intracellular release of phosphate from cells.[6]

Algorithm 17.1 Note 6 The mechanism of hypocalcemia in critical illness appears to be multifactorial, with sepsis being the most frequent. Proinflammatory cytokines tend to play an important role.[7] The magnitude of hypocalcemia correlates with the severity of the disease.

Video 17.5

Severe bone pain in a patient with hypocalcemia secondary to nutritional secondary hyperparathyroidism.

Video 17.6

Patient from Video 17.3 after recovery from tetany after administration of calcium gluconate.

ALGORITHM 17.1

Diagnostic approach to the patient with hypocalcemia.

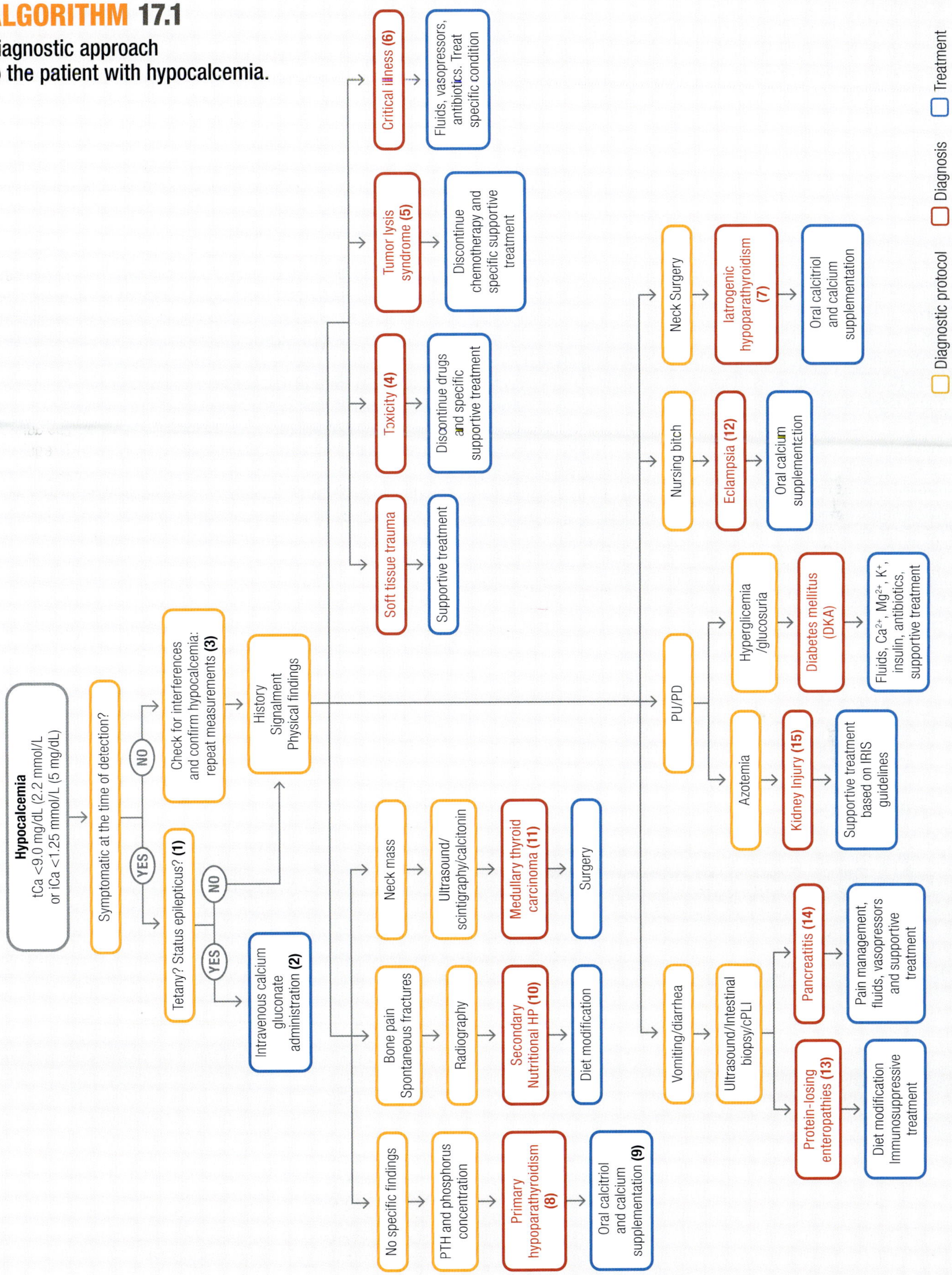

Algorithm 17.1 Note 7 The risk of developing postparathyroidectomy hypocalcemia can be predicted from presurgical calcium concentrations. Dogs with presurgical iCa concentrations higher than 1.75 mEq/L showed 7.5 times greater odds of becoming hypocalcemic postoperatively.[8]

Algorithm 17.1 Note 8 Primary hypoparathyroidism is an immune-mediated condition that leads to hypofunction of the parathyroid glands. Inappropriately low plasma PTH concentration to the extent of hypocalcemia, possibly associated with hyperphosphatemia, confirms the diagnosis.[9]

Algorithm 17.1 Note 9 Primary hypoparathyroidism (see chapter 31) requires oral calcium and vitamin D supplementation, usually lifelong. Calcitriol is the most potent form of vitamin D and also has the fastest maximum onset of action. Furthermore, calcitriol is a form of vitamin D that does not require renal activation, which is often compromised in hypoparathyroidism due to the lack of PTH. It is widely available in 0.25 µg capsules and can be given as a loading dose of 20 to 30 ng/kg/day for 2 to 4 days and adapted based on iCa (ideally) or tCa concentrations. There are numerous preparations with calcium salts, although calcium carbonate and calcium citrate are the most recommended. A dose of 25 to 50 mg/kg/day divided into two or three daily doses is recommended. The primary goal of long-term therapy is to maintain serum tCa concentration between 8.0 and 9.5 mg/dL or ionized calcium between 1.0 to 1.3 mmol/L, avoiding the risk of clinical signs of hypocalcemia and especially chronic hypercalcemia.[3] Because most commercially available pet food contains adequate calcium for daily needs, once a dog is stable, in some cases, calcium supplements can be phased off under the guidance of Ca measurements.

Algorithm 17.1 Note 10 Bone pain is the hallmark of NSP. Nutritional anamnesis, X-ray findings of reduced skeletal radiodensity (mainly vertebrae), weakening of the wall of long bones in dogs with bone pain, and normal-high plasma PTH concentration confirm the diagnosis. In some dogs with NSP, serum calcium is normal.

Algorithm 17.1 Note 11 Medullary thyroid carcinoma (MTC) is a tumor arising from the parafollicular cells of the thyroid gland that may cause hypocalcemia due to increased calcitonin secretion. The prevalence of MTC is probably underestimated, and only three published studies have been correlated with hypocalcemia.[10,11,14]

Algorithm 17.1 Note 12 Eclampsia occurs in small breed bitches between 1 and 3 weeks after parturition. Ossification of the skeleton and the poor source of calcium in the diet during pregnancy are the main mechanisms implicated. Moderate to severe clinical signs are observed.[12]

Algorithm 17.1 Note 13 Calcium/fatty acid complexes in the intestinal lumen, hypovitaminosis D and hypomagnesemia contributed to hypocalcemia in these patients. Hypoalbuminemia can interfere with the interpretation of serum tCa concentration.[1]

Algorithm 17.1 Note 14 Hypocalcemia occurring in dogs with acute pancreatitis is usually mild and subclinical. It is presumed to be due to increased calcitonin, calcium sequestration by peripancreatic fat, and free fatty acids.[4]

Algorithm 17.1 Note 15 Acute kidney injury is more likely to be symptomatic because the degree of hyperphosphatemia is usually greater than that seen in chronic kidney disease.[1] Decreased vitamin D activation is the main mechanism implicated in this type of hypocalcemia.

References

1. Schenck PA, Chew DJ, Nagode LA, et al. Disorders of calcium: hypercalcemia and hypocalcemia. In Dibartola SP (editor). Fluid, Electrolyte, and Acid-base Disorders in Small Animal Practice 4th edition. St. Louis, Elsevier Saunders, 2012, pp. 120-178.
2. Tørnqvist-Johnsen C, Schnabel T, Gow AG, et al. Investigation of the relationship between ionized and total calcium in dogs with ionized hypercalcemia. *Small Anim Pract* 61(4):247-252, 2020. doi:10.1111/jsap.13109.
3. Coady M, Fletcher DJ, Goggs R. Severity of ionized hypercalcemia and hypocalcemia is associated with etiology in dogs and cats. *Front Vet Sci* 6:276, 2019. doi:10.3389/fvets.2019.00276
4. Feldman EC. Hypocalcemia and primary hypoparathyroidism. In Feldman EC, Nelson RW, Reusch C, et al. Canine and Feline Endocrinology 4th edition. St. Louis, Elsevier Saunders, 2015, pp. 625-646.
5. Thrall MA, Grauer GF, Mero KN. Clinicopathologic findings in dogs and cats with ethylene glycol intoxication. *J Am Vet Med Assoc* 184(1):37-41, 1984.
6. Rahmani B, Patel S, Seyam O, et al. Current understanding of tumor lysis syndrome. *Hematol Oncol* 37(5):537-547, 2019. doi:10.1002/hon.2668
7. Holowaychuk MK. Hypocalcemia of critical illness in dogs and cats. *Vet Clin North Am Small Anim Pract* 43(6):1299-1317, 2013. doi:10.1016/j.cvsm.2013.07.008
8. Burkhardt SJ, Sumner JP, Mann S. Ambidirectional cohort study on the agreement of ultrasonography and surgery in the identification of parathyroid pathology, and predictors of postoperative hypocalcemia in 47 dogs undergoing parathyroidectomy due to primary hyperparathyroidism. *Vet Surg* 50(7):1379-1388, 2021. doi:10.1111/vsu.13707.
9. Russell NJ, Bond KA, Robertson ID. Primary hypoparathyroidism in dogs: a retrospective study of 17 cases. *Aust Vet J* 84(8):285-290, 2006. doi:10.1111/j.1751-0813.2006.00015.x.
10. Peterson ME, Randolph JF, Zaki FA, Heath H. Multiple endocrine neoplasia in a dog. *J Am Vet Med Assoc* 180(12):1476-1478, 1982.
11. Patnaik AK, Lieberman PH, Erlandson RA, Acevedo WM, Liu SK. Canine medullary carcinoma of the thyroid. *Vet Pathol* 15(5):590-599, 1978. doi:10.1177/030098587801500502.
12. Drobatz KJ, Casey KK. Eclampsia in dogs: 31 cases (1995-1998). *J Am Vet Med Assoc* 217(2):216-219, 2000. doi:10.2460/javma.2000.217.216.
13. Hume DZ, Drobatz KJ, Hess RS. Outcome of dogs with diabetic ketoacidosis: 127 dogs (1993-2003). *J Vet Intern Med* 20:547-555, 2006. doi:10.1111/j.1939-1676. 2006.tb02895.x
14. Teyssandier S, Campos M, Soler EA. Clinical and biochemical alterations associated with excess calcitonin in a dog with medullary thyroid carcinoma. Vet Rec Case Rep 12(3), 2023. doi:10.1002/vrc2.776.

CHAPTER 18

Hypercalcemia

Antonio Maria Tardo
DVM

Pathophysiology

Calcium plays a pivotal role in numerous physiological processes, encompassing muscle contraction, neurotransmission, hormone secretion, blood clotting, enzymatic reactions, and bone metabolism, among others. Almost all the calcium (99%) in the body is stored in bones and teeth in the form of hydroxyapatite ($Ca_{10}(PO_4)_6(OH)_2$). Only about 1% of the bone-calcium pool, present as amorphous crystals or in solution, is available for rapid diffusion into the extracellular fluid. The rest of the body calcium is distributed between the intracellular and extracellular compartments.[1]

Serum total calcium (tCa) exists in three forms: protein-bound (~35%), predominantly albumin; complexed with negatively charged ions (~10%), such as phosphate, bicarbonate, sulfate, citrate, and lactate; and ionized calcium (iCa).[3] iCa is the biologically active form and, in clinically healthy dogs, accounts for approximately 55% of the serum tCa concentration.[3] The protein-bound and complexed fractions act as a buffer, aiding in iCa regulation. Due to its critical role in essential biological processes, extracellular fluid iCa concentration is tightly maintained within a narrow range (approximately 1.2-1.4 mmol/L).[1]

Calcium homeostasis is complex and tightly regulated through the concerted actions of multiple organs and several hormones. Phosphate concentrations are controlled by the same systems that regulate calcium concentrations. The parathyroid glands, kidneys, bones, and intestine are key players in calcium-phosphate metabolism. The hormones involved include parathyroid hormone (PTH), vitamin D, and PTH-related protein (PTHrP).[2] Calcitonin, a calcium-lowering hormone produced by the thyroid gland, also impacts calcium-phosphate homeostasis, albeit to a lesser extent.[1]

PTH is synthesized in the parathyroid glands, and its release is modulated by extracellular iCa concentration. A steep inverse sigmoidal relationship exists between iCa and PTH, ensuring rapid PTH responses to minor declines in circulating iCa concentrations.[1] PTH increases calcium concentrations by enhancing renal tubular reuptake of calcium, mobilizing calcium from bones by increasing osteoclast activity and accelerating the formation of 1,25-dihydroxyvitamin D (calcitriol) in the kidneys. PTH also increases the rate of phosphaturia, thereby lowering serum phosphate concentrations (see chapter 29).

Calcitriol, the active form of vitamin D, enhances the intestinal absorption of calcium and phosphate and stimulates bone resorption, leading to an additional increase in circulating calcium concentrations. In contrast to humans, dogs lack the ability to synthesize vitamin D in their skin. Consequently, vitamin D, mainly in the form of cholecalciferol (vitamin D_3), must be derived from dietary sources. Once in the circulation, cholecalciferol is metabolized to 25-hydroxyvitamin D (calcidiol), the major circulating form of vitamin D, prior to further hydroxylation to calcitriol.

PTHrp is synthesized in various neoplastic cells and secreted locally. As such, it acts in a paracrine or autocrine manner. PTHrP shares the same biological activity as PTH and is often upregulated in neoplastic disease processes where normal negative feedback mechanisms are disrupted, leading to hypercalcemia. In veterinary medicine, PTHrP is best recognized for its role in the development of humoral hypercalcemia of malignancy (HHM) and is used as a "tumor marker".[2]

Hypercalcemia occurs when there is a derangement in calcium-regulating hormones (Table 18.1).

TABLE 18.1 Likely alterations in serum vitamin D, parathyroid hormone (PTH), and PTH-related protein (PTHrP) concentrations in dogs with disorders causing hypercalcemia.

	Vitamin D	PTH	PTHrP
Primary hyperparathyroidism	Normal or increased	Normal or increased	Normal
Humoral hypercalcemia of malignancy	Decreased, normal, or increased	Decreased	Normal or increased
Vitamin D toxicity	Increased	Decreased	Normal
Renal disease	Normal or decreased	Normal or increased	Normal
Hypoadrenocorticism	Normal	Normal or decreased	Normal
Granulomatous disease	Increased	Normal or decreased	Normal or increased
Non-malignant skeletal lesion	Normal or decreased	Decreased	Normal

Clinical signs

Hypercalcemia is a frequently encountered electrolyte abnormality in veterinary medicine. Its effects can be severe when it occurs, leading to considerable morbidity and mortality if not promptly recognized and addressed. The astute clinician must keep in mind that clinical manifestations of hypercalcemia are not always straightforward, as elevated blood calcium concentrations can either be a cause or a consequence of an underlying illness. Because calcium has an impact on every system in the body, signs of hypercalcemia are often vague and nonspecific. Clinical signs may vary depending on the magnitude of the hypercalcemia, its duration, and the rate of onset. Mild hypercalcemia may not be associated with owner-observed signs.[4] Even moderate to severe hypercalcemia, if it develops gradually, can be tolerated remarkably well.[4] Clinical signs are often more severe when the hypercalcemia develops rapidly, such as in vitamin D toxicosis and HHM.[4] The most common clinical signs in hypercalcemic dogs are polyuria/polydipsia, reduced appetite, weakness, lethargy, and decreased activity.[2] Less common signs include shivering/trembling, vomiting, constipation, diarrhea, weight loss, and stiff or painful gait.[2] Signs of lower urinary tract disease (pollakiuria, stranguria, and/or hematuria) can also be recognized and may be indicative of urolithiasis or urinary tract infection.[5] Owners of dogs with neoplastic diseases (anal sac neoplasia or lymphoma) may observe other related clinical signs, such as straining to defecate or ribbon-like feces.[4] Dogs with vitamin D toxicosis may appear seriously ill due to associated renal failure.[4] Although rare, potentially fatal complications of hypercalcemia include obtundation, seizures, coma, and arrhythmias.[2]

Physical examination of dogs with hypercalcemia can be unremarkable, but results are always critically important. Potential nonspecific findings include a low body condition score, generalized muscle atrophy, and weakness.[2] Since lymphoma is the most common cause of HHM in dogs, careful palpation of superficial lymph nodes should be systematically conducted.[2,4] Abdominal palpation may reveal hepatosplenomegaly or enlarged abdominal lymph nodes. Malignant (multiple myeloma) or non-malignant skeletal lesions (osteomyelitis, hypertrophic osteodystrophy, disuse osteoporosis) can cause lameness, reluctance to move, and generalized bone pain. Rectal palpation may help to identify anal sac neoplasia or enlarged retroperitoneal lymph nodes.[4]

In dogs with primary hyperparathyroidism, it is extremely unusual to palpate parathyroid nodules because they are small and covered by several muscle layers.[2] The presence of bradycardia in a dog with other evidence for hypovolemic shock (weak pulses, hypothermia, decreased capillary refill time) should raise concerns about the possibility of hypoadrenocorticism.

Diagnostic approach

Once hypercalcemia is recognized, clinicians are encouraged to determine the cause in order to establish an adequate therapeutic protocol and formulate a correct prognosis.

Algorithm 18.1 illustrates the approach to the hypercalcemic patient.[6]

Algorithm 18.1 Note 1 tCa is the most commonly used measure of calcium status in veterinary patients, even though it does not always correlate well with iCa, and changes in serum proteins may alter its concentration. Correction formulas have been developed to adjust tCa measurement relative to serum total protein or albumin. However, they are no longer used due to poor performance and increased availability of benchtop analyzers suitable for iCa measurement.[3] iCa should always be measured to assess calcium status accurately. When this is not possible, tCa should be interpreted with caution and in the context of serum albumin concentration.[2]

Algorithm 18.1 Note 2 When tCa concentration is increased, clinicians should measure iCa to determine whether the dog has ionized hypercalcemia. Serum can be used to measure iCa concentrations but should ideally be collected anaerobically. Exposure to air leads to loss of CO_2 from the sample, increased pH, and a falsely lowered iCa. Many benchtop analyzers perform iCa measurements on heparinized plasma or whole blood. iCa is less stable in whole or heparinized blood compared with serum and must be analyzed immediately. In addition, liquid heparin can dilute the sample and falsely decrease iCa concentration. Hence, commercially available syringes containing a premeasured quantity of dry heparin should be used. EDTA contamination should be avoided because EDTA chelates calcium, resulting in a falsely low iCa concentration.

Algorithm 18.1 Note 8 Diagnostic imaging plays a crucial role in investigating hypercalcemia. Abdominal ultrasound, thoracic and bone radiographs, and/or advanced imaging (computed tomography) should be evaluated for soft tissue masses, thoracic metastases, lytic lesions in the vertebrae or long bones, and organomegaly. These findings could indicate HHM and/or granulomatous diseases. Cervical ultrasound is the most relevant imaging exam to support the diagnosis of primary hyperparathyroidism (PHPTH) (see chapter 29). Soft tissue mineralization, generalized osteopenia, and urolithiasis can be observed in dogs with any hypercalcemic disorder.[2]

Algorithm 18.1 Note 9 PTHrp concentration is preferably measured in plasma using EDTA as an anticoagulant.[4] Similar to PTH, PTHrP is unstable, and it is recommended to maintain plasma samples under cold conditions until analysis. PTHrP concentration can be elevated in dogs with certain neoplastic diseases, with T-cell lymphoma and anal sac gland carcinoma being the most frequent ones.[7]

Algorithm 18.1 Note 13 Serum phosphorus concentration should always be evaluated in conjunction with calcium concentration and renal parameters. Hypophosphatemia, in the presence of adequate dietary phosphate and the absence of oral phosphate binders, is indicative of either PHPTH or HHM (Fig. 18.1). Hyperphosphatemia without azotemia suggests a non-parathyroid cause of hypercalcemia.

Algorithm 18.1 Note 14 Clinicians must adhere to their laboratory protocols regarding sample collection and processing. Proper handling of the sample is essential to an appropriate for an accurate diagnosis because PTH may degrade if exposed to warm temperatures.

Algorithm 18.1 Note 15 Serum PTH concentration must always be evaluated in relation to calcium concentration. In healthy dogs, as calcium concentration increases, PTH concentration decreases. Therefore, a serum PTH concentration within the reference range for a hypercalcemic dog is not normal. In dogs with PHPTH, serum PTH concentrations are typically high/normal to increased.[2]

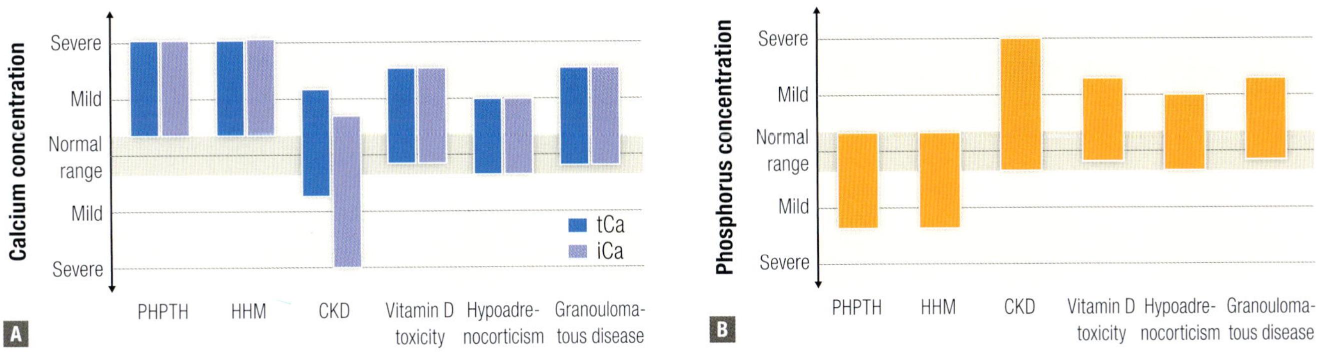

FIG. 18.1 The range in serum total calcium (tCa), ionized calcium (iCa), and phosphorus concentrations in dogs with disorders causing hypercalcemia. CKD, chronic kidney disease; HHM, humoral hypercalcemia of malignancy; PHPTH, primary hyperparathyroidism. Amended from: Feldman EC. Hypercalcemia and primary hyperparathyroidism. In Feldman EC, Nelson RW, Reusch CE, Scott-Moncrieff JCR, Behrend EN (editorss). Canine and Feline Endocrinology 4th edition. St Louis, Elsevier Saunders, 2015, p. 591.

Diagnosis

Algorithm 18.1 Note 5 Vitamin D toxicosis can be chronic, developing due to the ingestion of dietary supplements or topical antipsoriasis preparations for humans. Clinical signs and effects on mineral metabolism may require weeks to become obvious.[2] Overzealous dietary supplementation with marine oils, like cod liver or salmon oil, has been linked to hypercalcemia, as supplements designed for human consumption are often used.[4] Topical psoriasis preparations containing vitamin D analogs (calcipotriene, calcipotriol, and maxacalcitol) are the most common medications ingested by dogs presented for hypercalcemia, as these creams are often palatable.[4] The diagnosis of chronic vitamin D toxicosis relies on exposure history. An additional clue would be hypercalcemia associated with hyperphosphatemia in the absence of kidney disease.[2]

Algorithm 18.1 Note 6 Ingestion of vitamin D-based rodenticides is considered the most common cause of toxin-associated hypercalcemia in dogs.[2] Dosage as low as 0.1-0.5 mg/kg can cause clinical signs and hypercalcemia, respectively.[8] Lilies and *Cestrum diurnum* (day-blooming jessamine) are popular houseplants that should be considered sources of vitamin D toxicity in dogs because they contain active vitamin D metbolites.[2] Raisins or grapes, when ingested, can cause acute kidney injury (AKI) and hypercalcemia, though the exact mechanism remains unclear.[2] Dogs exposed to these toxins often develop kidney damage, leading to azotemia, which might distract the clinician from the primary cause of hypercalcemia.

Algorithm 18.1 Note 10 Malignancies are the leading cause of hypercalcemia in dogs.[2,4,9] In a study of 1,641 dogs with ionized hypercalcemia, lymphoma was identified as the most common underlying cause in about 38% of cases, followed by malignancies of unknown origin (22%) and anal sac gland carcinoma (12%).[10] In the same study, dogs with malignancy were more likely to have moderate to severe hypercalcemia.[10] Of lymphoma cases, T-cell phenotypes are more likely to induce hypercalcemia.[2] Various tumors such as multiple myeloma, carcinomas, thymoma, melanoma, bone tumors, and leukemia can also cause hypercalcemia.[2] Malignancies can lead to hypercalcemia through various mechanisms, including PTHrP and/or vitamin D secretion, cytokines, bone resorption due to hematologic malignancies in the bone marrow, and tumor metastasis to bones.[2] Therefore, a normal PTHrP concentration does not exclude HHM.[4]

Algorithm 18.1 Note 11 Macrophages within granulomatous tissue can produce calcitriol, leading to overt hypercalcemia. This phenomenon is well-established in human patients and has been reported in single-case reports in dogs.[4] Granulomatous diseases causing hypercalcemia in dogs have included blastomycosis, aspergillosis, coccidioidomycosis, hepatozoonosis, histoplasmosis, angiostrongylosis, nocardiosis, gastric phytiosis, panniculitis, and lymphadenitis.[2,4,9] Moreover, PTHrP-mediated hypercalcemia has been reported in two dogs with schistomiasis.[2]

Algorithm 18.1 Note 12 The presence of concurrent azotemia, hyperphosphatemia, and hypercalcemia might represent a diagnostic dilemma, as hypercalcemia could be the cause or the consequence of renal disease. Dogs with kidney disease might exhibit increased, decreased, or normal tCa levels. Ionized calcium concentrations can be increased in either AKI or, more frequently, chronic kidney disease (CKD).[2,4] Ionized hypercalcemia is reported to occur in approximately 10% of dogs with CKD, with most dogs having normal or low iCa concentrations.[2,4] When both hyperphosphatemia and azotemia are present, the clinician must rely on the history, physical examination, and additional tests (urinary protein-to-creatinine ratio, abdominal and cervical ultrasound, measurement of PTH and/or vitamin D) to determine the primary disorder leading to hypercalcemia.

Therapy

Algorithm 18.1 Note 3 Dogs with hypercalcemia of malignancy, vitamin D toxicosis, or other non-PHPTH causes of hypercalcemia may exhibit concerning clinical signs originating from both their underlying disorder and hypercalcemia. Treatment of the underlying disease may indirectly decrease serum calcium concentrations.[2] When removal of the underlying cause is not possible, prompt treatment for hypercalcemia should be initiated (refer to Algorithm 18.1 Note 4).

Algorithm 18.1 Note 4 Supportive treatment is often necessary to decrease serum calcium concentration to a less toxic level while awaiting a definitive diagnosis, definitive treatment to permanently reduce serum calcium concentration, or for the chronic management of hypercalcemia when the underlying cause cannot be eliminated. There is no single treatment protocol consistently effective for all causes of hypercalcemia. Consequently, regimens must be tailored for the individual patient.

ALGORITHM 18.1

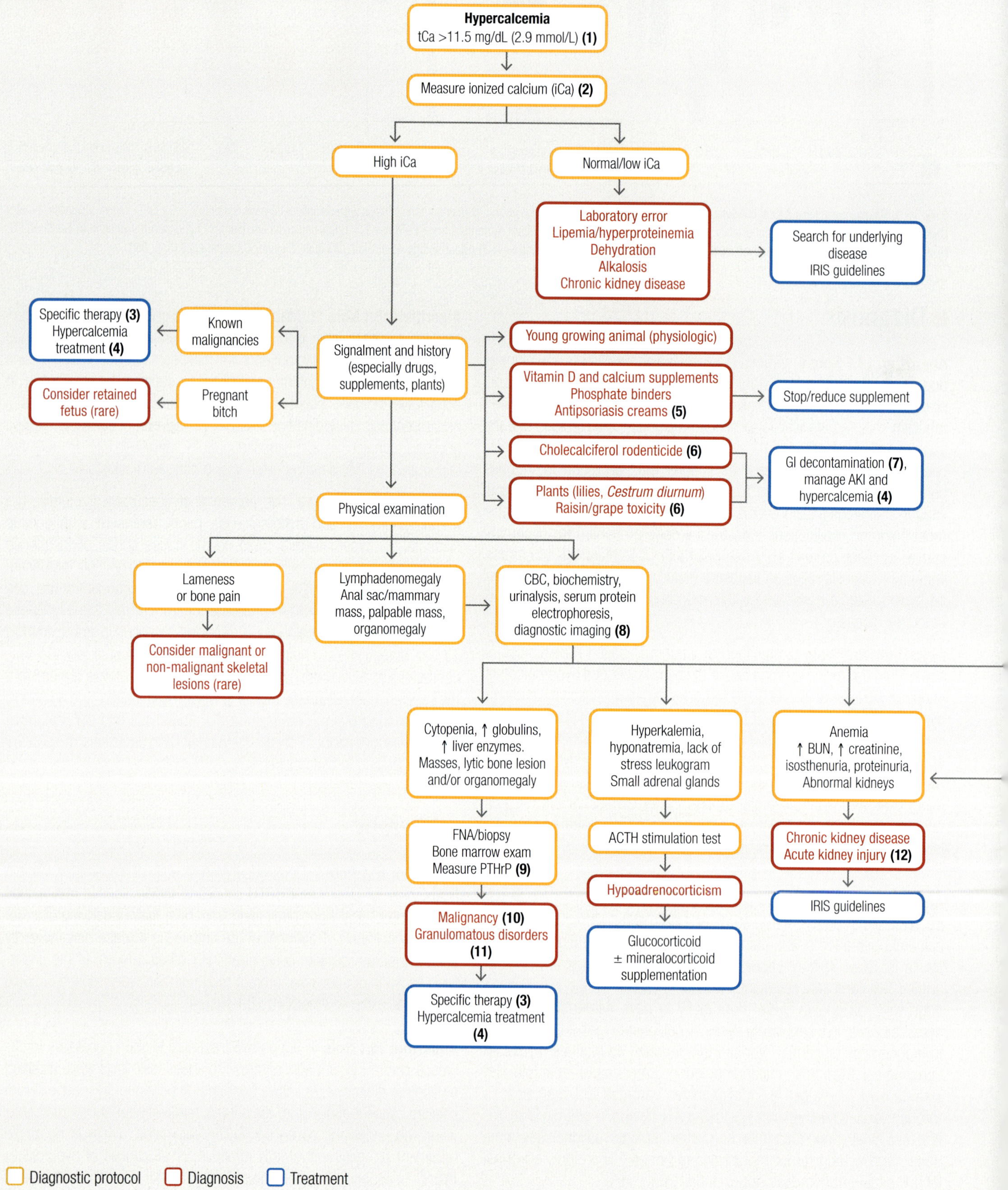

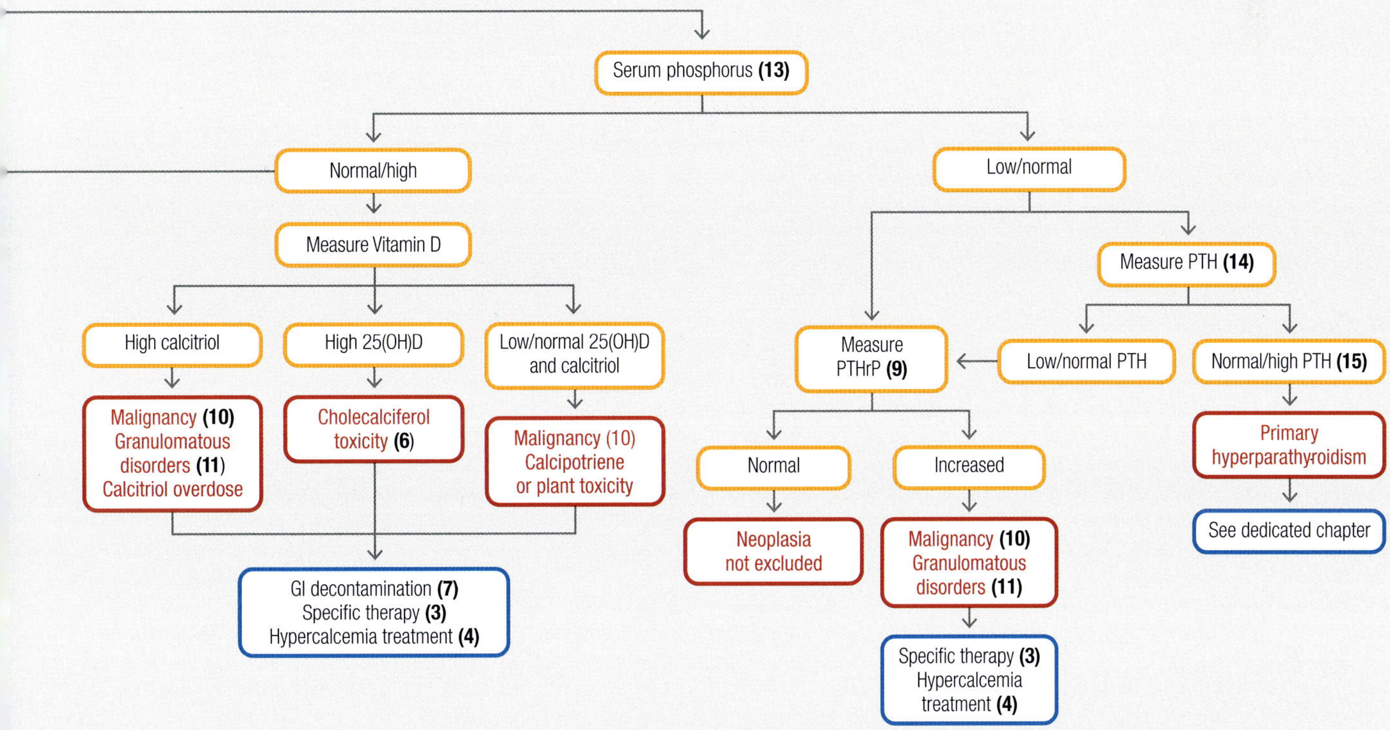
Serum phosphorus (13)
Normal/high
Low/normal
Measure Vitamin D
Measure PTH (14)
High calcitriol
High 25(OH)D
Low/normal 25(OH)D and calcitriol
Measure PTHrP (9)
Low/normal PTH
Normal/high PTH (15)
Malignancy (10) Granulomatous disorders (11) Calcitriol overdose
Cholecalciferol toxicity (6)
Malignancy (10) Calcipotriene or plant toxicity
Normal
Increased
Primary hyperparathyroidism
See dedicated chapter
Neoplasia not excluded
Malignancy (10) Granulomatous disorders (11)
GI decontamination (7) Specific therapy (3) Hypercalcemia treatment (4)
Specific therapy (3) Hypercalcemia treatment (4)

The goals of supportive treatment are to enhance renal excretion of calcium and to prevent calcium reabsorption from bone.[2] Parenteral fluid therapy is the first-line treatment in dogs with hypercalcemia. Fluid therapy should correct dehydration and induce diuresis once fluid volume and blood pressure have been restored.[2] Renal calcium excretion is enhanced by sodium. Thus, 0.9% sodium chloride (NaCl) is often the fluid of choice. In well-hydrated dogs, furosemide should be considered to promote additional calciuresis.[2] Glucocorticoids are effective therapy as they induce cytolysis, reduce bone resorption, decrease intestinal absorption, and increase calciuresis.[2] Glucocorticoid therapy should be avoided if a definitive diagnosis has not been established. Bisphosphonates may be used for chronic control of hypercalcemia, as they lower calcium by inhibiting osteoclast-mediated bone resorption.[7] Dehydration should be corrected before bisphosphonates are administered to lessen the chances of renal injury. Medical treatment options for hypercalcemia are outlined in Table 18.2.

Algorithm 18.1 Note 7 Decontamination via emesis or gastric lavage within 2-3 hours after exposure is recommended. In the case of cholecalciferol rodenticide ingestion, administration of multiple oral doses of activated charcoal is warranted (every 6 hours for the first 24 hours), since it enters the enterohepatic recirculation.[8]

TABLE 18.2 Specific treatments for hypercalcemia in dogs.

	Treatment	Dose	Indications	Comments
Volume expansion	■ SC 0.9% sodium chloride ■ IV 0.9% sodium chloride*	■ Small volumes ■ 100 to 125 mL/kg/day or "as needed"	■ Mild hypercalcemia ■ Moderate to severe hypercalcemia	■ Rarely indicated or beneficial ■ Careful in patients with congestive heart failure or hypertension
Diuretics	■ Furosemide	■ 2-4 mg/kg every 8 to 12 hours, IV, SC, or PO	■ Moderate to severe hypercalcemia	■ Use only after the patient is fully rehydrated
Alkalinizing agent	■ Sodium bicarbonate	■ 1 mEq/kg IV slow bolus; may continue at 0.3 × base deficit × weight in kg/day	■ Severe hypercalcemia	■ Useful in patients who remain acidotic despite adequate rehydration. Requires close monitoring
Glucocorticoids	■ Prednisolone ■ Dexamethasone	■ 1-2 mg/kg every 12 to 24 hours OS, SC, or IV ■ 0.1-0.2 mg/kg every 12 hours IV or SC	■ Moderate to severe hypercalcemia	■ Use only after the diagnosis has been obtained
Bone resorption inhibitors	■ Salmon calcitonin	■ 4 to 6 IU/kg as IV infusion and then SC every 8 or 12 hours	■ Hypervitaminosis D ■ Severe hypercalcemia	■ Should be considered instead of glucocorticoids when a definitive diagnosis has not been obtained. Response may be short-lived; vomiting and anorexia may occur
Bisphosphonates	■ Pamidronate ■ Zoledronate ■ Alendronate	■ 1-2 mg/kg in 250 mL 0.9% NaCl IV over 2 hours every 2-4 weeks. ■ 0.1-0.25 mg/kg in 60 mL 0.9% NaCl IV over 15 minutes every 2-4 weeks. ■ 5 to 20 mg orally every 7 days	■ Moderate to severe hypercalcemia	■ Use only after the patient is fully rehydrated. Pamidronate and zolendronate are expensive, and use in dogs is limited. ■ Poor intestinal absorption. Must ensure complete passage of medication into stomach to avoid esophagitis

*Potassium supplementation might be necessary.

References

1. Graves TK. Hypercalcemia. In Feldman EC, Fracassi F, Peterson ME (editors). Feline Endocrinology. Milan, Edra, 2019, pp. 319-334.
2. Feldman EC. Hypercalcemia and primary hyperparathyroidism. In Feldman EC, Nelson RW, Reusch CE, Scott-Moncrieff JCR, Behrend EN (editors). Canine and Feline Endocrinology 4th edition. St Louis, Elsevier Saunders, 2015, pp. 580-624.
3. Schenck PA, Chew DJ. Calcium: total or ionized? *Vet Clin North Am Small Animal Pract* 38(3): 497-502, 2008.
4. Skelly BJ. Control of calcium metabolism and investigation of hypo- and hypercalcemia. In Moneey CT, Peterson ME, Shiel RE (editors). BSAVA Manual of Canine and Feline Endocrinology 5th edition. British Small Animal Veterinary Association, 2023, pp. 97-107.
5. Feldman EC, Hoar B, Pollard R, et al. Pretreatment clinical and laboratory findings in dogs with primary hyperparathyroidism: 210 cases (1987-2004). *J Am Vet Med Assoc* 227(5): 756-761, 2005.
6. Arenas C. Hypercalcemia. In Fracassi F (editor). Diagnostic and Therapeutic Algorithms in Internal Medicine for Dogs and Cats. Milan, Edra, 2022, pp. 137-140.
7. Bailey DB. Paraneoplastic syndromes. In Vail DM, H.Thamm D, Liptak JM (editors). Withrow & MacEwen's Small Animal Clinical Oncology. Missouri, Elsevier, 2020, pp. 98-112.
8. Lee JA. Chemical toxicoses. In Ettinger SJ, Feldman EC, Côté E (editors). Textbook of Veterinary Internal Medicine. Missouri, Elsevier, 2017, pp. 1660-1670.
9. Galvao JB, Schenck P, Chew D. A quick reference on hypercalcemia. *Vet Clin North Am Small Anim Pract* 47:241-248, 2017.
10. Coady M, Fletcher DJ, Goggs R. Severity of ionized hypercalcemia and hypocalcemia is associated with etiology in dogs and cats. *Front Vet Sci* 6:276, 2019.

CHAPTER 19

Proteinuria

Tim Williams
MA, VetMB, PhD, AFHEA, FRCPath, DECVCP, MRCVS

Pathophysiology

The normal urine of animals contains only a small amount of albumin and other proteins because the glomerulus is selectively permeable, which minimizes protein filtration and excretion. Large and/or negatively charged proteins are less readily filtered by the normal glomerular barrier than small and electroneutral or positively charged proteins. Most proteins that are filtered and enter the urine are reabsorbed in the renal proximal convoluted tubules by pinocytosis.

Proteinuria can be physiological (also termed functional) or pathological. Physiological proteinuria is transient and can be associated with strenuous exercise, stress, extreme heat or cold, pyrexia, or seizures. The mechanism for physiological proteinuria is unclear, although it has been suggested that it could occur secondary to renal vasoconstriction, ischemia, congestion, conformational changes in proteins associated with hyperlactatemia which increase the permeability of proteins through the glomerular barrier, and increased permeability of the glomerular capillary membrane associated with increased sympathetic nervous system activity. Pathological proteinuria is only diagnosed if persistence of proteinuria (usually over a >2-week period) is demonstrated.

Pathological proteinuria can be categorized as follows:

- Systemic diseases associated with proteinuria. Proteinuria is associated with increased circulating concentrations of acute phase proteins, suggesting systemic inflammation *per se* might cause proteinuria. Usually, this is associated with low magnitude proteinuria (urinary protein to creatinine ratio (UPCR) <1), although occasionally, cases with moderate to marked proteinuria (UPCR >2) are seen. Proteinuria is a relatively common feature in dogs with hypercortisolism (44-75% of cases) and in dogs with diabetes mellitus (28-44%), which is likely to reflect increased renal excretion of albumin and other proteins (including IgG, RBP, and NAG),[1,2] although larger studies are needed to confirm this hypothesis. Increased proteinuria in diabetes mellitus probably reflects a combination of increased glomerular permeability (renal glomerular proteinuria) and decreased tubular reabsorption of protein (renal tubular proteinuria). Proteinuria has also been reported in dogs with hypertension, which appears to be secondary to albuminuria, presumably secondary to glomerular hypertension and hyperfiltration,[3] and in dogs with lymphoma,[4] although the nature of the proteinuria associated with lymphoma has not been investigated to date.
- Prerenal proteinuria. This type of proteinuria is caused by increased circulating blood concentrations of small proteins (e.g., myoglobin, free hemoglobin, or paraproteins produced by plasma cells), which can freely pass through the normal glomerular barrier. When the filtered quantity of these proteins exceeds the reabsorptive capacity of the renal tubular cells, proteinuria will occur. This is a relatively uncommon cause of proteinuria in animals and is associated with conditions such as rhabdomyolysis, intravascular hemolysis, and multiple myeloma.
- Renal glomerular proteinuria. This form of proteinuria occurs when circulating blood concentrations of proteins are normal, but there is reduced selectivity of the glomerular barrier. Hence, an increased proportion of the circulating proteins are filtered across the glomerular membrane and into the Bowman's space. The increased quantity of filtered proteins overwhelms the normal reabsorptive capacity of the renal tubular cells, and this leads to proteinuria. This type of proteinuria is associated with diseases of the glomeruli, such as glomerulonephritis, amyloidosis, or other glomerulonephropathies.
- Renal tubular proteinuria. This type of proteinuria occurs when the glomerular barrier is functioning normally. However, due to damage or dysfunction of the renal tubular epithelial cells, there is reduced reabsorption of the normal filtered protein load by the tubular cells, and proteinuria occurs.
- Postrenal proteinuria. This is the most common cause of proteinuria in animals. It occurs due to the excretion of proteins from the urinary (or reproductive) tract in response to inflammation and/or infection and can cause proteinuria of any magnitude. Therefore, when assessing proteinuria, it is important to check the urine sediment and dipstick to rule out urinary tract inflammation, which might falsely increase the UPCR.

Clinical signs

Most animals with mild to moderate proteinuria (UPCR <2) may not present with any clinical signs. However, where proteinuria is secondary to renal disease, then other clinical signs of renal disease, such as polydipsia, polyuria, weight loss, and reduced appetite, may be apparent. Otherwise, clinical signs may be associated with diseases that cause proteinuria (e.g., clinical signs of lower urinary tract disease if proteinuria is due to postrenal proteinuria associated with urinary tract inflammation, clinical signs of hypercortisolism, and others).

Marked proteinuria associated with renal glomerular proteinuria can lead to hypoalbuminemia, which if marked (<15 g/L), can lead to peripheral edema and body cavity effusion formation.

Diagnostic approach

Algorithm 11.1 shows the diagnostic approach to proteinuria. Urine dipstick protein results can be used as an initial screening test for proteinuria. However, false positive and false negative results are possible (Table 19.1). Hence, the most accurate way to assess for proteinuria is to measure UPCR.

Algorithm 19.1 Note 1 UPCR >0.5 in dogs is defined as overtly proteinuric, and UPCR between 0.2-0.5 is defined as borderline proteinuric.[5] Thus, pathological renal proteinuria can be diagnosed if the UPCR is persistently >0.5, provided that systemic diseases associated with proteinuria and prerenal or postrenal causes of proteinuria have been excluded.

Algorithm 19.1 Note 2 Postrenal proteinuria is probably the most common cause of proteinuria and can be excluded by evaluation of urine sediment; if there is evidence of hematuria or pyuria on urine sediment, then postrenal proteinuria is likely to occur. For this reason, urine dipstick and sediment examination should always be performed alongside the measurement of UPCR. The correlation between bacteriuria (without active sediment) and proteinuria is controversial, with some studies reporting no association[6,7] but other studies identifying significant associations between positive urine culture and proteinuria (defined as UPCR >0.5) in dogs with inactive sediment.[8] Hence, a urine culture may also be required to fully exclude postrenal causes of proteinuria.

TABLE 19.1 Causes of error in diagnostic methods for proteinuria.

Urine dipstick protein	**Causes of false positive results:** ■ Positive result on dipstick may be normal if urine is concentrated. If the urine dipstick is negative for protein, then significant proteinuria is unlikely to be present (sensitivity 94% in dogs[13] if ≥ trace protein dipstick result is considered positive). However, specificity is relatively low (51%). ■ Highly alkaline urine (pH >8.0) ■ Gross hematuria and pigmenturia ■ Chlorhexidine contamination of sample ■ Contamination of sample by some disinfectants
	Causes of false negative results: ■ Urine dipsticks are less sensitive to positively charged or cellular protein detection. Hence, light chain proteinuria may be missed using dipstick analysis alone
Urine protein to creatinine ratio (UPCR)	**Causes of false positive results:** ■ Marked blood contamination (>250 RBCs/400× field)[14]

Algorithm 19.1 Note 3 Proteinuria can be associated with the administration of corticosteroids and tyrosine kinase inhibitors, so these should be excluded based on clinical history. Other diseases that can be associated with proteinuria should be excluded next; if serum acute phase protein concentrations are high and the UPCR is only mildly increased (UPCR <1-2), then systemic inflammation may be the cause of proteinuria and UPCR should be re-evaluated once the systemic inflammation has been resolved, diabetes mellitus can be excluded based on serum glucose concentrations (± fructosamine) and, depending on clinical suspicion, further testing for hypercortisolism could be considered (see relevant chapters). Pancreatitis may also be associated with proteinuria, so serum lipase/cPLI and abdominal ultrasound could be measured. Thoracic and abdominal imaging (± cytology) should also be performed to exclude neoplasia, particularly lymphoma.

Prerenal causes of proteinuria can be excluded by measurement of serum globulin concentrations, serum CK activity (to exclude significant myocyte injury), and consideration of hematology results (regenerative anemia, ghost cells, or other evidence of intravascular hemolysis). If multiple myeloma/B-cell lymphoproliferative disorder and the presence of circulating paraproteins (M proteins) is suspected, then serum protein electrophoresis (with immunofixation) could also be performed since 10% of cases with circulating M proteins have normal serum globulin concentrations. Urine protein electrophoresis to evaluate for Bence-Jones proteinuria could also be considered.

Algorithm 19. 1 Note 4 Once postrenal, prerenal, and systemic diseases associated with proteinuria have been excluded, then pathological renal proteinuria can be suspected. The magnitude of proteinuria will enable the distinction between renal glomerular proteinuria (UPCR >2) and renal tubular proteinuria (UPCR <2, but often <1). In both glomerular and renal proteinuria, abdominal ultrasound would be beneficial to identify architectural changes that might be associated with neoplasia or chronic kidney disease.

Algorithm 19.1 Note 5 If renal glomerular proteinuria is suspected, then testing for infectious diseases that can be associated with glomerulonephritis (leishmaniasis, anaplasmosis, ehrlichiosis, borreliosis, hepatozoonosis, and leptospirosis) should be considered, based on the risk of infection. A renal biopsy could also be considered in patients with marked proteinuria (UPCR >3.5) or in patients that do not respond to standard therapy (see below). It is recommended that personnel experienced in obtaining, handling, and interpreting renal biopsies should undertake this procedure in order to maximize the diagnostic yield.[9]

ALGORITHM 19.1

Diagnostic approach to proteinuria.

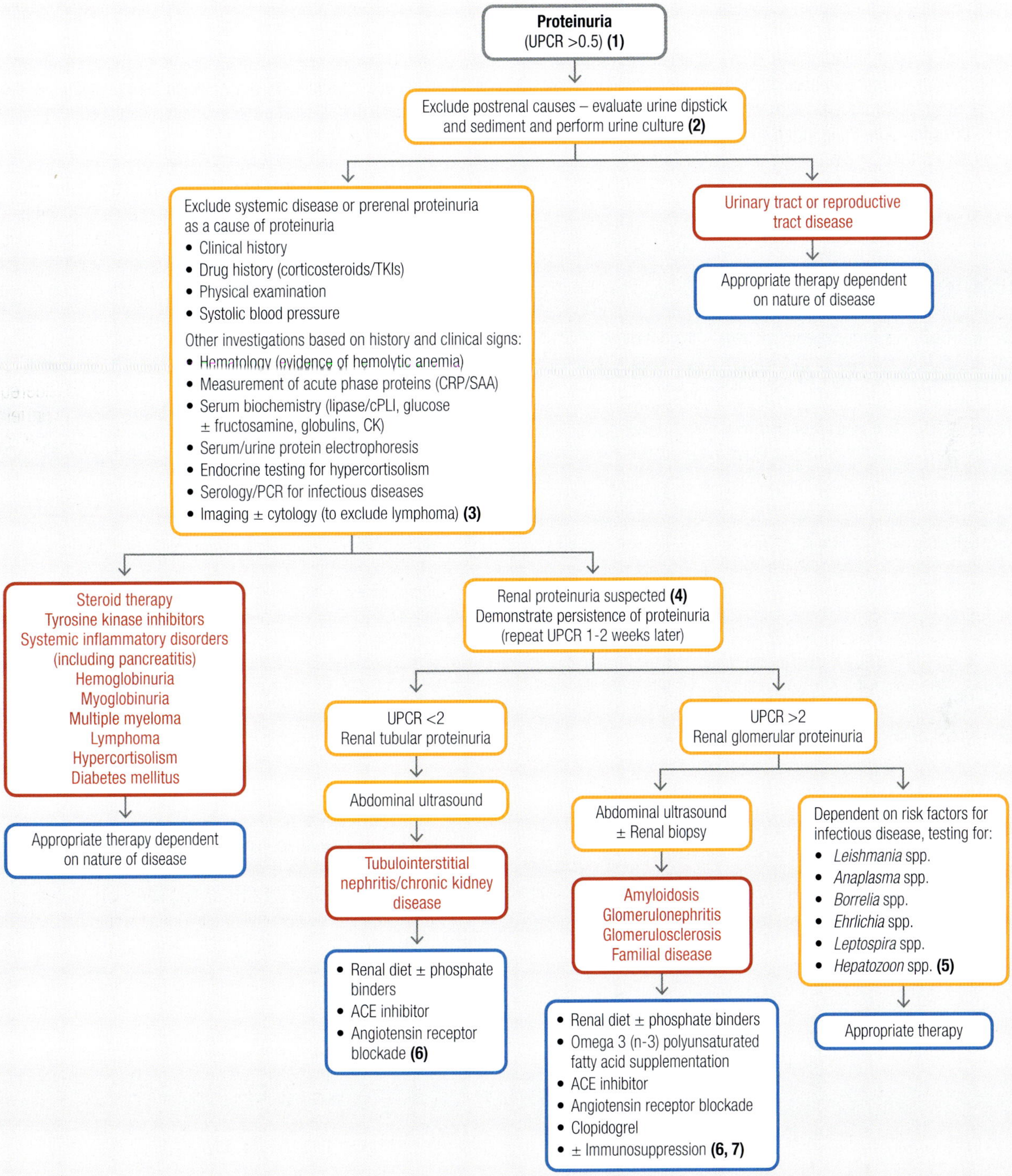

Diagnostic protocol | Diagnosis | Treatment

Treatment

Algorithm 19.1 Note 6 For patients with renal glomerular and tubular proteinuria, the feeding of a prescription renal diet is recommended, along with antiproteinuric therapy (ACE inhibitors ± angiotensin receptor blockers).[5]

Algorithm 19.1 Note 7 Patients with renal glomerular proteinuria are also at risk of thromboembolism. Hence, antithrombotic therapy with clopidogrel should be instituted. It is also recommended that dogs with renal glomerular proteinuria should receive omega-3 polyunsaturated fatty acid supplementation.[10] Immunosuppression is indicated in patients with severe, persistent, or progressive glomerular disease for which there is renal biopsy evidence of an immune-mediated etiology (and no contraindication to immunosuppression).[11] Immunosuppression can also be cautiously considered if dogs with severe azotemia (serum creatinine concentrations >3 mg/dL; >265 µmol/L), progressive azotemia, or severe hypoalbuminemia (serum albumin concentrations <20 g/L) which fail to respond to standard therapy, provided that familial disease or amyloidosis are not suspected to be the cause of proteinuria.[12]

References

1. Smets PM, et al. Long-term follow-up of renal function in dogs after treatment for ACTH-dependent hyperadrenocorticism. *J Vet Intern Med* 26(3) 565-574, 2012.
2. Marynissen SJ, et al. Long-term follow-up of renal function assessing serum cystatin C in dogs with diabetes mellitus or hyperadrenocorticism. *Vet Clin Pathol* 45(2):320-329, 2016.
3. Bacic A, et al. Evaluation of albuminuria and its relationship with blood pressure in dogs with chronic kidney disease. *Vet Clin Pathol* 39(2):203-209, 2010.
4. Di Bella A, et al. Proteinuria in canine patients with lymphoma. *J Small Anim Pract* 54(1):28-32, 2013.
5. Lees GE, et al. Assessment and management of proteinuria in dogs and cats: 2004 ACVIM Forum Consensus Statement (small animal). *J Vet Intern Med* 19(3):377-385, 2005.
6. Grimes M, et al. Characteristics associated with bacterial growth in urine in 451 proteinuric dogs (2008-2018). *J Vet Intern Med* 34(2):770-776, 2020.
7. Meindl AG, et al. Relationships among urinary protein-to-creatinine ratio, urine specific gravity, and bacteriuria in canine urine samples. *J Vet Intern Med* 33(1):192-199, 2019.
8. Broadbridge C, Williams TL. Evaluation of haem dipstick pad, urine protein, urine pH and urine protein:creatinine ratio results as a marker of bacteriuria in dogs and cats with inactive urine sediment. *J Small Anim Pract* 64(8):493-498, 2023.
9. Littman MP, et al. Consensus recommendations for the diagnostic investigation of dogs with suspected glomerular disease. *J Vet Intern Med* 27 Suppl 1:S19-26, 2013.
10. Brown S, et al. Consensus recommendations for standard therapy of glomerular disease in dogs. *J Vet Intern Med* 27 Suppl 1:S27-43, 2013.
11. Segev G, et al. Consensus recommendations for immunosuppressive treatment of dogs with glomerular disease based on established pathology. *J Vet Intern Med* 27 Suppl 1:S44-54, 2013.
12. Pressler B, et al. Consensus guidelines for immunosuppressive treatment of dogs with glomerular disease absent a pathologic diagnosis. *J Vet Intern Med* 27 Suppl 1:S55-9, 2013.
13. Zatelli A, et al. Evaluation of a urine dipstick test for confirmation or exclusion of proteinuria in dogs. *Am J Vet Res* 71(2):235-240, 2010.
14. Vientós-Plotts AI, et al. Effect of blood contamination on results of dipstick evaluation and urine protein-to-urine creatinine ratio for urine samples from dogs and cats. *Am J Vet Res* 79(5):525-531, 2018.

Blood pressure measurements

Paula García San José
DVM, PhD

María Dolores Pérez Alenza
DVM, PhD

Blood pressure (BP) is the pressure the circulating blood exerts against the blood vessels' walls. It is the product of the cardiac output and the vascular resistance, measured in millimeters of mercury (mmHg). The term "blood pressure" usually refers to systemic arterial BP, and it is usually divided into systolic BP (maximum BP in one heartbeat), diastolic BP (minimum BP between two heartbeats), and mean BP (diastolic + [(systolic-diastolic)/3]).[1,2] In dogs, there are many endocrine diseases associated with either hypotension or hypertension, such as hypercortisolism, hypoadrenocorticism, pheochromocytoma, hyperaldosteronism, hypothyroidism, and diabetes mellitus.[1,3,4] Therefore, it is crucial to know the available methods to determine blood pressure as well as their advantages and disadvantages.

Blood pressure measurement techniques

Blood pressure methodology can be classified as invasive or direct, and noninvasive or indirect measurement. The gold standard method to determine BP is the invasive technique, which involves catheterization of an artery and is mainly performed in anesthetized or critically ill animals.[3] A noninvasive BP measurement approach is more commonly used in daily clinical practice for screening and therapy monitoring.

Video 20.1

Placement of an arterial catheter in the dorsopedal artery of a small dog undergoing general anesthesia to provide continuous blood pressure monitoring. (Courtesy of the Anesthesia and Analgesia Service of the Veterinary Teaching Hospital Complutense)

Video 20.2

Flushing of the plastic tube with heparinized saline, connection between the transducer (placed at the same height as the right atrium) and the arterial catheter, and calibration of the transducer to atmospheric pressure ("zeroed") (Courtesy of the Anesthesia and Analgesia Service of the Veterinary Teaching Hospital Complutense).

When measuring BP in dogs, it is essential to follow standardized protocols and use equipment appropriate for the size of the animal. Additionally, consider factors such as the dog's temperament, stress level, and overall health, as these can influence BP readings. All these factors, as well as cuff size and site placement, the animal's position, values, and the meaning of the values considered valid (and the reasons to exclude any value) need to be recorded.[3,5]

Blood pressure measurement can be a spot measurement (in a certain moment, e.g., during a clinical examination) or continuous (i.e., during an anesthetic procedure or in a hospitalized animal), and either direct or indirect methods can be used.[3]

Invasive or direct technique

The invasive or direct technique provides repeatable and accurate BP results. However, technical skills and equipment requirements make this procedure less commonly applied than the indirect BP measurements. The invasive BP measurement is most commonly used when continuous BP measurements are needed rather than one single evaluation.[3]

This procedure involves the catheterization of an artery with a catheter attached to a pressure transducer, which converts the pressure signal into an electric signal that can be registered and displayed as a pressure wave. The preferred options for applying this technique are the dorsal metatarsal, femoral, and coccygeal arteries (Video 20.1). When used for an acute evaluation, a needle can be used instead of a catheter. The catheter or needle is connected to the transducer using a plastic tube filled with heparinized saline (1-2 UI/mL). The transducer must be calibrated ("zeroed") before connecting it to the patient to atmospheric pressure and placed at the same height as the right atrium (Video 20.2).[3]

When used in awake animals, local anesthesia is recommended to increase the tolerability of the procedure. The restraint and the discomfort associated with an arterial puncture might falsely increase BP results. Hypotension, on the other hand, can be reliably detected. After removing the needle or catheter, it is necessary to apply pressure in the puncture for at least 5 minutes,

TABLE 20.1 ACVIM guidelines protocol for blood pressure measurement (BP).

- Semiannual calibration of the blood pressure (BP) devices is mandatory.
- The procedure must be standardized and any events (barking, excessive stress, …), BP measurement technique, cuff size and body position need to be recorded.
- Blood pressure measurement needs to be performed after a 5-10 minute acclimation period, before any other procedure is performed, without sedation and in an isolated environment and away from other animals. Generally, it is useful that the owner is present.
- Measurements will only be recorded when the patient is calm and motionless.
- The animal should be placed ideally in ventral or lateral recumbency to avoid an excessive distance from the heart base to the cuff (if more than 10 cm, a correction factor of +0.8 mm Hg/cm below or above the heart base can be applied). However, it is important to apply minimum restrain and place the animal in a comfortable position.
- The cuff width should be approximately 30%-40% of circumference of the cuff placement site. This can be placed on a limb or the tail.
- The first measurement should be discarded and a total of 5-7 consecutive consistent values should be recorded. If there is a consistent downward trend BP will be measured as many times as necessary until 5-7 consecutive consistent readings are available.
- If inconsistent values are obtained the procedure needs to be repeated, including changing the cuff and the cuff site until consistent readings are obtained.
- Individuals performing these techniques need to be trained.

Modified and adapted Acierno, MJ, Brown, S, Coleman, AE, et al. ACVIM consensus statement: guidelines for identifying, evaluating, and managing systemic hypertension in dogs and cats. *J Vet Intern Med* 32:1803-1822, 2018.

Video 20.3

Blood pressure measurement technique in a Boxer using an oscillometric device with minimum restrain. The measurements should be repeated until 5-7 consecutive consistent readings are obtained (Courtesy of the Emergency and Critical Care Service of the Veterinary Teaching Hospital Complutense).

and it is recommended to monitor the patient for approximately 1 hour in order to detect any complication associated with the formation of a hematoma.[3]

Noninvasive or indirect techniques

The indirect techniques for BP measurement include oscillometry, high-definition oscillometry, and Doppler ultrasonography.[5]

To maximize reliability, it is important to be strict when following the recommendations to perform these measurements and use devices that have undergone validation following the standards for dogs and cats.[5]

Protocol for blood pressure measurements using indirect techniques

The ACVIM consensus statement of 2018 describes the standard protocol that should be followed when indirect techniques are used in awake animals (Table 20.1, Video 20.3).[5]

Significant intraindividual variation is demonstrated when using different indirect devices.[6] Thus, when repeated BP measurements are obtained, the procedure should be performed using the same device and identical cuff, cuff size, and body position.[5]

Methods to measure noninvasive blood pressure

Oscillometry

Arterial BP measurements rely on detecting oscillations in the cuff pressure caused by the pulsatile flow of blood during each cardiac cycle. This method uses an automatic detection system and a cuff placed over an artery of the limbs or tail (Fig. 20.1). It is important to place the center of the inflatable chamber over the artery (usually indicated in the cuffs).

The device automatically inflates the cuff until the artery is occluded and then deflated slowly in a pulsatile way. The system detects the changes in the vessel wall when the pressure is released; the pressure at which oscillations are maximal is considered the mean BP. Depending

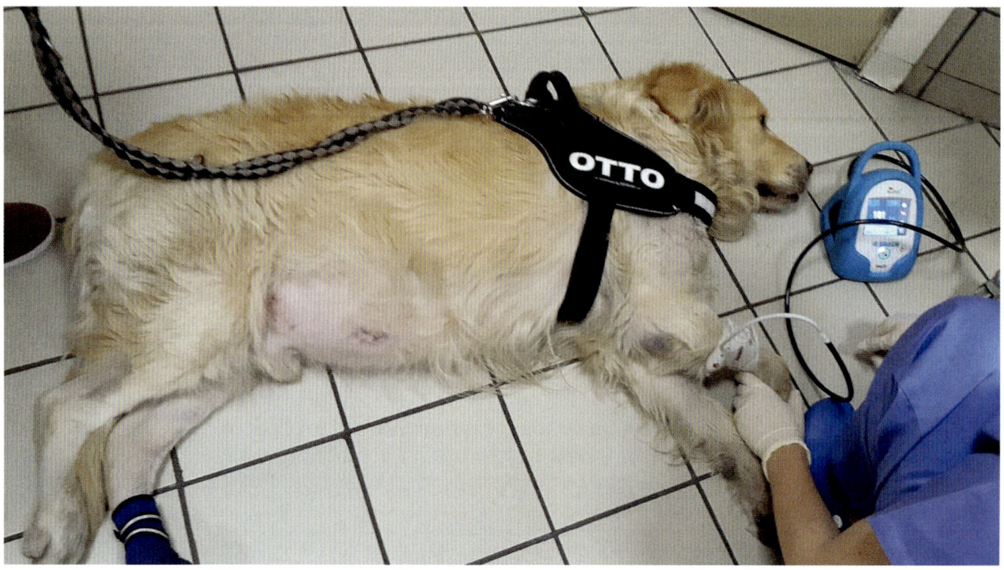

FIG. 20.1 Blood pressure measurement using an oscillometric device in the forelimb of a 12-year-old male Golden Retriever with hypercortisolism using minimum restrain.

on the device, the system usually calculates systolic and diastolic BP using different algorithms. These algorithms typically consider the first detected oscillations as those closer to the systolic BP, and when the device detects a sudden decrease in the amplitude of the oscillations, it uses this value to calculate the diastolic BP.[3]

Oscilometry can be imprecise when the artery is small (i.e., in small dogs). The results might be nonreliable if the patient is moving (including trembling or panting) or when the pulse is weak. Furthermore, systolic BP can be underestimated with this method.[3,5]

High definition oscillometry

When compared to oscillometry, the high-definition oscillometry system allows linear deflation of the cuff, and the algorithms used are specifically designed for animals. This method also might be able to detect a wider range of BPs, measure blood pressure at higher heart rates, and detect arrhythmia. Attempts to compare this method with traditional oscillometric devices or Doppler ultrasonography have rendered variable results. Therefore, high-definition oscillometry does not seem to be more reliable than the other noninvasive methods.[3]

Doppler ultrasonography

This method detects ultrasonic flow in a peripheral artery by detecting frequency changes between ultrasound waves that bounce off blood cells moving within the blood vessel. The frequency variations are converted to audible signals and BD reading.

The steps to perform this procedure are:

- A cuff of an appropriate size, as previously explained, is connected to a sphygmomanometer and placed around an extremity (mid-radius in the forelimb or proximal to the hock in the hindlimb) or around the tail (Fig. 20.2).
- The Doppler ultrasound probe is placed on an artery distal to the cuff, applying ultrasound gel. If necessary, the hair of the zone can be previously clipped. The most common arteries used are the superficial palmar arterial arch in the forelimb, the dorsal pedal artery in the hindlimb, and the coccygeal artery in the ventral aspect of the tail.
- The probe is gently adjusted until the pulse waves are clearly audible. Some animals might be sensitive to the sound of the pulse waves. In these cases, the use of headphones can improve the tolerability of the procedure; however, this does not usually result in lower BP results.
- The probe needs to be in the same position during all the measurements; thus, it can be held or fixed with adhesive tape if the patient allows it.
- The cuff is inflated 20-40 mmHg over the point where the pulse waves are no longer heard.
- Then, the cuff slowly deflates until the Doppler signal is again audible. This is recorded as the systolic BP.
- The cuff is further deflated until the Doppler signal changes in pitch or becomes muffled. This is recorded as the diastolic BP. However, this is subjective, and these changes might not be audible, especially in small or rigid vessels.
- The cuff is completely deflated, and the procedure is repeated as many times as necessary.

This technique is the most operator-dependent among all the indirect measurement techniques, especially for diastolic BP, and accuracy improves when performed by a well-trained operator. Before inflating the cuff, it is necessary to have a clearly audible, strong pulse wave to obtain reliable BP results. This technique is less influenced by movement, arrhythmias, and hypotension. The BP can be overestimated when using Doppler ultrasonography; therefore, it is necessary to repeat the procedure to avoid spurious results.[3,5]

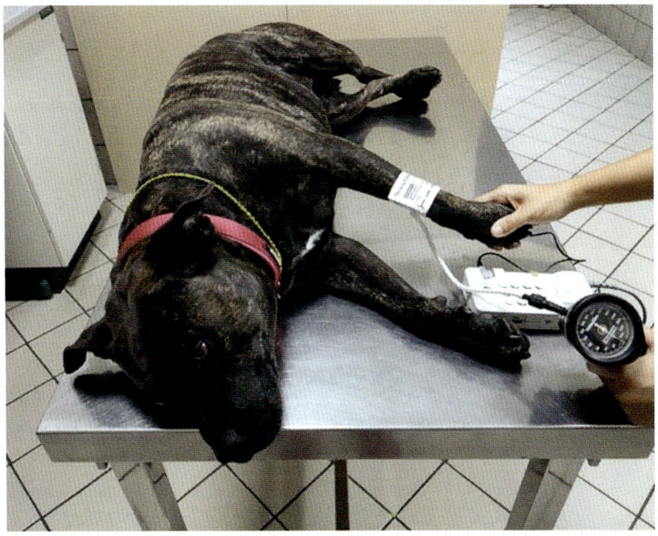

FIG. 20.2 Blood pressure measurement using a Doppler ultrasound device in the forelimb of a 10-year-old female American Staffordshire Terrier with hypercortisolism.

Wrist blood pressure monitors for human use

A white coat effect is unavoidable when measuring BP in clinics. Therefore, wrist blood pressure monitors designed for human use were tested at home in a dog's natural environment. However, the results were inaccurate, so this approach is not recommended.[8]

Indications for blood pressure measurement

The assessment of BP should be performed in every patient with a suspicion of an alteration of BP, in all animals with a condition known to affect BP, and during the monitoring of anesthetized and hospitalized patients. It can also be evaluated as part of the routine evaluation of every patient, especially in senior dogs, in order to obtain a baseline for an individual patient.[3,5]

Endocrine diseases associated with systemic hypertension include hypercortisolism, hyperaldosteronism, diabetes mellitus, pheochromocytoma, and hypothyroidism.[4,5] Hypoadrenocorticism is most commonly associated with hypotension. Interestingly, hyperkalemia due to hypoaldosteronism can cause bradycardia instead of tachycardia, even in hypotensive patients, and this discrepancy must alert the clinician of hypoadrenocorticism.[1]

Treatment options are discussed in detail in chapters dedicated to the above-mentioned conditions.

KEY POINTS

- Many endocrine diseases of dogs are associated with hypotension or hypertension, like hypercortisolism, hypoadrenocorticism, pheochromocytoma, hyperaldosteronism, hypothyroidism, and diabetes mellitus.
- The gold standard technique to measure blood pressure is invasive, which requires catheterization of an artery.
- Noninvasive or indirect techniques include oscillometry, high-definition oscillometry, and Doppler ultrasonography.
- Blood pressure measurements must follow standardized protocols and appropriate equipment to warrant reliability.

References

1. Waddell LS. Systemic hypotension. In Ettinger S, Feldman EC, Côté E (editors). Textbook of Veterinary Internal Medicine 8th edition. St. Louis, Elsevier, 2017, pp. 671-675.
2. Schauvliege S. Patient monitoring and monitoring equipment. In Duke-Novakowski T, de Vries M, Seymour C (editors). BSAVA Manual of Canine and Feline Anesthesia and Analgesia, 3rd edition. Gloucester, BSAVA, 2016, pp. 77-96.
3. Stepien R. Blood pressure measurement. In Ettinger S, Feldman EC, Côté E (editors). Textbook of Veterinary Internal Medicine 8th edition. St. Louis, Elsevier, 2017, pp. 377-380.
4. Chalhoub S, Palma D. Pathophysiology and clinical manifestations of systemic hypertension. In Ettinger S, Feldman EC, Côté E (editors). Textbook of Veterinary Internal Medicine 8th edition. St. Louis, Elsevier, 2017, pp. 659-665.
5. Acierno MJ, Brown S, Coleman AE, et al. ACVIM consensus statement: guidelines for the identification, evaluation, and management of systemic hypertension in dogs and cats. *J Vet Intern Med* 32(6):1803-1822, 2018.
6. Marynissen S, Schils G, Stammeleer L, et al. Systolic blood pressure measurements with Doppler ultrasonic flow detector and high-definition oscillometry are comparable on population level but show large intra-individual differences in apparently healthy elderly dogs. *J Am Vet Med Assoc* 261(7):1-8, 2023.
7. Koo ST, Carr AP. Comparison of home blood pressure and office blood pressure measurement in dogs and cats. *Can J Vet Res* 86:203-208, 2022.
8. Martinelli E, Ferriani R, Zanaboni A, et al. Use of a human wrist blood pressure monitor for arterial blood pressure measurements in normotensive conscious dogs in comparison to veterinary high-definition oscillometry. *Vet Med Sci* 8:1429-1433, 2022.

CHAPTER 21

Glucose monitoring

Francesca Del Baldo
DVM, MRCVS, PhD, DECVIM-CA (Internal Medicine)

Measuring blood glucose (BG) concentration (BGc) plays a crucial role in making diagnostic and therapeutic decisions, especially in patients with diabetes mellitus (DM) and with conditions that can lead to hypoglycemia. Glucose monitoring is also applicable to nondiabetic patients at risk of experiencing altered glucose homeostasis, including critical care cases and pediatric patients. The gold standard for determining BGc is automated chemistry analyzers utilizing the hexokinase method. However, due to practical limitations, alternative methods for monitoring BG have been developed over time. Portable blood glucose meters (PBGMs) and implantable glucose sensors, known as continuous glucose monitoring systems (CGMSs), are two such advancements.

Measurement of blood glucose using automated chemistry analyzers

Glucose concentration in blood can be measured using various enzymatic techniques, including glucose hexokinase, glucose oxidase, or glucose dehydrogenase assays.[1] The hexokinase method is the most commonly employed and is considered the gold standard for quantifying glucose concentration in blood. In this method, glucose is converted to glucose-6-phosphate by hexokinase, and then glucose-6-phosphate is further oxidized by glucose-6-phosphate dehydrogenase, resulting in the production of NADH. The amount of NADH produced is directly proportional to the glucose concentration in the blood and is quantified using spectrophotometry.

Improper blood sample handling can give a false decrease (5-10% per hour)[1] in glucose concentration since erythrocytes and leucocytes within a blood sample will carry on metabolizing glucose after collection. Therefore, if the sample is not analyzed immediately, centrifuged to remove cells, or collected into a fluoride oxalate tube to prevent additional glucose utilization by cells, the glucose concentration measured results spuriously low. The impact of this phenomenon is more pronounced in samples with elevated white blood cell or red blood cell counts, as well as in cases of bacterial contamination or infections.

The hexokinase method has several limitations, including the requirement for a relatively large blood volume, longer turnaround time for obtaining results, limited availability, and elevated costs.

Use of portable blood glucose meter devices

Portable blood glucose meter devices

Portable blood glucose meters (PBGMs) are small devices designed for humans with diabetes mellitus to self-monitor BGc. They allow faster, cheaper, and easier BG measurement compared to laboratory methods and simultaneously require a small sample volume. Nowadays, these devices are used either to generate blood glucose curves or single glucose measurements in diabetic patients. In addition, they can routinely be used to screen patients for hyperglycemia or hypoglycemia. Over time, several new PBGMs from various manufacturers have appeared on the market. Many of them possess various new qualities, such as greater precision, faster measurements, decreased blood volume required to obtain the results, and reduced dependence on operator technique.

These systems quantify glucose by using an enzymatic reaction, which occurs after matching the sample with a disposable test strip containing glucose oxidase-like enzymes. Measurements can be obtained using either a reflectometric technique or an impedenziometric assay. In reflectometric devices, a drop of blood is placed on a test strip, and an oxidative reaction occurs in the reaction layer, resulting in the production of gluconic acid and hydrogen peroxide. The peroxide then reacts with the enzyme peroxidase, causing oxidation of a reactive dye on the strip. The resulting color intensity corresponds to the glucose concentration, which is automatically converted into a glucose measurement. In impedenziometric devices, the plasma diffuses into an internal layer of the test strip containing enzymes (glucose oxidase or glucose dehydrogenase) and electrodes. The enzymes catalyze the conversion of glucose to gluconic acid, generating electrons that produce a current calibrated to measure the glucose concentration in the specimen.

Currently, a wide range of PBGM is available on the market, most of which are intended for human use. Some models require coding or calibration by inserting a code strip or number into the meter when using new test strips. Incorrect coding can lead to inaccurate readings. Other models feature "no coding technology", automatically calibrating and coding with each test strip insertion. Given the high number of PBGMs commercially available, when considering PBGMs for clinical use in dogs, it is essential to select devices assessed in independent quality control studies. Nowadays, the accuracy of PBGMs is assessed based on the criteria outlined by the International Standards Organization (ISO 15197:2013), which specify acceptable ranges for glucose measurements compared to reference methods (Fig. 21.1).[2] These criteria are specifically intended for use in human medicine and are characterized by strict standards. Consequently, a certain level of deviation from the reference method can be allowed. When applied to dogs, the accuracy of commercially available PBGM devices designed for humans varies significantly. Some PBGMs are sufficiently accurate and precise for monitoring the BGc in dogs. However, most of these devices tend to underestimate the actual BGc compared to the laboratory reference method.[3,4] This underestimation occurs because most PBGMs designed for humans are plasma-calibrated (i.e., by using a formula, they display a glucose concentration as if it was derived from plasma and not from capillary whole blood) in order to facilitate comparison between laboratory and PBGM measurements.[3] Since the amount of glucose within the red blood cells compared to the glucose in plasma in dogs is lower than in humans (7% vs. 50%), those PBGMs may underestimate the "true" BGc.

To date, AccuChek Aviva Nano (Roche Diagnostics)[4] and Accu-Chek Performa (Roche Diagnostics)[5] are among the most accurate human PBGM for use in dogs. The AlphaTRAK (Abbott Animal Health) is specifically developed for veterinary use and is considered the most suitable PBGM for use in dogs. This device is plasma-calibrated, taking into account the different glucose distribution between whole blood and plasma. The AlphaTRAK demonstrates higher accuracy and precision compared to PBGMs designed for humans.[3] Moreover, it offers additional advantages, such as requiring a small sample volume (0.3 mL) and having an extended measurement range (20-750 mg/dL; [1.1-41.6 mmol/L]). However, glucose readings obtained with AlphaTRAK may exhibit significant deviations from the reference method, with differences increasing as the BGc increases. In contrast to many human PBGMs, which usually give BG values that are lower than the reference method, the AlphaTRAK may either under (55% of BG measurements) or overestimate (43% of BG measurements) the "true" glucose concentration.[3] Because of this lack of consistency, caution should be used in interpreting the results obtained with AlphaTRAK. If there is any doubt regarding the accuracy of a BGc result, the measurement should be repeated with the same meter and, ideally, with the laboratory reference method.

There are many potential sources of error in the determination of BGc using these systems, and these sources may vary slightly from one device to another.[6] These sources include operator-related factors such

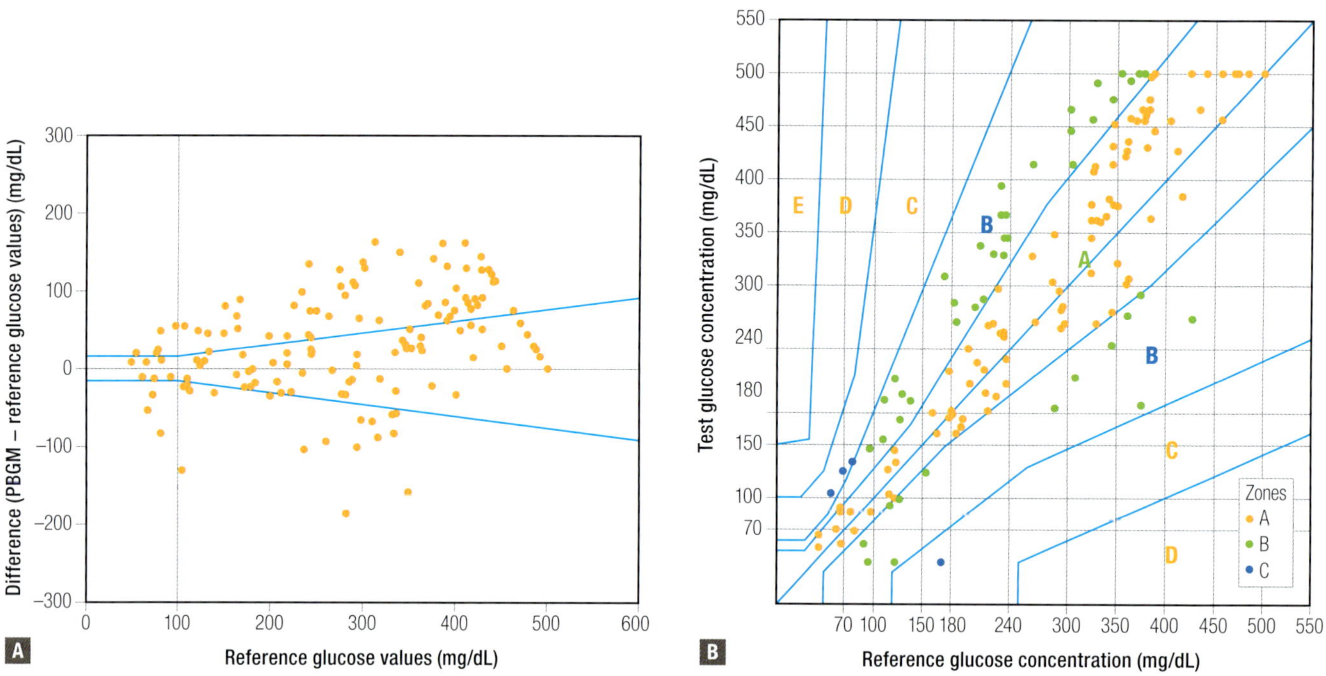

FIG. 21.1 ISO 15197:2013ISO criteria used to assess the accuracy of portable blood glucose meters. (A) Bland-Altman plots: on the x-axis are the reference glucose values, plotted against the differences between the two techniques. The standard required limits are defined by the symmetric lines: at ±15 mg/dL from the reference value for glucose determinations <100 mg/dL and at ± 15% from the reference for glucose ≥100 mg/dL. At least 95% of the PBGM glucose measurements should fall within ±15 mg/dL (0.84 mmol/L) of the reference method at blood glucose concentrations <100 mg/dL (5.6 mmol/L) and within ±15% of the reference method at blood glucose concentrations ≥100 mg/dL.[1] (B) Error grid analysis: the reference glucose values on the x-axis are plotted against the blood glucose values obtained by the glucose meter (y-axis). The EGA categorizes errors in blood glucose measurements based on their potential clinical risk. The grid is divided into five zones as follows: zone A results will not have an effect on clinical action; zone B results will alter clinical action, but the action will have minimal effect on the clinical outcome; zone C results will prompt clinical action that is likely to affect the clinical outcome; zone D results will cause errors in treatment that could pose a substantial medical risk to the patient; and zone E results will cause severe treatment errors that could have dangerous consequences for the patient. ISO 15197:2013 requires that 99% of the values fall within zones A + B for a device to be considered accurate.

as improper machine calibration, the use of outdated reagent strips, and incorrect blood droplet size or placement. Environmental factors such as temperature, altitude, and humidity can also influence the accuracy of the measurements.[6] Other factors that may affect BG determination include patient hematocrit (HCT),[6] blood oxygen pressure, blood pH, plasma concentrations of substances like triglycerides and bilirubin, and concurrent drug administration.[6] The impact of HCT on PBGM readings is particularly noteworthy, especially in critical care patients who often have conditions leading to abnormal erythrocyte count. In animals with low HCT, PBGMs consistently overestimate BGc,[7] while an increased HCT can result in a decrease in the measured BGc.[7] This effect is believed to be caused by altered diffusion rates of plasma to the test strip reagent pad due to abnormal RBC counts.[7]

Sampling and lancing devices

Capillary blood samples for glucose measurements can be obtained from various sites, including the ear, oral mucosa, and paw pads (Fig. 21.2). According to several studies, BG values obtained from the various sample sites do not differ significantly.[8,9] Therefore, the best site to collect the blood samples is the one that the animal tolerates the best and consistently yields an adequate blood sample. In the author's experience, the inner aspect of the pinna is one of the best sampling sites in dogs (Fig. 21.2A). Blood sampling from the oral mucosa is another option in dogs (Fig. 21.2B). If using this site, it is recommended to dry the buccal mucosa with dry gauze before sampling to avoid obtaining falsely low results. Paw pads can also provide excellent blood samples; however, collecting from the metacarpal, metatarsal, or digital pads can be uncomfortable and carries a risk of contamination. Using the wrist pad (Fig. 21.2C) on the forelimb can alleviate these issues and is generally well tolerated.

After the puncture and collection of the blood drop, no pressure is usually required as no bleeding is expected after capillary sampling. Different lancing devices are available for collecting capillary blood samples. These devices, equipped with spring-loaded lancets, provide controlled skin penetration at various depths. They come in different gauge sizes and offer various depth settings. The choice of whether and which lancing device to use depends on individual preference. Alternatively, a hypodermic needle can be used.

Continuous glucose monitoring systems

Continuous glucose monitoring systems use transcutaneous or subcutaneous sensors to measure interstitial glucose (IG) concentration (IGc). These devices typically consist of a sterile single-use sensor, a glucose monitor that records data, and a communication device for data download. In addition, wireless devices utilize a transmitter to distribute information from the sensor to the monitor. The first-generation systems allowed only a retrospective analysis of the glucose concentrations after disconnecting the sensor and uploading the data (retrospective CGMS), whereas the newest-generation devices measure and display the data immediately, allowing direct intervention (real-time CGMS). These systems detect glucose using technologies similar to those of the PBGM.

When using these devices, it is important to consider that the systems measure IG, not BG. The relationship between interstitial and plasma glucose levels is explained by a two-compartment model, where the capillary wall acts as a barrier to the diffusion of glucose between plasma and interstitial fluid (ISF).[10] The changes in ISF glucose concentration are influenced by the rate of glucose diffusion across the capillary wall and the glucose clearance rate from the ISF. Glucose clearance from the ISF depends on insulin-mediated uptake by surrounding cells, which is proportional to ISF glucose concentration and cellular uptake rate. When cellular uptake is negligible, and the diffusion rate remains constant, a steady-state relationship exists between interstitial and plasma glucose concentrations.[10] However, there is a delay in glucose diffusion from plasma to ISF, resulting in a lag phase between rapid changes in BG and IG. The delay has been estimated to be 5 to 12 minutes in dogs.[10] The lag phase can also be affected by the diffusion of glucose from the ISF into the sensor. However, available CGMSs have digital filters designed to compensate for this delay.

Several human CGMSs are currently available, and some of them have been studied for use in dogs: Guardian Real Time® (Medtronic), MiniMed Gold® (Medtronic), GlucoDay® (Menarini diagnostic), FreeStyle Libre® (Abbott), and Eversense® (Senseonics).[10] Most of these CGMSs have some defects which limit their clinical use. They require regular calibration two to three times a day by measuring the BGc with a PBGM; therefore, capillary blood sampling is still necessary. The recording range is usually 40-400 mg/dL (2.2-22 mmol/L); data outside this range are correctly recorded but need to be downloaded to be visualized.

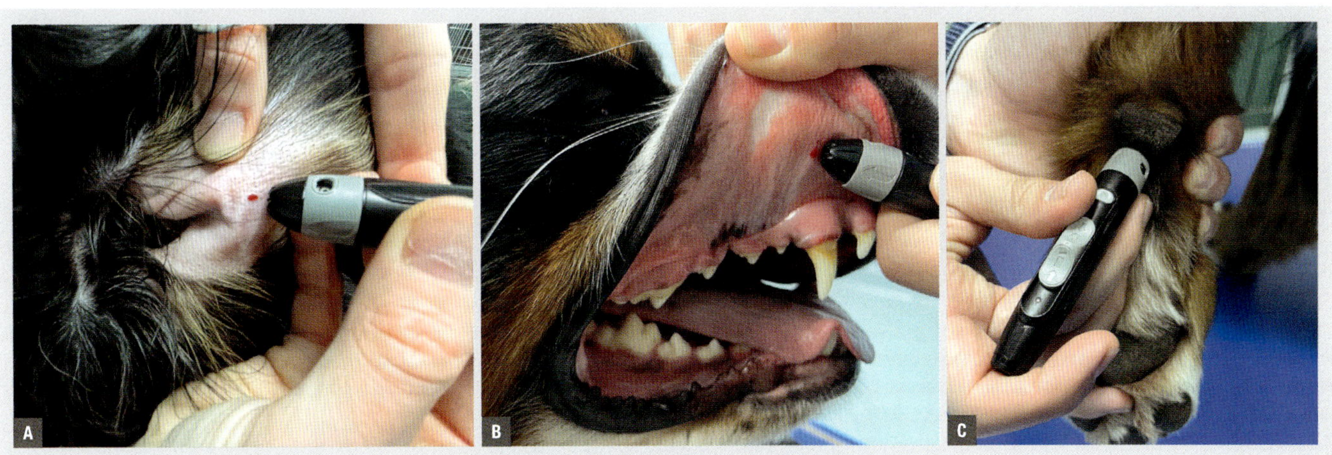

FIG. 21.2 (A) Capillary blood sampling using a lancing device on the inner aspect of the pinna, (B) oral mucosa, and (C) wrist-pad.

Furthermore, if the BGc is outside this range, the system cannot be calibrated, and calibration has to be postponed until the BG is in the working range. Lastly, the sensor is expensive and can only be used for a few days.

Flash glucose monitoring systems

The main difference between FGMSs and CGMSs is that, with a CGMS, the IGc is displayed on a monitoring device automatically or transmitted by Bluetooth to a cell phone or other device. On the other hand, an FGMS only shows IG readings when the sensor is scanned by a reader or a mobile phone with a compatible app. The Abbott FreeStyle Libre® is currently the only FGMS studied in dogs. FreeStyle Libre® 1 consists of a small, lightweight disc-shaped sensor (35 mm × 5 mm) that measures IGc using a small subcutaneous catheter (0.4 mm × 5 mm). It provides comprehensive glucose data without requiring calibration and can be worn continuously for up to 14 days. Glucose detection is based on wired enzyme technology, which consists of both enzymatic (glucose oxidase) and amperometric (electrodes) systems.[10] The reduction of glucose by glucose oxidase results in the generation of an electric current, the intensity of which is proportional to the IGc. The detection limits of the sensor are between 20 and 500 mg/dL (1.1 and 27.75 mmol/L); measurements outside this range are recorded as "LO" and "HI," respectively. The FreeStyle Libre is currently the most commonly used CGMS in veterinary medicine. Up to now, all the studies performed on dogs have used FreeStyle Libre 1.

The FreeStyle Libre 2 was developed some years later. The shape is identical to FreeStyle Libre 1, which shares most of its characteristics. The main difference and the most significant improvement is Bluetooth connectivity, which means that the FreeStyle Libre 2 has the ability to provide optional alerts for high and low BG readings. The FreeStyle Libre 3 has recently received a European conformity mark for people with diabetes in Europe. This is the world's smallest, thinnest glucose sensor (70% smaller than the previous systems). This next-generation system provides the same benefits as FreeStyle Libre 2, including 14-day accuracy and optional glucose alarms. However, it has been improved with new features, such as continuous real-time glucose readings automatically delivered to the smartphone every minute and a sensor that is easy to apply using a one-piece applicator. The FreeStyle Libre 3 application and the necessary materials and equipment are shown in Video 21.1. Fig. 21.3 shows how to obtain real-time IG data by scanning the sensor with the reader or with the FreeStyle LibreLink mobile app, available for both Android and iOS operating systems. Fig. 21.4 shows a practical guide for the use of the LibreView system. LibreView is a free, secure, cloud-based diabetes management system provided by Abbott. The system generates summary glucose reports from the uploaded sensor data and provides a secure repository for data. Furthermore, this system allows the glucose data to be easily shared with healthcare professionals.

Video 21.1

Demonstration of FreeStyle Libre 3 flash glucose monitoring system application in a diabetic dog.

Accuracy of FreeStyle Libre 1 in dogs

The device is usually well-tolerated in dogs,[11-15] even if a greater risk of sensor failure might occur in dogs weighing <10 kg.[15] A mild erythema at the site of the sensor application has been the only complication recorded.[11-15] The device has adequate clinical accuracy in dogs with DM. The mean ± SD differences from the reference hexokinase method were

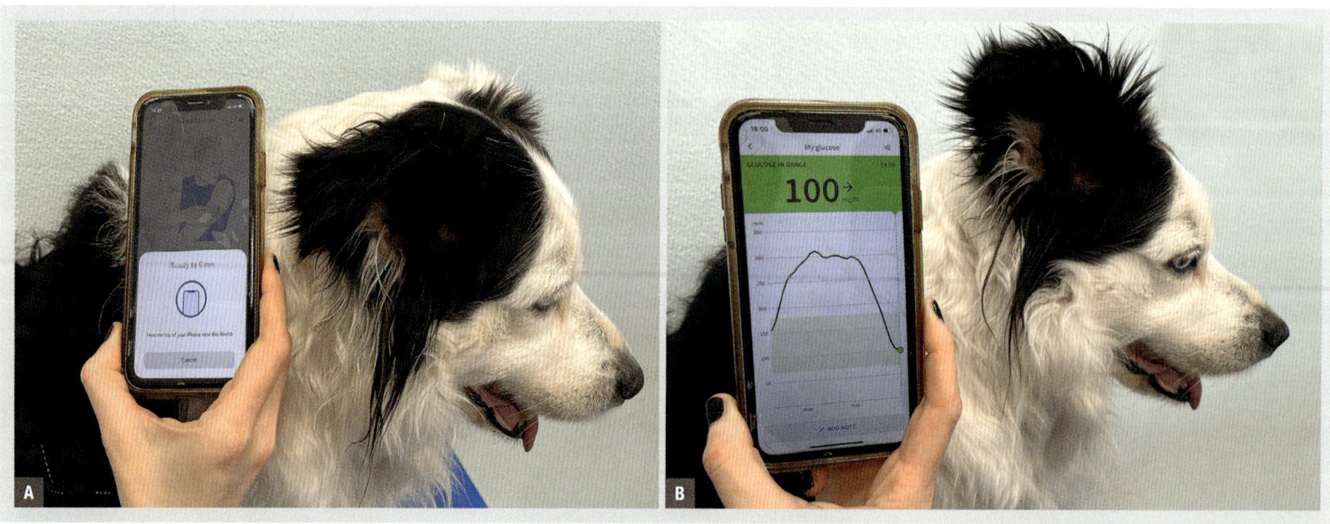

FIG. 21.3 Images showing how to obtain interstitial glucose data in real-time. (**A**) The IG concentrations are transferred from the sensor to the phone (*) with the compatible FreeStyle LibreLink app when the user brings the phone into close proximity to the sensor. Scanning can be performed as often as is needed to measure the current IG concentration; otherwise, the measurements are automatically recorded and stored on the sensor (every 15 minutes) and displayed on the reader/phone when scanned (#). (**B**) After the scan, the phone displays the current sensor IG concentration, an IG trend arrow, and the IG concentrations over the preceding 8 hours.

* With FreeStyle Libre 1 and 2 scanning can be performed also with the proper reader. The reader stores the data for 90 days. The reader can be reused with a new sensor at the end of the recording period. A USB port on the reader can be used to charge it and download all the data onto a computer using the LibreView system. # With the use of FreeStyle Libre 3 and FreeStyle Libre 2 with version 2.10 of the FreeStyle LibreLink app, glucose readings are streamed directly to the smartphone every minute without the need to scan the sensor.

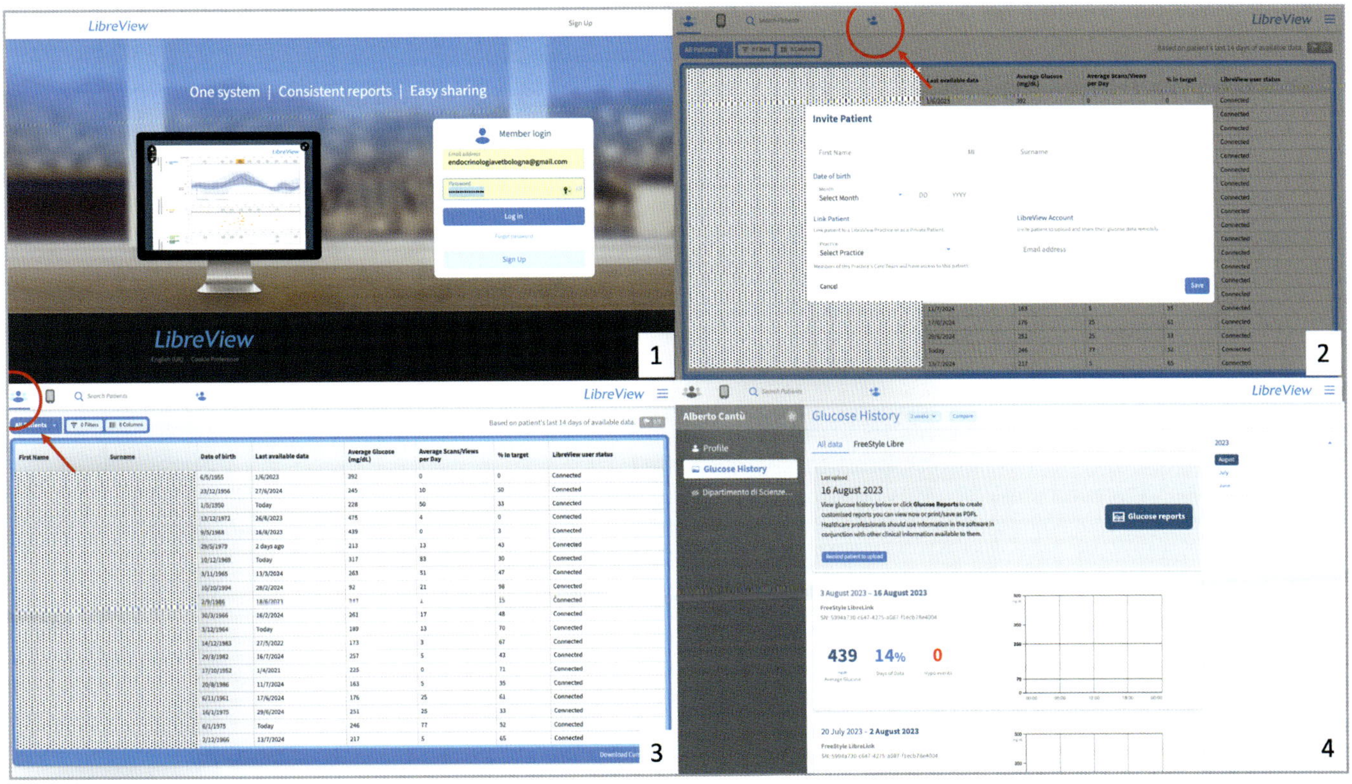

FIG. 21.4 Practical guide to using Libre view: (**1**) Log in to LibreView (www.libreview.com)or register if you are using it for the first time; (**2**) Invite the animal's owner (using the email with which he/she subscribed to the "LibreLink" app) by clicking the icon highlighted with the red circle; (**3**) Access the "Patient Dashboard" by clicking the icon highlighted with the red circle and select the desired patient; (**4**) By selecting glucose reports, a list of different data views will appear on the left. Among the various available reports, one of the most useful is the Daily Log, which displays 24-hour glucose fluctuations during the monitoring period (see Fig. 39.4).

2.3 ± 46.8 mg/dL (0.13 mmol/L ± 2.6 mmol/L)[11] and 17.2 ± 39.3 mg/dL (0.95 mmol/L ± 2.18 mmol/L).[15] However, the FGMS readings were less accurate for glucose concentrations <70 mg/dL (3.8 mmol/L).[11]

Despite the lower accuracy in the hypoglycemic range, overall, the Consensus Error Grid Analysis (EGA) results showed adequate clinical accuracy, with 99% of the IG readings falling in zones A and B.[11] In the hypoglycemic range (reference method BG <100 mg/dL; [5.5 mmol/L]), the mean absolute difference between the FGMS and the reference hexokinase method was 22.3 mg/dL (1.24 mmol/L).[16] The proportions of IG readings within ± 15 mg/dL (0.83 mmol/L) of the reference BG was only 39.1%, well below the >95% minimum mandated by the ISO 15197:2013 criteria. The Consensus EGA showed that only 80.1% of paired glucose values were in zones A and B.[16] Moreover, FGMS was not reliable in detecting rapid changes in the BGc.[16]

Changes in metabolic variables that occur in dogs with diabetic ketoacidosis (ketosis, acidosis, hyperlactatemia) did not affect the accuracy of the device;[12] however, in dehydrated animals, the FGMS was less accurate.[14] Hematocrit, hemolysis, icterus, or lipemia did not affect FGMS readings.[15] In contrast, skin thickness can affect FGMS accuracy because dogs with thinner skin showed less accurate measurements as compared to dogs with thicker skin (>5 mm).[17]

New technologies

Eversense® (Senseonics) is a novel long-term implantable CGMS consisting of a subcutaneously inserted sensor, a wearable transmitter, and a mobile application for displaying glucose information on a handheld device. The main advantage of Eversense XL is its extended sensor lifespan, allowing CGMS wear time of up to 180 days. Furthermore, this device may provide additional ease of use over transcutaneous CGMSs since frequent sensor insertions through the skin are not needed, and the transmitter can be easily removed without the need for sensor replacement. However, unlike transcutaneous CGMSs, the sensor requires a minimally invasive surgical procedure performed by a healthcare professional for implantation and removal. An abiotic (non-enzyme) fluorescent glucose-indicating polymer is grafted to the poly(methyl methacrylate) shell of the sensor. Glucose binding leads to increased fluorescence intensity, which is measured by the optical components of the sensor. The overlying wearable transmitter powers the sensor, employing an inductive link, receiving the fluorescence intensity data and converting it into glucose data, which is then transmitted via Bluetooth for display on the mobile app.

To date, clinical use of Eversense® has been documented in only three diabetic dogs.[18] Device insertion and use were well-tolerated. Eversense® glucose measurements showed a significant correlation with those obtained by FGMS (r = 0.85) and a validated PBGM (rs = 0.81).[18] The device demonstrated acceptable clinical accuracy, with 95.5% of IG readings in zones A and B of EGA. However, analytical accuracy criteria were not satisfied (44% within ISO limits).[18] Limitations associated with the use of the device include excessive movement of the sensor, the need for daily calibrations, high costs, and limited availability.[18] Before considering its routine clinical use, further studies to assess the clinical and analytical accuracy of this device are necessary.

KEY POINTS

- Regular monitoring of the blood glucose concentration (BGc) plays a crucial role in successfully controlling diabetic patients as well as patients with conditions that can lead to hypoglycemia.
- The gold standard for determining BGc is automated chemistry analyzers utilizing the hexokinase method. However, due to several limitations that make this method impractical, over time, many "patient-side" BG monitoring methods have been developed: portable blood glucose meters (PBGMs) and continuous glucose monitoring systems (CGMSs) are two such advancements.
- Portable blood glucose meters (PBGMs) allow a fast, cheap, and easy blood glucose measurement and, at the same time, require a small sample volume. These devices are nowadays used either to generate blood glucose curves in diabetic patients or to screen patients for hyperglycemia or hypoglycemia. Given the high number of PBGMs commercially available, only devices evaluated in independent quality control studies should be considered for clinical use in dogs. Up to date, the most accurate PBGM for dogs is AlphaTRAK (Abbott Animal Health).
- Continuous glucose monitoring systems (CGMSs) emerged as an innovative technology with the potential to revolutionize diabetes management. These systems consist of wearable non/minimally-invasive devices that measure interstitial glucose concentration almost continuously for several consecutive days/weeks, mitigating the need for repeated venipuncture and greatly increasing information regarding glucose fluctuations and trends. Nowadays, the Abbott FreeStyle Libre® flash glucose monitoring system is the most commonly used CGMS. In dogs, the device has adequate clinical accuracy, even if, in the hypoglycemic range, the accuracy is lower.

References

1. Stockham SL, Scott MA. Glucose, ketoamines, and related regulatory hormones. In Stockham SL, Scott MA (editors). Fundamentals of Veterinary Clinical Pathology 2nd edition. Blackwell Ames, 2008, pp.708-731.
2. International Organization for Standardization. In vitro diagnostic test systems—requirements for blood-glucose monitoring systems for self-testing in managing diabetes mellitus (ISO 15197:2013). EN ISO 15197:2015.
3. Cohen TA, Nelson RW, Kass PH, et al. Evaluation of six portable blood glucose meters for measuring blood glucose concentration in dogs. *J Am Vet Med Assoc* 235(3):276-280, 2009. doi:10.2460/javma.235.3.276.
4. Brito-Casillas Y, Figueirinhas P, Wiebe JC, et al. ISO-based assessment of accuracy and precision of glucose meters in dogs. *J Vet Intern Med* 28(5):1405-1413, 2014. doi: 10.1111/jvim.12397.
5. Kang MH, Kim DH, Jeong IS, Choi GC, Park HM. Evaluation of four portable blood glucose meters in diabetic and non-diabetic dogs and cats. *Vet Quart* 36(1):2-9, 2016. doi:10.1080/01652176.2015.1092617.
6. Gerber KL, Freeman KP. ASVCP guidelines: quality assurance for portable blood glucose meter (glucometer) use in veterinary medicine. *Vet Clin Pathol* 45(1):10-27, 2016. doi: 10.1111/vcp.12310.
7. Paul AE, Shiel RE, Juvet F, et al. Effect of hematocrit on accuracy of two point-of-care glucometers for use in dogs. *J Am Vet Med Assoc* 72(9):1204-1208, 2011. doi:10.2460/ajvr.72.9.1204.
8. Zeugswetter FK, Karlovitz S. Bukkale Glukosemessung beim Hund unter Probengewinnung mit Sicherheitslanzetten [Buccal glucose measurements in dogs using safety lancets for blood sampling]. *Tierarztl Prax Ausg K Kleintiere Heimtiere* 42(3):174-179, 2014.
9. Borin-Crivellenti S, Crivellenti LZ, Tinucci-Costa M. The carpal pad as an alternative sampling site for blood glucose testing in dogs. *J Small Anim Pract* 53(12):684-686, 2012. doi:10.1111/j.1748-5827.2012.01299.x.
10. Del Baldo F, Fracassi F. Continuous glucose monitoring in dogs and cats: application of new technology to an old problem. *Vet Clin North Am Small Anim Pract* 53(3):591-613, 2023. doi:10.1016/j.cvsm.2023.01.008.
11. Corradini S, Pilosio B, Dondi F, et al. Accuracy of flash glucose monitoring system in diabetic dogs. *J Vet Intern Med* 30(4):983-988, 2016. doi:10.1111/jvim.14355.
12. Malerba E, Cattani C, Del Baldo F, et al. Accuracy of flash glucose monitoring system in dogs with diabetic ketoacidosis. *J Vet Intern Med* 34:83-91, 2020. doi:10.1111/jvim.15657.
13. Del Baldo F, Canton C, Testa S, et al. Comparison
14. between a flash glucose monitoring system and a portable blood glucose meter for monitoring dogs with diabetes mellitus. *J Vet Intern Med* 34(6):2296-305, 2020. doi:10.1111/jvim.15930.
15. Silva DD, Cecci GRM, Biz G, et al. Evaluation of a flash glucose monitoring system in dogs with diabetic ketoacidosis. *Dom Anim Endocrinol* 74:106525, 2021. doi:10.1016/j.domaniend.2020.106525.
16. Shea EK, Hess RS. Assessment of postprandial hyperglycemia and circadian fluctuation of glucose concentrations in diabetic dogs using a flash glucose monitoring system. *J Vet Intern Med* 35(2):843-52, 2021. doi:10.1111/jvim.16046.
17. Howard LA, Lidbury JA, Jeffery N, et al. Evaluation of a flash glucose monitoring system in nondiabetic dogs with rapidly changing blood glucose concentrations. *J Vet Intern Med* 35(6):2628-2635, 2021. doi:10.1111/jvim.16273.
18. Del Baldo F, Diana A, Canton C, et al. The influence of skin thickness on flash glucose monitoring system accuracy in dogs with diabetes mellitus. *Animals (Basel)* 11(2):408, 2021. doi:10.3390/ani11020408.
19. Tardo AM, Irace C, Del Baldo F, et al. Clinical use of a 180-day implantable glucose monitoring system in dogs with diabetes mellitus: a case series. *Animals (Basel)* 12(7):860, 2022. doi:10.3390/ani12070860.

CHAPTER 22

Hormone measurements

Peter A. Graham
BVMS, PhD, CertVR, DECVCP, SFHEA, MRCVS

The diagnosis and monitoring of canine endocrinopathies depend heavily on measuring hormone concentrations in biological fluids such as serum, plasma, urine, and saliva. The methods used to generate hormone results should be carefully considered to improve the chances of correct diagnoses and patient management decisions.

Types of assays

Immunoassay

The routine measurement of hormones for veterinary clinical purposes is performed by immunoassay. In this method, antibodies that react with the hormone of interest are an integral part of the analytical process. The analytical performance of immunoassays can vary according to the antibodies used, the way the assay is optimized and calibrated, the detection systems used, and whether the assay method has been designed to take account of physiological factors such as protein binding or assay interferences.

Antibodies

Antibodies raised against the hormone of interest are the basic component of an immunoassay. As a product of a biological process, they can have widely varying properties. Antibodies will have different binding characteristics (affinities and avidities) with the hormone with which they are meant to interact, and they may additionally interact with molecules that are structurally like the hormone of interest (cross-reactivity).

Assays may depend on polyclonal antisera raised in individual live animals or monoclonal antibodies generated by laboratory hybridoma or phage display techniques. Polyclonal implies that multiple plasma cell clones have contributed antibodies that react with different epitopes of the molecule (hormone) of interest. Monoclonal antibodies react with a single epitope. There are advantages and disadvantages to each type. Monoclonal antibodies allow for longer useful working life on an assay, while in polyclonal assays, the original antibody pool may exhaust more quickly and require manufacturers to reformulate the assay method. This is relevant for any veterinary hormone measurement that relies on commercial assays from human diagnostics because a reformulated polyclonal human assay may no longer have the performance characteristics in veterinary samples that its predecessor version had. Veterinary laboratories must be particularly vigilant for changes in assay effectiveness by using their own internal independent control samples and by maintaining suspicion about any change in the method components.

The antibodies used will determine how specific the assay is for the hormone and whether it suffers interference from similar molecules. For example, most commercial cortisol assays are based on antibodies that will cross-react with prednisolone, resulting in assay interference. For peptide hormones, there is the added complication of species variation. If a peptide structure is well conserved across species, it is likely that an antibody that works well for one species could work for another too, although this is by no means always the case. Also, there may be sufficient cross-reactivity to use the assay in another species but with less good analytical characteristics, as the antibody may have a lower affinity for the equivalent hormone in a different species.

Immunoassay formats

Immunoassays have been developed in many different formats (Table 22.1). The interaction between patient hormones and antibodies that form the basis of immunoassays needs to be detected in some way. This is possible by combining a detection technology (e.g., gamma counter, luminometer, spectrophotometer) with a signal generation technology (e.g., tracer, labeled antibody, labeled hormone) and calibration based on the signals generated by sample(s) of known concentration. In most systems, there is a separation mechanism so those assay components that have not interacted with antibodies or hormones of interest can be removed before the detection step.

The system may depend on the detection of radiation (radioimmunoassay; RIA), color change (spectrophotometry), or light (luminescence and fluorescence), which is achieved by labeling a hormone or antibody with a radiochemical or an enzyme. Enzyme labels catalyze reactions to induce a color change, luminescence, or fluorescence. For example, in an enzyme-linked immunosorbent assay (ELISA) or lateral flow device, an enzyme (e.g., horseradish peroxidase) catalyzes a color change

TABLE 22.1 Example hormone immunoassay technologies.

Assay platform	Detection	Principle
Siemens Immulite	Chemiluminescence	Alkaline phosphatase catalyzed adamantyl dioxetane phosphate luminescence, coated beads allow centrifuge-assisted wash separation step
IDEXX Snap	Color change	Horseradish peroxidase catalyzed 3,3',5,5'-tetramethylbenzidine color generation. Bidirectional lateral flow and separation wash step
IDEXX Catalyst	Color change	Multilayered slide including a bound monoclonal antibody layer, Horseradish peroxidase catalyzed 3,3',5,5'-tetramethylbenzidine color generation detected by reflectance spectrophotometry
Tosoh AIA	Fluorescence	Alkaline phosphatase catalyzed 4-methyl umbelliferyl phosphate fluorescence. Coated magnetic beads facilitate wash separation
Zomedica Truforma	Bulk acoustic wave	Hormone interaction with antibody labeled with enzyme which catalyzes the generation of insoluble products that induce detectable resonance frequency shift on hormone or antibody-coated acoustic wave resonance sensor. Wash separation step prior to enzyme-substrate addition.
Thermo Microgenics DRI (T_4)	Color change	T_4-conjugated glucose-6-phosphate dehydrogenase catalyzed NAD/NADH color change. Free antibody inhibits G6PDH unless bound competitively to patient T_4 rather than conjugate T_4. Homologous assay, no wash separation step required.
Zoetis Vetscan T_4	Color change	T_4-conjugated glucose-6-phosphate dehydrogenase catalyzed NAD/NADH color change. Free antibody inhibits G6PDH unless bound competitively to patient T_4 rather than conjugate T_4. Homologous assay, no wash separation step required.
Fujifilm AU10	Surface plasmon-enhanced fluorescence	Antibody or hormone-bound fluorescent particle. Laser excitation fluorescence signal generation only from particles interacting with gold film sensor. No wash separation step required

that can be detected spectrophotometrically. In the Siemens Immulite™ systems, alkaline phosphatase catalyzes the luminescence reaction. As a metalloenzyme, it is likely that this enzyme's function would be adversely affected for samples that had been exposed to the chelating agent EDTA and misleading results generated.

The differences between detection systems will affect their resilience against interfering factors, their suitability for automation, and the risks of reagent deterioration. There may be patient-related or other factors that can interfere with color/light generation or detection, but these factors cannot interfere with radiation.

In (heterologous) assays that require a separation step, detection antibodies could be bound to the walls of reaction tubes or wells or to beads that will allow the unbound components to be washed away, leaving only the successful hormone-antibody interaction to be detected (Fig. 22.1). Precipitation and centrifugation could be another option. There are a few (homologous) assays in common use that are designed such that they do not require a wash/separation step (Fig. 22.2).

Regardless of the signal or detection technology, many assays are designed on a competitive principle. In these, a labeled hormone competes with the patient hormone for available antibody binding sites. In a situation of low patient hormone concentrations, there will be a strong signal detected and vice versa. An alternative format that may be commonly used for peptide hormones relies on two antibodies, one bound to a surface that "captures" the hormone and another labeled antibody that binds to the captured hormone. In this two-site immunometric setup, the higher the patient's hormone concentration, the stronger the signal.

In veterinary diagnostic endocrinology, RIA techniques have long been considered the gold standard because of their resilience against interferences and the ability of specialist laboratories to independently tweak and optimize their assays. However, there is no measurement platform technology that is uniformly superior in all circumstances. Whether an individual assay for a particular hormone is useful in a veterinary context will depend on the combination of antibody, assay design and calibration, as well as detection system. A particular detection platform may be very good at measuring one hormone of veterinary interest but not good at measuring another. For example, the Siemens Immulite™ system is used successfully in many veterinary laboratories to measure common measurements, but it cannot be applied for canine parathyroid hormone (PTH) detection.[3]

Signal data processing, optimization, and calibration

In the development stages of an assay, it is possible to optimize it for a specific purpose by adjusting sample volumes, antibody concentrations, reaction temperatures, incubation times, buffer content, etc. Assays may also be optimized to measure a particular range of concentrations or species of hormone. For example, assays that measure salivary cortisol have been optimized for a different concentration range than those that measure serum cortisol, and assays for thyroxine in canine serum are optimized (or modified in the laboratory) to be able to accurately measure the lower concentrations observed in canine serum compared to humans.

Because of the way in which antibodies interact with antigens, the dose-response relationship is usually curvilinear. Such a calibration curve can be somewhat "straightened" by log transformation to make a mathematical estimation of dose from response easier. Radioimmunoassay standard curves will usually contain five or six samples of known concentration across the range of expected values. Some assay systems with sufficiently stable reaction conditions may have curves "in-built" to platform software that is adjusted by one or two calibration samples.

In peptide hormone assays where calibration standards are assigned values based on the human hormone and where the purified veterinary

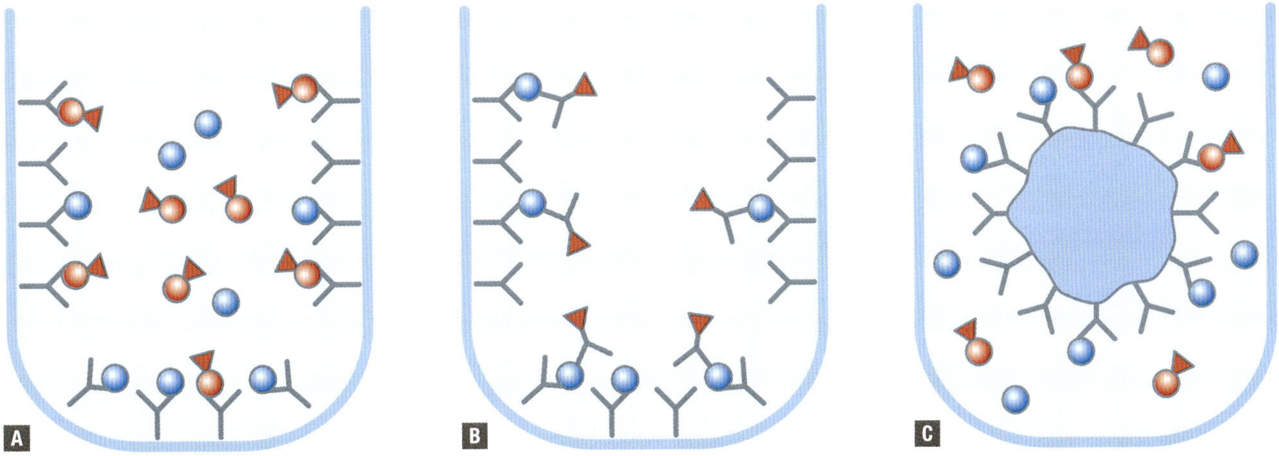

FIG. 22.1 Example immunoassay formats dependent on a wash separation step. The patient's hormone of interest (blue circles) competes for the antibody site with a labeled (red triangle) version in a competitive immunoassay (**A**) or creates a sandwich between two antibodies (immunometric assay) (**B**). Competitive immunoassays have a negative dose-response curve, and immunometric assays have a positive one. Antibodies are depicted bound to the wall of a reaction vessel to facilitate wash separation (**A**), (**B**), or bound to beads (**C**), but alternative substrates (paper, membranes) are possible.

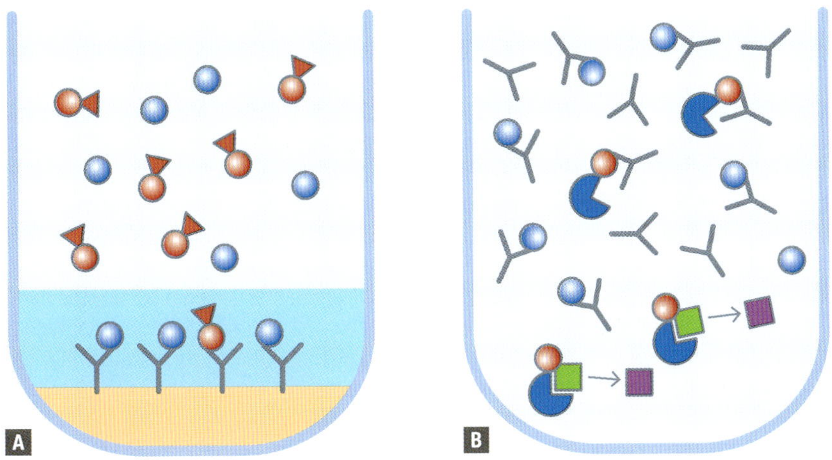

FIG. 22.2 Example immunoassay formats not dependent on a wash separation step. In bulk acoustic wave and plasmon-enhanced surface immunofluorescence (**A**), only the antibody-hormone interactions occurring on or near (shaded) the sensor (yellow) are detected. In the DRI assay format (**B**), enzyme activity catalyzing a color change is blocked by the antibodies unless antibody sites are occupied by the patient hormone (blue circles).

equivalent is not easily available, the combination of the species of the standard and the antibody affinity and cross-reactivity for the veterinary hormone means that in some peptide assays the veterinary result is technically an "equivalent immunoreactivity" in assay units (e.g., ng/mL) rather a true weight by volume of the veterinary hormone. It is this concept that is responsible for the need for different reference intervals for the same peptide analyte across different methods and why sometimes a laboratory will need to alter its reference interval if its assay method (manufacturer, antibody, or standards) changes even though, clearly, the actual serum concentrations of the hormone in the healthy population will not have changed.

Because assays are optimized to perform well across a particular range of measured concentrations, it is not uncommon that outside these ranges, results are reported as ">" or "<". In an assay that needs to use a log-transformed standard curve, the "0" concentration standard cannot be plotted, and estimation of results below the lowest plottable standard is, therefore, inherently difficult. "Less-than" results might also be generated for values below the limit of quantification, that is, the lowest value at which the assay can produce results with acceptable imprecision.

Non-immunological assays

In recent years a small number of veterinary laboratories have started to implement non-immunological assay systems for hormones. These are generally chromatographic methods coupled with a detection system, and increasingly, that detection system is tandem mass spectrometry (e.g., LC-MSMS). These systems do not suffer the variation in antibody binding and cross-reactivity problems of immunoassays and are likely to become more common. That said, although the potential for greater harmonization of results between laboratories exists for this technology, in current practice, this is not achieved yet.

Binding proteins and free hormone measurement

Hormones that are significantly protein-bound may require sample pretreatment before an immunoassay procedure. For example, steroids may be solvent-extracted before analysis to make the molecule more available for interaction with detection antibodies. However, this step has been largely lost from most commercial routine methods for common veterinary steroids (e.g., cortisol). Extraction methodology is still employed in the measurement of IGF-1, and the methods chosen will affect the reliability of IGF-1 measurement in veterinary samples.[4] In the case of total T_4 measurement, T_4 is displaced from binding proteins to enable antibody interactions using aniline naphthalene sulphonic acid (ANS).

Some hormones' biological activities correlate better with their free rather than total concentration. The most relevant canine example is free T_4. The accurate and reliable measurement of free T_4 poses some challenges. It is important that the assay reagent components, including antibodies, binding proteins, and labeled hormones, do not interfere disruptively with the equilibrium between bound and free hormones in the sample. Detection antibody binding capacities have to be low to avoid "stripping" extra T_4 from serum binding proteins, buffer components (e.g., albumin) should have limited impact on the free faction, and the labeled T_4 (analog) should not interact with serum binding proteins despite being able to interact with detection antibodies. Anything that disturbs the equilibrium too much will mean that a free T_4 assay behaves more like a total T_4 assay and loses the advantages that free T_4 measurement should bring. One effect of non-thyroidal illness is to lower thyroid hormone binding capacity in serum, and assays need to be constructed in such a way that they still function well in situations of such lowered thyroid binding capacity.

There are three main categories of free T_4 methods: 1) equilibrium dialysis, 2) two-step immunoassay, and 2) one-step (analog) methods. The first two are less likely to be subject to interference from, e.g., altered serum binding capacity in non-thyroidal illness. In the first, T_4 equilibrates in a dialysate buffer across a membrane that "removes" binding proteins from the subsequent measurement reactions. In the second, patient serum is washed from the antibody-coated reaction tube before labeled T_4 is added, limiting the influence of binding proteins and in the third, patient serum, including binding proteins labeled T_4 and detection antibodies are incubated in one step, making the interactions between patient hormone and detection antibodies more susceptible to the influence of T_4-binding proteins.

Free hormone methods require a different validation interpretation approach compared with total hormone methods. A common part of immunoassay validation protocols would be serial dilution (see below). The equilibrium kinetics of highly bound hormones (e.g., T_4) are such that low magnitude dilutions should not cause a change in result. That is, although we expect the result of a 1 in 4 dilution to generate a result of 25% of the undiluted serum in a total hormone assay, in a free T_4 assay, we would not expect to see a change. This can be a simple way of determining whether a particular free T_4 assay is likely to be a true free hormone method (rather than one that mimics total T_4 interpretation). Additionally, any "method comparison" approach to determine accuracy needs to use serum samples from patients with a wide range of hormone binding capacities as well as varying hormone concentrations.

Video 22.1

Endocrine immunoassay quality. The process of understanding the reliability of endocrine laboratory results.

Validation, verification, and quality

It is important that assays used in endocrinology publications and for diagnostic and therapeutic monitoring decisions are fit for their intended purpose. Commercial methods developed for human use applied to veterinary samples should be "validated," and those developed and marketed for veterinary use should be "verified."

A validation protocol should include evaluation of imprecision, accuracy, specificity, and sensitivity and would often be enhanced by the generation of reference intervals, diagnostic thresholds, and investigation of common interferents (Video 22.1).

Imprecision is usually assessed by repeated measures of a sample of clinically relevant concentrations (close to decision thresholds) and is expressed as the analytical coefficient of variation ($CVA\% = 100 \times$ standard deviation/mean).

Accuracy (or bias) is the difference between results generated and the "true value," and it can be assessed in a variety of ways, including spike/recovery of purified hormone in samples or by method comparison with an established, validated method,[2] or external quality assessment reports.

Specificity is a measure of whether closely related substances will be detected in the assay and falsely attributed to the hormone of interest. Commercially produced methods will usually have a list of related compounds that have been assessed in their instructions for use, e.g., dexamethasone or prednisolone in a cortisol assay and fludrocortisone in an aldosterone assay. Specificity can also be assessed by dilutional parallelism of patient results with the standard curve.

Sensitivity has been variably defined as the smallest change in concentration that can be detected or the smallest concentration that can be discerned from zero. This may be established as a limit of detection (LoD) by multiple repeat analyses of serum that does not contain the hormone of interest (expressed as mean + 2× standard deviation of results) or as a limit of quantification (LoQ) the lowest concentration that can be measured with acceptable imprecision.

When a completely untried method is proposed, a cost-effective preliminary investigation can be achieved with a small sample mixture study to determine whether it will be worth progressing to full validation. Two individual (or pools of) serum samples with expected low or high concentrations of the hormone of interest are mixed together 50:50, and the subsequently created samples can be mixed further with the starting samples to create sets of three, five, or nine samples that should have concentrations that lie on a straight line when plotted equidistantly (Fig. 22.3). Methods that yield results that have a curvilinear relationship or do not land on a straight line will have some limitation in one or more of the performance evaluation metrics above.

Benefits and implications of validation/verification

The data arising from a validation or verification study may be helpful in multiple ways. Knowledge of CVA, especially combined with published biological variation data, allows for an understanding of the degree of "grey zone" a method has around a cutoff value (e.g., a cortisol CVA of 15% around a cortisol cutoff of 40 nmol/L represents a threshold range of 28-52 nmol/L. The CVA will also help calculate a reference change value,[5] and determine whether results generated by repeat analysis of the sample are the "same as" or "different" from the first result.[1]

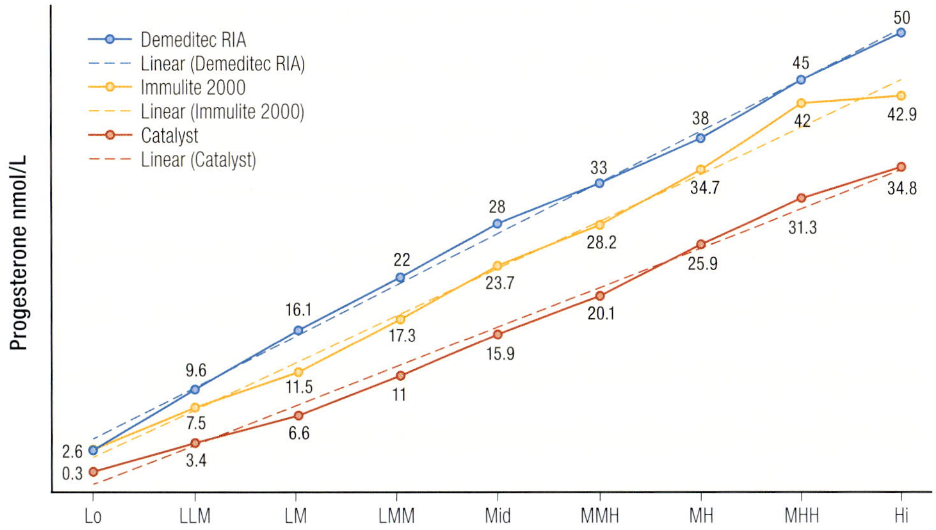

FIG. 22.3 Preliminary comparison of three methods for serum progesterone. Samples were created by mixing pools of canine serum of low (Lo) and high (Hi) progesterone concentration in 50:50 proportions to create an equidistant concentration. All nine samples were analyzed by three methods. The three methods generated a range of results that could generate discordant interpretations if the same interpretive guidance was used (e.g., for timed mating)

The combination of CVA and bias allows for the calculation of the total error, which can be compared with the medically acceptable error, which in turn allows for the establishment of the most appropriate quality control approach and the concept of "controllable error". That is, if the best that the QC system can achieve is that it will only notice an assay deterioration if it causes a 30% change in results and the diagnostic thresholds and clinical decisions are based on an expectation that error is less than 20%, errors of interpretation will occur.

Interferences

An element of method validation/verification is understanding the susceptibility of the method to generate misleading results in the presence of interfering factors. The potential interference of lipemia, icterus, and hemolysis and the impact of sample type (e.g., gel tubes, EDTA plasma) are usually studied. For protein-bound hormones, interference that affects the free fraction needs to be understood (e.g., free fatty acids and furosemide as positive interferents for free T_4).
Given immunoassays' reliance on laboratory antibodies, the presence of patient antibodies against assay components (e.g., anti-mAb) or hormones of interest will cause misleading results. Whether results are falsely elevated or decreased depends on how the assay method has been designed. Examples in veterinary applications include T_4 cross-reacting antithyroglobulin antibodies and anti-insulin antibodies.

Transferability of results

The variation in laboratory results is likely greater for non-conserved peptides and glycoproteins. However, even when molecular structure is conserved (e.g., cortisol, T_4), different methods may yield different results, and the same method might yield different results when implemented in different laboratories. Therefore, method-specific and/or locally derived reference intervals and diagnostic thresholds are important. Not all published diagnostic thresholds will transfer well to all laboratories and methods.
The European Society for Veterinary Endocrinology External Quality Assessment Scheme (ESVE EQAS), established in 2012, highlights this variation (Fig. 22.4 and Fig. 22.5).
Furthermore, sample collection and handling can influence the results. The handling recommendations of large veterinary endocrinology laboratories are provided in Table 22.2.

Cortisol

	n	Mean	StDev	%CV
Method 1	1	69		
Method 2	5	88	10.8	12.2
Method 3	5	101	2.9	2.9
Method 4	3	90	1.9	2.1
Method 5	1	107		
Method 6	2	56	10.2	18.3
Method 7	1	58		
Method 8	1	95		
Method 9	17	106	12.8	12.1
Method 10	35	96	8.2	8.5
Method 11	1	42		
Method 12	1	125		
		Trimmed	*Adjusted*	
All Methods	**73**	**97**	**12.6**	**13.0**

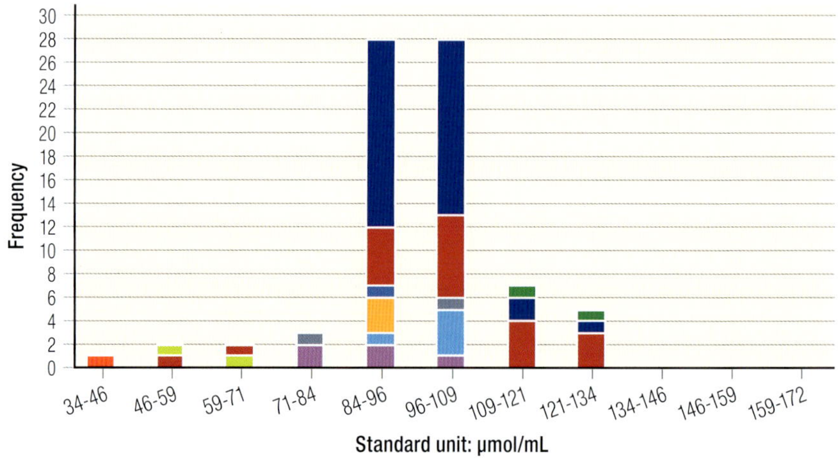

Note: reported results ranged from 42 to 126 nmol/L.
Although method 11 yielded a low result compared to the consensus, it is reported against a lower reference range than most other labs. Methods 7 and 8 were in-clinic analyzers.

FIG. 22.4 Interlaboratory variation in cortisol results in an external quality assessment scheme. Comparison of results generated by 73 veterinary laboratories for canine cortisol in the ESVE EQA scheme.

Insulin

	n	Mean	StDev	%CV
Method 1	1	19.0		
Method 2	1	15.8		
Method 3	6	25.1	1.89	7.5
Method 4	1	23.6		
Method 5	3	39.3	2.52	6.4
Method 6	1	54.7		
Method 7	1	1.0		
Method 8	6	1.3	0.65	51.1
Method 9	1	23.3		
Method 10	2	25.9	1.32	5.1
Method 11	1	25.0		
Method 12	0			
		Trimmed	*Adjusted*	
All Methods	**24**	**19.8**	**15.09**	**76.2**

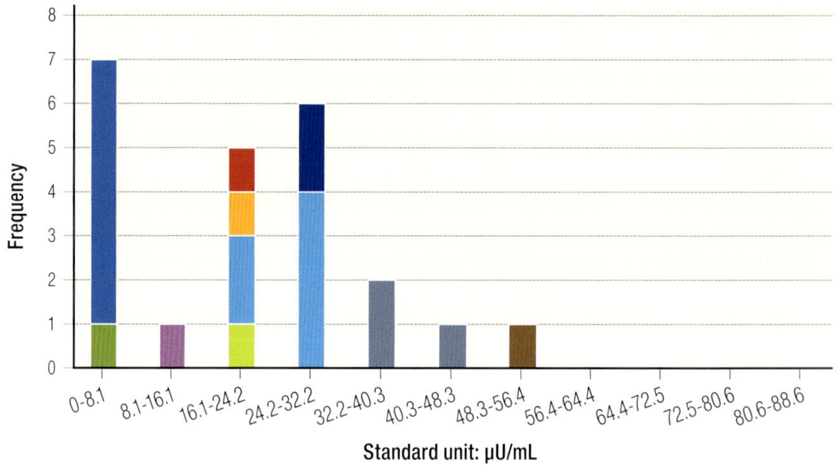

Note: reported results ranged from below the limit of detection to 54.7 µU/mL. Methods 7 and 8 were Siemens Immulite.

FIG. 22.5 Interlaboratory variation in insulin results in an external quality assessment scheme. Comparison of results generated by 24 veterinary laboratories for canine insulin in the ESVE EQA scheme. The Siemens Immulite methods generated lower results for insulin than other methods.

TABLE 22.2 Sample type and handling recommendations for veterinary hormone measurement.

Test	Sample required	Special shipping and handling
Adrenocorticotropic hormone	EDTA plasma	■ Freeze; ship on ice or frozen via overnight courier ■ Must arrive below 16°C
Aldosterone	EDTA or heparin plasma or serum	■ Refrigerate or freeze; ship on ice. Should arrive either overnight or the next day ■ Separate EDTA plasma samples within 30 minutes of collection ■ No special sample handling
Anti-Müllerian hormone	Serum or heparin plasma	■ No special sample handling
Cortisol	Serum or heparin plasma	■ Refrigerate or freeze; ship on ice. Should arrive either overnight or the next day ■ Separate samples within 30 minutes of collection ■ No special sample handling
Erythropoietin	Serum	■ No special sample handling
Gastrin	Serum	■ Refrigerate or freeze; ship on ice during hot months
17-alpha-hydroxyprogesterone	Serum or heparin plasma	■ No special sample handling
Insulin	Serum	■ Refrigerate or freeze; ship on ice ■ Animal should be fasted before collection ■ No special sample handling
Insulin-like growth factor-1	Serum or heparin plasma	■ Refrigerate or freeze; ship on ice ■ No special sample handling
Insulin antibodies	Serum	■ No special sample handling
Metanephrines (blood)	EDTA plasma	■ Freeze; ship on dry ice
Metanephrines (urine)	Urine	■ Acidified ■ Plain ■ Acidification not required (UU) ■ Freeze; ship on ice
Estradiol	Serum or heparin plasma	■ No special sample handling
Parathyroid hormone	Serum or EDTA plasma	■ Refrigerate or freeze; ship on ice or frozen via overnight courier ■ Must arrive below 16°C ■ Avoid lipemia and hemolysis
Parathyroid hormone-related protein	EDTA plasma	■ Freeze; ship on ice or frozen via overnight courier ■ Must arrive below 16°C ■ Avoid lipemia and hemolysis ■ Do not send an EDTA tube without separating the plasma
Progesterone	Serum or heparin plasma No gel tubes	■ Refrigerate or freeze; ship on ice. Should arrive either overnight or the next day ■ No special sample handling
Relaxin	Heparin plasma	■ No special sample handling
Renin	EDTA plasma	■ Freeze; ship frozen by overnight courier
Testosterone	Serum or heparin plasma	■ Refrigerate or freeze; ship on ice ■ No special sample handling
Thyroglobulin and thyroid hormone autoantibodies	Serum or heparin plasma	■ Avoid hemolysis and lipemia ■ No special sample handling
Thyrotropin (thyroid-stimulating hormone) (canine)	Serum or heparin plasma	■ Avoid hemolysis and lipemia ■ No special sample handling
Thyroxine (total)	Serum or heparin plasma	■ Avoid hemolysis and lipemia ■ No special sample handling

The handling recommendations are generally compiled from Michigan State University –Veterinary Diagnostic Laboratory (USA), NationWide Laboratories (UK), and Utrecht University (NL) guidance. Note the variation in sample handling requirements for individual hormones. This emphasizes the need to refer to the individual laboratory being used.

Modified with permission from Mooney CT, Peterson ME, Shiel RE (editors). BSAVA Manual of Canine and Feline Endocrinology 5th edition, BSAVA.

KEY POINTS

- The diagnosis and management of canine endocrinopathies relies heavily on laboratory results.
- An understanding of the methodology employed, its limitations, and common errors helps prevent inappropriate clinical decisions.
- Immunoassay remains the most common method for hormone measurement, but there are many formats of this technology available, particularly for more common endocrine investigations.
- Different assays and even different laboratories applying the same assay can give variable results.
- It is important to know whether the laboratory or in-clinic analytical method has been validated and whether it is appropriate for the clinical purpose for which it is being put.
- No one signal detection method is uniformly superior to other methods. Multiple factors will determine an assay method's suitability for a particular hormone in a particular species, including the detection system, antibodies, format, calibration, optimization, and analytical range.
- Non-immunological methods of hormone measurement are becoming more accessible; these have the potential to improve aspects of veterinary hormone measurement and harmonization.

References

1. Graham PA. Principles of interpreting endocrine test results. In Mooney CT, Peterson, ME, Shiel RE (editors). BSAVA Manual of Canine and Feline Endocrinology, 2023, pp. 22-28. 10.22233/9781910443866.4
2. Jensen AL, Kjelgaard-Hansen M. Method comparison in the clinical laboratory. *Vet Clin Pathol* 35:276-286, 2006. https://doi.org/10.1111/j.1939-165X.2006.tb00131.x
3. Mooney CT, Shiel RE, Fawcett K, Matthews E, Gunn E. A comparison of canine whole and intact parathyroid hormone concentrations as measured by different assays. *J Small Anim Pract* 60:507-513, 2019. https://doi.org/10.1111/jsap.13006.
4. Tschuor F, Zini E, Schellenberg S, Wenger M, Boretti FS, Reusch CE. Evaluation of four methods used to measure plasma insulin-like growth factor 1 concentrations in healthy cats and cats with diabetes mellitus or other diseases. *Am J Vet Res* 73(12):1925-1931, 2012. doi: 10.2460/ajvr.73.12.1925.
5. Walton RM. Subject-based reference values: biological variation, individuality, and reference change values. *Vet Clin Pathol* 41(2):175-181, 2012. doi:10.1111/j.1939-165X.2012.00414.x

Hypothalamus and pituitary gland: anatomy and physiology

Roberto Chiocchetti
DVM, PhD

Anatomy

Hypothalamus

The hypothalamus forms the floor of the diencephalon and includes the optic chiasm, the tuber cinereum, which continues in the shape of a funnel with the infundibulum (pars proximalis of the neurohypophysis), and a bilobated mammillary body (corpus mamillare).[1] The hypothalamus is crossed by numerous fibers and is made up of numerous small nuclei of functionally important nerve cells.[2] Three hypothalamic regions are recognized: caudal, intermediate, and rostral. The caudal region acts on the sympathetic system, while the intermediate and rostral regions involve the parasympathetic and endocrine systems. The balance between these different structures ensures the maintenance of homeostasis, which is essential for the survival of the individual.[2]

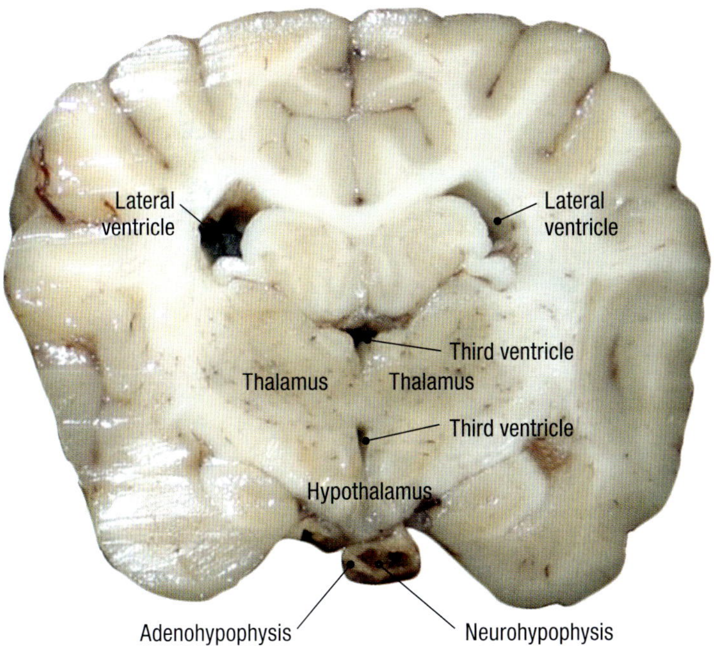

FIG 23.1 Cross section of the formalin-fixed brain of a 1-year-old dog (Great Dane). Original preparation.

Pituitary gland

The pituitary gland is located in the ventral part of the diencephalon (Fig. 23.1 and Fig. 23.2A), housed in the hypophyseal fossa (fossa hypophysialis), a depression of the basisphenoid bone called the sella turcica, caudally limited by the dorsum sellae.
The pituitary gland is surrounded by a doubling of the dura mater, which forms the diaphragma sellae around its peduncle (pituitary stalk), which anatomically and functionally connects the pituitary to the hypothalamus.
The pituitary gland (glandula pituitaria) has a dual embryological origin reflected in a dual structure (adenohypophysis and neurohypophysis) which has distinct functions.[1]

Adenohypophysis

The adenohypophysis (anterior pituitary) is composed of three parts: 1) pars distalis, which forms the greater part of the adenohypophysis (Fig. 23.2A); 2) pars intermedia, the inner part of the adenohypophysis, and 3) pars tuberalis, a tubular sheath extending upwards from the pars distalis, surrounding the infundibulum (neurohypophysis) and part of the hypothalamic median eminence. The hypophyseal portal vessels are found in this space.[1,3]
The pars distalis mainly comprises hormone-producing cells grouped in acini delineated by a basement membrane and capillaries. Endocrine cells show a topological distribution and a numerical organization and may be classified according to their specific secretory products: corticotropic cells (secreting adrenocorticotropic hormone [ACTH], 10-20%) and thyrotropic cells (secreting thyroid-stimulating hormone [TSH], 10%) are more densely distributed in the central portion of the gland, whereas somatotropic cells (secreting GH, 50%), prolactin cells (secreting PRL, 10-20%) and gonadotropic cells (secreting luteinizing hormone [LH] and follicle-stimulating hormone [FSH], 10%) are distributed more laterally. Some cells are multifunctional and can secrete two different hormones (for instance, GH/TSH and FSH/LH). The pars intermedia contains corticotropic cells and melanotropic cells, which produce ACTH and alpha-melanocyte stimulating hormone (α-MSH), respectively.[4] For the most part, the pars tuberalis contains gonadotropic and thyrotropic cells.[5]

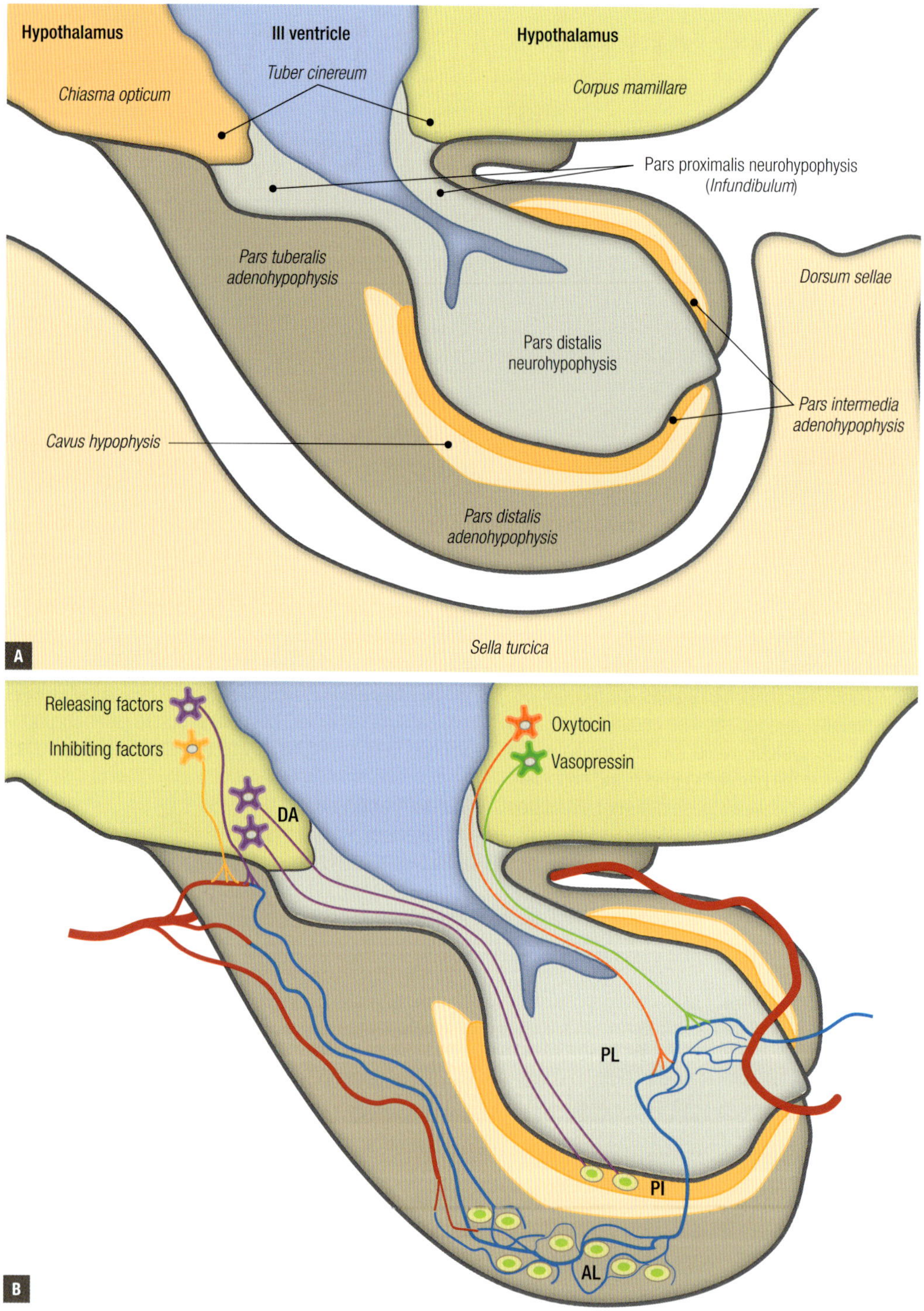

FIG 23.2 (A) Schematic lateral view of the hypothalamus and hypophysis of a dog harbored in the sella turcica of the basisphenoid bone. The schematic drawing shows the different parts of the hypothalamus and hypophysis. (B) Schematic representation of the relationship of the hypothalamus and the pituitary gland. The hypothalamus exerts control over the cells of the anterior lobe (AL) by means of releasing and inhibiting factors that reach the AL cells via the pituitary portal system. The pars intermedia (PI) is under direct neurotransmitter (dopamine, DA) control. The posterior lobe (PL) of the pituitary is the downward projection of the hypothalamus, the neurons that produce, transport, and release vasopressin and oxytocin in the PL. (Adapted from Rijnberk and Kooistra, 2010).

Neurohypophysis

The neurohypophysis (posterior pituitary) consists of two parts: 1) the infundibulum, a funnel-shaped descending projection of the hypothalamus, and 2) the compact pars distalis neurohypophysis, which represents the major portion of the neurohypophysis.[1]

The neurohypophysis is where ADH and oxytocin are stored; they are produced by separate neurons in the hypothalamic nuclei and travel across the infundibulum and the pars distalis neurohypophysis.[6]

Physiology

The functions of the hypothalamus are so basic that its structure and organizational patterns are conserved throughout the mammalian spectrum. In 1929, Dr. Harvey Cushing wrote the following regarding the hypothalamus: “Here in this well-concealed spot, almost to be covered with a thumbnail, lies the very mainspring of primitive existence –vegetative, emotional, reproductive– on which, with more or less success, man has come to superimpose a cortex of inhibitions”. Almost every

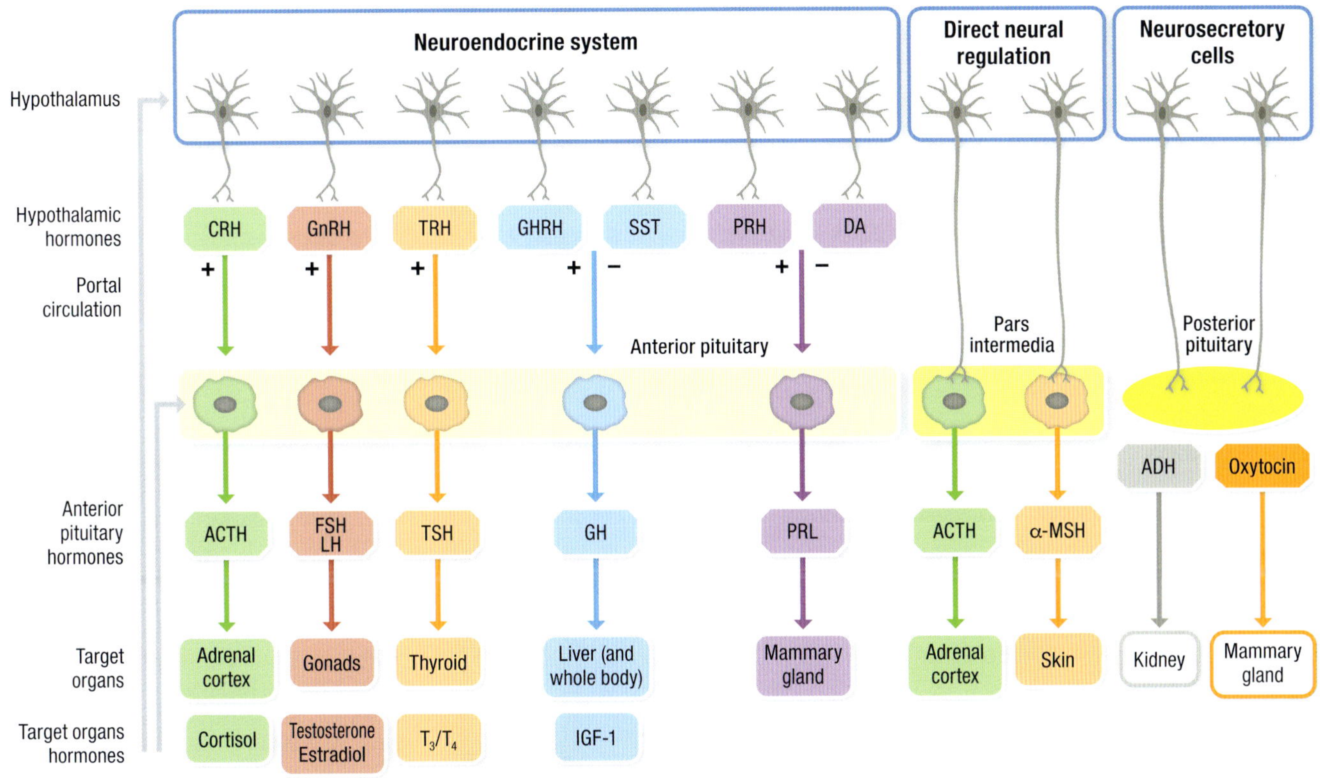

FIG. 23.3 Simplified diagram of the three mechanisms (neuroendocrine system in the anterior pituitary, direct neuronal regulation of the pars intermedia, and neurosecretory cells in the posterior lobe) that regulate the secretion of the hormones in the pituitary gland. ACTH, adrenocorticotropic hormone; ADH, antidiuretic hormone or vasopressin; CRH, corticotropin-releasing factor; DA, dopamine; FSH, follicle-stimulating hormone; GH, growth hormone; GHRH, growth hormone-releasing hormone; GnRH, gonadotropin-releasing hormone; IGF-1, insulin-like growth factor 1; LH, luteinizing hormone; α-MSH, α-melanocyte-stimulating hormone; PRH, prolactin-releasing hormone; PRL, prolactin; SST, somatostatin; TRH, thyrotropin-releasing hormone; TSH, thyroid-stimulating hormone; T_3, tri-iodothyronine; T_4, tetraiodothyronine or thyroxine; +, stimulation; –, inhibition.

major subdivision of the central nervous system communicates with the hypothalamus and is subject to its influence. The hypothalamus, which is at the center of the relationship between the nervous system and the endocrine system, communicates with the peripheral organ system by converting synaptic information to humoral signals; this function is possible thanks to the presence of neuroendocrine cells, which convert a nervous stimulus into an endocrine secretion.[7]

The hypothalamus exerts its control over the endocrine system by means of three main mechanisms:[3,6]

1. Neurosecretory pathway: the magnocellular neuroendocrine cells in the paraventricular and supraoptic nuclei send their axons directly to the neurohypophysis, where they release vasopressin (antidiuretic hormone [ADH]) and oxytocin from their terminals (Fig. 23.2B).
2. Neuroendocrine system: the parvicellular neuroendocrine cells contain hormones that are secreted into the hypothalamo-hypophyseal portal circulation in order to control the adenohypophysis. These hormones are corticotropin-releasing factor (CRF), thyrotrophin-releasing hormone (TRH), and gonadotropin-releasing hormone (GnRH), which stimulate the secretion of the corresponding pituitary hormones, which, in turn, regulate the function of the adrenal and the thyroid glands, and the gonads, respectively. Other neuroendocrine cells produce hormones that stimulate or inhibit the secretion of growth hormone (GH) and prolactin (PRL); GH-releasing hormone (GHRH) and somatostatin stimulate and inhibit, respectively, the secretion of GH, while dopamine inhibits the secretion of PRL (Fig. 23.3).
3. Direct neuronal regulation: the pars intermedia is poorly penetrated by blood vessels and is controlled by nerve fibers that arise from the hypothalamic dopaminergic neurons and make synaptic contacts with corticotrophs and melanotrophs (Fig. 23.2B). These cells synthesize a major precursor protein called proopiomelanocortin (POMC), which generates, by means of proteolytic cleavage, several biologically active peptides, including ACTH, corticotropin-like intermediate-lobe peptide (CLIP), α-MSH and β-endorphin. The secretion of ACTH- and POMC-derived peptides is under negative regulation by dopamine, which acts on D2 receptors. Other receptors are expressed by corticotrophs (somatostatin receptors SSTR2 and SSTR5) and melanotrophs (β-adrenergic receptors).[8]

In addition, the hypothalamus also exerts influence over the endocrine system by means of autonomic innervation of the endocrine organs. Both sympathetic and parasympathetic innervation of the pancreas, for example, can influence the secretion of insulin and glucagon.[9]

The production and secretion of the six hormones of the anterior lobe (ACTH, TSH, GH, FSH, LH, and PRL) are generally regulated via multiple (long, short, and ultrashort) feedback regulatory loops. These control mechanisms are made possible by the presence of the receptors for various pituitary hormones in the hypothalamus and the adenohypophysis. During ultra short-loop feedback, secretory products from cell feedback to the same cell modify the function of the cell itself (autocrine regulation).

KEY POINTS

- The hypothalamus is composed of the caudal, intermediate, and rostral regions.
- The caudal region acts on the sympathetic system, while the intermediate and rostral regions involve the parasympathetic and endocrine systems. The balance between the three structures ensures the maintenance of homeostasis.
- The pituitary gland is composed of the adenohypophysis and the neurohypophysis. It is involved in the secretion of hormones (ACTH, TSH, GH, FSH, LH, and PRL).

References

1. Hullinger R. The endocrine system In Hermanson JW, de Lahunta A, Evans HE. Miller's Anatomy of the Dog 4th edition. St. Louis, Elsevier Saunders, pp. 406-411, 2013.
2. Barone R. Anatomia comparata dei mammiferi domestici, vol. 6. Neurologia. Casa Editrice Edagricole, pp. 342-356, 2006.
3. Meij BP, Kooistra HS, Rijnberk A. Hypothalamus-pititary system. In Rijnberk A, Kooistra HS (editors). Clinical Endocrinology of Dogs and Cats. Hannover, Schlütersche, 2010, pp. 13-44.
4. Halmi NS, Peterson ME, Colurso GJ, et al. Pituitary intermediate lobe in dog: two cell types and high bioactive adrenocorticotropin content. *Science* 211(4477):72-74, 1981. doi:10.1126/science.6255564.
5. El Etreby MF, Fath El Bab MR. Localization of gonadotrophic hormones in the dog pituitary gland. A study using immunoenzyme histochemistry and chemical staining. *Cell Tissue Res* 183(2):167-75, 1977. doi:10.1007/BF00226617.
6. Goff JP. The endocrine system. In Erickson HH (editor). Duke's Physiology of Domestic Animals. John Wiley & Sons, 2015, pp. 617-725.
7. Card JP, Swanson LW, Moore RY. The hypothalamus: an overview of regulatory systems. In Zigmond MJ, Bloom FE, Landis SC, Roberts JL, Squire LR (editors). Fundamental Neuroscience. San Diego, Academic Press, 1999, pp. 1013-1026.
8. Sato A, Hara Y. Protein expression of somatostatin receptor 2, somatostatin receptor 5 and dopamine D2 receptor in normal pituitary gland and ACTH-secreting pituitary adenoma in dogs. *Res Vet Sci* 119:61-66, 2018. doi:10.1016/j.rvsc.2018.04.015.
9. Havel PJ, Mundinger TO, Taborsky GJ. Pancreatic sympathetic nerves contribute to increased glucagon secretion during severe hypoglycemia in dogs. *Am J Physiol* 270(1 Pt 1):E20-26, 1996. doi:10.1152/ajpendo.1996.270.1.E20.

CHAPTER 24

Growth hormone disorders

Federico Fracassi
DVM, PhD, DECVIM (SAIM)

Annemarie M.W.Y. Voorbij
DVM, PhD, DECVIM-CA (Internal Medicine)

Growth hormone (GH), a single-chain polypeptide, is produced in the somatotropic cells of the pituitary gland. Although its amino acid sequence differs substantially between species, the sequence of canine GH is identical to that of porcine GH.[1]

Similar to other pituitary hormones, GH secretion is pulsatile in nature. Pituitary GH secretion is regulated primarily by two hypothalamic hormones with opposing actions: the stimulatory growth hormone-releasing hormone (GHRH) and the inhibitory somatostatin (Fig. 24.1).

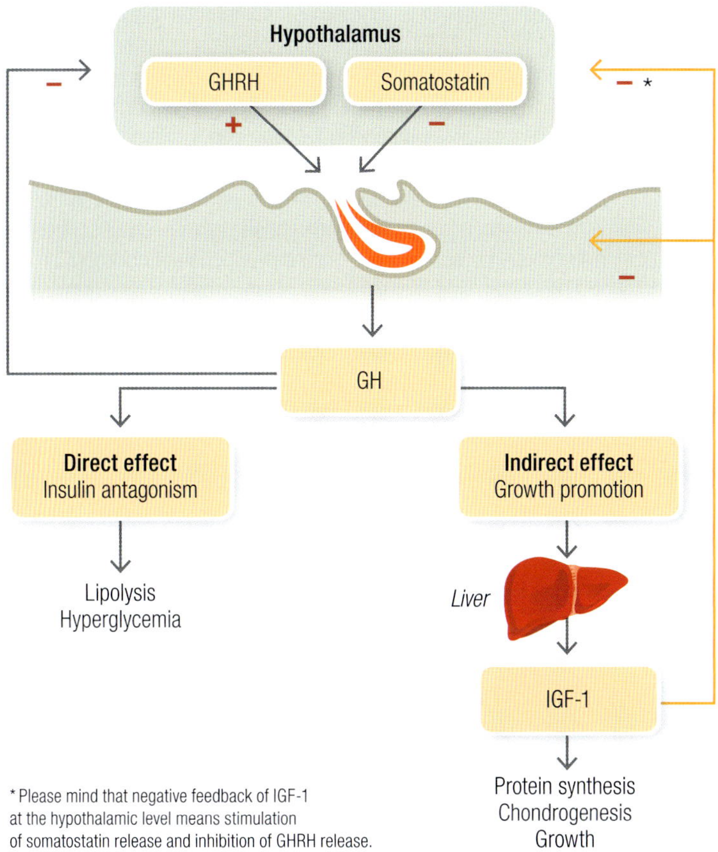

FIG. 24.1 Schematic illustration of the regulation of pituitary growth hormone secretion. *GH*, growth hormone; *GHRH*, growth hormone releasing hormone; *IGF-1*, insulin-like growth factor 1; *+*, stimulation; –, inhibition. (Modified from Meij et al., 2010)[19]

In addition, insulin-like growth factor 1 (IGF-1) exerts an indirect inhibitory effect on GH release by stimulating the release of somatostatin and by a direct inhibitory influence at the pituitary level.[2] Growth hormone itself also has a negative feedback effect at the hypothalamic level.[3] Furthermore, the frequency and amplitude of GH secretory pulses are influenced by many factors such as age, gender, nutrition, body composition, physical exercise, and several other hormones, such as thyroid hormone, progesterone, glucocorticoids, and ghrelin. In young dogs, ghrelin is an even more potent GH secretagogue than GHRH.[4] The main function of ghrelin, however, is stimulation of food intake, and the circulating ghrelin concentration will, therefore, be increased in a fasted state.[5] Episodic GH release can also be induced by synthetic GH-secretagogues, which act through the same receptor as ghrelin.[6,7]

Physiologic effect

Unlike most pituitary hormones, the effects of GH are not confined to a single target tissue. Growth hormone has both rapid catabolic and slow (long-lasting) hypertrophic effects. The acute catabolic effects, like enhanced lipolysis in fat cells, gluconeogenesis, and restriction of glucose transport across the cell membrane of fat and muscle cells are mainly due to anti-insulin activity and promote hyperglycemia. The slow anabolic effects are mainly mediated via IGF-1. The primary source of circulating IGF-1 is the liver. However, this hormone is also produced in many peripheral tissues, where it has a local (paracrine or autocrine) growth-promoting effect. Unlike insulin, circulating IGF-1 is largely bound to binding proteins (IGFBPs). Therefore, the half-life of IGF-1 is prolonged, which contributes to its long-term growth-promoting actions. Insulin-like growth factor 1 is an important regulator of body size through protein synthesis, chondrogenesis, and growth stimulation. There is a strong linear correlation between plasma IGF-1 concentrations and body size. Furthermore, an IGF-1 single-nucleotide polymorphism haplotype has been reported as an important factor in determining the final body size of dogs.[8] Increasing evidence shows that

GH itself directly promotes growth through stimulation of target cells and that GH itself may be a major determinant of body size. It appears that young dogs of large breeds go through a longer period of high GH release (i.e., juvenile hypersomatotropism) compared to young dogs of small breeds.[9]

Hypersomatotropism (acromegaly)

Acromegaly is a chronic endocrine disorder characterized by overgrowth of soft tissue and/or bony structures and insulin resistance due to GH overproduction in adulthood. Since not all dogs with "acromegaly" have typical clinical signs, the term hypersomatotropism might be more appropriate to define such condition. Unlike the situation in humans and cats, hypersomatotropism due to a pituitary adenoma is rare in dogs; it has been described in only five dogs so far.[10-14] In dogs, circulating GH is not only derived from the pituitary gland but also originates from the mammary gland. Mammary GH is stimulated by progesterone, which is a physiologic event that occurs in all intact bitches. Hypersomatotropism in dogs is more frequently related to the production and secretion of mammary GH. This production occurs in middle-aged or elderly bitches during the luteal phase of the estrus cycle as a consequence of high levels of progesterone in the blood or as the result of treatment with progestins (e.g., medroxyprogesterone acetate). The high concentrations of plasma progesterone during the luteal phase induce the secretion of GH from foci of hyperplastic columnar epithelium in the mammary glands. The high circulating levels of GH induced by hyperprogesteronemia can lead to hypersomatotropism, particularly in elderly bitches during diestrus when the synthesis of progesterone is maximal. This condition has also been described in pregnant bitches; the concentrations of plasma progesterone during pregnancy are the same as those during diestrus.

Furthermore, it has recently been observed that mammary tumors in dogs can secrete GH independently from direct progesterone stimulation.[15,16]

Signalment

Pituitary somatotroph adenoma has so far been described in male, mainly large breed dogs (Doberman Pinscher, Dalmatian, Samoyed, Labrador Retriever, Border Terrier), with age ranges between 5 and 10 years.[10-14] Spontaneous progesterone-induced hypersomatotropism and hypersomatotropism due to exogenous progestin application occur in elderly intact females and have been reported in different dog breeds of different sizes, including Beagles, Dachshunds, English Cocker Spaniels, Dalmatians, Golden Retrievers, German Shepherd dogs, Bouviers, and mixed breed dogs.[17,18] A case-control study reported that spontaneous progesterone-induced hypersomatotropism is more commonly observed in German Shepherd dogs. In this study, the incidence of the disease within the intact female German Shepherd dog population was 1.65% and was significantly higher than that in the overall intact female population (0.15%).[16]

Clinical signs

The clinical signs of excess secretion of GH tend to develop gradually. Clinical signs mainly result from the anabolic, growth-promoting actions of GH and IGF-1, together with the diabetogenic actions of GH. Some dogs only reveal the typical physical changes of hypersomatotropism; some predominantly show clinical signs of diabetes mellitus, while others have both categories of symptoms. Dogs with hypersomatotropism of mammary origin are often presented three to five weeks after estrus. The symptoms initially tend to regress following diestrus; however, they become more severe with successive estrus cycles. The mildest forms and earliest stages of the disease are usually characterized by polyuria, polydipsia, sometimes polyphagia, excessive panting (Video 24.1), and weakness. Other reported signs are respiratory stridor, weight gain, macroglossia, widened interdental spaces (Fig. 24.2), broadening of the head, enlargement of the abdomen due to visceromegaly, enlargement of the paws, weight gain, exophthalmos, and mammary nodules.[16-19] Various degrees of hyperkeratosis and hyperplasia of the epidermis and dermis, sometimes associated with a certain amount of hypertrichosis, have been described. Dermal hyperplasia is caused by increased production of collagen, an increase in fibroblasts, and accumulation of mucopolysaccharides, which give the tissues a dense, compact, and thickened appearance, and can be associated with diffuse mucinous degeneration (myxedema). The signs of canine hypersomatotropism due to a GH-secreting pituitary adenoma are the same as those of hypersomatotropism of mammary origin. A Dalmatian dog with hypersomatotropism due to a pituitary tumor also had gait abnormalities (Video 24.2) consisting of chronic progressive

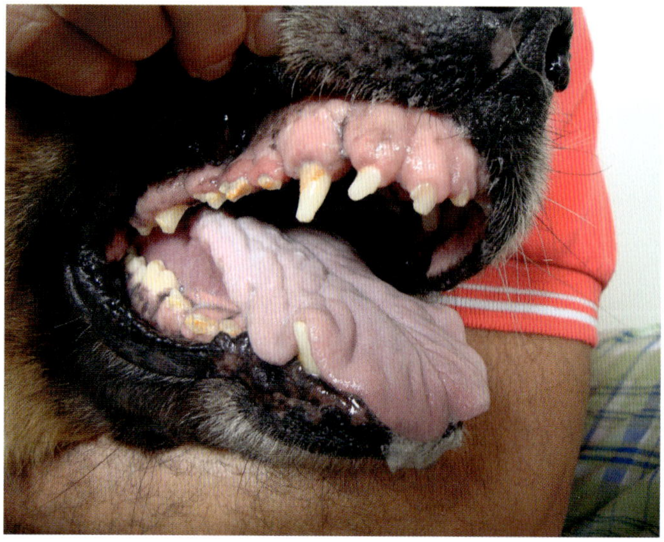

FIG. 24.2 Photograph of a 10-year-old intact female German Shepherd dog with hypersomatotropism: notice the enlarged interdental spaces.

Video 24.1

A 10-year-old intact female German Shepherd Dog with hypersomatotropism: notice the overt resting panting.

Video 24.2

A 10-year-old male Dalmatian dog with hypersomatotropism due to a pituitary adenoma: notice the overall increase in body size, redundant skin with many folds on head and neck. The gait is characterized by stiff movements.

stiffness, difficulty turning and standing up, and neck rigidity, which were caused by proliferation of joint cartilage, and severe spondylosis deformans with osteophytes.[11] Overt diabetes mellitus develops in a substantial percentage of dogs with hypersomatotropism and is associated with polyuria and polydipsia. However, mild to moderate polyuria and polydipsia may also be present without diabetes and are probably related to either exogenous progestins and/or GH excess.[18]

Clinical pathology

In dogs with hypersomatotropism, the blood glucose concentration may be normal, mildly elevated (e.g., between 120 mg/dL and 180 mg/dL [6.7 mmol/L and 10 mmol/L]), or severely elevated. Increased serum fructosamine concentration and glycosuria may or may not be present depending on the degree of hyperglycemia. Other common clinicopathological abnormalities observed in dogs with hypersomatotropism are an increase in serum alkaline phosphatase, creatine kinase, triglyceride, and phosphate. Hematocrit, blood urea nitrogen, sodium and chloride concentrations, and urinary specific gravity are often low.[16]

Diagnosis

The tentative diagnosis of excess GH is based on the presence of characteristic clinical signs in association with diestrus or a history of prolonged administration of progestins. The definitive diagnosis requires the documentation of GH excess. GH assays are problematic; in fact, GH should be determined using a canine-specific radioimmunoassay that is not widely available. Furthermore, a high level of plasma GH may be the result of a secretory pulse in a healthy animal. Therefore, plasma GH is recommended to be determined in three to five blood samples collected at 10-minute intervals. In a study of a group of bitches with spontaneous hypersomatotropism and progestin-induced hypersomatotropism, the concentrations of plasma GH ranged from 11 to 1476 ng/mL.

Other ways to increase the diagnostic accuracy of plasma GH determination are using the somatostatin suppression test and the glucose tolerance test. The somatostatin suppression test is performed by collecting blood samples for plasma GH determination before and 15, 30, 45, 60, and 90 minutes after the intravenous administration of 10 µg/kg body weight of somatostatin. This test should result in no or a minimally decreased plasma GH concentration in dogs with hypersomatotropism. The glucose tolerance test can be performed in dogs without concurrent diabetes mellitus and allows the detection of insulin resistance and demonstration that plasma GH concentrations are inappropriately high. The test is performed by giving a 50% glucose solution intravenously (1 g/kg body weight) and measuring plasma concentrations of GH, insulin, and glucose at 0, 15, 30, 60, and 90 minutes after glucose administration. This test should result in no or a minimally decreased plasma GH concentration in dogs with hypersomatotropism. Furthermore, basal plasma insulin is usually high in dogs with hypersomatotropism, and a delayed return to normal plasma glucose levels can be observed in these animals. As described above, IGF-1 directly reflects GH activity as it is synthesized in the liver (and other tissues) under the control of GH. The plasma concentrations of IGF-1 are much less subject to fluctuations, and a single random blood sample is considered appropriate. Measurement of IGF-1 is routinely used to screen for hypersomatotropism in humans, and high IGF-1 levels are sensitive markers for GH excess. Plasma IGF-1 can be measured using assays designed for humans, and many laboratories perform this analysis. The size and age of the animal should be taken into consideration since IGF-1 levels are directly proportional to the subject's mass and age. In dogs with hypersomatotropism, IGF-1 levels are often highly increased (e.g., two to three times the upper limit of normal).

It is important to remember that dogs with primary hypothyroidism have elevated plasma GH and IGF-1 concentrations as well and, therefore, similar clinical signs as hypersomatotropism. Obviously, dogs suspected of hypersomatotropism should be tested for primary hypothyroidism first. In rare cases of hypersomatotropism of pituitary origin, CT or MRI can reveal a pituitary mass.

Treatment

Hypersomatotropism induced by progestin can be solved by withdrawal of the hormone treatment. Progesterone-induced hypersomatotropism is treated via ovariectomy/ovariohysterectomy, which should be performed as soon as possible after the diagnosis is made.

Circulating GH and IGF-1 concentrations normalize rapidly after ovariectomy/ovariohysterectomy but more slowly after discontinuation of progestin. This causes a reduction in soft tissue volume, in particular that of the oropharynx. In contrast, the bone changes are irreversible. The clinicopathological abnormalities resolve or markedly improve after the ovariectomy/ovariohysterectomy.[16]

In dogs with progesterone-induced hypersomatotropism and diabetes mellitus, the ovariectomy/ovariohysterectomy should be performed as soon as possible, even before knowing the serum IGF-1 concentration. This is to limit the deleterious effects of glucose toxicity on β-cell function, thereby improving the chance of diabetic remission. Insulin therapy is initiated immediately in all dogs with moderate to highly increased blood glucose concentrations (>140 mg/dL [7.8 mmol/L]); the insulin dose depends on the severity of hyperglycemia and ranges between approximately 0.10 to 0.25 U/kg q12h, SC. During surgery and the following days to weeks, close blood glucose monitoring should be performed. Insulin requirements usually decrease rapidly due to the cessation of insulin resistance, and hypoglycemia may occur if insulin doses are not amended.[18] If ovariectomy/ovariohysterectomy cannot be performed immediately in these animals or when long-acting exogenous progestins have been administered, treatment with aglepristone, a progesterone receptor antagonist, is suggested. Aglepristone is administered at a dose of 10 mg/kg SC q24h for 2 consecutive days. After ovariectomy/ovariohysterectomy, aglepristone is no longer needed. In diabetic dogs where ovariectomy/ovariohysterectomy is not possible or permitted, aglepristone should be continued at the dose of 10 mg/kg SC once weekly. In progesterone-induced hypersomatotropism, aglepristone can be discontinued when the measurement of serum progesterone indicates the end of diestrus. This approach is empirical and based on the study of Bhatti et al.[20] and the author's experience. An optimal protocol has not yet been established. Mammary tumors should be removed surgically because they may be a source of GH/IGF-1 production.[15,16]

In dogs with hypersomatotropism due to a pituitary tumor, either radiation therapy[14] or hypophysectomy should be considered. A case report describes the treatment of an 8-year-old castrated male Border Terrier dog with hypersomatotropism due to a GH-secreting pituitary tumor; the dog also had concurrent diabetes mellitus. The treatment with radiation therapy and the somatostatin analog pasireotide resulted in the remission of diabetes mellitus, a decrease in serum IGF-1 concentration, and a reversal of some of the hypersomatotropism-associated soft tissue changes.[13]

Prognosis

The prognosis of progesterone-induced hypersomatotropism is good with regard to all the potentially reversible clinical signs, except the development of diabetes mellitus, which may not regress. A 7-year-old male castrated Labrador Retriever with hypersomatotropism due to a GH-producing pituitary tumor was treated with radiation therapy and survived for two and a half more years.[14]

Pituitary dwarfism

Etiology

Any defect in the development of the pituitary gland may result in a form of isolated or combined pituitary hormone deficiency. Congenital GH deficiency or pituitary dwarfism is the best-known example of such a deficiency. Pituitary dwarfism has been described in several dog breeds, such as Czechoslovakian Wolfdogs, Saarloos Wolfdogs, Karelian Bear Dogs, and Tibetan Terriers, but is most commonly encountered in German Shepherd Dogs. German Shepherd dwarfs have a combined deficiency of GH, thyroid-stimulating hormone (TSH), and prolactin, as well as impaired release of gonadotropins. By contrast, adrenocorticotropic hormone (ACTH) secretion is preserved in these animals.[21]

Pituitary dwarfism in German Shepherd Dogs was originally thought to be caused by pressure atrophy of the pituitary anterior lobe by cyst formation in Rathke's pouch.[22] Although most dwarfs of this breed do have pituitary cysts, young dwarfs may have no or only small cysts. The size of these cysts is unlikely to be able to cause pressure atrophy.[21] Furthermore, the unaffected ACTH secretion in German Shepherd dwarfs argues against cyst formation in Rathke's pouch as the primary cause of pituitary dwarfism. Therefore, cyst formation in Rathke's pouch is most likely a consequence of the underlying genetic defect rather than the cause of pituitary dwarfism in affected dogs.

Pituitary dwarfism is described as a simple, autosomal recessive inherited disorder in all the breeds mentioned above.[23-27]

Pituitary dwarfism in German Shepherd Dogs and related breeds, e.g., Czechoslovakian Wolfdogs and Saarloos Wolfdogs, is associated with mutations in the gene encoding for the transcription factor LHX3. Analysis of intron 5 of *LHX3* revealed that dwarfs have a deletion of one of six 7-basepair repeats. This small intron size is associated with defective splicing of *LHX3*.[23,24] More recently, an identical *LHX3* mutation was identified in Tibetan Terriers with pituitary dwarfism.[25]

Screening of a large group of clinically healthy Saarloos and Czechoslovakian Wolfdogs revealed that the percentage of carriers of the mutated allele was 31% and 21%, respectively.[24] This shows pituitary dwarfism is a relevant disorder in these breeds and emphasizes the need for genetic screening. Pituitary dwarfism and the associated DNA defects most likely render individuals so weak that they either die in the uterus or shortly after birth, which would explain why the condition is not encountered in the clinic more often.

Congenital GH deficiency may also be due to genetic defects other than an *LHX3* mutation. In Karelian Bear Dogs, for example, pituitary dwarfism is associated with a *POU1F1* gene defect.[27] The transcription factor POU1F1, also known as PIT-1, is essential for the differentiation of the thyrotroph, lactotroph, and somatotroph cell lineages and subsequent expression of the *TSH-β*, *prolactin*, and *GH1* genes.[28] Therefore, Karelian Bear Dog dwarfs are expected to have a combined deficiency of TSH, prolactin, and GH. Furthermore, a 6-month-old female Chihuahua was reported with proportionate dwarfism, retained puppy hair coat, and hypoglycemia. The deficiency in this Chihuahua was ascribed to a 6-basepair deletion in exon 5 of the growth hormone gene, *GH1*.[29]

Growth hormone and IGF-1 are known to be involved in renal development, and a deficiency of these hormones may result in glomerular maldevelopment. Therefore, the renal function of pituitary dwarfs may be impaired as a result of a decreased glomerular filtration rate, due to GH and thyroid hormone deficiency.[30-32]

As in humans, the *LHX3* mutation is associated with malformations of the atlantoaxial joint in dogs as well, leading to instability and dynamic compression of the cervical spinal cord.[33]

Clinical signs

Pituitary dwarfism is a serious illness, and clinical signs are not limited to physical appearance (Table 24.1). The range of clinical features is wide and may vary between dwarfs.[34,35] During the first weeks after birth, pituitary dwarfs may be of similar size as their littermates. However, affected animals develop proportionate growth retardation after this period, and unlike their healthy littermates, pituitary dwarfs retain their puppy hair coat (retention of lanugo or secondary hairs and lack primary or guard hairs). The dwarfs gradually develop bilateral symmetrical alopecia, starting at the points of wear and sparing the head and the extremities (Fig. 24.3). Their skin becomes progressively hyperpigmented and scaly, and secondary bacterial infections are quite common. Pituitary dwarfs often also have a pointed muzzle and relatively long pointy ears, resembling the face of a fox (Fig. 24.4).

Pituitary dwarfism has no sex predilection. In male dwarfs, unilateral or bilateral cryptorchidism is often observed. In female dwarfs, persistent estrus of more than four weeks duration is a common finding, characterized by swelling of the vulva, bloody vaginal discharge, and attractiveness to male dogs. Due to the absence of an LH surge, ovulation does not occur, and circulating progesterone concentration remains low, often below 3 nmol/L.

German Shepherd dwarfs and dwarfs of related breeds may also be presented with neurological signs indicating a cervical spinal cord disorder (Video 24.3).[33]

Furthermore, physical examination may reveal a continuous heart murmur, due to a patent ductus arteriosus.[21]

During the first years of their lives, pituitary dwarfs are usually bright and alert little dogs. However, especially when these animals don't receive proper treatment, they develop inappetence and become less active with time. This usually occurs at 2-3 years of age and has been ascribed to secondary hypothyroidism and impaired renal function.[19]

Clinical pathology

Except for an increased plasma creatinine concentration, no other significant abnormalities are usually noted on a standard complete blood count and biochemistry panel.

Thyroid hormone and thyroid-stimulating hormone

In most pituitary dwarfs, the plasma thyroxine concentration is below the reference interval. However, instead of an elevated plasma TSH concentration, as expected with primary hypothyroidism, TSH concentrations are often at or close to the lower limit of the TSH assay, due to decreased pituitary TSH secretion. Interestingly, plasma thyroxine concentration can be within the reference range in some pituitary dwarfs.

TABLE 24.1 Clinical manifestations and postmortem findings associated with pituitary dwarfism in dogs.

Musculoskeletal	Dermatologic	Reproduction
■ Stunted growth ■ Thin skeleton ■ Changes in ossification centers ■ Delayed closure of growth plates ■ Delayed dental erupture ■ Fox-like facial features ■ Muscle atrophy ■ Abnormal position dens axis ■ Atlantoaxial instability ■ Dynamic compression spinal cord by dorsally displaced dens axis	■ Soft, wooly hair coat ■ Retention of lanugo hairs ■ Lack of guard hairs ■ Isolated patches of guard hair ■ Bilateral symmetrical alopecia at trunk, neck, and proximal extremities ■ Hyperpigmentation of the skin ■ Thin, fragile skin ■ Wrinkles ■ Scales ■ Seborrhea sicca ■ Comedones ■ Papules ■ Pyoderma	■ Cryptorchidism ■ Flaccid penile sheath ■ Failure to have estrus cycles
Neurological	**Other signs**	**Postmortem findings**
■ Tetraparesis or paresis posterior ■ Proprioceptive ataxia of limbs ■ Opisthotonos ■ Hypermetria ■ Painful passive neck movements	■ Shrill, puppy-like bark ■ Signs of secondary hypothyroidism ■ Mental dullness ■ Impairment of renal function	■ Pituitary cysts ■ Atrophy adenohypophysis ■ Hypoplasia thyroid gland ■ Persistent ductus arteriosus ■ Incomplete ossifications suture lines C1 ■ Fibrous and cartilaginous tissue in dorsal and lateroventral clefts C1 ■ Wallerian degeneration spinal cord

Modified from Nelson and Della Maggiore, 2020.[34]

Video 24.3

Neurologic examination of an 8-month-old female intact Czechoslovakian Wolfdog with pituitary dwarfism and atlantoaxial malformation and instability.

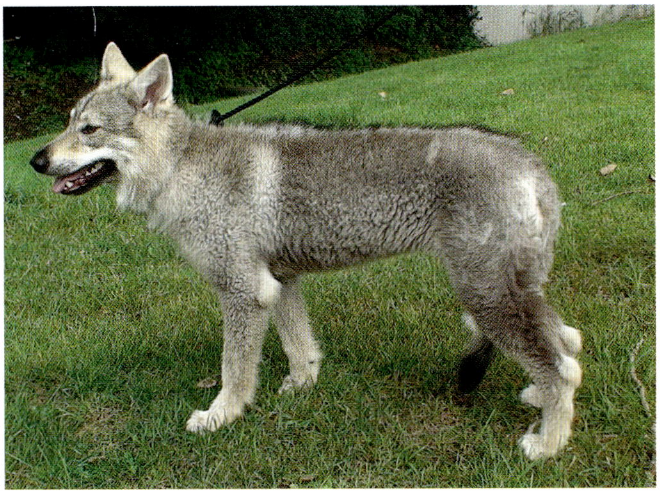

FIG. 24.3 Photograph of an 8-month-old female intact Czechoslovakian Wolfdog with pituitary dwarfism. Note the proportionate growth retardation and retention of its puppy hair coat with isolated patches of adult hair.

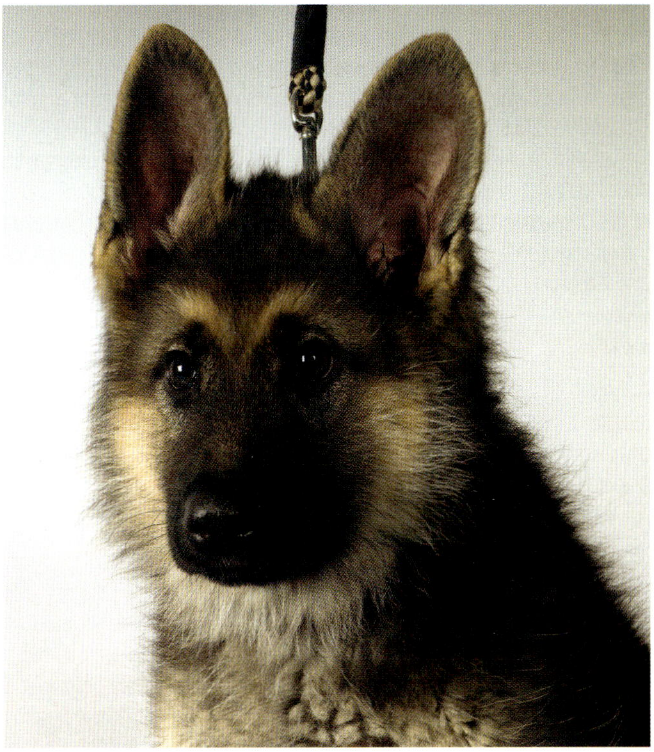

FIG. 24.4 Photograph of a German Shepherd dwarf with the characteristic fox-like facial features.

Growth hormone

Because GH is secreted in rhythmic pulses and intervening troughs, basal circulating GH concentrations may be low in healthy animals. Therefore, a definite diagnosis of GH deficiency cannot rely upon a low circulating GH concentration alone. As described above, due to the variety of the amino acid sequence of GH between species, a species-specific homologous radioimmunoassay is needed to measure plasma GH. Alas, assays for measuring canine GH are not widely available.

Insulin-like growth factor I

Because GH deficiency results in a low circulating IGF-1 concentration, measurement of the plasma IGF-1 concentration can be used to assess the GH status of an animal indirectly. Fortunately, the amino acid sequence of IGF-1 is less species-specific than that of GH. Therefore, IGF-1 can be measured using a heterologous (human) assay. Other advantages of IGF-1 are its long half-life and lack of pulsatile secretion. Circulating IGF-1 concentrations are low in pituitary dwarfs, even when age and body size are considered. The mean (± SEM) plasma IGF-1 concentration in German Shepherd dwarfs (8.1 ± 1.3 nmol/L) has been reported to be considerably lower than the mean plasma IGF-1 concentrations in healthy, adult (36.7 ± 3.0 nmol/L) and immature German Shepherd Dogs (45.2 ± 6.6 nmol/L).[21] Nevertheless, IGF-1 measurements do not provide a definitive diagnosis as there may be some overlap between the circulating IGF-1 concentrations of dwarfs and that of healthy animals.

Diagnostic imaging

In dogs with pituitary dwarfism, a CT or MRI of the pituitary area often reveals the presence of pituitary cysts that gradually enlarge during life. In most young dwarfs, the pituitary is quite small, compatible with pituitary hypoplasia, i.e., a lack of endocrine cells in the pituitary anterior lobe.[21,36] Because pituitary cysts are not unusual in healthy dogs, especially in brachycephalic breeds, the presence of pituitary cysts cannot be used to diagnose pituitary dwarfism.

In German Shepherd dwarfs and dwarfs of related breeds, diagnostic imaging of the cranial neck and skull may identify abnormal positioning of the dens axis and incomplete ossification of the suture lines between the ossification centers of the atlas with concurrent atlantoaxial instability and dynamic compression of the spinal cord by the dens axis.[33]

Diagnosis

Although the clinical signs of pituitary dwarfism may be obvious, the diagnosis must be substantiated. A definitive diagnosis of pituitary dwarfism should be based on the results of a pituitary stimulation test or genetic testing.

Pituitary stimulation tests

To test the responsiveness of the somatotropic cells of the pituitary, GH stimulants such as GHRH (1 µg/kg IV) or α-adrenergic drugs, such as clonidine (10 µg/kg IV) or xylazine (100 µg/kg IV), can be used. Growth hormone concentrations should be determined immediately before and 20-30 minutes after intravenous administration of the stimulant. In healthy dogs, circulating GH concentrations should increase at least 2-to-4 fold after stimulation. In dogs with pituitary dwarfism, no significant rise in circulating GH concentrations is expected. Administration of xylazine or clonidine may cause sedation, bradycardia, hypotension, or vomiting.

An alternative method to diagnose GH deficiency is the ghrelin stimulation test. Human ghrelin is administrated in a dose of 2 µg/kg IV. A circulating GH concentration of more than 5 µg/L 20 minutes after stimulation excludes pituitary dwarfism.[37]

To test the secretory capacity of the other hormone-secreting pituitary cells, the adenohypophysis can be concurrently stimulated with corticotropin-releasing hormone (CRH, 1 µg/kg IV), thyrotropin-releasing hormone (TRH, 10 µg/kg IV), and gonadotropin-releasing hormone (GnRH, 10 µg/kg IV).[38]

Genetic testing

Genetic tests are available to identify pituitary dwarfs and carriers of the *LHX3* or *POU1F1* mutation.[23,24,27] If all breeding animals of affected breeds were genetically tested for the presence of mutations reported to cause dwarfism in those breeds and an appropriate breeding policy implemented, this disease could be eradicated completely.

Therapy

Unfortunately, canine GH is not commercially available. Because of the differences in amino acid sequence between canine and human GH, dogs can develop antibodies directed against human GH. Therefore, it cannot be used to treat canine dwarfs.[39] Fortunately, the amino acid sequence of porcine GH is identical to that of canine GH and will not result in antibody formation.[1] Alas, legislation forbids its use in most European countries. The recommended starting dose for porcine GH is 0.1-0.3 IU/kg SC, 3 times per week. Because this treatment may result in GH excess, side effects such as diabetes mellitus may occur. Therefore, monitoring circulating GH and glucose concentrations in these animals every 3 weeks is recommended. Long-term dose rates should be determined based on the measurement of circulating IGF-1. The status of the growth plates at the beginning of treatment determines whether the administration of porcine GH will lead to linear growth. Improvement of the skin and hair coat usually occurs within 6 to 8 weeks after the start of therapy. The hairs that grow back are typically lanugo hairs. The growth of guard hairs is variable.

In dogs, progestins induce the expression of the GH gene in the mammary gland with subsequent secretion of this mammary GH into the systemic circulation.[40] Therefore, progestin can be used to treat pituitary dwarfs as well. Medroxyprogesterone acetate (MPA) should be administered in doses of 2.5-5 mg/kg SC, initially at 3-week intervals and subsequently at 6-week intervals. Administration of MPA may lead to increased body size, development of a complete adult hair coat, and increased circulating IGF-1 and GH concentrations.[36] Alternatively, proligestone could be used.[41]

Unfortunately, progestin treatment is associated with several side effects, including recurrent periods of pruritic pyoderma, skeletal maldevelopment, mammary tumors, and diabetes mellitus. Therefore, monitoring GH, IGF-1, and glucose circulating concentrations is paramount. Treated animals may develop acromegalic features without circulating GH concentrations exceeding the upper limit of the reference range. In these cases, but certainly when the plasma IGF-1 concentration approaches 200 µg/L, treatment should be discontinued for a few months. In bitches, an ovariohysterectomy should be performed before progestin treatment is started to prevent cystic endometrial hyperplasia.

In addition to GH replacement, thyroid hormone replacement should be started as soon as there is evidence of secondary hypothyroidism. Levothyroxine is administered orally, with a 15 µg/kg starting dose q12h. The plasma thyroxine concentration should be monitored closely because the absorption and metabolism of levothyroxine are variable. The dosage may have to be adjusted several times before a satisfactory clinical response is reached.

Prognosis

Without proper treatment, the long-term prognosis of pituitary dwarfs is usually poor. By 3-5 years of age, affected animals are usually bald, thin, and dull. These changes are likely due to progressive loss of pituitary function, continuing expansion of pituitary cysts, and progressive renal failure. Furthermore, due to atlantoaxial instability, dwarfs can display progressive neurological deficits, and even sudden death may occur following sudden neck movements.[19,33] Although the prognosis improves significantly when dwarfs are adequately treated with either porcine GH or progestins and levothyroxine, their prognosis remains guarded.

KEY POINTS

Hypersomatotropism

- Hypersomatotropism is a chronic endocrine disorder characterized by overgrowth of soft tissue and/or bony structures and insulin resistance due to growth hormone (GH) overproduction in adulthood.
- Hypersomatotropism in dogs is more frequently related to the production and secretion of mammary GH.
- Hypersomatotropism due to a pituitary adenoma is rare in dogs.
- The clinical signs are polyuria, polydipsia, sometimes polyphagia, excessive panting, weakness, respiratory stridor, weight gain, macroglossia, widened interdental spaces, broadening of the head, enlargement of the abdomen due to visceromegaly, enlargement of the paws, weight gain, exophthalmos, and mammary nodules.
- Progesterone-induced hypersomatotropism is treated via ovariectomy/ovariohysterectomy.

Pituitary dwarfism

- Pituitary dwarfism is an inherited disorder, most commonly encountered in German Shepherd Dogs and related breeds, but has also been described in other dog breeds.
- In most of these breeds, it results in a combined deficiency of GH, thyroid-stimulating hormone (TSH), prolactin, and gonadotropins. In contrast, the secretion of adrenocorticotropic hormone (ACTH) is preserved in these animals.
- The main clinical manifestations are proportionate growth retardation, retention of their puppy hair coat with a lack of primary guard hairs, and bilateral alopecia starting at the points of wear.
- Definite diagnosis should rely on pituitary function tests or genetic test results.
- Although the prognosis improves significantly when dwarfs are properly treated with levothyroxine and either porcine GH or progestins, their prognosis remains guarded.

References

1. Ascacio-Martinez JA, Barrera Saldana HA. A dog growth hormone cDNA, codes for a mature protein identical to a pig growth hormone. *Gene* 143:277-280, 1994.
2. Ceda GP, et al. The growth hormone (GH)-releasing hormone (GHRH)-GH-somatomedin axis: evidence for rapid inhibition of GHRH-elicited GH release by insulin-like growth factors I and II. *Endocrinology* 120:1658, 1987.
3. Lanzi R, et al. Time course and mechanism of growth hormone's negative feedback effect on its own spontaneous release. *Endocrinology* 130:780, 1992.
4. Bhatti SFM, De Vliegher SP, Van Ham L, Kooistra HS. Effects of growth hormone-releasing peptides in healthy dogs and in dogs with pituitary-dependent hyperadrenocorticism. *Mol Cell Endocrinol* 197, 97-103, 2002.
5. Bhatti SF, Hofland LJ, Van Koetsveld P, et al. Effects of food intake and food withholding on plasma ghrelin concentrations in healthy dogs. *Am J Vet Res* 67:1557-1563, 2006b.
6. McKee KK, et al. Molecular analysis of rat pituitary and hypothalamic growth hormone secretagogue receptors. *Mol Endocrinol* 11:415, 1997.
7. Kojima M, Hosoda H, Date Y, et al. Ghrelin is a growth-hormone-releasing acylated peptide from stomach. *Nature* 402:656-660, 1999.
8. Sutter NB, Bustamante CD, Chase K, et al. A single IGF1 allele is a major determinant of small size in dogs. *Science* 316, 112-115, 2007.
9. Favier RP, Mol JA, Kooistra HS, et al. Large body size in the dog is associated with transient GH

excess at a young age. *J Endocrinol* 170:479-484, 2001.
10. Van Keulen LJ, et al. Diabetes mellitus in a dog with a growth hormone-producing acidophilic adenoma of the adenohypophysis. *Vet Pathol* 33:451, 1996.
11. Fracassi F, et al. Acromegaly due to a somatotroph adenoma in a dog. *Domest Anim Endocrinol* 32:43, 2007.
12. Johnstone T, et al. Hypothyroidism associated with acromegaly and insulin-resistant diabetes mellitus in a Samoyed. *Aust Vet J* 92:437, 2014.
13. Zublena F, et al. Radiotherapy and pasireotide treatment of a growth hormone-producing pituitary tumor in a diabetic dog. *Can Vet J* 59:1089, 2018.
14. Reusch C, et al. Acromegaly due to a pituitary tumor in a dog –diagnosis, therapy and long-term follow-up. *Schweiz Arch Tierheilkd* 161:319, 2019.
15. Murai A, et al. GH-producing mammary tumors in two dogs with acromegaly. *J Vet Med Sci* 74:771, 2012.
16. Fracassi F, et al. Spontaneous acromegaly: a retrospective case-control study in German Shepherd dogs. *Vet J* 202:69, 2014.
17. Rijnberk A, et al. Acromegaly associated with transient overproduction of growth hormone in a dog. *J Am Vet Med Assoc* 177:534, 1980.
18. Reusch CE. Disorders of growth hormone. In Feldman EC, Nelson RW, Reusch CE, Scott-Moncrieff JCR, Behrend E (editors). Canine and Feline Endocrinology 4th edition. St. Louis, Elsevier, 2015, pp. 37-76.
19. Meij B, Rijnberk A, Kooistra HS. Hypothalamus-pituitary system. In Rijnberk A, Kooistra HS (editors). Clinical Endocrinology of Dogs and Cats 2nd edition. Hannover, Schlütersche Verslagsgeselschaft mbH & Co, 2010, pp. 13-54.
20. Bhatti SF, et al. Treatment of growth hormone excess in dogs with the progesterone receptor antagonist aglepristone. *Theriogenology* 66:797, 2006.
21. Kooistra HS, Voorhout G, Mol JA and Rijnberk A. Combined pituitary hormone deficiency in German Shepherd dogs with dwarfism. *Domest Anim Endocrinol* 19:177-190, 2000.
22. Müller-Peddinghaus R, El Eltebry MF, Siefert J and Ranke M. Hypophysärer Zwergwuchs beim Deutschen Schäferhund. *Vet Pathol* 17:406-421, 1980.
23. Voorbij AM, Van Steenbeek FG, Vos-Loohuis M, et al. A contracted DNA repeat in LHX3 intron 5 is associated with aberrant splicing and pituitary dwarfism in German shepherd dogs. *PLOS One* 6, 2011. doi:10.1371/journal.pone.0027940
24. Voorbij AM, Leegwater PA and Kooistra HS. Pituitary dwarfism in Saarloos and Czechoslovakian wolfdogs is associated with a mutation in LHX3. *J Vet Intern Med* 28:1770-1774, 2014.
25. Thaiwong T, et al. Dwarfism in Tibetan Terrier dogs with an LHX3 mutation. *J Vet Diagn Invest* 33:740, 2021.
26. Andresen E, Willeberg P. Pituitary dwarfism in German Shepherd dogs: additional evidence of simple, autosomal recessive inheritance. *Nordisk Vet Med* 28:481-486, 1976.
27. Kyöstilä, et al. Intronic variant in POU1F1 associated with canine pituitary dwarfsm. *Human Genetics* 140:1553, 2021.
28. Fang Q, George AS, Brinkmeier ML, Mortensen AH, Gergics P, Cheung LY, Daly AZ, Ajmal A, Perez Millan MI, Ozel AB, Kitzman JO, Mills RE, Li JZ, Camper SA. Genetics of combined pituitary hormone deficiency: roadmap into the genome era. *Endocr Rev* 37:636-675, 2016. https://doi.org/10.1210/er.2016-1101
29. Lio A, Maeda S, Yonezawa T, Momoi Y, Motegi T. Isolated growth hormone deficiency in a Chihuahua with a GH1 mutation. *J Vet Diagn Invest* 32:733-736, 2020.
30. Falkheden T, et al. Renal function and kidney size following hypophysectomy in man. *Acta Endocrinol* 48:348, 1965.
31. Feld S, et al. Growth hormone, the insulin-like growth factor system, and the kidney. *Endocr Rev* 17:423, 1996.
32. Haylor J, et al. Renal function and morphometry in the dwarf rat following a reduction in renal mass. *Nephrol Dial Transplant* 11:643, 1996.
33. Voorbij AM, Meij BP, Van Bruggen LW, et al. Atlanto-axial malformation and instability in dogs with pituitary dwarfism due to an LHX3 mutation. *J Vet Intern Med* 29:207-213, 2015.
34. Nelson RW, Della Maggiore AM. Disorders of the hypothalamus and pituitary gland. In Nelson RW, Couto CG (editors). Small Animal Internal Medicine 6th edition. St. Louis, Mosby Elsevier, 2020, 740-757.
35. Voorbij AM, Kooistra HS. Pituitary dwarfism in German shepherd dogs. *J Vet Clin Sci* 2:4-11, 2009.
36. Kooistra HS, Voorhout G, Selman PJ, Rijnberk A. Progestin-induced growth hormone (GH) production in the treatment of dogs with congenital GH deficiency. *Domest Anim Endocrinol* 15:93-102, 1998.
37. Bhatti SFM, De Vliegher SP, Mol JA, et al. Ghrelin-stimulation test in the diagnosis of canine pituitary dwarfism. *Res Vet Sci* 81:24-30, 2006c.
38. Meij BP, Mol JA, Hazewinkel HAW, Bevers MM, Rijnberk A. Assessment of a combined anterior pituitary function test in beagle dogs: rapid sequential intravenous administration of four hypothalamic releasing hormones. *Domest Anim Endocrinol* 13:161-170, 1996.
39. Van Herpen H, Rijnberk A, Mol JA. Production of antibodies to biosynthetic human growth hormone in the dog. *Vet Rec* 134:171, 1994.
40. Selman PJ, Mol JA, Rutteman GR et al. Progestin-induced growth hormone excess in the dog originates in the mammary gland. *Endocrinology* 134:287-292, 1994.
41. Knottenbelt CM, Herrtage ME. Use of proligestone in the management of three German shepherd dogs with pituitary dwarfism. *J Small Anim Pract* 43:164-170, 2002.

CHAPTER 25

Vasopressin-related disorders of water homeostasis

Hans S. Kooistra
DVM, PhD, DECVIM-CA
(Internal Medicine)

It is quite remarkable that animals, including humans and dogs, are able to maintain water homeostasis. Despite the oral intake of water, with a very low osmolality, and food, with a very high osmolality, dogs are able to maintain plasma osmolality at an almost constant level of about 300 mOsm/kg. One of the main mechanisms to achieve this is urine production with a strongly fluctuating osmolality, indicating that the kidneys play a central role in water homeostasis.

In a healthy adult dog with a body weight of around 10 kg, about 36 liters of primary urine is produced each day. However, such a dog will only produce a few hundred milliliters of urine, meaning that the vast majority of the water in the primary urine has to be reabsorbed. More than 80% of the filtered water in the primary urine is reabsorbed in the proximal tubules, where water passively follows the active reabsorption of sodium, potassium, glucose, etc. (Fig. 25.1). The remaining water in the primary urine reaches the descending limb of the loop of Henle, located in the renal medulla. This part of the loop of Henle is permeable to water, and water will go from the inside of the tubule to the hypertonic renal medulla. The reabsorption of water in the first half of the nephron is hardly regulated. In contrast, water reabsorption in the second part of the nephron is very well regulated. The adjustments of water reabsorption needed to maintain the water (and electrolyte) balance in the distal convoluted tubules and the collecting ducts mainly depend on the hormones aldosterone, stimulating sodium reabsorption and potassium excretion, and the antidiuretic hormone vasopressin (VP), also known as antidiuretic hormone (ADH).

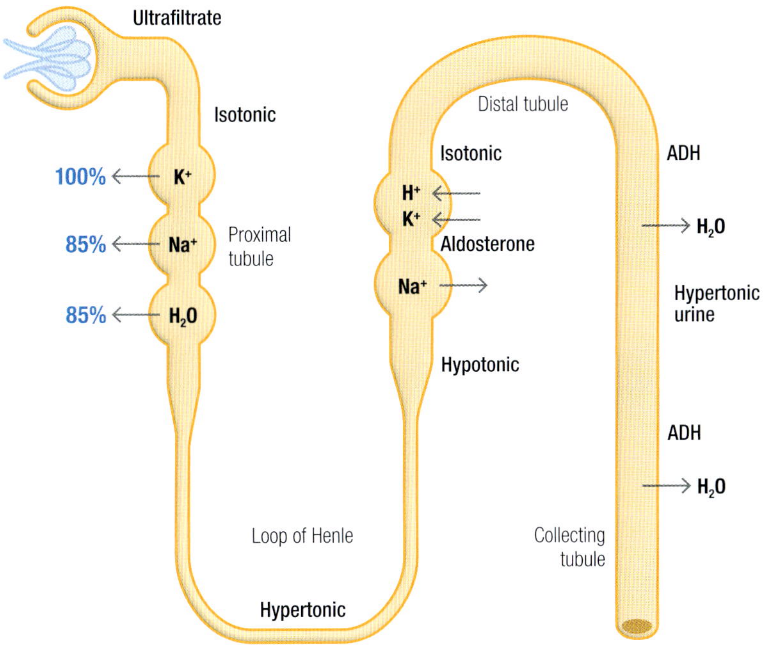

FIG. 25.1 Regulation of the water balance in the nephron.

Vasopressin plays a vital role in water homeostasis. It is produced by neurons located in the hypothalamus. After the production of the hormone, VP is transported along the nerve fibers and stored in secretory vesicles in the terminal ends of these nerve fibers located in the neurohypophysis. It can be released into the systemic circulation in response to appropriate stimuli.[1]

Like other pituitary hormones, VP is secreted in a pulsatile fashion (Fig. 25.2).[2] The major determinant of its release is plasma osmolality. Specialized neurons called "osmosensors" or "osmoreceptors" are concentrated in the anterior hypothalamus. Osmotic stimulation increases both basal and pulsatile VP secretion.[2] Significant changes in circulating blood volume and blood pressure, detected by baroreceptors, also influence VP release.

The anterior hypothalamus not only contains osmoreceptors regulating VP secretion but also thirst osmoreceptors. The control of VP secretion and thirst sensation is partially interwoven in that drinking not only leads to the satiation of thirst but also to the cessation of VP secretion. In addition to systemic signals, i.e., plasma osmolality (Posm) and blood volume/blood pressure, the water balance is regulated by presystemic signals. In dogs, drinking induces volume-dependent oropharyngeal signals that inhibit thirst and VP secretion well before the ingested water has left the stomach.

Three receptor subtypes mediate the effects of VP:

- V1 receptors on blood vessels. Stimulation of the V1 receptors results in vasoconstriction, which is the reason the hormone is called vasopressin.
- V2 receptors on renal collecting duct epithelial cells. Stimulation of the V2 receptors results in water reabsorption, which is the reason the hormone is called antidiuretic hormone.

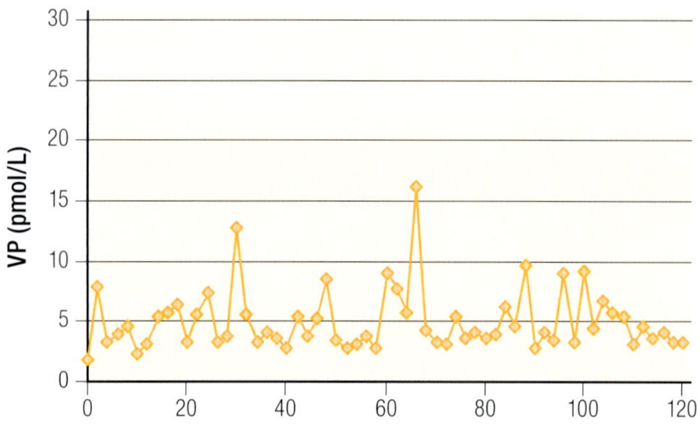

FIG. 25.2 Pulsatile secretion pattern of vasopressin (VP) in a 6-year-old Beagle dog. Blood samples were collected every 2 minutes for 2 hours (Modified from Van Vonderen et al., 2004a).

- V3 receptors mediate the secretion of adrenocorticotropic hormone from the adenohypophysis.

The cellular mechanism of VP activity in the renal tubule involves binding to specific contraluminal V2 receptor sites on the serosal surface of the collecting duct cell, an adenylate cyclase response, and phosphorylation of proteins that lead to transient insertion of water channels (aquaporins) in the luminal membrane of the collecting duct cell (Fig. 25.3). Several different aquaporins (AQPs) in the kidney have been characterized, each correlating with well-defined segmental permeabilities in the nephron. AQP-3 and AQP-4 are localized in the basolateral membrane of the collecting duct and permit water to pass from the cell to the interstitium. AQP-2 is the major ADH-regulated water channel.[3] Within a few minutes, VP can increase the water permeability of the collecting duct cells by stimulating the translocation of AQP-2 from an intracellular reservoir to the luminal membrane. After VP withdrawal, AQP-2 is redistributed into the cell by endocytosis, and water permeability decreases. During stimulation by VP, a small percentage of AQP-2 is excreted into the urine. This urinary AQP-2 excretion closely reflects changes in VP exposure and has been proposed as a marker for collecting duct responsiveness in polyuric dogs.[4]

Cations, drugs, and hormones can influence the action of VP, thereby causing polyuria. For example, hypercalcemia is associated with decreased activity of adenylate cyclase, AQP-2 downregulation, and reduced insertion of AQP-2 in the luminal membrane of the collecting duct cell. Glucocorticoids also interfere with the action of VP, although in dogs, loss of reactivity of the osmoreceptor system also contributes to corticosteroid-induced polyuria.

In this chapter, the main VP-related disorders will be discussed, including the syndrome of inappropriate ADH release (SIAD) and diabetes insipidus (DI). In addition, primary polydipsia and primary adipsia will be discussed, as they both affect water homeostasis.

Syndrome of inappropriate ADH release

Etiology and pathophysiology

Elevated or normal VP (i.e., ADH) secretion is inappropriate in the presence of low plasma osmolality. Reduced suppressibility of VP release causes water retention and may lower plasma osmolality to the extent of causing clinical manifestations of cellular overhydration. In principle, this condition is associated with highly concentrated urine, but in humans, there is also a variant with resetting of the osmostat in which VP secretion can be fully suppressed, resulting in dilute urine at low plasma sodium concentrations. Only a few cases of syndrome of inappropriate ADH release (SIAD) have been described in dogs, and there also appear

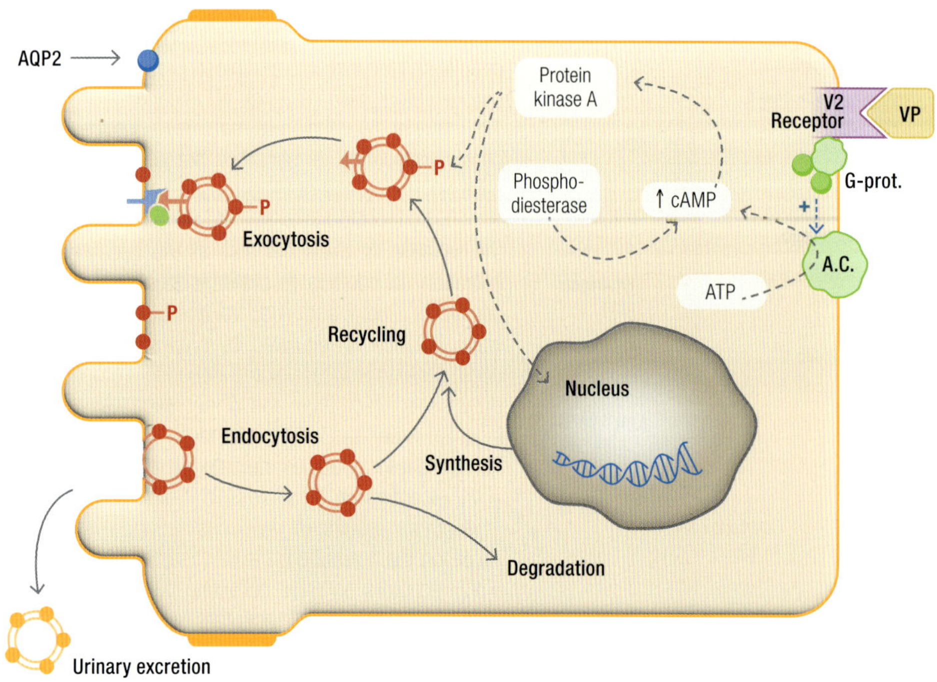

FIG. 25.3 Regulation of aquaporin-2 (AQP2) trafficking and expression in collecting duct cell. AC, adenylate cyclase; ATP, adenosine triphosphate; cAMP, cyclic adenosine monophosphate; VP, vasopressin. Modified after Nielsen et al., 1999.[13]

to be two forms, with and without polyuria. However, the diagnosis of SIAD in dogs with polyuria can be questioned, taking into account that hypersecretion of VP has also been reported in some dogs with primary polydipsia.[5]

SIAD is known to occur in humans as a complication of trans-sphenoidal resection of pituitary adenomas. The syndrome may arise as a consequence of uncontrolled VP release from surgically damaged hypothalamic centers. Hyponatremia due to SIAD has also been diagnosed after hypophysectomy in dogs with pituitary-dependent hypercortisolism. Furthermore, SIAD in dogs has been related to trauma due to bite wounds,[6] histiocytic sarcoma,[7] and several inflammatory disorders.

In addition to endogenous VP excess, similar abnormalities may be produced by excessive administration of synthetic VP. Particularly, dogs with primary polydipsia incorrectly treated with desmopressin seem to be at risk of developing the hypotonicity syndrome.

Clinical manifestations

In principle, both defective water excretion and increased water intake may lead to plasma hypotonicity, which is essentially hyponatremia. In hyponatremia, two-thirds of the relative water surplus is intracellular, making generalized cellular edema the hallmark of acute hypotonia. Unlike extracranial tissues that can expand freely, the distending brain is compressed against the unyielding cranium, provoking cerebral edema syndrome. This syndrome includes weakness, lethargy, and nausea and may culminate in resting tremors, generalized seizures, and coma. In addition to neurological manifestations, some of the reported cases included polyuria, which seems paradoxical in presumed VP excess. In these cases, primary polydipsia should be considered.

Diagnosis

SIAD can only be diagnosed after the exclusion of other potential causes of hypotonicity, such as hypoadrenocorticism, hypothyroidism, recent diuretic use, and hospital-acquired fluid imbalance. Then, at least three of the following criteria should be fulfilled:

- Plasma hypotonicity (Posm <280 mOsm/kg).
- Inappropriately high urine concentration in the presence of plasma hypotonicity.
- Plasma VP concentration inappropriately high relative to Posm.
- Improvement after fluid restriction.

Treatment

The therapy for SIAD focuses on the correction of hyponatremia and treatment of the underlying disease if identified. Fluid restriction is an important part of the therapy.

Severe hyponatremia (<120 mmol/L) should be corrected with intravenous fluid therapy using conventional crystalloid solutions (e.g., 0.9% saline) to raise plasma sodium concentration at a rate of less than 12 mmol/L/day. Hypertonic saline (3-5%) should be avoided, as it may raise the plasma sodium concentration too rapidly. Too rapid correction of (chronic) hyponatremia can result in osmotic demyelination syndrome due to brain dehydration as free water moves out of the brain and into the relatively hypertonic plasma. Clinical signs of osmotic demyelination syndrome usually occur 3-4 days after (too) rapid correction of hyponatremia, are neurologic in nature (lethargy, ataxia, hypermetria, paresis), and may be fatal.

Once plasma sodium concentration has been corrected to >125 mmol/L, water intake may be restricted to a volume less than urine output to promote free water loss and restore normal body fluid volume.

Chronic management of SIAD is directed at treating the underlying cause. If this is not possible, plasma hypo-osmolality and hyponatremia should be prevented by water restriction. This may be less effective in cases in which there is high urine concentration.

Receptor-specific V2 antagonists, so-called aquaretic agents, may block the action of VP in the collecting duct cells and thus promote water excretion specifically. However, these antagonists are expensive, and there is little experience with their use in dogs with SIAD.

Diabetes insipidus

The term diabetes insipidus (DI) is derived from the Greek *diabainein* (passing through) and the Latin *insipidus* (without taste). It is characterized by large volumes of urine with an osmolality lower than that of blood plasma and so dilute that it is almost tasteless. From a pathophysiological point of view, two fundamentally different pathogenetic categories of DI can be distinguished:

- A disturbance of the hypothalamic-pituitary system causing insufficient VP release (central diabetes insipidus).
- A disease or functional change of the kidneys, leading to insufficient response to VP (nephrogenic diabetes insipidus).

Central diabetes insipidus

Etiology and pathophysiology

Central diabetes insipidus (CDI) is characterized by three primary findings: 1) dilute urine despite strong osmotic stimuli for VP secretion, 2) absence of renal disease, and 3) a rise in urine osmolality following the administration of synthetic VP. Both complete and partial CDI have been recognized in dogs. In complete CDI, there is very little increase in urine osmolality with increasing plasma osmolality. The animal is essentially devoid of releasable VP. In partial CDI, there is a release of VP with increasing plasma osmolality, but in subnormal amounts.

Among the possible causes of impaired VP release, an intracranial tumor is possible in middle-aged and elderly dogs, most often a primary pituitary neoplasm. There are two possible mechanisms for the impaired release in case of a pituitary tumor: 1) the enlarging pituitary adenoma in the anterior lobe compresses the posterior lobe, resulting in pressure atrophy of the posterior lobe and reduced VP release, 2) large pituitary tumors with suprasellar extension can compress the hypothalamic nuclei, impairing VP synthesis (probably via degeneration of the hypothalamic neurons). Both mechanisms can contribute to VP deficiency and the inability to react adequately to osmotic stimuli. It may be difficult to diagnose CDI in dogs in which a pituitary corticotroph adenoma has caused hypercortisolism (Cushing's disease). CDI may be overlooked because of the polyuria caused by glucocorticoid excess. In these cases, CDI may become apparent when the hypercortisolism has been eliminated by treatment.

Neoplastic non-pituitary lesions reported to cause CDI include meningioma and malignant lymphoma.[8] A non-neoplastic cause of CDI is the trauma and subsequent inflammation of larva migrans. CDI has also been described in association with congenital pituitary anomalies.[9] Severe head injury is also known to be a cause of CDI. CDI can also occur as a complication of pituitary surgery, i.e., hypophysectomy, most often performed to treat Cushing's disease. CDI appears immediately following hypophysectomy and quite often disappears spontaneously after days to months. If the pituitary stalk is sectioned so high as to induce retrograde degeneration of the hypothalamic neurons, the CDI can be permanent.

There remains the possibility of the so-called idiopathic form of CDI. This term is used in cases in which there is no evident lesion in the hypothalamus or pituitary. This may be the case, especially in young animals, although the subsequent course of the disease, diagnostic imaging, or autopsy may eventually reveal a lesion that could not be identified initially. It may also be due to immune-mediated destruction of VP-producing neurons.

Clinical manifestations

The major clinical manifestations are polyuria, polydipsia, and a near-continuous demand for water. In severe cases, water intake and urine volume may be huge, requiring micturition almost every hour throughout the day and night. Although in partial CDI, water intake and urine volume may be only moderately increased, in severe cases of complete CDI, water intake may be so enormous as to interfere with food intake and thus result in weight loss. In dogs in which a large neoplasm is the underlying cause, there may be additional neurological symptoms and endocrine deficiencies. CDI caused by head trauma may not only be associated with soft tissue and skeletal lesions, but damage to the hypothalamus-pituitary region may cause additional hormone deficiencies, such as secondary hypothyroidism.

If water is withheld from an animal with complete CDI, life-threatening hypertonic encephalopathy occurs within a few hours (plasma sodium concentration >170 mmol/L; Posm >375 mOsm/kg), initially manifested by ataxia and sopor. This can also occur when the causative lesion extends to the thirst center, and adipsia develops.

Diagnosis

Both urine specific gravity (Usg) and urine osmolality (Uosm) will be below that of plasma: Usg <1.010 and Uosm <290 mOsm/kg, although in mild cases, Uosm may be up to 600 mOsm/kg. Blood examination usually reveals no abnormalities except for (slight) hypernatremia and a (slightly) elevated Posm due to inadequate replenishment of the excreted water.

For some time, the water deprivation test combined with synthetic VP administration, i.e., the modified water deprivation test, has been used to diagnose CDI. However, this test is difficult to perform correctly, is unpleasant for the animal, relies heavily on emptying the bladder at each urine collection, and is indirect because changes in urine concentration are used as an index of VP release. Furthermore, the stimulus to VP release is a combination of hypertonicity and hypovolemia, especially near the end of the period of dehydration.

Protocol water deprivation test

In this indirect test of VP secretory capacity, plasma osmolality is increased by water deprivation to stimulate VP release. The effect of endogenous VP is determined by measurements of urine osmolality (Uosm) or specific gravity (Usg). The test is indicated to differentiate between diabetes insipidus and primary polydipsia.

Following 12 hours of fasting, water is withheld, and Uosm (or Usg) is measured every 2 hours (or more frequently when the polyuria is severe). The bladder has to be emptied every 2 hours. When the loss of body weight, measured every 2 hours, is more than 5% of the initial body weight, the test is stopped.

In primary polydipsia, Uosm (or Usg) gradually rises to more than 1000 mOsm/kg during water deprivation. In the case of diabetes insipidus, Uosm remains below 1000 mOsm/kg during water deprivation. Differentiation between central and nephrogenic diabetes insipidus relies on the effect of administration of synthetic vasopressin.

A more direct way to diagnose CDI is by measuring plasma VP concentrations during osmotic stimulation by hypertonic saline infusion, but this is a cumbersome procedure that can only be performed in specialized institutions. Moreover, a VP assay is not widely available.

Increasingly, the diagnostic procedure starts with serial Uosm measurements in urine samples collected by the owner at home. The owner then administers desmopressin (DDAVP, synthetic VP) for 4-5 days and collects another series of urine samples during the last day of desmopressin treatment. In both complete and partial CDI, polyuria and polydipsia cease after administration of desmopressin, and Uosm rises from low values to >1000 mOsm/kg. CDI is unlikely if Uosm remains well below 1000 mOsm/kg.

When there is a history of head trauma or suspicion of a pituitary lesion/tumor that might cause additional pituitary deficiencies, the adenohypophyseal function should be studied, and the pituitary area should be visualized by CT and/or MRI scan. The neurohypophysis can be visualized with dynamic CT. In the presence of a pituitary adenoma, the neurohypophysis can be displaced or no longer be visible. However, in only a small proportion of cases, does a pituitary tumor interfere with VP release sufficiently to cause CDI.

Treatment

The VP analog desmopressin or DDAVP (1-diamino, 9-D-arginine vasopressin) is the drug most commonly used for treatment. It is available for use in humans in ampoules for parenteral injection (4 µg per ampoule), intranasal solution (100 µg per mL), and tablets (0.1, 0.2, and 0.4 mg). One drop of the intranasal solution (= 1.5-4 µg DDAVP) administered in the conjunctival sac twice daily sufficiently controls the polyuria in most dogs with CDI. With the administration of three drops/day, urine production usually returns to normal, but some owners (in part for financial reasons) administer it only twice daily. The starting dose of the desmopressin tablets is 0.1 mg twice daily. If additional pituitary deficiencies have been revealed as a result of head trauma, pituitary tumor, or hypophysectomy, they should be treated as required with thyroxine and/or glucocorticoids.

Nephrogenic diabetes insipidus

Etiology, pathophysiology, and clinical manifestations

In nephrogenic diabetes insipidus (NDI), the kidneys are unable to concentrate urine despite adequate plasma VP concentrations. The condition may be congenital or acquired, but the congenital form appears to be extremely rare. In contrast, acquired or secondary NDI is the most common cause of polyuria in dogs. The polyuria may be the result of the downregulation of AQP-2 and/or reduced delivery of AQP-2 to the luminal membrane of the collecting duct cell.

In dogs, acquired chronic renal failure associated with polyuria is also considered a form of NDI. The polyuria may not be the iatrotropic problem that causes the owner to consult the veterinarian.

Juvenile-onset renal diseases have been reported to occur as familial diseases but also as isolated cases of renal failure. Various underlying

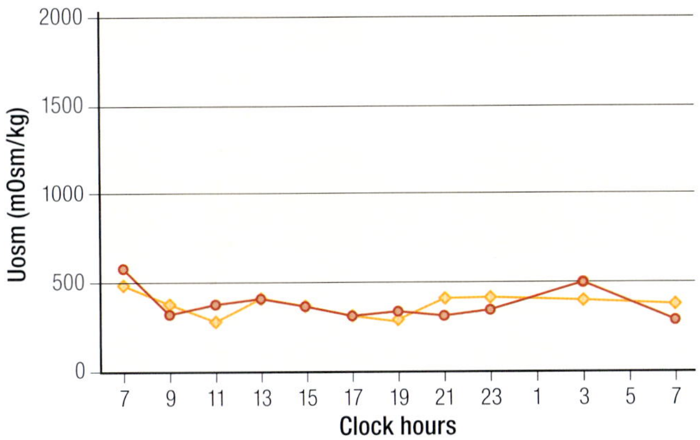

FIG. 25.4 Results of serial measurements of urine osmolality (Uosm) in two dogs with nephrogenic diabetes insipidus (NDI).

abnormalities have been reported in familial renal disease, such as amyloidosis, glomerular basement disorders, and polycystic kidney disease. These animals usually develop chronic renal insufficiency and consequently may be presented with polyuria due to isosthenuria.

Diagnosis

Usually, NDI leads to isosthenuria (Usg 1.008-1.012). However, with tubular changes and fibrosis in the renal medulla, Usg may be below that of isosthenuria.

Serial measurements of Uosm reveal it to be low with only minor fluctuations (Fig. 25.4). Water deprivation does not result in normalization of the concentration of the urine. Administration of desmopressin has little or no effect, but this does not necessarily mean that the primary abnormality is renal, for poor response to desmopressin may also occur in conditions causing VP resistance, such as hypercortisolism.

NDI should only be diagnosed if other causes of polyuria, in particular those abnormalities resulting in decreased sensitivity of the collecting duct cells to VP, such as hypercalcemia, pyometra, hypercortisolism, hyperaldosteronism, etc., have been ruled out.

Treatment

For most dogs with NDI, a treatment to resolve the polyuria is not available. In a few dogs with NDI, relatively high doses of desmopressin may decrease the polyuria. If this is not effective, oral administration of hydrochlorothiazide (2-4 mg/kg twice daily) and a low-sodium diet may be considered. The latter treatment has decreased urine volume in a few dogs with NDI, usually without a significant change in urine osmolality. It has been proposed that the thiazide diuretic and a low-sodium diet cause extracellular volume contraction. As a result, the glomerular filtration rate decreases, and proximal tubular reabsorption of sodium and water increases. Consequently, less sodium and water are delivered to the collecting ducts, and urinary volume is reduced but not normalized.[10] However, there is increasing evidence that sodium depletion and increased proximal tubular water reabsorption do not solely account for the antidiuretic effect. Hydrochlorothiazide can also directly increase water permeability in the medullary collecting ducts, possibly by inducing AQP-2 expression independent of VP.[11]

Primary polydipsia

Etiology, pathophysiology, and clinical manifestations

Although primary polydipsia is not primarily a VP-related disorder, the facts that the main clinical manifestation, i.e., polyuria and polydipsia, may mimic that of DI and that primary polydipsia can result in changes in VP release warrant inclusion in this chapter.

Primary polydipsia is characterized by a marked increase in water intake that cannot be explained as a compensatory mechanism for excessive fluid loss. There is no urinary concentrating defect, and at various times during the day, the dog may produce either highly diluted urine or concentrated urine. Important to note is that marked fluctuations in Uosm may also occur even though the owner observes nothing remarkable in the dog's drinking behavior. In a series of 89 healthy pet dogs, Uosm in morning urines ranged from 273 to 2620 mOsm/kg (Usg 1.009 to >1.050) with a mean (+/- SD) of 1541 (+/- 527 mOsm/kg (Usg 1.035 +/- 0.010).[12] In none of these dogs was the sometimes marked variation in water intake and urine volume considered by the owners to be associated with abnormal drinking.

Dogs with more pronounced primary polydipsia may be presented to the veterinarian because of polyuria and polydipsia. This is said to be the case in hyperactive young dogs that are left alone for many hours during the day or have undergone important changes in their environment. Placing these dogs in a completely different environment, as during hospitalization, has sometimes stopped the problem. The problem may also develop later in life, such as in the excitement of the anticipated pleasure of going for a walk. In the past, this was often referred to as psychogenic polydipsia, but primary polydipsia is a more correct term as it also includes physical causes of polydipsia. Transient primary polydipsia has also been reported to occur in association with gastrointestinal disease, in which case water intake was more than the fluid losses via diarrhea and vomiting.

As mentioned earlier in this chapter, satiation of thirst occurs in dogs during drinking before any detectable change in plasma osmolality, plasma volume, or blood pressure as a result of absorption of the water. Oropharyngeal signals inhibiting thirst normally prevent the dog from drinking an amount of water in excess of its physiological need. Nevertheless, water consumption has been shown to fluctuate with food intake and exercise: dogs consumed 40% of their total daily water intake 2 hours after eating dry food, and after treadmill running for 30 minutes, water intake was higher than the water losses during the exercise. These factors, together with other environmental factors and/or moments of intense interactions in some dogs, seem to bring about a complex of signals that override the oropharyngeal and osmotic signals that normally result in appropriate water intake.

Diagnosis

The results of routine blood examinations are usually unremarkable, except for Posm and plasma sodium concentration, which may be at or just below the lower limit of their respective reference ranges.

Marked fluctuations in Uosm in serial urine samples collected at frequent intervals and some values >1000 mOsm/kg provide the diagnosis of primary polydipsia (Fig. 25.5). However, the fluctuations are not so pronounced in all dogs with primary polydipsia and in some dogs with primary polydipsia, Uosm fluctuates between about 200 and 600 mOsm/kg. In such cases, a water deprivation test can be helpful to diagnose the

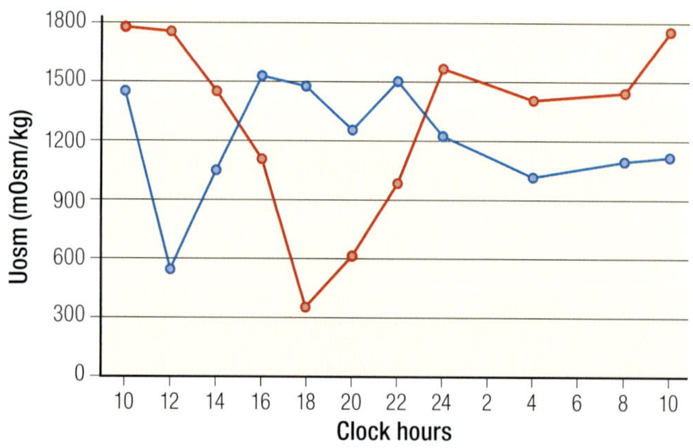

FIG. 25.5 Results of serial measurements of urine osmolality (Uosm) in two dogs with primary polydipsia.

disorder. With water deprivation, Uosm should exceed 1000 mOsm/kg with weight loss ≤3% and only slight increases in Posm and plasma sodium concentration. The plasma VP concentration measured during the water deprivation test in dogs with primary polydipsia remains low.[5] During hypertonic saline infusion, abnormalities in VP release may include episodes of hypersecretion as well as delayed and low responses to plasma hypertonicity.[5] It is not clear whether the latter indicates a primary disturbance in osmoreceptor function and regulation of ADH secretion or that it is the result of chronic overhydration downregulating VP release in response to hypertonicity. The occasionally observed "hyperresponses" might represent erratic secretory bursts but might also reflect the pulsatile release pattern induced by the hypertonicity.

Treatment

Dogs with strong fluctuations in Uosm at set times during the day are difficult to treat. The water bowl can be removed during periods when excessive water intake can be expected, and the conditioned behavior can be discouraged. Some caution is warranted in dogs with less pronounced spontaneous fluctuations in Uosm at low values but in which water deprivation leads to Uosm >1000 mOsm/kg in <8 h. In some of these dogs, Posm may not be low, and water restriction, although effective, may increase Posm and lead to severe sensations of thirst, reducing the dog's quality of life. Treatment with VP analog desmopressin or DDAVP (1-diamino, 9-D-arginine vasopressin) may decrease polyuria/polydipsia in a few dogs with primary polydipsia. One drop of the intranasal solution (= 1.5-4 μg DDAVP) administered in the conjunctival sac thrice daily may control the polyuria. The dose of the desmopressin tablets is 0.1 mg twice daily.

Primary adipsia

Etiology, pathophysiology, and clinical manifestations

Primary adipsia or hypodipsia is a rare, congenital, or acquired condition associated with an absent or decreased sensation of thirst, even in the presence of body water depletion. It can occur as the result of a disorder in the hypothalamic-pituitary region (including the thirst center). It may be due to an intracranial tumor but may also be present without physical changes in imaging studies. Moreover, adipsia can result from pituitary surgery (e.g., hypophysectomy).

History taking regarding the quantity of fluid intake may reveal the lack of thirst, pointing to adipsia. Clinical signs may include lethargy, muscle weakness, and, in severe cases, even coma. On physical examination, loss of skin turgor and dry, reddish mucous membranes may be found.

Diagnosis

Adipsia results in hemoconcentration and a high plasma osmolality. Besides an increase in the hematocrit and the plasma osmolality, laboratory investigation in patients with adipsia may reveal hypernatremia (hypernatremic dehydration), elevated plasma concentrations of urea and creatinine, and elevated serum protein concentrations. Brain imaging studies, such as CT or MRI scans, are indicated if the underlying cause for adipsia needs to be determined.

Treatment

Patients affected by adipsia lack the ability to sense thirst. The only available "treatment" is to increase the animal's water intake. These patients must maintain a strict daily water intake schedule. Usually, the best way to ensure sufficient water intake is to add water to the food. Chronic hypernatremia in animals with adipsia should not be corrected too rapidly to avoid cerebral edema. The plasma sodium concentration should not decrease more than 0.5 mmol/L per hour.

KEY POINTS

- The neurohypophysis releases vasopressin in response to increased plasma osmolality and, to a lesser degree, reduced blood volume/low blood pressure.
- Vasopressin binds to specific V2 receptors at the renal collecting duct cells. Activation of these receptors results in the insertion of water channels (aquaporins) in the luminal membrane of the cell, leading to increased water reabsorption from the lumen of the duct into the hypertonic renal medulla, resulting in urine concentration.
- Inappropriate VP release (SIAD) causes water retention and may lower plasma osmolality to the extent of causing clinical manifestations of cellular overhydration. Unlike extracranial tissues that can expand freely, the distending brain is compressed against the unyielding cranium, provoking cerebral edema syndrome.
- Central diabetes insipidus (CDI) results from a lack of hypothalamic production or pituitary release of VP secondary to immune-mediated destruction of VP-producing neurons, cerebral trauma (head injury), intracranial neoplasia (often a pituitary tumor), or other hypothalamic/pituitary lesions. In dogs, hypercortisolism and hyperaldosteronism may also result in less VP secretion.
- In nephrogenic diabetes insipidus (NDI), the kidneys are unable to concentrate urine despite adequate circulating levels of VP. Frequently, the cause of inadequate VP action remains unknown. NDI may also be secondary to other disorders, such as hypercortisolism, hypercalcemia, or pyometra.

References

1. Rijnberk A, Kooistra HS. Hypothalamus-pituitary system. In Rijnberk A, Kooistra HS (editors). Clinical Endocrinology of Dogs and Cats 2nd edition. Hannover, Schlütersche Verslagsgeselschaft mbH & Co, 2010, pp. 13-54.
2. Van Vonderen IK, Wolfswinkel J, Oosterlaken-Dijksterhuis MA, Rijnberk A, Kooistra HS. Pulsatile secretion pattern of vasopressin under basal conditions, after water deprivation, and during osmotic stimulation in dogs. *Domest Anim Endocrinol* 27:1-12, 2004a.
3. Schrier RW. Body water homeostasis: clinical disorders of urinary dilution and concentration. *J Am Soc Nephrol* 17:1820-1832, 2006.
4. Van Vonderen IK, Wolfswinkel J, van den Ingh TSGAM, Mol JA, Rijnberk A, Kooistra HS. Urinary aquaporin-2 excretion in dogs: a marker for collecting duct responsiveness to vasopressin. *Domest Anim Endocrinol* 27:141-153, 2004b.
5. Van Vonderen IK, Kooistra HS, Timmermans-Sprang EPM, Rijnberk A. Disturbed vasopressin release in four dogs with so-called primary polydipsia. *J Vet Intern Med* 13:419-425, 1999.
6. Cilli NM, Bellis T. Syndrome of inappropriate antidiuretic hormone secretion secondary to trauma in a dog. *J Vet Emerg Crit Care (San Antonio)* 32:135-140, 2022.
7. Barrot AC, Bédard A, Dunn M. Syndrome of inappropriate antidiuretic hormone secretion in a dog with a histiocytic sarcoma. *Can Vet J* 58:713-715, 2017.
8. Nielsen L, Thompson H, Hammond GJ, Chang YP, Ramsey IK. Central diabetes insipidus associated with primary focal B cell lymphoma in a dog. *Vet Rec* 162:124-126, 2008.
9. Ramsey IK, Dennis R, Herrtage ME. Concurrent central diabetes insipidus and panhypopituitarism in a German Shepherd dog. *J Small Anim Pract* 40:271-274, 1999.
10. Magaldi AJ. New insights into the paradoxical effect of thiazides in diabetes insipidus therapy. *Nephrol Dial Transplant* 15:1903-1905, 2000.
11. Kim GH, Lee JW, Oh YK, Chang HR, Joo KW, Na KYEarm JH, Knepper MA, Han JS. Antidiuretic effect of hydrochlorothiazide in lithium-induced nephrogenic diabetes insipidus is associated with upregulation of aquaporin-2, NaCl cotransporter, and epithelial sodium channel. *J Am Soc Nephrol* 15:2836-2843, 2004.
12. Van Vonderen IK, Kooistra HS, Rijnberk A. Intra- and interindividual variation in urine osmolality and urine specific gravity in healthy pet dogs of various ages. *J Vet Intern Med* 11:30-35, 1997.
13. Nielsen S, Kwon TH, Christensen BM, Promeneur D, Frokiaer J, Marples D. Physiology and pathophysiology of renal aquaporins. *J Am Soc Nephro* 10:647-663, 1999.

CHAPTER 26

Anatomy and physiology of the thyroid gland

Lisa Stammeleer
DVM, DECVIM-CA
(Internal Medicine)

The human thyroid was first illustrated by Leonardo da Vinci in 1500, whereas the first anatomical description of the human thyroid dates from 1543 by Vesalius. Actual thyroid hormones were first isolated by Eugen Baumann in 1896. He boiled the thyroid glands of a thousand sheep and named the precipitate "iodithyrin".[1]

Anatomy

The thyroid consists of two lobes, each on one side of the trachea. Ectopic thyroid tissue is a relatively common finding in dogs; it is found in about 50% of adult dogs at necropsy examination. This tissue can be located anywhere from the tongue to the diaphragm. The cranial and caudal thyroid arteries provide blood supply to the thyroid. These arteries originate from the carotid and brachiocephalic artery, respectively. On a microscopic level, each thyroid lobe consists of follicles containing a homogeneous staining substance, colloid. The epithelial cells delineating the follicles are cuboidal in shape when thyroid hormone secretion is basal, while their shape is columnar in case of upregulated hormone production. The parafollicular cells (or C-cells) are dispersed in the interstitium and produce calcitonin (Fig. 26.1).[2]

Physiology

Ingested iodine is converted to iodide in the intestinal tract before entering the circulation. The follicular cells trap iodide via the sodium-iodide symporter. This step is mediated by the thyroid-stimulating hormone (TSH). Iodide molecules bind to the tyrosine ring of thyroglobulin in the colloid. One or two iodide molecules can attach to one thyroglobulin molecule, resulting in monoiodotyrosine (MIT) or diiodotyrosine (DIT), respectively. This process is referred to as iodination or organification. Two tyrosine residues couple to form either triiodothyronine (T_3, one MIT, and one DIT) or tetraiodothyronine (T_4, two DIT). Thyroid hormones are stored in the colloid upon secretion. Thyroglobulin and its attached MIT, DIT, T_3, and T_4 must pass through the follicular cell for cleavage by lysosomal enzymes before secretion into circulation is achieved. Only a small amount of thyroglobulin also enters circulation. Thyroid peroxidase (TPO) facilitates oxidation of I^-, organification of thyroglobulin, and coupling of iodinated tyrosine residues (Fig. 26.2).

Thyroid hormones are lipophilic and mostly protein-bound in circulation. Only the unbound or "free" fraction (less than 1% of the total T_3 and T_4 concentrations) is biologically active. Sixty percent of circulating thyroid hormones

FIG. 26.1 Illustration of the microscopic structure of the thyroid gland.

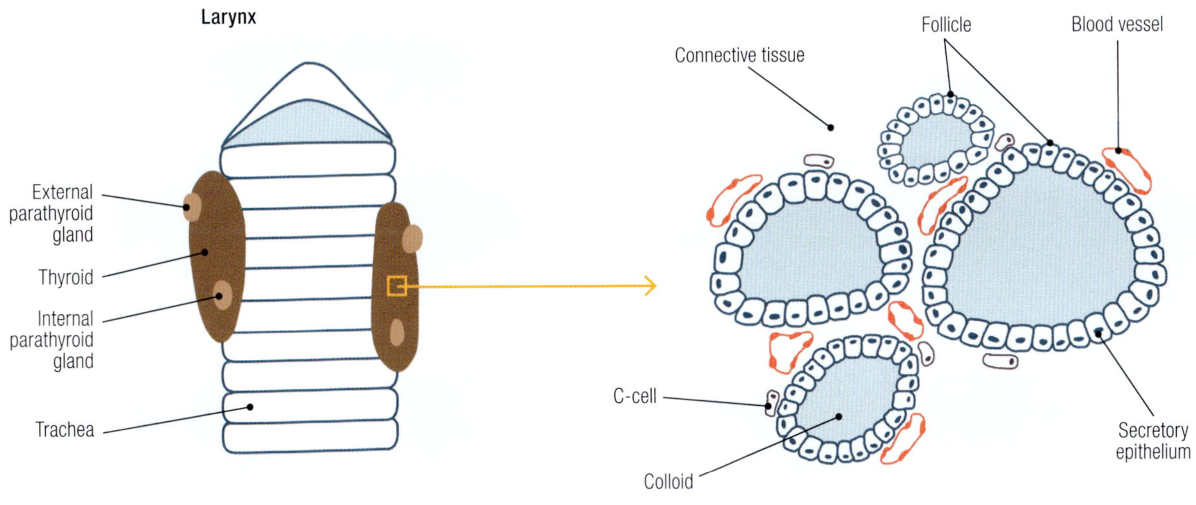

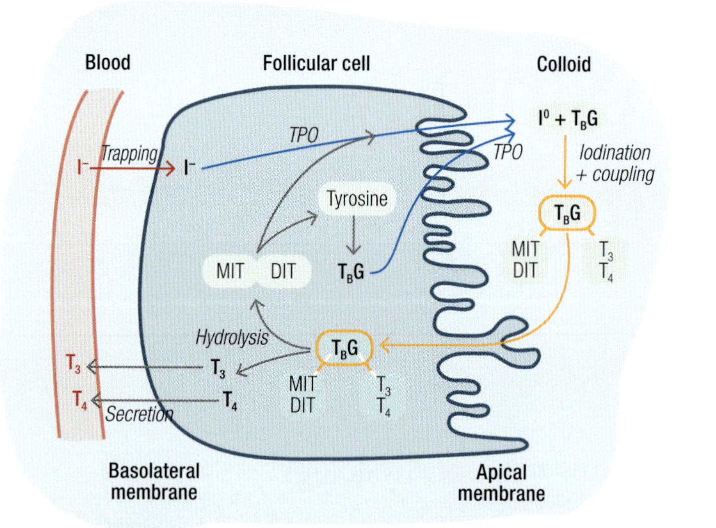

FIG. 26.2 Thyroid hormone synthesis. Iodide (I^-) is trapped by the follicular cells and oxidized to I_0 (mediated by thyroid peroxidase; TPO). Thyroglobulin (T_BG), produced in the follicular cells, is transported into the colloid. Oxidized I^0 is bound to the tyrosine residues of T_BG (organification). The iodinated tyrosine residues (monoiodotyrosine and diiodotyrosine; MIT and DIT, respectively) remain bound to the thyroglobulin molecule and undergo oxidative condensation to triiodothyronine (T_3) and tetraiodothyronine (T_4). Thyroglobulin and the attached T_3, T_4, MIT, and DIT enter the follicular cells where T_3, T_4, MIT, and DIT are released from the thyroglobulin molecule by hydrolysis. The thyroid hormones T_3 and T_4 are released into circulation. Iodide and tyrosine are recycled from the MIT and DIT molecules.

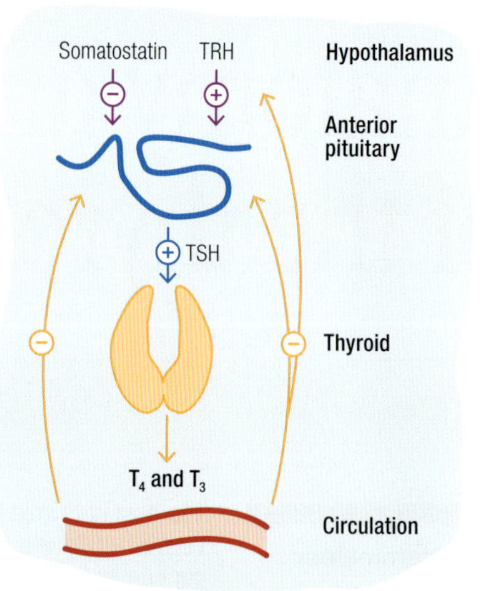

FIG. 26.3 Schematic representation of the hypothalamic-pituitary-thyroid axis. Somatostatin limits the release of thyrotropin or thyroid-stimulating hormone (TSH) while thyrotropin-releasing hormone (TRH) promotes the synthesis and release of TSH. Thyrotropin, in turn, stimulates the synthesis of T_3 and T_4. Both triiodothyronine (T_3) and tetraiodothyronine (T_4) provide negative feedback to the anterior pituitary, limiting the production of TSH. Mostly T_3 provides negative at the level of the hypothalamus.

are bound to thyroxine-binding globulin. Other binding proteins include thyroxine-bound prealbumin, transthyretin, albumin, and various lipoprotein fractions. Due to the high affinity for plasma proteins, the serum half-life of T_4 (10-16 hours) and T_3 (5-6 hours) is longer compared to other hormones. Triiodothyronine (T_3) is three to four times more potent than T_4. Triiodothyronine is produced both in the thyroid gland (40% of the total T_3 production) and in the periphery by outer ring monodeiodination of T_4. Inner ring deiodination results in metabolically inactive reverse T_3 (rT_3). Thyroid hormone production is regulated by a negative feedback system, where both T_3 and T_4 provide negative feedback to the anterior hypophysis (Fig. 26.3). The most important sites for elimination (by removal of iodide molecules or by conjugation) are the liver and the kidneys. Iodide molecules are recycled in both the thyroid gland and via the enterohepatic cycle after secretion in bile.

Thyroid hormones are the primary determinants of basal metabolism and have a large array of physiological effects. They stimulate calorigenesis, erythropoiesis, bone turnover, protein and enzyme synthesis, and almost all parts of carbohydrate and lipid metabolism (synthesis, mobilization, and degradation). Both T_3 and T_4 have positive inotropic and chronotropic effects and are necessary for the normal function of the respiratory center. Thyroid hormones are essential during fetal development, especially for the neural and skeletal system.[2,3,4,5]

KEY POINTS

- The thyroid gland is the only production site of T_4. Triiodothyronine (T_3) is produced intra- and extrathyroidally.
- Both T_4 and T_3 are highly protein-bound in circulation. Only the "free" or unbound fraction is biologically active.
- Thyroid peroxidase is the main enzyme catalyzing thyroid hormone production in the thyroid gland.
- Both T_4 and T_3 provide negative feedback to the anterior pituitary, resulting in decreased production of TSH and, subsequently, T_4 and T_3.
- Thyroid hormones are the main determinants of basal metabolism.

References

1. Niazi AK, Kalra S, Irfan A, Islam A. Thyroidology over the ages. *Indian J Endocrinol Metabolism* 15(Suppl 2):121-126, 2011.
2. Hall JE, Guyton AC (editors). Guyton and Hall Textbook of Medical Physiology 14th edition. Philadelphia, Elsevier Saunders, 2020.
3. Scott-Moncrieff CJ. Hypothyroidism. In Feldman EC, Nelson RW, Reusch CE, Scott-Moncrieff JCR (editors). Canine and Feline Endocrinology 4th edition. Missouri Elsevier Saunders, 2015, pp. 77-80.
4. Greco DS, Stabenfeldt GH. The endocrine system. In Klein BG (editor). Cunningham's Textbook of Veterinary Physiology 6th edition. Missouri, Elsevier Health Sciences Division, 2019, pp. 378-393.
5. Melmed S, Koenig R, Rosen CJ, Auchus RJ, Goldfine AB. Williams Textbook of Endocrinology 14th edition. Missouri, Elsevier Health Sciences Division, 2019.

CHAPTER 27

Canine hypothyroidism

Andrea Corsini
DVM, PhD, DECVIM-CA
(Internal Medicine)

Tera Pijnacker
DVM, DECVIM-CA
(Internal Medicine)

Hypothyroidism results from decreased production of thyroid hormones. It is by far the most common thyroid disease in dogs, with an estimated prevalence between 0.07% and 0.23% and an annual incidence risk of 0.04%.[1-5] These percentages are merely indicative because many factors can affect the prevalence and the incidence in a given population (e.g., geographical distribution, breed predisposition, referral, or general population). In addition, it is likely that canine hypothyroidism is an overdiagnosed condition due to the inherent difficulties in obtaining a definitive diagnosis.

Etiology

Canine hypothyroidism may be acquired or congenital, and both forms can be classified as primary, secondary, or tertiary. Primary hypothyroidism is due to diseases affecting the thyroid gland, secondary hypothyroidism is due to decreased or absent thyroid-stimulating hormone (TSH) secretion from the pituitary gland, and tertiary hypothyroidism is caused by decreased or absent thyrotropin-releasing hormone (TRH) secretion from the hypothalamus. The term central hypothyroidism includes both secondary and tertiary hypothyroidism. Primary hypothyroidism accounts for the vast majority of the cases, while central hypothyroidism is rare in dogs.

Acquired hypothyroidism

Primary hypothyroidism

Acquired primary hypothyroidism is the most common form of naturally occurring hypothyroidism in adult dogs. The typical histologic lesions described in adult hypothyroid dogs are lymphocytic thyroiditis or idiopathic thyroid atrophy, with equal frequency.[6]

Lymphocytic thyroiditis is an autoimmune disease characterized by lymphoplasmacytic infiltration of the thyroid gland with progressive destruction of functional thyroid tissue (Fig. 27.1). Antibodies directed against thyroid tissue, usually antithyroglobulin antibodies (TgAAs) and, less commonly, anti-TPO antibodies, may be detected in the serum of affected dogs in the initial phase.[7] Dogs with early thyroiditis are extremely unlikely to be detected at this stage because they have no clinical signs or clinicopathologic abnormalities, and thyroid function tests are normal. As the disease progresses and functional thyroid tissue decreases to less than 40-50%, dogs develop subclinical hypothyroidism, which is characterized by a compensatory increase in serum TSH concentration that allows maintenance of a normal serum total T_4 concentration, and therefore absence of clinical signs. Finally, clinical hypothyroidism develops when at least 75% of the functional tissue is destroyed. At this stage, dogs show clinical signs, have decreased serum thyroid hormone concentrations, and may be antibody-positive (antibody-positive overt hypothyroidism) or antibody-negative (noninflammatory atrophic hypothyroidism).[8]

An association between antibody-positive hypothyroidism and specific major histocompatibility complex (MHC) dog leucocyte antigen (DLA) haplotypes has been described in Doberman Pinschers, Rhodesian Ridgebacks, and English Setters but not in other breeds predisposed to hypothyroidism (e.g., Boxers).[9] The rate of progression of lymphocytic thyroiditis can vary greatly and is higher in predisposed breeds. It has been estimated that approximately one in five dogs with subclinical thyroiditis will develop thyroid dysfunction within a year, and not all affected dogs will eventually develop clinical hypothyroidism.[10]

Idiopathic thyroid atrophy is characterized by a loss of thyroid follicles replaced by fibrous or adipose tissue, often without clear signs of inflammation. These findings support the assumption that idiopathic thyroid atrophy may be both the end stage of lymphocytic thyroiditis or a primary degenerative disease.[6] It is likely that the progression of the disease will be similar to that described for lymphocytic thyroiditis in dogs that develop hypothyroidism due to idiopathic thyroid atrophy. Other less common causes of acquired thyroid failure in dogs include iodine deficiency, which can lead to goitrous hypothyroidism, thyroid gland destruction due to neoplasia, and iatrogenic hypothyroidism due to surgical thyroidectomy, radioactive iodine treatment, medical treatment with antithyroid drugs or a prolonged course of sulfonamides.[4,5,11]

Autoimmune polyendocrine syndrome

Acquired primary hypothyroidism due to lymphocytic thyroiditis can be associated with other autoimmune diseases, sometimes affecting other endocrine organs.

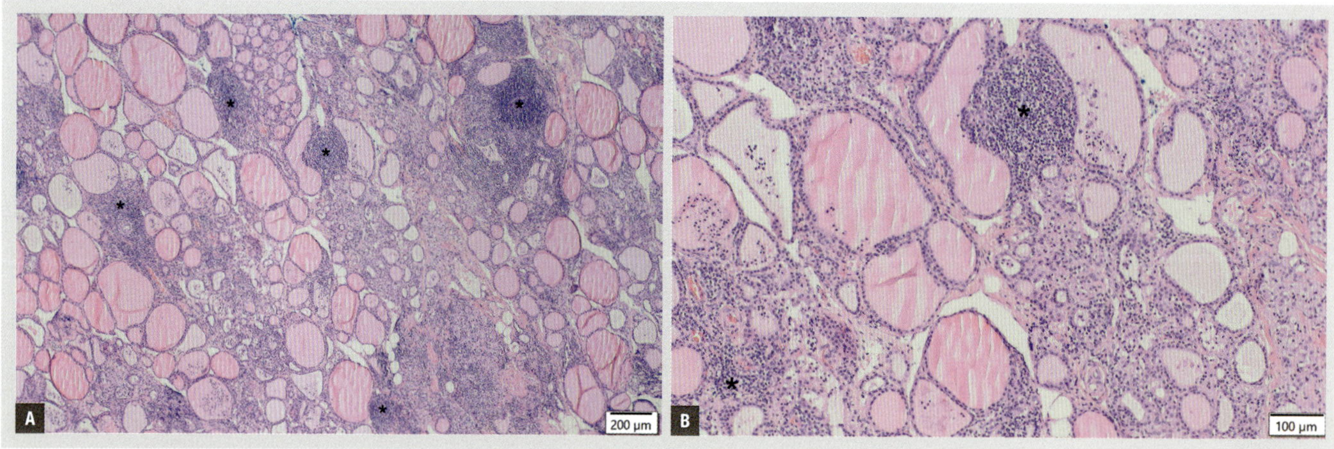

FIG. 27.1 Microscopic appearance of the thyroid gland in a dog with lymphocytic thyroiditis and hypothyroidism. Note the mononuclear cell infiltration (asterisks), disruption of the normal architecture, and loss of colloid-containing follicles. Images courtesy of Dr. W. Bergmann, Utrecht University.

Autoimmune polyendocrine syndromes (APS) are well described in humans as a clustering of at least two autoimmune endocrine diseases in a single patient. Although uncommonly, the clustering of endocrine disorders allegedly sharing immune-mediated etiology has also been described in dogs, with the most frequent combinations being hypothyroidism and hypoadrenocorticism, hypothyroidism and diabetes mellitus, and hypoadrenocorticism and diabetes mellitus.[12] These presentations closely resemble Schmidt syndrome, a combination of Addison's disease with autoimmune hypothyroidism and/or type 1 diabetes mellitus, which is part of a larger syndrome in humans defined as APS type 2. Clinicians should suspect polyendocrine syndromes in dogs with multiple endocrine gland failure, but the diagnosis of hypothyroidism must be assessed carefully in these patients because both uncontrolled diabetes mellitus and untreated hypoadrenocorticism can affect thyroid testing in dogs (see Endocrine testing later).

Central hypothyroidism

Central hypothyroidism is characterized by TRH deficiency (tertiary hypothyroidism) or TSH deficiency (secondary hypothyroidism), both of which result in decreased thyroid hormone synthesis and secretion and ultimately, atrophic degeneration of the thyroid gland. Acquired secondary hypothyroidism is the most common form of central hypothyroidism but is estimated to account for less than 5% of adult hypothyroid dogs. It may be due to suppression of pituitary function or destruction of the pituitary gland. Hypercortisolism, either endogenous or iatrogenic, and malnutrition are common causes of suppression of TSH secretion, although in most cases, they are not associated with clinical hypothyroidism.[13] Destruction of the pituitary gland is rare and is mainly due to invasive pituitary or brain neoplasia. It can be iatrogenic (e.g., radiation therapy, hypophysectomy) or sporadically seen in cases of head trauma, lymphocytic adenohypophysitis, or intracranial hemorrhage.[14]

Tertiary hypothyroidism is considered extremely rare in dogs and has only been described in one case report.[15]

Congenital hypothyroidism

Congenital hypothyroidism is considered rare in dogs, with only 3.6% of cases of hypothyroidism diagnosed in dogs <1 year of age. The true prevalence is unknown, considering there are no recent epidemiologic data and, most importantly, mild cases can go unnoticed, and severe cases are likely to die at birth undiagnosed.[16] In humans, congenital primary hypothyroidism can be caused by a variety of mechanisms involving the hypothalamic-pituitary axis or the thyroid hormone receptor. In dogs, all cases described to date have been caused by dyshormonogenesis or thyroid dysgenesis and occur either as a sporadic or familial disease. Iodine deficiency during pregnancy has been suggested as a possible cause of congenital hypothyroidism in litters, based on cases reported in humans, but there are no published cases in dogs. Dyshormonogenesis is caused by inborn defects in any step of thyroid hormone biosynthesis and, in most cases, results in congenital hypothyroidism with goiter (CHG). In dogs with dyshormonogenesis, the hypothalamic-pituitary-thyroid axis and TSH receptors are intact. Therefore, elevated serum TSH concentrations result in thyroid hyperplasia and goiter. Autosomal recessive mutations of the TPO gene preventing the synthesis of functional TPO have been described as the cause of CHG in toy Fox Terriers, Rat Terriers, Tenterfield Terriers, Spanish Water dogs, and a French Bulldog.[17-19] A different mutation leading to a defect in the activity of the sodium/iodide symporter (NIS), a protein that mediates the transport of iodide in the thyroid gland, has recently been described in a family of Shi Tzu dogs with CHG.[20] Thyroid dysgenesis is associated with aplasia, hypoplasia, or ectopia of the thyroid gland, resulting in nongoitrous congenital hypothyroidism. It has been described in four pups, but the molecular genetic defects have not been identified in any of these dogs. Congenital central hypothyroidism, apparently due to isolated TSH deficiency, has been described in a family of Giant Schnauzers and a Boxer. Congenital adenohypophyseal hypoplasia associated with central hypothyroidism has been described in a 2-week-old Portuguese Water Dog.[4,5] Central hypothyroidism was confirmed in seven Miniature Schnauzers, suggesting a genetic background in this breed. Of these dogs, only three had disproportionate dwarfism, a hallmark of congenital hypothyroidism, while the remaining four dogs were not dwarfs and were diagnosed between 5 and 8 years of age, suggesting that mild TSH deficiency may allow for normal growth. Alternatively, these dogs may have had different forms of central hypothyroidism.[21] TSH deficiency is also implicated in the combined pituitary hormone deficiency caused by the LHX3 gene mutation, which is responsible for the pituitary dwarfism described in German Shepherds and related breeds and recently reported in Tibetan Terrier dogs (see chapter 25).[22]

Clinical features

Acquired hypothyroidism

Signalment

Hypothyroidism can occur in any dog, but purebred dogs are at increased risk.[3,23] The perception of which breeds are predisposed to hypothyroidism may be influenced by many factors (e.g., geographic differences, breed popularity, criteria used to diagnose hypothyroidism), and many breeds are described in published studies. Doberman Pinschers, Golden Retrievers, Irish Setters, Rhodesian Ridgebacks, Giant Schnauzers, Cocker Spaniels, and Boxers have been consistently reported as predisposed among different studies.[3,8,16,23,24] A recent study of a large population of dogs under primary veterinary care in the United Kingdom also found a very high predisposition in Tibetan Terriers and Shetland Sheepdogs, while Pugs, Yorkshire Terriers, Shi Tzus, and Jack Russell Terriers were the most protected breeds.[3] Hypothyroidism is typically a disease of middle-aged dogs, with a median age of first diagnosis of about 7 years, but it can be diagnosed at any age. However, it is an uncommon diagnosis in dogs younger than 2 years of age.[2,3] It seems that breeds predisposed to lymphocytic thyroiditis are more likely to develop hypothyroidism at a younger age.[8] Neutering has been associated with an increased risk of hypothyroidism both in male and female dogs, but there is no definitive evidence supporting a causal correlation between sex and/or neutering and the development of hypothyroidism.[1-3,16,25]

Clinical signs

Adult hypothyroid dogs can present with a wide range of clinical signs because thyroid hormones influence the function of almost every organ system. The typical clinical presentation includes metabolic and dermatologic signs, while neuromuscular, reproductive, and cardiovascular manifestations are less common.

Video 27.1

A 6-year-old male Belgian Sheepdog suffering from primary hypothyroidism: the dog presented rarefaction of hair on the entire trunk and limbs, the hair was dry and dull, and the body condition score was increased. Courtesy of Prof. F. Fracassi, University of Bologna.

Metabolic signs are described in about 70-80% of the cases and are due to a decreased general metabolic rate. Lethargy, exercise intolerance/weakness, and weight gain, often associated with obesity, are common.[1,2,26,27] Of note, the vast majority of obese dogs are not hypothyroid. Less commonly, hypothyroid dogs may have cold intolerance and hypothermia. Metabolic signs can be subtle in onset and slow in progression, and it is common for owners not to recognize these signs until they become severe or resolve with the treatment. Long-standing untreated hypothyroidism can result in myxedema coma, an extremely rare but potentially fatal complication characterized by abnormal mental status, profound weakness, severe hypothermia, bradycardia, and shock. Hypothyroidism also causes an increase in serum growth hormone (GH) and insulin-like growth factor 1 (IGF-1) concentrations that lead to insulin resistance that may worsen pre-existing diabetes mellitus and, rarely, result in acromegalic features.[28,29]

Dermatologic abnormalities occur in up to 80% of the cases and are usually easier for owners to recognize. Thyroid hormones are required to maintain normal hair growth, so hypothyroid dogs typically exhibit dry and brittle hair coats, or "endocrine" alopecia (Video 27.1). This is nonpruritic alopecia, which is bilaterally symmetric and mainly localized at areas of friction or pressure such as the neck, flanks, ventral abdomen, tail base, and tail ("rat tail"); the head and distal extremities are usually spared (Fig. 27.2A, Fig. 27.2B and Fig. 27.2C). Failure to regrow hair after clipping, skin hyperpigmentation, and seborrhea are also common. The term myxedema is also used to define the thickening of the skin with nonpitting edema caused by accumulation of glycosaminoglycans and hyaluronic acid in the dermis, which contributes to the typical "tragical facial expression" (Fig. 27.2D). Hypothyroidism is responsible for decreased immune function, predisposing to recurrent otitis or pyoderma, which may cause pruritus.[1,2,26,27] The prevalence of metabolic and dermatological signs reported in hypothyroid dogs in major published studies is summarized in Table 27.1.

Various neuromuscular manifestations have been described in dogs with hypothyroidism, including CNS diseases, cranial nerve deficits (e.g., trigeminal or facial nerve paralysis), central and peripheral vestibular dysfunction, generalized peripheral neuropathies, laryngeal paralysis, megaesophagus, and myasthenia gravis.[33,34] The relationship between hypothyroidism and neurologic manifestations may be causal, merely represent a concurrence of diseases, or, at least in some cases, reflect nonthyroidal illness syndrome rather than hypothyroidism.

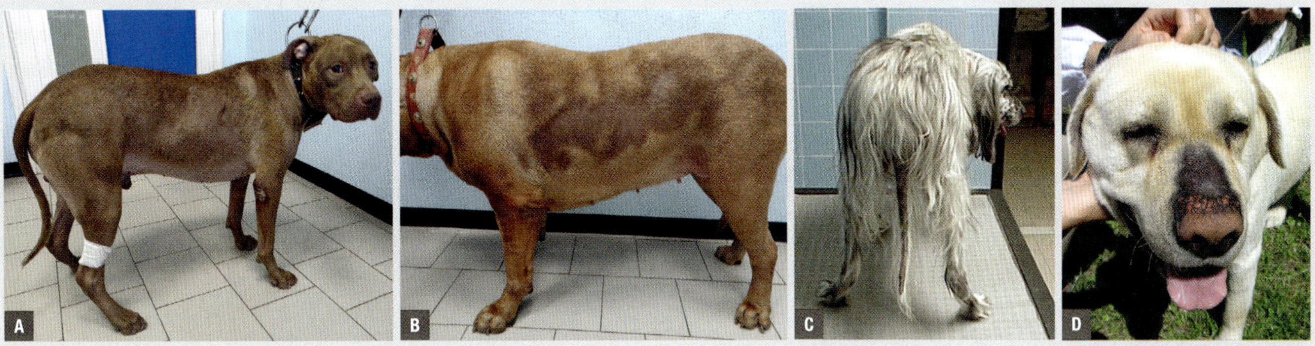

FIG 27.2 (A) A 6-year-old intact male mixed-breed dog with hypothyroidism with hair thinning and mild bilateral symmetric alopecia. (B) An 8-year-old intact female Dogue de Bordeaux with hypothyroidism, with marked alopecia of the flanks and increased body condition score. (C) A 5-year-old female Irish Setter dog with primary hypothyroidism showing characteristic alopecia of the tail called "rat tail". (D) A 5-year-old male Labrador Retriever with hypothyroidism. The myxedema is evident, contributing to the typical "tragical facial expression". Nasal hyperpigmentation and alopecia are also noticeable. Images (C) and (D) courtesy of Prof. F. Fracassi, University of Bologna.

TABLE 27.1 Clinical signs described in different studies in dogs with hypothyroidism.

Study referenced	Number of hypothyroid dogs	Metabolic signs (% of dogs)				Dermatological signs (% of dogs)	
		Lethargy	Obesity or weight gain	Exercise intolerance	Cold intolerance	Alopecia	Other
Kaelin, et al., 1986[30]	16	68	68			75	
Panciera, et al., 1994[1]	66	21	41	20		26	50
Dixon, et al., 1999[2]	50	76	44	24	10	56	80
Le Traon, et al., 2009[31]	35	77	77	63		74	97
Jaillardon, et al., 2011[26]	220	54	69			60	79
Van Dijl, et al., 2014[32]	10	70	90	60	0	80	100
Corsini, et al., 2021[27]	40	65	42	67	2	70	82

An experimental model of hypothyroidism failed to reproduce peripheral neuropathy in dogs but demonstrated subclinical myopathy.[35,36] Notably, neuromuscular signs do not consistently improve with the treatment of hypothyroidism. Thyroid hormone deficiency has anecdotally been associated with behavioral problems and increased aggressiveness, but published studies failed to demonstrate a correlation.[37]

Detrimental effects of hypothyroidism on reproduction in female dogs include increased periparturient mortality and decreased puppy weight at birth, and there is weak evidence that it may decrease fertility and interfere with normal estrous cycles (e.g., prolonged interestrous interval, weak or silent estrous cycle). In intact female dogs, hypothyroidism causes hyperprolactinemia, which may rarely result in galactorrhea.[38] Thyroid hormone deficiency is considered a rare cause of infertility in male dogs, and experimentally induced hypothyroidism did not cause reproductive dysfunction in males.[4,5]

Cardiovascular function is strongly influenced by thyroid hormones, but clinical signs associated with cardiovascular dysfunction are relatively uncommon in hypothyroid dogs. Atrial fibrillation, bradycardia, and hypokinetic cardiomyopathy, which may mimic dilated cardiomyopathy (DCM), have been associated with hypothyroidism (Video 27.2).[39] The latter is usually mild and asymptomatic and typically resolves with a few months of treatment of hypothyroidism. Of note, thyroid hormone deficiency by itself is unlikely to cause heart failure rather than worsening a pre-existing heart disease. Studies evaluating hypothyroidism and DCM in Doberman Pinschers have not found a causal relationship between the diseases, which most likely occur independently.[40] Hypothyroid dogs have an increased risk of atherosclerosis, and there are reports of aortic thrombosis, but a predisposition to cardiovascular events is unclear.[41]

Uncommonly, hypothyroidism may cause constipation in dogs, while diarrhea has been reported, but it is likely due to other diseases. Corneal lipid deposits (arcus lipoides) as a result of hyperlipidemia are another rare manifestation. Hypothyroidism does not cause polyuria/polydipsia (PU/PD) in dogs, and whenever PU/PD is reported in a dog with clinical signs suggestive of hypothyroidism (e.g., dermatologic abnormalities, lethargy), it should raise suspicion for a different diagnosis, such as hypercortisolism, or other diseases.

Video 27.2

A 5-year-old female Maremma Shepherd affected by primary hypothyroidism. Echocardiographic images (long axis view) before therapy (A) and 2 months after levothyroxine supplementation (B). An increase in heart rate and fractional shortening is evident after treatment. Courtesy of Prof. F. Fracassi, University of Bologna.

Congenital hypothyroidism

Thyroid hormones affect virtually every system in the body and their deficiency early in life results in a wide range of possible clinical signs that are only partially similar to those described in adult hypothyroid dogs. Among their many functions, thyroid hormones are essential for central nervous system (CNS) maturation, bone growth, and chondrogenesis. Since normal thyroid hormone concentrations are required for physical and mental development, the hallmarks of congenital hypothyroidism are growth retardation with disproportionate dwarfism and impaired mental development, which is why congenital hypothyroidism is also called cretinism. This presentation differs markedly from dogs with combined pituitary hormone deficiency, which presents with proportionate dwarfism and normal mental status. Puppies with congenital hypothyroidism have normal or, in the case of prolonged gestation, large birth weight, followed by aberrant and delayed growth. The first signs of abnormal growth compared to healthy littermates appear at 2-3 weeks of age but are usually difficult to detect at this time. Failure to thrive is typically obvious to owners by 8-12 weeks of age, and abnormal body proportions become striking in the following months. Disproportionate dwarfism is characterized by a short and broad skull, shortened mandible and ears, enlarged or protruding tongue, short thick neck, wide/square trunk, and shortened limbs (Fig. 27.3A, Fig. 27.3B, and Fig. 27.3C).[4,5,17,21] The delayed and abnormal skeletal development is caused by delayed epiphyseal maturation and epiphyseal dysgenesis, which is easily seen on radiographs of the spine and appendicular skeleton since the vertebral bodies and the long bones are the most affected skeletal sections; these abnormalities may eventually lead to degenerative joint disease (Fig. 27.4).[42] Hypothyroid puppies are mentally dull, lethargic, lack playfulness compared to healthy littermates or normal puppies, and show impaired learning and, sometimes, inability to eat independently (Video 27.3). Some dogs may present with neuromuscular signs such as weakness, hyporeflexia,

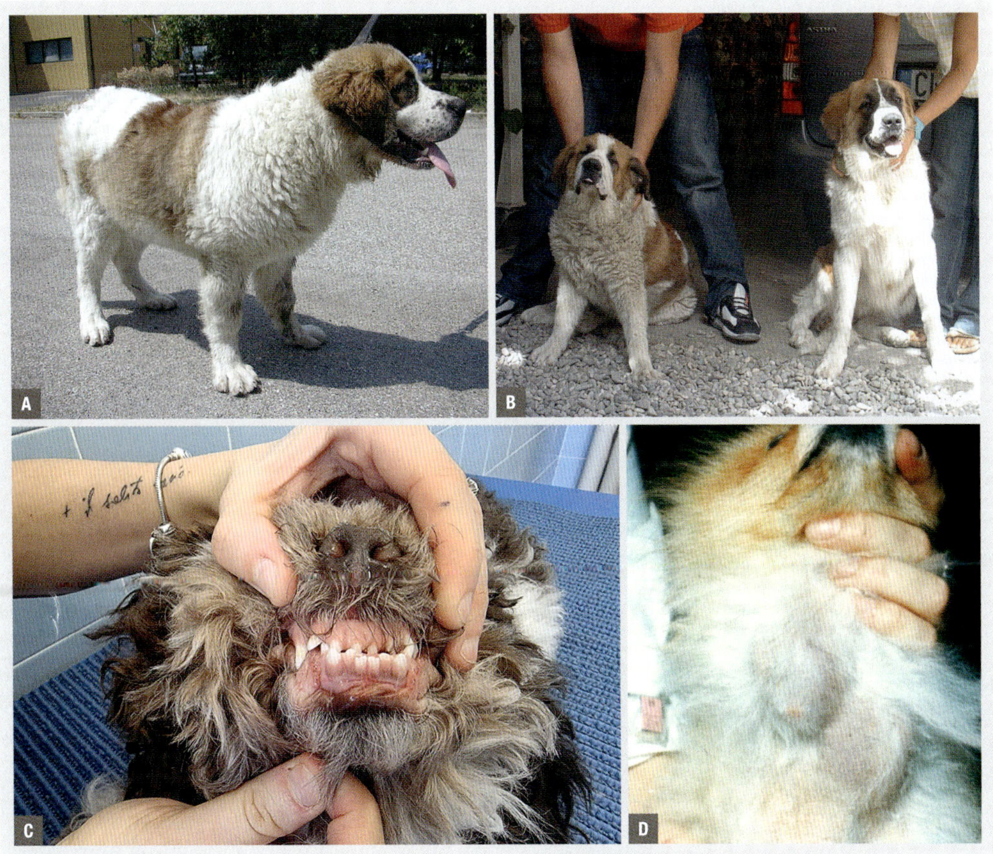

FIG. 27.3 (**A**) A 6-month-old male Saint Bernard dog with congenital hypothyroidism showing a broad face, short thick neck, and shortened limbs; the hair coat is fluffy with a typical "puppy" appearance. (**B**) Disproportionate dwarfism features are evident when compared to the littermate. (**C**) A 9-month-old male Lagotto Romagnolo with congenital hypothyroidism showing abnormal eruption of teeth. (**D**) Appearance of a goiter in a young dog with congenital goitrous hypothyroidism. Images courtesy of Prof. F. Fracassi, University of Bologna (**A, B, C**) and Prof. H.S. Kooistra, Utrecht University (**D**).

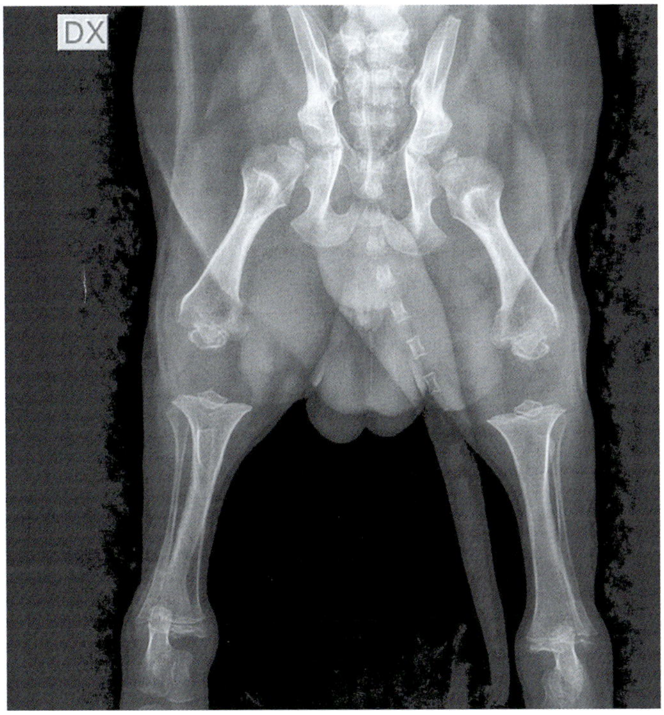

FIG. 27.4 Radiography of the appendicular skeleton (pelvic limbs) of a 9-month-old male Lagotto Romagnolo (same as Fig. 27.3C) showing delayed epiphyseal maturation and epiphyseal dysgenesis. Courtesy of the Diagnostic Imaging Section, Department of Veterinary Clinical Sciences, University of Bologna.

muscle tremors, and abnormal proprioception, likely due to abnormal cerebellar development, hypomyelination, and reduction of axons in CNS.[4,5] They retain a peculiarly soft and fluffy "puppy" hair coat with thick skin, and over time, they develop diffuse truncal thinning of the hair, which may progress to complete alopecia with hyperpigmentation and seborrhea; recurrent episodes of otitis externa have also been reported. Other clinical signs associated with congenital hypothyroidism are delayed eruption of deciduous and permanent teeth, kyphosis, abdominal distension, constipation, hypothermia, and inappetence. Goiter can be or not be present depending on the underlying mechanism causing hypothyroidism (Fig. 27.3D).[4,5]

The vast majority of dogs with congenital hypothyroidism present with clear symptoms. However, in the case of dyshormonogenesis, the defect may vary in severity, and if mild, the dog may grow normally, and clinical signs may be subtle or not apparent until months or years after birth; the same may occur in dogs with mild TSH deficiency.[20,21]

Video 27.3

A 6-month-old male Caucasian Shepherd dog with congenital hypothyroidism. The dog appears mentally dull and lethargic. Courtesy of Prof. F. Fracassi, University of Bologna.

TABLE 27.2 Clinicopathological abnormalities described in different studies in dogs with hypothyroidism.

Study referenced	Number of dogs	Percentage of dogs									
		↓HCT	↑CHOL	↑TRI	↑ALP	↑ALT	↑AST	↑CK	↑Crea	↑SDMA	↑Fructosamine
Kaelin, et al., 1986[30]	16	42	71	/	/	/	/	42	/	/	/
Panciera, et al., 1994[1]	66	32	73	/	30	/	/	18	/	/	/
Dixon, et al., 1999[2]	50	40	78	88	/	/	15	35	/	/	43
Reusch, et al., 2002[46]	11	/	/	/	/	/	/	/	/	/	81
Le Traon, et al., 2009[31]	35	40	80	83	/	/	/	/	/	/	/
Di Paola, et al., 2021[50]	24	39	91	/	/	/	/	/	33	50	/
Corsini, et al. 2021[27]	40	33	81	75	/	51	26	/	13	/	/

HCT, hematocrit; CHOL, cholesterol; TRI, triglycerides; ALP, alkaline phosphatase; ALT, alanine transaminase; AST, aspartate aminotransferase; CK, creatine kinase; Crea, creatinine; SDMA, symmetric dimethylarginine.

Clinicopathological findings

Overview

Routine laboratory examination may reveal several hematological and biochemical alterations in dogs with hypothyroidism. Before discussing these abnormalities, it is important to note that none of them is specific to hypothyroidism. Although some –mainly biochemical– alterations can strengthen the suspicion of hypothyroidism, routine clinicopathologic analysis is especially useful in detecting or suspecting nonthyroidal illness (NTI).

Complete blood count

The most common hematologic abnormality found in hypothyroid dogs is a mild nonregenerative anemia due to decreased hematopoiesis (Table 27.2).[1,2,43,44] Other reported changes include a decreased neutrophil count, an elevated platelet count, and an increased red cell distribution width.[2,43,45]

Routine serum biochemistry

Elevated triglyceride and cholesterol levels are one of the most consistent findings in canine hypothyroidism, reported in about 80% of dogs (Table 27.2).[1,2] This is the result of decreased lipid degradation, as thyroid hormones are essential players in lipid metabolism. A large increase in cholesterol concentration is more typical of hypothyroidism than of NTI, which can aid in differentiating between the two.[2]

An increased activity of the muscle enzyme creatine kinase is found in 18-35% of dogs with primary hypothyroidism but only rarely exceeds twice the upper limit of the reference interval.[1,2] This increase might be the result of the myopathy that is described in hypothyroidism.[35] Mild increases in liver enzyme activity occur in approximately 20-30% of hypothyroid dogs, the suggested cause for this being mild hepatic lipid deposition.[1,2]

Serum fructosamine concentrations are reported to be elevated in 43-82% of hypothyroid dogs.[2,46] The underlying mechanism seems to be a reduced protein turnover, not significantly prolonged hyperglycemia.[46]

Renal parameters of serum creatinine and symmetric dimethylarginine (SDMA) were found to be elevated in some hypothyroid dogs. Thyroid hormone is an important regulator of glomerular filtration rate (GFR), which explains the reduced GFR in hypothyroid dogs.[47] Also, renal blood flow is reduced in hypothyroidism as a result of decreased cardiac output.[48,49] Serum creatinine concentration has been reported to be mildly above the reference range in 33% of hypothyroid dogs.[50] Concentrations of SDMA were above the reference range in 50% of dogs when using a reference interval of <14 μg/dL but only in 4% of dogs when using the recently suggested higher cutoff value of 18 μg/dL.[50]

The mean serum potassium concentration of hypothyroid dogs is mildly but significantly higher than that of euthyroid dogs and increases significantly during exercise. This can be explained by the severe reduction of the Na^+-, K^+-ATPase capacity in the skeletal muscle pool.[51]

Other clinicopathological findings

Increased circulating GH and IGF-1 concentrations have been reported in dogs with hypothyroidism.[28] This is mainly due to decreased hypothalamic somatostatin secretion and a paradoxical response of GH to TRH.

Endocrine testing

Overview

Accurately diagnosing canine hypothyroidism can be challenging, proof of which is presented in the widespread overdiagnosis –and unnecessary treatment– of the disease. Different tests are available, among which are basal hormone measurements but also dynamic function tests and diagnostic imaging. All tests lack 100% diagnostic accuracy, which emphasizes the need for only testing dogs with compatible clinical signs and clinicopathologic alterations. Many diseases and therapies influence the result of thyroid testing, and their effects must be considered before interpreting thyroid function tests or perhaps even before performing thyroid testing (Fig. 27.5).

Basal hormone tests

Total triiodothyronine

The total serum triiodothyronine (T_3) concentration may remain within its reference interval in several hypothyroid dogs.[52] Because of this, the measurement of total T_3 for diagnosing hypothyroidism lacks sensitivity. The fact that total T_3 concentration remains within the reference interval could be the result of a preference of the thyroid gland for secretion of T_3 over T_4 when thyroid function declines. Another hypothesis

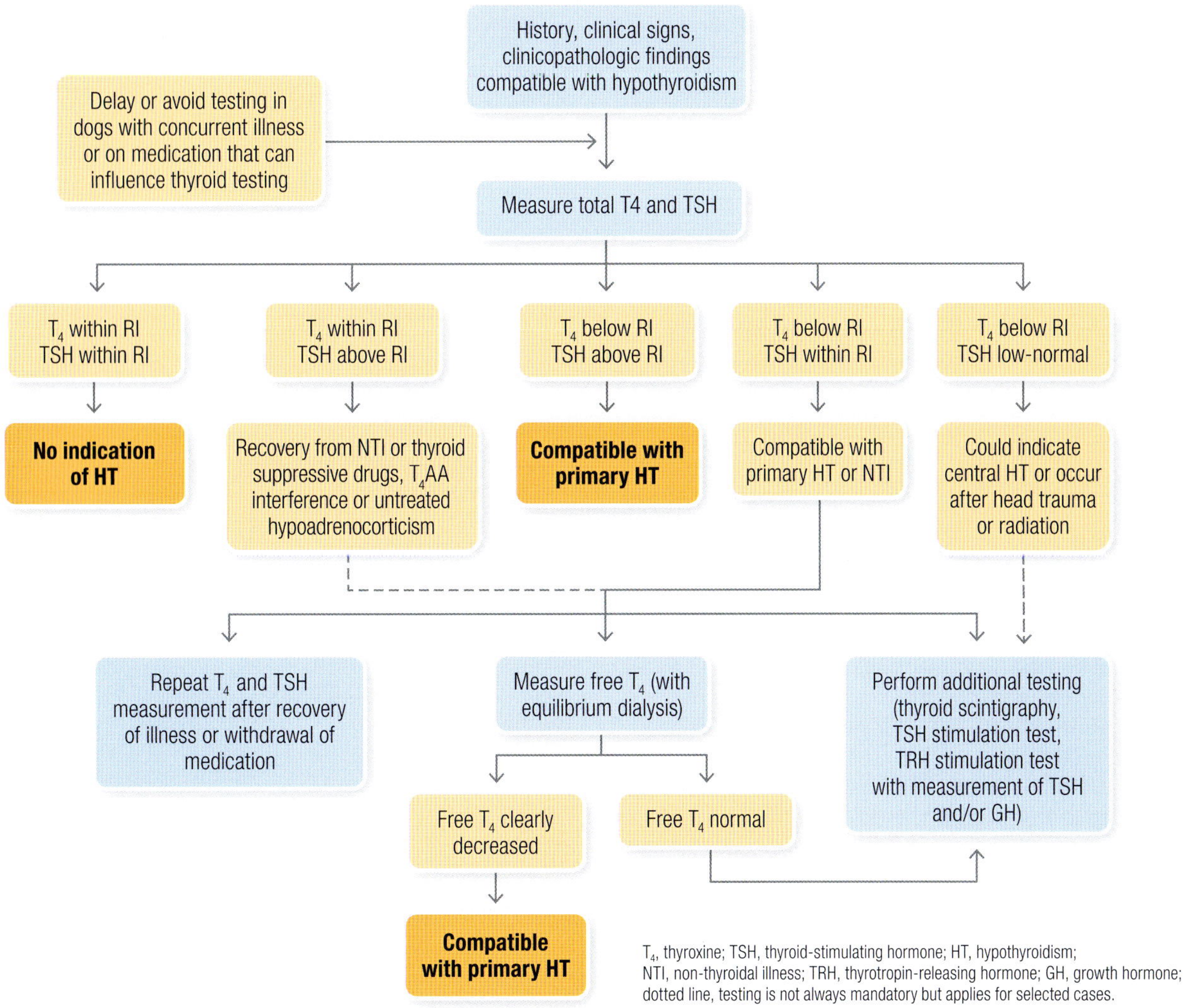

FIG. 27.5 Diagnostic approach to a dog suspected of having hypothyroidism.

is that an increased peripheral conversion of T_4 to the biologically more potent T_3 occurs in hypothyroidism. Both are beneficial mechanisms for the individual when thyroid function is reduced. Another explanation for total T_3 concentrations that do not decrease below the reference interval in hypothyroid dogs could be the presence of T_3 autoantibodies (T_3AA), which falsely increases measured concentrations in approximately 6% of dogs.[53] Also, T_3 concentrations will decrease in non-thyroidal illness, further limiting their use in the diagnosis of primary hypothyroidism.

Total thyroxine

The first step in diagnosing canine hypothyroidism is usually measuring the total thyroxine (T_4) concentration. Total T_4 includes both protein-bound T_4 and unbound T_4 (called "free thyroxine", [fT_4]).

The vast majority of hypothyroid dogs have very low to undetectable serum total T_4 concentrations, and the reported sensitivity of total T_4 as a diagnostic test has been reported to be more than 90%.[52,54]

Approximately 2% of dogs suspected of having hypothyroidism have autoantibodies against T_4 (T_4AA) that can falsely increase the measured total T_4 concentration, which is, in part, an explanation for the imperfect sensitivity.[53]

The major drawback of total T_4 in the diagnosis of hypothyroidism is the pronounced lack of specificity due to many nonthyroidal factors that can result in a subnormal total T_4 concentration in euthyroid dogs.[54] The result of this poor specificity is that a diagnosis of hypothyroidism cannot be made based solely on a low total T_4 concentration.

Due to these test specifics, it is recommended to postpone measuring total T_4 in dogs with concurrent illness or those being treated with medications known to influence the serum total T_4 concentration.

Free thyroxine

The only metabolically active form of T_4 is free thyroxine (fT_4), as it is able to leave the circulation and enter cells. In hypothyroid dogs, fT_4 concentrations are expected to be decreased.

Concentrations of fT_4 are less affected by NTI or T_4 autoantibodies, resulting in a higher specificity (78-94%) than total T_4. However, the sensitivity of fT_4 (80-98%) is slightly lower than that of total T_4.[52,54]

Currently, equilibrium dialysis and ultrafiltration-based methods are considered the gold standard for measuring fT_4 (fT_4-ED) concentrations because interference from circulating T_4 autoantibodies or other binding proteins is eliminated by dialysis. These assays are time-consuming and relatively expensive. Another type of assay being marketed is the semiautomated chemiluminescent immunoassay (CLIA) method, which is less labor-intensive and requires less technical training. Unfortunately, the results of this assay are less valuable as they are influenced by the presence of T_4 autoantibodies and can result in normal fT_4 concentrations in up to 25-38% of hypothyroid dogs.[55] Also, fT_4 concentrations, measured via CLIA, decreased with increased severity of non-thyroidal illness in a manner similar to total T_4.[56] The added value of measuring fT_4 by CLIA alongside total T_4 is low.[57]

Thyroid-stimulating hormone

In dogs with primary hypothyroidism, plasma thyroid-stimulating hormone (TSH) concentration is expected to be increased due to a lack of negative feedback by thyroid hormones. TSH is, therefore, often measured alongside total T_4 to increase specificity. A low total T_4 concentration combined with a clearly elevated TSH concentration is highly suggestive of primary hypothyroidism.

However, 24-42% of hypothyroid dogs have a plasma TSH concentration within the reference range, reducing its sensitivity as a diagnostic test.[52,54,58,59] Consequently, a low serum total T_4 concentration in combination with a plasma TSH concentration within the reference interval does not distinguish between hypothyroidism and NTI.

The causes that have been hypothesized by current literature to explain a normal TSH in a hypothyroid dog are:

- Some of these hypothyroid dogs may have secondary instead of primary hypothyroidism.
- A decreased pituitary secretion of TSH could occur in chronic hypothyroidism, as was seen in a study investigating TSH concentrations in dogs with experimentally induced hypothyroidism.[29]
- Another explanation might be that the pulsatile secretion of TSH could result in TSH concentrations that will intermittently be within the reference interval.[60]
- Yet another possibility is that in dogs with chronic hypothyroidism, isoforms of TSH are produced that are not measured by the currently available TSH assays.[52]

The specificity of elevated TSH concentrations is high, as a high TSH concentration is only rarely encountered in euthyroid dogs.[59] High TSH values, when found in dogs with normal total T_4 concentrations, could indicate silent or subclinical hypothyroidism. It can also occur in dogs with untreated hypoadrenocorticism or in animals that recover from nonthyroidal illness.[8,61] The currently available TSH assays fail to detect low TSH concentrations, which limits its use as a basal hormone measurement in diagnosing central hypothyroidism.

Autoantibody measurement

In lymphocytic thyroiditis, antithyroglobulin antibodies (TgAAs) can be formed. This is the result of an autoimmune response to thyroglobulin, the major protein in the colloid of the thyroid gland. TgAAs are one of several types of antibodies that are produced in thyroiditis. A high percentage of hypothyroid dogs form TgAAs, and this can be a sign of autoimmune thyroiditis in these patients.[62] However, euthyroid dogs may also have TgAAs, but only a minority of them will go on to develop primary hypothyroidism.[10] So, the detection of TgAAs provides no information on thyroid function. Therefore, the presence of TgAA can not be used as a diagnostic test to detect primary hypothyroidism. A positive result could suggest a thyroid pathology, some of which could evolve into primary hypothyroidism.

Growth hormone

An interesting observation is that hypothyroidism in dogs is associated with increased release of GH.[28] This has been shown to occur both in hypothyroid dogs with elevated TSH concentrations and hypothyroid dogs with TSH concentrations within the reference range.[63] Basal plasma GH concentrations in hypothyroid dogs are significantly higher than in dogs with NTI.[63] Also, basal GH concentrations have only minimal overlap between hypothyroid dogs and dogs with NTI, suggesting this could be a useful diagnostic criterion to differentiate the two.[63] The higher circulating GH concentration is mainly due to a decreased hypothalamic somatostatin secretion and a paradoxical response of GH to TRH.[29] Unfortunately, the current unavailability of a reliable commercial GH assay limits its use outside of a research setting.

Stimulation tests for diagnosing primary hypothyroidism

TSH stimulation test

When basal total T_4, fT_4, and TSH concentrations are inconclusive but suspicion of primary hypothyroidism remains, a TSH stimulation test can be performed. This test and thyroid scintigraphy are considered the gold standard for the diagnosis of canine hypothyroidism. Stimulation with exogenous TSH evaluates the reserve capacity of the thyroid glands.

Recombinant human TSH (rhTSH) is currently used in the TSH stimulation test. As the vials of this rhTSH are expensive and one vial is more than is needed for one test, aliquots of rhTSH can be prepared and stored at 4°C for 4 weeks and at −20°C for up to 12 weeks without loss of biological activity, allowing for several tests per ampule.[64,65] It is the author's experience that stability at −20°C is much higher than 3 months, but further studies will be necessary to quantify the exact duration of storage allowed.

Test protocol

Blood is collected before (T = 0) and 6 hours after (T = 6h) the intravenous injection of a fixed dose of rhTSH, and serum total T_4 concentrations are measured in both samples.[66] Most studies reported a fixed dose of 75 µg per dog, but both higher (150 µg and 100 µg) and lower dosages (50 µg) of rhTSH per dog have been described.[27,67,68] A recent publication using 75 µg per dog that included dogs with systemic illness and dogs receiving medications found excellent diagnostic accuracy.[27]

Interpretation

Poststimulation levels of total T_4 above 21.9 nmol/L (1.7 µg/dL) ruled out hypothyroidism with a negative predictive value of 100% when the test is performed using 75 µg per dog of rhTSH, while poststimulation total T_4 below 16.7 nmol/L (1.3 µg/dL) has a positive predictive value of 95%. (Fig. 27.6).[27] Previous studies suggest that in euthyroid dogs, plasma total T_4 rises above 32 nmol/L (2.5 µg/dL) and is at least 1.5 times the basal T_4 concentration, while post-TSH T_4 values below 20 nmol/L (1.5 µg/dL) and less than 1.5 times the basal T_4 concentration point to hypothyroidism. Test results not matching with either euthyroid status or a clear diagnosis of hypothyroidism remain unresolved. This can occur in severe systemic illness or with medication that can affect thyroid function.[66]

Thyrotropin-releasing hormone stimulation test

The thyrotropin-releasing hormone (TRH) stimulation test, with the measurement of total T_4 concentrations before and after stimulation, is considered a less reliable test than the TSH stimulation test. Contrary to what would be expected, there is frequently no significant increase in

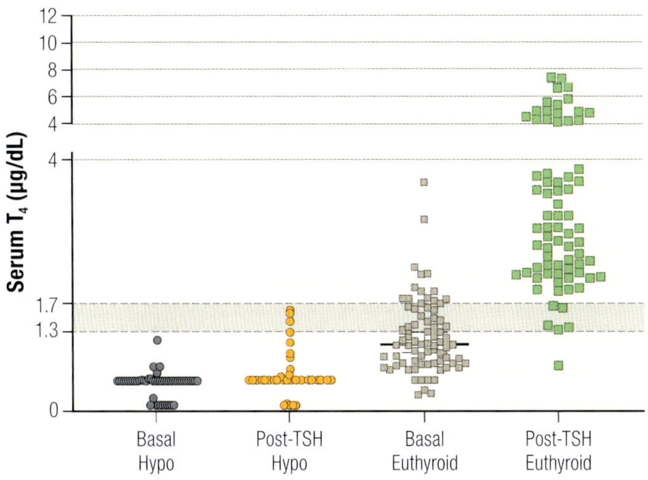

FIG. 27.6 Dot plots comparing serum T_4 concentrations before and after stimulation with 75 µg/dog of rhTSH in euthyroid (green squares) and hypothyroid (orange circles) dogs. The horizontal lines represent the 25th, 50th (median), and 75th percentile. The horizontal dotted lines represent the optimal cutoffs suggested to confirm (<1.3 µg/dL; 16.7 nmol/L) or rule out (>1.7 µg/dL; 21.9 nmol/L) hypothyroidism, with a grey zone in between. Adapted from: Corsini A, Faroni E, Lunetta F, Fracassi F. Recombinant human thyrotropin stimulation test in 114 dogs with suspected hypothyroidism: a cross-sectional study. *J Small Anim Pract* 62(4):257-264, 2021.

plasma total T_4 after TRH stimulation in euthyroid dogs. A strong increase in total T_4 after stimulation excludes hypothyroidism.[69]

TRH stimulation tests, measuring TSH or GH before and after stimulation, offer a promising alternative.[63] A blood sample is collected at baseline, and then 10 µg per kg body weight of TRH is administered intravenously. Next, a blood sample is collected at 45 minutes. Hypothyroid dogs are expected to have a TRH-induced increase in GH concentration and a lack of increase in TSH concentration. Euthyroid dogs are expected to increase TSH concentration following TRH administration but lack an increase in GH concentration (Fig. 27.7).

Diagnosis of central hypothyroidism

In dogs with secondary hypothyroidism, the serum total T_4 concentration is below the reference range, and the TSH concentration is very low or even below the detection limit. Secondary hypothyroidism can be diagnosed if repeated intravenous administration of rhTSH during 3 consecutive days results in an increase of the serum total T_4 concentration or reactivates thyroid uptake of 99mTcO$_4$ in scintigraphy (see below). In dogs with secondary hypothyroidism, stimulation with TRH does not result in an increase in serum TSH concentration, differentiating it from dogs with NTI. In one reported case of a dog with tertiary hypothyroidism, the serum total T_4 concentration was below the reference range, and the TSH concentration was within the reference range. The diagnosis was based on TSH and TRH response testing with both tests resulting in >1.5-fold increase of the total T_4 concentration. TRH stimulation also resulted in increased TSH concentrations.[15]

Some dogs with central hypothyroidism also have a deficiency in GH, prolactin, or gonadotropins and can show morphological alterations when the pituitary area is imaged.[70] A well-known example is German Shepherd dogs with an LHX3 mutation.[71]

Factors influencing thyroid hormone concentration

Normal thyroid hormone fluctuations

Thyroxine concentrations are known to show episodic variation in euthyroid dogs, with an average of 3.3 "peaks" per 24-hour period.[72] This could result in periodically reduced total T_4 concentration in dogs without thyroid dysfunction. In cases where hypothyroidism is not suspected, retesting at a later time could potentially avoid an unnecessary subsequent diagnostic pathway.

Body size, age, and gender

Mean serum total T_4 concentrations are higher in small dogs than in medium and large dogs. Total T_4 concentrations decline with increasing age and could result in values below the reference interval in some cases. Gender does not seem to affect thyroid hormone concentrations.[73]

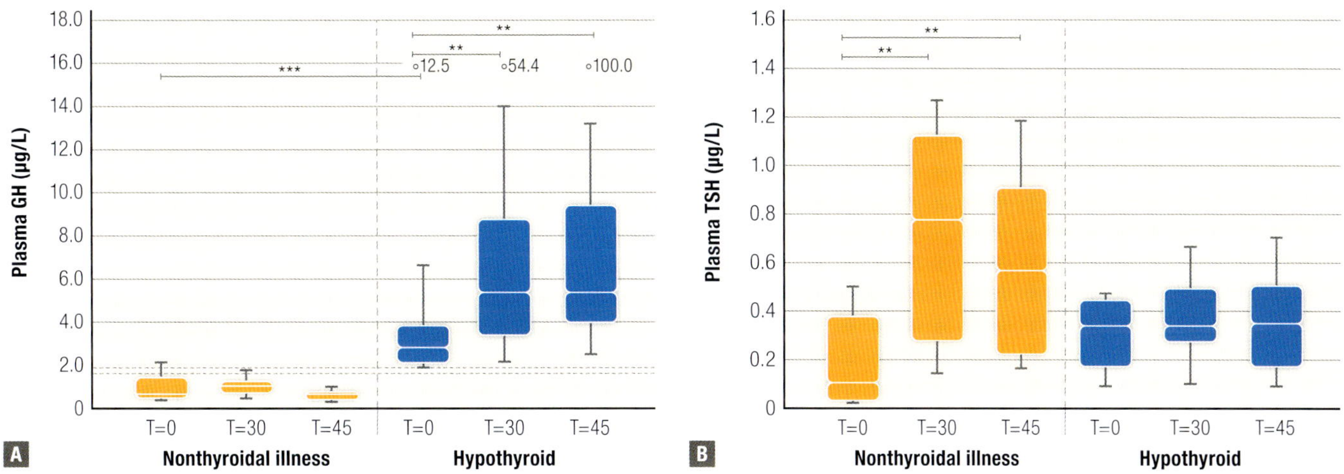

FIG. 27.7 Boxplots showing (**A**) plasma GH concentrations (µg/L) and (**B**) plasma TSH concentrations (µg/L) at baseline and at 30 and 45 minutes after TRH administration in 10 dogs with NTI and 11 dogs with hypothyroidism. One outlier is plotted individually. Double asterisks (**) indicate significant (p<0.01) difference. Triple asterisks (***) indicate significant (p<0.001) difference in baseline plasma GH concentrations between groups. The dotted lines in (**A**) represent cutoff levels (1.95 µg/L for T30 and 1.75 µg/L for T45). At T30 and T45, there was no overlap between hypothyroid dogs and dogs with NTI. Adapted from: Pijnacker T, Kooistra HS, Vermeulen CF, van der Vinne M, Prins M, Galac S, Mol JA. Use of basal and TRH-stimulated plasma growth hormone concentrations to differentiate between primary hypothyroidism and nonthyroidal illness in dogs. *J Vet Int Med* 32(4):1319-1324, 2018.

Breed

Numerous sighthound breeds have a lower total T_4 concentration, often below the standard reference interval. Among them are Greyhounds, Basenji dogs, Sloughis, Salukis, and Whippets. Also, when tested before the race, racing sled dogs have lower to subnormal total T_3, T_4, and free T_4 concentrations. Bordeaux dogs have also been shown to have significantly lower total T_4 concentrations; 56% of healthy Bordeaux dogs were reported to have a total T_4 below the standard reference interval.[4,5,74]

Nonthyroidal illness

One of the most important influences on thyroid hormone concentrations and interpretation of thyroid testing is the presence of an NTI. With increasing severity of any illness, the likelihood of finding a decreased total T_3, total T_4, and fT_4 becomes higher.[75,76] Plasma TSH concentration is likely to remain within its reference interval in sick dogs.[76] One important exception to this is primary hypoadrenocorticism, in which 37% of dogs at the time of diagnosis have an increased TSH concentration, with only 7% of dogs having a decreased total T_4 concentration.[61]

Drugs

Another important factor to consider in dogs suspected of primary hypothyroidism is the influence of several drugs on thyroid hormone concentrations (Table 27.3).[77] Among these are the frequently prescribed glucocorticoids, carprofen, phenobarbital, and sulfonamide-containing antibiotics. The latter requires particular consideration because they have been associated with the induction of hypothyroidism by (reversibly) inhibiting the enzyme TPO. This results in laboratory values indistinguishable from spontaneous primary hypothyroidism, with total T_4 and fT_4 concentrations below reference and an increased TSH concentration. Another important drug known to have an effect on thyroid hormone concentrations and stimulation tests is levothyroxine (L-T_4). Recent research showed that in dogs treated with L-T_4 levothyroxine for a short term (16 weeks), a withdrawal period of 1 week was sufficient to restore normal T_4 and TSH levels. However, considering that a longer period of L-T_4 treatment can lead to a different response, at least a 6-week withdrawal period is recommended before thyroid testing should be performed.[78]
Drugs that are investigated and have been shown to have no influence on circulating concentrations of total T_4, fT_4, and TSH are potassium bromide, imepitoin, propranolol (TSH not measured), ketoprofen, and deracoxib.[79,80]

TABLE 27.3 The influence of several drugs on thyroid hormone concentrations.

	Total T_4	Free T_4	TSH
Aspirin	↓	↓ or =	=
Carprofen	↓ or =	=	= or ↓
Clomipramine	↓	↓	=
Dexamethasone	↓ or =		=
Phenobarbital	↓ or =	↓ or =	= or ↑
Prednisone/prednisolone	↓ or =	↓ or =	=
Potentiated sulfonamides	↓ or =	↓ or =	↑
Toceranib	=	↓	↑
Trilostane[13]	=	↓	↑

Diagnostic imaging

Thyroid imaging can be subdivided into functional and morphologic diagnostic imaging. Functional diagnostic imaging can be used as a diagnostic tool, as is the case in thyroid scintigraphy. Other imaging modalities, such as ultrasound, CT, and MRI, only provide information on gross morphology.

Scintigraphy

Thyroid scintigraphy makes use of the uptake of radioactive pertechnetate ($99mTcO_4^-$) by the sodium-iodine symporters of the thyrocytes, as the pertechnetate ion has a size and charge similar to iodine. In dogs, the pertechnetate is injected intravenously, and uptake is measured by a gamma camera after 45-60 minutes. The normal canine thyroid lobes appear as two uniformly intense, symmetric ovals in the mid-cervical area. They are slightly smaller than the salivary glands, which also take up pertechnetate. The ratio between the thyroid- and salivary glands is 1:1 in euthyroid dogs (Fig. 27.8A). In hypothyroid dogs, the pertechnetate uptake in the thyroid gland is decreased or even absent (Fig. 27.8B).[81] Thyroid scintigraphy using pertechnetate for diagnosing canine hypothyroidism has high diagnostic accuracy. In almost all cases, a clear difference in thyroidal uptake of pertechnetate between hypothyroid dogs and dogs with NTI can be appreciated.[82] The "percentage uptake of pertechnetate" can be calculated by most diagnostic imaging software. One study reported that in dogs with hypothyroidism, percentage uptake at 60 minutes ranged from 0.03 to 0.26% of the injected dose and, in the dogs with NTI, from 0.39 to 1.86%, thus showing no overlap between these two groups.[82] Unfortunately, this diagnostic aid is only available in a few referral centers since specialist equipment and radiation-isolation facilities are needed.

Ultrasonography

Ultrasonography can be of help in the diagnosis of canine hypothyroidism. With ultrasonography, an experienced operator can measure the thyroid volume and the maximal cross-sectional area of the thyroid. Both were reported to be significantly smaller in dogs with hypothyroidism when compared to control dogs. Also, dogs with NTI had normal thyroid volumes and cross-sectional areas, which could aid in differentiating these patients from true hypothyroid dogs.[83]

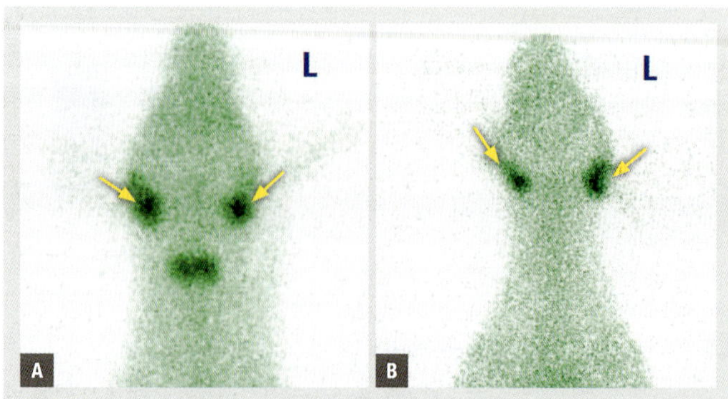

FIG. 27.8 (A) Scintigraphy of normal canine thyroid lobes, which appear as two uniformly intense, symmetric ovals in the mid-cervical area. The salivary glands (arrows) take up pertechnetate. (B) Scintigraphy of a hypothyroid dog, the pertechnetate uptake is decreased or even absent. The salivary glands are still visible.

The echogenicity (hypoechoic compared to the surrounding musculature), shape (round to oval-shaped thyroid lobes in the transverse imaging plane), and pattern (more heterogeneous) were also reported to be altered in hypothyroid dogs when compared to euthyroid dogs.[84,85] All these changes can be valuable adjunctive tests, especially when trying to differentiate between hypothyroid and euthyroid dogs with NTI. However, a final diagnosis cannot be based on thyroid ultrasonography alone. Also, the reliability is highly dependent on the skill and experience of the ultrasonographer.

Computed tomography and magnetic resonance imaging scan

The appearance of the normal thyroid gland in healthy dogs has been described for both computed tomography (CT) scans and magnetic resonance imaging (MRI) scans.[86,87] However, no literature concerning CT and MRI studies in dogs with primary hypothyroidism has been published yet. The cost of these imaging modalities is currently limiting their use in diagnosing hypothyroidism. With the prospect of reduced costs of CT and MRI when the availability of these techniques in veterinary medicine becomes more widespread, this might change in the future.

Treatment

Thyroid hormone replacement

Hypothyroidism requires lifelong thyroid hormone replacement treatment (THRT) with L-T_4 supplementation; there are several brand-name synthetic L-T_4 products approved for use in dogs. The suggested starting daily dose is 20 µg/kg, with the dosage (20 µg/kg once daily or 10 µg/kg twice daily) that depends on the L-T_4 formulation (oral solution or tablets, respectively), although once daily regimens are effective in many dogs regardless the formulation.[31,32,88] The starting dose is approximately ten times higher than in humans because the bioavailability of orally administered L-T_4 in dogs is poor and can be affected by many factors. The bioavailability is approximately 50% higher when L-T_4 is administered in a fasted dog compared to administration with food, so L-T_4 should be given 2 hours before a meal.[89] However, this may be unpractical for some owners, and administration with food is acceptable, provided that the timing of feeding and oral dosing is standardized for each dog; a consistent diet is also recommended to reduce variability in absorption. Although different brand name L-T_4 products have comparable efficacy, they may have different pharmacokinetics and bioavailability, and the clinician should consistently use the same formulation in the same dog; products approved for use in dogs should be preferred.[89,90] Other factors that may affect L-T_4 absorption from the gastrointestinal tract in dogs include concurrent medications, concurrent diseases, and physiological conditions such as age or body condition score. For all these reasons, the final L-T_4 dose may vary and must be titrated in each dog based on monitoring. Adequate treatment should lead to complete resolution of clinical or clinicopathological signs related to hypothyroidism (Fig. 27.9). Lethargy and other metabolic signs, including clinicopathological anomalies, are the first to improve, resolving within days to weeks; obesity may take longer. Dermatological signs may require 2 to 4 months to resolve, even if improvement is expected within some weeks; frequently, hair conditions worsen before improving.[88] Neurological signs and reproductive anomalies may require up to 6 months to resolve.

Treatment of dogs with hypothyroidism and concurrent diseases

Starting L-T_4 treatment in newly diagnosed hypothyroid dogs with concurrent diabetes mellitus usually results in a significant decrease in insulin resistance. Therefore, close blood glucose monitoring is suggested, and a 10-20% decrease in insulin dose may be considered to avoid the risk of hypoglycemia. Some authors suggest that in dogs with severe concurrent diseases (e.g., cardiac diseases), THRT should be introduced gradually, decreasing the starting dose by 25-50%. However, this recommendation was made considering higher starting doses (e.g., 20 µg/kg twice daily), and probably it is not necessary when the starting dose is 10 µg/kg twice daily.[5]

Therapeutic monitoring

Response to THRT is assessed mainly on clinical response, along with clinicopathological and hormonal testing. The first therapeutic monitoring is scheduled 4 weeks after the beginning of treatment and then 4 weeks after any dose adjustment or change of formulation. Once the final L-T_4 dose is achieved and the dog is clinically stable, monitoring should be performed at 3 months and then every 6 to 12 months. Therapeutic monitoring is based on serum total T_4 measured 4 to 6 hours after L-T_4 administration and serum TSH can be monitored for normalization in dogs in which TSH was increased at the time of diagnosis. Measurement of serum fT_4 is not recommended for monitoring because it gives no advantages compared with total T_4 and markedly increases the cost for the owners. In dogs with anti-T_4 autoantibodies, which can interfere with total T_4 monitoring, fT_4-ED may be considered. On the day of monitoring, the owner must be instructed to strictly adhere to the normal therapeutic routine (e.g., give L-T_4 and feed the dog at the same time and with the same amount and type of food) and the time interval of serum total T_4 measurement must be standardized in each dog. Serum total T_4 concentration should be in the upper half of the reference range or slightly elevated (up to approximately 6.0 µg/dL [77 nmol/L]). Adequately treated dogs had a mean total T_4 concentration of approximately 4.3 µg/dL (55 nmol/L).[31,32,88] In dogs with an inadequate clinical response and total T_4 values below 2.7 µg/dL (35 nmol/L), the dose should be increased by 50%. Persistently increased TSH concentration is also a possible predictor of an increased therapeutic requirement.[88] Clinical signs of thyrotoxicosis, such as PU/PD, polyphagia, panting, weight loss, restlessness, and hyperthermia, may appear with tT_4 values above 7.0 µg/dL (90 nmol/L), but are uncommon since dogs are quite resistant to L-T_4 overdose. The thyrotoxicosis promptly resolves with THRT discontinuation.

Failure to respond

Failure to achieve an adequate clinical response in a dog with serum total T_4 concentrations well within the therapeutic range and normal serum TSH concentration should prompt a re-evaluation of the diagnosis of hypothyroidism, especially if it was performed without gold standard testing (see Endocrine testing). The presence of a concurrent disease responsible for the clinical signs is another possible explanation.

Prognosis

The prognosis for adult-onset hypothyroidism is excellent, and the disease-specific survival is considered long. The prognosis for congenital hypothyroidism depends on prompt diagnosis and treatment and can be excellent if THRT is started early in life.

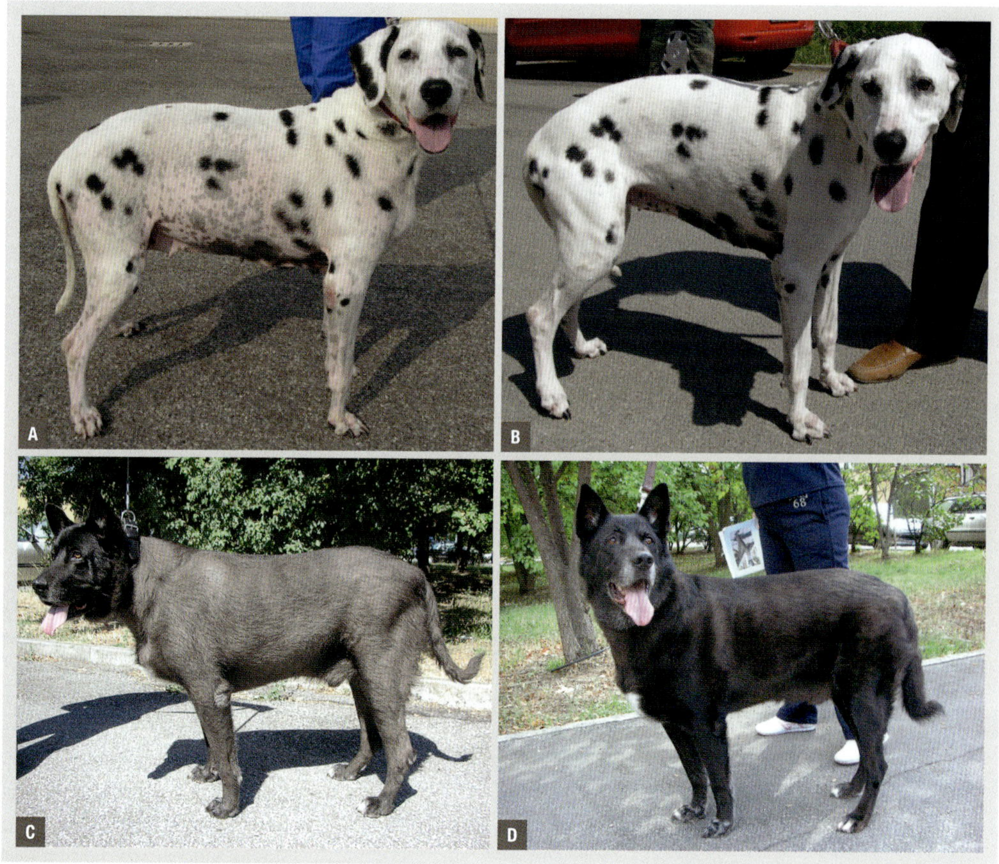

FIG. 27.9 A 4-year-old Dalmatian dog with hypothyroidism. (**A**) Before treatment, the dog tended to gain weight and showed bilateral symmetrical alopecia. (**B**) After 4 months of therapy, weight loss and resolution of the dermatological alterations were observed. (**C**) A 6-year-old male Belgian Sheepdog suffering from primary hypothyroidism presented at the diagnosis with rarefaction of hair on the entire trunk and limbs, dry and dull hair, and increased body condition score. (**D**) The same dog 8 months after the start of levothyroxine supplementation showing complete hair regrowth and normalization of the body condition score. Images courtesy of Prof. F. Fracassi, University of Bologna.

KEY POINTS

- Canine hypothyroidism is a common endocrinopathy and the most common thyroid disease in dogs.
- The most common form is acquired primary hypothyroidism, while central hypothyroidism and congenital hypothyroidism are rare.
- The typical clinical presentation includes metabolic (e.g., lethargy, exercise intolerance, weight gain) and dermatologic (e.g., dull hair coat, alopecia, recurrent otitis, or pyoderma) signs, which are described in around 70-80% of hypothyroid dogs.
- The diagnosis should be based on compatible clinical features and basal thyroid (total T_4 and TSH) testing. Stimulation testing or thyroid imaging techniques can aid in reaching a final diagnosis.
- A serious concern is overdiagnosis when based solely on total T_4 concentration, as many diseases and drugs can decrease thyroxine concentrations.
- Treatment is based on lifelong L-T_4 supplementation, which usually results in a complete resolution of clinical signs and clinicopathological abnormalities. Adequate monitoring is required to titrate the dose.

References

1. Panciera DL. Hypothyroidism in dogs: 66 cases (1987-1992). *J Am Vet Med Assoc* 204(5):761-767, 1994.
2. Dixon M, Reid SWJ, Mooney CT. Epidemiological, clinical, haematological and biochemical characteristics of canine hypothyroidism. *Vet Rec* 145(17):481-487, 1999.
3. O'Neill DG, Khoo JSP, Brodbelt DC, Church DB, Pegram C, Geddes RF. Frequency, breed predispositions and other demographic risk factors for diagnosis of hypothyroidism in dogs under primary veterinary care in the UK. *Canine Med Genet* 9(1):1-14, 2022.
4. Scott-Moncrieff JC. Canine hypothyroidism. In Reusch C, Nelson RW, Feldman EC, J. Moncrieff JC (editors). Canine and Feline Endocrinology 4th edition. St. Louis, Elsevier, 2014.
5. Mooney CT. Canine hypothyroidism. In Ettinger SJ, Feldman EC, Côté E (editors). Textbook of Veterinary Internal Medicine 8th edition. St. Louis, Elsevier, 2016.
6. Gosselin SJ, Capen CC, Martin SL. Histologic and ultrastructural evaluation of thyroid lesions

associated with hypothyroidism in dogs. *Vet Pathol* 18(3):299-309, 1981.

7. Skopek E, Patzl M, Nachreiner RF. Detection of autoantibodies against thyroid peroxidase in serum samples of hypothyroid dogs. *Am J Vet Res* 67(5):809-814, 2006.
8. Graham PA, Refsal KR, Nachreiner RF. Etiopathologic findings of canine hypothyroidism. *Vet Clin North Am Small Anim Pract* 37(4):617-631, 2007.
9. Kennedy LJ, Quarmby S, Happ GM, Barnes A, Ramsey IK, Dixon RM, et al. Association of canine hypothyroidism with a common major histocompatibility complex DLA class II allele. *Tissue Antigens* 68(1):82-86, 2006.
10. Graham P. A 12-month prospective study of 234 thyroglobulin antibody-positive dogs which had no laboratory evidence of thyroid dysfunction. *J Vet Intern Med* 15:298, 2001.
11. Yun T, Na Y, Lee D, Koo Y, Chae Y, Nam H, et al. Case report: technetium 99m pertechnetate scintigraphy findings in a dog with Iodine Deficiency-Induced Goitrous Hypothyroidism. *Front Vet Sci* 9:1-5, 2022.
12. Blois SL, Dickie E, Kruth SA, Allen DG. Multiple endocrine diseases in dogs: 35 cases (1996-2009). *J Am Vet Med Assoc* 238(12):1616-1621, 2011.
13. Kenefick SJ, Neiger R. The effect of trilostane treatment on circulating thyroid hormone concentrations in dogs with pituitary-dependent hyperadrenocorticism. *J Small Anim Pract* 49(3):139-143, 2008.
14. Murtagh K, Arrol L, Goncalves R, Granger N, German AJ, Smith PM. Hypothalamic-anterior pituitary hormone deficiencies following traumatic brain injury in dogs. *Vet Rec* 176(1):20, 2015.
15. Shiel RE, Acke E, Puggioni A, Cassidy JP, Mooney CT. Tertiary hypothyroidism in a dog. *Ir Vet J* 60(2):88, 2007.
16. Milne KL, Hayes HM. Epidemiologic features of canine hypothyroidism. *Cornell Vet* 71(1):3-14, 1981.
17. Dodgson SE, Day R, Fyfe JC. Congenital hypothyroidism with goiter in Tenterfield Terriers. *J Vet Intern Med* 26(6):1350-1357, 2012.
18. Fyfe JC, Lynch M, Olsen J, Louër E. A thyroid peroxidase (TPO) mutation in dogs reveals a canid-specific gene structure. *Mamm Genome Off J Int Mamm Genome Soc* 24(3-4):127-133, 2013.
19. Major S, Pettigrew RW, Fyfe JC. Molecular genetic characterization of thyroid dyshormonogenesis in a French Bulldog. *J Vet Intern Med* 29(6):1534-1540, 2015.
20. Soler Arias EA, Castillo VA, Garcia JD, Fyfe JC. Congenital dyshormonogenic hypothyroidism with goiter caused by a sodium/iodide symporter (SLC5A5) mutation in a family of Shih-Tzu dogs. *Domest Anim Endocrinol* 65:1-8, 2018.
21. Voorbij AMWY, Leegwater PAJ, Buijtels JJCWM, Daminet S, Kooistra HS. Central hypothyroidism in Miniature Schnauzers. *J Vet Intern Med* 30(1):85-91, 2016.
22. Thaiwong T, Corner S, Forge S La, Kiupel M. Dwarfism in Tibetan Terrier dogs with an LHX3 mutation. *J Vet Diagn Invest* 33:740-743, 2021.
23. Bellumori TP, Famula TR, Bannasch DL, Belanger JM, Oberbauer AM. Prevalence of inherited disorders among mixed-breed and purebred dogs: 27,254 cases (1995-2010). *J Am Vet Med Assoc* 242(11):1549-1555, 2013.
24. Ringstad NK, Lingaas F, Thoresen SI. Breed distributions for diabetes mellitus and hypothyroidism in Norwegian dogs. *Canine Med Genet* 9(1):1-10, 2022.
25. Sundburg CR, Belanger JM, Bannasch DL, Famula TR, Oberbauer AM. Gonadectomy effects on the risk of immune disorders in the dog: A retrospective study. *BMC Vet Res* 12(1):1-10, 2016.
26. Jaillardon L, Martin L, Nguyen P, Siliart B. Serum insulin-like growth factor type 1 concentrations in healthy dogs and dogs with spontaneous primary hypothyroidism. *Vet J* 190(2):e95-e99, 2011.
27. Corsini A, Faroni E, Lunetta F, Fracassi F. Recombinant human thyrotropin stimulation test in 114 dogs with suspected hypothyroidism: a cross-sectional study. *J Small Anim Pract* 62(4):257-264, 2021.
28. Lee WM, Diaz-Espineira M, Mol JA, Rijnberk A, Kooistra HS. Primary hypothyroidism in dogs is associated with elevated GH release. *J Endocrinol* 168(1):59-66, 2001.
29. Diaz-Espiñeira MM, Mol JA, Van Den Ingh TSGAM, Van Der Vlugt-Meijer RH, Rijnberk A, Kooistra HS. Functional and morphological changes in the adenohypophysis of dogs with induced primary hypothyroidism: loss of TSH hypersecretion, hypersomatotropism, hypoprolactinemia, and pituitary enlargement with transdifferentiation. *Domest Anim Endocrinol* 35(1):98–111, 2008.
30. Kaelin S, Watson ADJ, Church DB. Hypothyroidism in the dog: a retrospective study of sixteen cases. *J Small Anim Pract* 27(8):533-539, 1986.
31. Le Traon G, Brennan SF, Burgaud S, Daminet S, Gommeren K, Horspool LJI, et al. Clinical evaluation of a novel liquid formulation of L-thyroxine for once daily treatment of dogs with hypothyroidism. *J Vet Intern Med* 23(1):43-49, 2009.
32. van Dijl IC, Le Traon G, van de Meulengraaf BDAM, Burgaud S, Horspool LJI, Kooistra HS. Pharmacokinetics of total thyroxine after repeated oral administration of levothyroxine solution and its clinical efficacy in hypothyroid dogs. *J Vet Intern Med* 28(4):1229-1234, 2014.
33. Jaggy A, Oliver JE, Ferguson DC, Mahaffey EA, Jun TG. Neurological manifestations of hypothyroidism: A retrospective study of 29 dogs. *J Vet Intern Med* 8(5):328-336, 1994.
34. Higgins MA, Rossmeisl JH, Panciera DL. Hypothyroid-associated central vestibular disease in 10 dogs: 1999-2005. *J Vet Intern Med* 20(6):1363-1369, 2006.
35. Rossmeisl JH, Duncan RB, Inzana KD, Panciera DL, Shelton GD. Longitudinal study of the effects of chronic hypothyroidism on skeletal muscle in dogs. *Am J Vet Res* 70(7):879-889, 2009.
36. Rossmeisl JH. Resistance of the peripheral nervous system to the effects of chronic canine hypothyroidism. *J Vet Intern Med* 24(4):875-881, 2010.
37. Hrovat A, De Keuster T, Kooistra HS, Duchateau L, Oyama MA, Peremans K, et al. Behavior in dogs with spontaneous hypothyroidism during treatment with levothyroxine. *J Vet Intern Med* 33(1):64-71, 2019.
38. Diaz-Espiñeira MM, Mol JA, Rijnberk A, Kooistra HS. Adenohypophyseal function in dogs with primary hypothyroidism and nonthyroidal illness. *J Vet Intern Med* 23(1):100-107, 2009.
39. Guglielmini C, Berlanda M, Fracassi F, Poser H, Koren S, Baron Toaldo M. Electrocardiographic and echocardiographic evaluation in dogs with hypothyroidism before and after levothyroxine supplementation: A prospective controlled study. *J Vet Intern Med* 33(5):1935-1942, 2019.
40. Beier P, Reese S, Holler PJ, Simak J, Tater G, Wess G. The role of hypothyroidism in the etiology and progression of dilated cardiomyopathy in Doberman Pinschers. *J Vet Intern Med* 29(1):141-149, 2015.
41. Hess RS, Kass PH, Van Winkle TJ. Association between diabetes mellitus, hypothyroidism or hyperadrenocorticism, and atherosclerosis in dogs. *J Vet Intern Med* 17(4):489-494, 2003.
42. Saunders HM, Jezyk PK. The radiographic appearance of canine congenital of canine congenital hypothyroidism: skeletal changes with delayed delayed treatment. *Vet Radiol* 32(4):171-177, 1991.
43. Sullivan P, Gompf R, Schmeitzel L, Clift R, Cottrell M, McDonald TP. Altered platelet indices in dogs with hypothyroidism and cats with hyperthyroidism. *Am J Vet Res* 54(12):2004-2009, 1993.
44. Cline MJ, Berlin NI. Erythropoiesis and red cell survival in the hypothyroid dog. *Am J Physiol-Leg Content* 204(3):415-418, 1963.
45. Martinez C, Mooney CT, Shiel RE, Tang PK, Mooney L, O'Neill EJ. Evaluation of red blood cell distribution width in dogs with various illnesses. *Can Vet J* 60(9):964-971, 2019.
46. Reusch CE, Gerber B, Boretti FS. Serum fructosamine concentrations in dogs with hypothyroidism. *Vet Res Commun* 26(7):531-536, 2002.
47. Panciera DL, Lefebvre HP. Effect of experimental hypothyroidism on glomerular filtration rate and plasma creatinine concentration in dogs. *J Vet Intern Med* 23(5):1045-1050, 2009.
48. Gold M, Scott J, Spitzer J. Myocardial metabolism of free fatty acids in control, hyperthyroid, and hypothyroid dogs. *Am J Physiol-Leg Content* 213(1):239-244, 1967.
49. Taylor RR, Covell JW, Ross J. Influence of the thyroid state on left ventricular tension-velocity relations in the intact, sedated dog. *J Clin Invest* 48(4):775-784, 1969.
50. Di Paola A, Carotenuto G, Dondi F, Corsini A, Corradini S, Fracassi F. Symmetric dimethylarginine concentrations in dogs with hypothyroidism before and after treatement with levothyroxine. *J Small Anim Pract* 62(2):89-96, 2021.
51. Schaafsma IA, Van Emst MG, Kooistra HS, Verkleij CB, Peeters ME, Boer P, et al. Exercise-induced hyperkalemia in hypothyroid dogs. *Domest Anim Endocrinol* 22(2):113-125, 2002.

52. Peterson ME, Melián C, Nichols R. Measurement of serum total thyroxine, triiodothyronine, free thyroxine, and thyrotropin concentrations for diagnosis of hypothyroidism in dogs. *J Am Vet Med Assoc* 211(11):1396-1402, 1997.
53. Nachreiner RF, Refsal KR, Graham PA, Bowman MM. Prevalence of serum thyroid hormone autoantibodies in dogs with clinical signs of hypothyroidism. *J Am Vet Med Assoc* 220(4):466-471, 2002.
54. Dixon RM, Mooney CT. Evaluation of serum free thyroxine and thyrotropin concentrations in the diagnosis of canine hypothyroidism. *J Small Anim Pract* 40(2):72-78, 1999.
55. Randolph JF, Lamb SV, Cheraskin JL, Schanbacher BJ, Salerno VJ, Mack KM, et al. Free thyroxine concentrations by equilibrium dialysis and chemiluminescent immunoassays in 13 hypothyroid dogs positive for thyroglobulin antibody. *J Vet Intern Med* 29(3):877-881, 2015.
56. Bennaim M, Shiel RE, Evans H, Mooney CT. Free thyroxine measurement by analogue immunoassay and equilibrium dialysis in dogs with non-thyroidal illness. *Res Vet Sci* 147:37-43, 2022.
57. Rasmussen SH, Andersen HH, Kjelgaard-Hansen M. Combined assessment of serum free and total T_4 in a general clinical setting seemingly has limited potential in improving diagnostic accuracy of thyroid dysfunction in dogs and cats. *Vet Clin Pathol* 43(1):1-3, 2014.
58. Scott-Moncrieff JC, Nelson RW, Bruner JM, Williams DA. Comparison of serum concentrations of thyroid-stimulating hormone in healthy dogs, hypothyroid dogs, and euthyroid dogs with concurrent disease. *J Am Vet Med Assoc* 212(3):387-391, 1998.
59. Boretti FS, Reusch CE. Endogenous TSH in the diagnosis of hypothyroidism in dogs. *Schweiz Arch Für Tierheilkd* 146(4):183-188, 2004.
60. Kooistra HS, Diaz-Espineira M, Mol JA, Van Den Brom WE, Rijnberk A. Secretion pattern of thyroid-stimulating hormone in dogs during euthyroidism and hypothyroidism. *Domest Anim Endocrinol* 18(1):19-29, 2000.
61. Reusch CE, Fracassi F, Sieber-Ruckstuhl NS, Burkhardt WA, Hofer-Inteeworn N, Schuppisser C, et al. Altered serum thyrotropin concentrations in dogs with primary hypoadrenocorticism before and during treatment. *J Vet Intern Med* 31(6):1643-1648, 2017.
62. Dixon RM, Mooney CT. Canine serum thyroglobulin autoantibodies in health, hypothyroidism and non-thyroidal illness. *Res Vet Sci* 66(3):243-246, 1999.
63. Pijnacker T, Kooistra HS, Vermeulen CF, van der Vinne M, Prins M, Galac S, et al. Use of basal and TRH-stimulated plasma growth hormone concentrations to differentiate between primary hypothyroidism and nonthyroidal illness in dogs. *J Vet Intern Med* 32(4):1319-1324, 2018.
64. Daminet S, Fifle L, Paradis M, Duchateau L, Moreau M. Use of recombinant human thyroid-stimulating hormone for thyrotropin stimulation test in healthy, hypothyroid and euthyroid sick dogs. *Can Vet J* 48(12):1273-1279, 2007.
65. Roover KD, Duchateau L, Carmichael N, Van Geffen C, Daminet S. Effect of storage of reconstituted recombinant human thyroid-stimulating hormone (rhTSH) on thyroid-stimulating hormone (TSH) response testing in euthyroid dogs. *J Vet Intern Med* 20(4):812-817, 2006.
66. Boretti FS, Sieber-Ruckstuhl NS, Favrot C, Lutz H, Hofmann-Lehmann R, Reusch CE. Evaluation of recombinant human thyroid-stimulating hormone to test thyroid function in dogs suspected of having hypothyroidism. *Am J Vet Res* 67(12):2012-2016, 2006.
67. Boretti FS, Sieber-Ruckstuhl NS, Wenger-Riggenbach B, Gerber B, Lutz H, Hofmann-Lehmann R, et al. Comparison of 2 doses of recombinant human thyrotropin for thyroid function testing in healthy and suspected hypothyroid dogs. *J Vet Intern Med* 23(4):856-861, 2009.
68. Sauve F, Paradis M. Use of recombinant human thyroid-stimulating hormone for thyrotropin stimulation test in euthyroid dogs. *Can Vet J* 41(3):215, 2000.
69. Frank L. Comparison of thyrotropin-releasing hormone (TRH) to thyrotropin (TSH) stimulation for evaluating thyroid function in dogs. *J Am Anim Hosp Assoc* 32(6):481-487, 1996.
70. Kooistra HS, Voorhout G, Mol JA, Rijnberk A. Combined pituitary hormone deficiency in German Shepherd dogs with dwarfism. *Domest Anim Endocrinol* 19(3):177-190, 2000.
71. Voorbij AMWY, van Steenbeek FG, Vos-Loohuis M, Martens EECP, Hanson-Nilsson JM, van Oost BA, et al. A contracted DNA repeat in LHX3 intron 5 is associated with aberrant splicing and pituitary dwarfism in German shepherd dogs. *PLoS One* 6(11), 2011.
72. Kemppainen RJ, Sartin JL. Evidence for episodic but not circadian activity in plasma concentrations of adrenocorticotrophin, cortisol and thyroxine in dogs. *J Endocrinol* 103(2):219-226, 1984.
73. Reimers TJ, Lawler DF, Sutaria PM, Correa MT, Erb HN. Effects of age, sex, and body size on serum concentrations of thyroid and adrenocortical hormones in dogs. *Am J Vet Res* 51(3):454-457, 1990.
74. Lavoué R, Geffré A, Braun JP, Peeters D, Trumel C. Breed-specific biochemical reference intervals for the adult Dogue de Bordeaux. *Vet Clin Pathol* 42(3):346-359, 2013.
75. Mooney C. Canine hypothyroidism: A review of aetiology and diagnosis. *N Z Vet J* 59(3):105-114, 2011.
76. Kantrowitz LB, Peterson ME, Melián C, Nichols R. Serum total thyroxine, total triiodothyronine, free thyroxine, and thyrotropin concentrations in dogs with nonthyroidal disease. *J Am Vet Med Assoc* 219(6):765-769, 2001.
77. Bolton TA, Panciera DL. Influence of medications on thyroid function in dogs: An update. *J Vet Intern Med* 17(4):463, 2023.
78. Ziglioli V, Panciera DL, Troy GC, Monroe WE, Boes KM, Refsal KR. Effects of levothyroxine administration and withdrawal on the hypothalamic-pituitary-thyroid axis in euthyroid dogs. *J Vet Intern Med* 31(3):705-710, 2017.
79. Daminet S, Croubels S, Duchateau L, Debunne A, Van Geffen C, Hoybergs Y, et al. Influence of acetylsalicylic acid and ketoprofen on canine thyroid function tests. *Vet J* 166(3):224-232, 2003.
80. Panciera DL, Refsal KR, Sennello KA, Ward DL. Effects of deracoxib and aspirin on serum concentrations of thyroxine, 3,5,3'-triiodothyronine, free thyroxine, and thyroid-stimulating hormone in healthy dogs. *Am J Vet Res* 67(4):599-603, 2006.
81. Kintzer PP, Peterson ME. Nuclear medicine of the thyroid gland. Scintigraphy and radioiodine therapy. *Vet Clin North Am Small Anim Pract* 24:587-605, 1994.
82. Espineira MMD, Mol JA, Peeters ME, Pollak YWEA, Iversen L, Dijk JE, et al. Assessment of thyroid function in dogs with low plasma thyroxine concentration. *J Vet Intern Med* 21(1):25-32, 2007.
83. Reese S, Breyer U, Deeg C, Kraft W, Kaspers B. Thyroid sonography as an effective tool to discriminate between euthyroid sick and hypothyroid dogs. *J Vet Intern Med* 19(4):491-498, 2005.
84. Brömel C, Pollard RE, Kass PH, Samii VF, Davidson AP, Nelson RW. Ultrasonographic evaluation of the thyroid gland in healthy, hypothyroid, and euthyroid Golden Retrievers with nonthyroidal illness. *J Vet Intern Med* 19(4):499-506, 2005.
85. Taeymans O, Daminet S, Duchateau L, Saunders JH. Pre- and post-treatment ultranography in hypothyroid dogs: ultrasound in hypothyroid dogs including follow-up. *Vet Radiol Ultrasound* 48(3):262-269, 2007.
86. Taeymans O, Dennis R, Saunders JH. Magnetic resonance imaging of the normal canine thyroid gland. *Vet Radiol Ultrasound* 49(3):238-242, 2008.
87. Taeymans O, Schwarz T, Duchateau L, Barberet V, Gielen I, Haskins M, et al. Computed tomographic features of the normal canine thyroid gland: computed tomographic features of the normal canine thyroid gland. *Vet Radiol Ultrasound* 49(1):13-19, 2008.
88. Dixon RM, Reid SWJ, Mooney CT. Treatment and therapeutic monitoring of canine hypothyroidism. *J Small Anim Pract* 43(8):334-340, 2002.
89. Le Traon G, Burgaud S, Horspool LJI. Pharmacokinetics of total thyroxine in dogs after administration of an oral solution of levothyroxine sodium. *J Vet Pharmacol Ther* 31(2):95-101, 2008.
90. Simpson C, Devi JL, Whittem T. Bioavailability of two L-thyroxine formulations after oral administration to healthy dogs. *Aust Vet J* 91(3):83-88, 2013.

CHAPTER 28

Thyroid tumors and hyperthyroidism

Sylvie Daminet
DVM, PhD, DECVIM-CA (Internal Medicine), DACVIM

Miguel Campos
DVM, PhD, DECVIM-CA (Internal Medicine)

Etiology

Thyroid tumors are common endocrine tumors in dogs. They represent approximately 1-4% of all canine neoplasms and 10-15% of all head and neck neoplasms.[1] Canine thyroid tumors are locally invasive and rapidly metastasizing.

Classification of thyroid tumors

Most canine thyroid tumors detected clinically are carcinomas. Although thyroid adenomas do occur, they are usually small and nonfunctional; hence, they are not detected clinically unless during necropsy or incidentally during CT or MRI of the neck region.[2,3] Canine thyroid carcinomas can be classified as either follicular cell thyroid carcinomas (FTCs), which arise from thyroid follicular cells, or medullary thyroid carcinomas (MTCs), which arise from the parafollicular cells (C-cells).[4]
FTCs account for approximately ⅔ of canine thyroid carcinomas, while MTCs represent the other third.[5,6] In most veterinary studies, the prevalence of MTC is likely underestimated as these tumors may be difficult to distinguish from FTC of compact type by microscopic observation alone. In the absence of follicular architecture, follicular cell origin can be confirmed with immunohistochemistry for thyroglobulin, while C-cell origin can be confirmed with immunohistochemistry for calcitonin or markers of neuroendocrine tissue (e.g., chromogranin A, synaptophysin).[5,6] Although the clinical presentation of FTCs and MTCs is similar, distinguishing both tumor types could play a role when considering therapeutic options.[7]
During embryogenesis, failed migration of the thyroid gland primordium along the normal pathway may result in the development of ectopic thyroid tissue in abnormal locations from the base of the tongue to the heart.[8] Ectopic thyroid tissue behaves in the same physiological and pathological manner as normal thyroid tissue, and on rare occasions it can become neoplastic.[9] Ectopic thyroid carcinomas represent 1% of all cardiac tumors and 7% of all sublingual tumors in dogs[9] (Fig. 28.1).

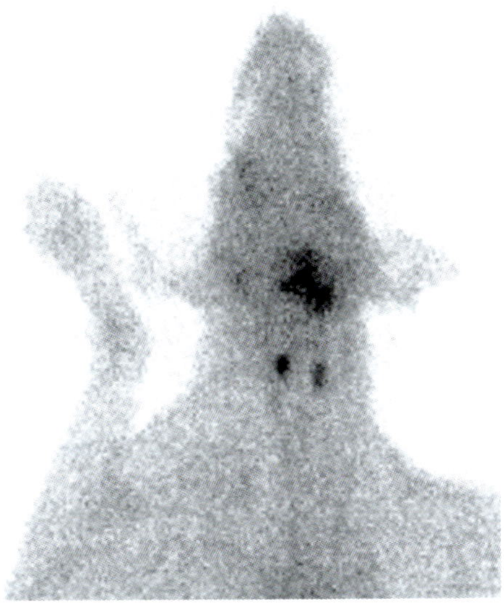

FIG. 28.1 Ventrodorsal view of a thyroid planar technetium-99 (99mTc) scintigraphy of a dog with ectopic sublingual thyroid carcinoma with heterogenous uptake pattern. Courtesy of Gustavo Cobucci, Nuclear Medicine Department, Gamma Vet.

Pathogenesis

The pathogenesis of canine thyroid cancer remains largely unknown. Studies in people have shown an association between thyroid neoplasia and iodine deficiency or excess, chronic stimulation by thyrotropin, ionizing radiation, and many genetic alterations. Lymphocytic thyroiditis and exposure to ionizing radiation have both been reported as predisposing factors in dogs.[10,11]
Mutations in the tumor suppressor gene p53 are uncommon in both human and canine thyroid cancer.[12] Similar to humans, approximately 60% of canine thyroid tumors are DNA-aneuploid. However, in dogs, more than 80% of aneuploid thyroid tumors are hypodiploid, while hypodiploidy is rare in humans.
Activating missense mutations in K-RAS described in human thyroid cancer are uncommon in dogs. No functional mutations were found in the sequenced regions of H-RAS, N-RAS, PIK3CA, BRAF, RET, and PTEN, demonstrating that those mutations most frequently associated with human thyroid neoplasia are rare in dogs.[13]
In humans, several genetic alterations lead to activation of the MAPK and/or the PI3K/Akt signaling pathways, which play a predominant role in human thyroid gland oncogenesis and are most likely involved in dogs as well.[13,14]
In people, thyroid tumors are part of the multiple endocrine neoplasia (MEN) syndrome type 2, which is a genetic disorder caused by germline mutations in the RET proto-oncogene and is associated with a high lifetime

risk of developing MTC. Large pathology studies have shown that MEN syndromes are rare in dogs.[15]

Thyrotoxicosis

Thyrotoxicosis corresponds to the clinical syndrome caused by excessive thyroid hormones in circulation, irrespective of the source, while hyperthyroidism refers specifically to increased thyroid hormone secretion from the thyroid gland.[16] True hyperthyroidism occurs in approximately 20% of canine thyroid carcinomas.

Another important cause of thyrotoxicosis in dogs is the consumption of meat-based products (BARF [biologically appropriate raw food] or treats, e.g., dried gullet) containing thyroid tissue and, therefore, excessive amounts of thyroid hormones.[17] When the suspicion of thyrotoxicosis arises due to the presence of typical clinical signs (e.g., weight loss, polyuria, polydipsia, polyphagia), a complete anamnesis (including dietary history) and a thorough physical examination including cervical palpation is essential in identifying the underlying cause.

Clinical features

Signalment

Thyroid tumors usually develop in middle-aged to older dogs.[4] There is no gender predilection. Beagles, Golden Retrievers, Boxers, and Siberian Huskies are at increased risk.[4]

Clinical signs

Most dogs are presented due to the incidental detection of a palpable mid-cervical mass by the owner or because of clinical signs resulting from compression or invasion of surrounding tissues by a large or invasive mass. Weight loss is present in approximately 30% of dogs, 20% present with cough, 19% present with polyuria polydipsia, and around 10% present with dyspnea or stridor due to large or invasive tumors.[6,18] With advanced disease, dysphagia and dysphonia can also be noticed.

Around 60-70% of dogs have unilateral tumors, 10-20% have bilateral tumors, and 10% have ectopic tumors.[6,18] Ectopic thyroid tumors are commonly located ventrally to the larynx (sublingual), invading the hyoid bone, but can potentially be located anywhere from the base of the tongue to the base of the heart.[9,18,19]

Dogs with functional FTC usually present with clinical signs of hyperthyroidism, such as polyuria, polydipsia, weight loss, panting, aggressiveness, vomiting, and diarrhea. Rarely, dogs may also present with clinical signs of hypothyroidism, which could be present prior to the development of thyroid neoplasia (see above thyroiditis as a predisposing factor) or be due to extensive destruction of healthy thyroid tissue in cases of bilateral thyroid neoplasia.

Video 28.1

The owner or veterinarian might be more easily able to detect a large thyroid mass in a small breed with short hair than in a larger breed with long hair. Evaluation of "mobility" can be clinically misleading, as larger masses are easily classified clinically as "fixed" and "unresectable". The video shows a patient with a large but "movable" mass that is amenable to thyroidectomy.

Physical examination

Although palpation (Video 28.1) is an important first step to assess whether a thyroid mass is "mobile" or "fixed" there are two important limitations. Firstly, only about half of thyroid tumors that feel "fixed" at palpation have macroscopic evidence of local invasiveness during surgery or necropsy.[6] Secondly, only about half of the tumors considered "fixed or partially fixed" at palpation will actually have imaging evidence of capsule disruption, while masses considered "mobile" at palpation can still exhibit imaging signs of capsule disruption. In conclusion, palpation is not an accurate predictor of local invasiveness.[20] Therefore, advanced imaging techniques (CT or MRI) should be recommended for best treatment planning. Regional peripheral lymph nodes should also be palpated for any sign of enlargement.

In hyperthyroid dogs, tachycardia with or without cardiac arrhythmias is frequent.

Clinicopathological findings

As expected, leukocytosis and mild nonregenerative anemia can be present with neoplasia. Despite MTCs arising from calcitonin-producing C-cells, hypocalcemia has been rarely reported in these patients.[5,6] Paraneoplastic ionized hypercalcemia due to the production of parathyroid hormone-related protein (PTH-rp) has been reported in dogs with thyroid carcinoma. Urinalysis is usually unremarkable.

The majority of dogs with thyroid neoplasia are euthyroid.[18] Between 10 and 30% of dogs are hyperthyroid, and some have decreased serum/plasma total thyroxine (T_4) concentrations, mostly due to nonthyroidal illness and rarely due to hypothyroidism.[6,21] In hyperthyroid dogs, endogenous thyroid-stimulating hormone (TSH) concentrations are expected to decrease.

Clinicians can also encounter increased T_4 concentrations when investigating canine hypothyroidism. This can be attributed to the presence of antiT_4 autoantibodies in dogs with thyroiditis and their interference with the T_4 immunoassay. In hypothyroid dogs, TSH concentrations are most commonly increased.

For the diagnostic approach to hypothyroidism, please refer to the corresponding chapter.

Diagnostic imaging

Imaging plays an essential role in the management of dogs with thyroid tumors. It is important to assess local invasiveness, especially considering the limitations of palpation (see above), and to evaluate for the presence of metastasis. As part of treatment planning, thyroid scintigraphy or single-photon emission computed tomography (SPECT) can play an important role, especially when treatment with radioiodine is contemplated.

Evaluation of local invasiveness

Although thyroid ultrasound is a rapid and noninvasive modality, clinicians should interpret ultrasound findings of thyroid tumors with caution, as local invasiveness can be underestimated. Compared to CT and MRI, ultrasonography has a lower sensitivity and specificity to correctly identify the thyroid origin of a cervical mass and, most importantly, lower sensitivity in detecting tumor capsule disruption.[20] MRI scan was the most sensitive imaging modality to detect local invasiveness and may be crucial in selected patients to determine the best treatment option.

Still, in difficult cases with large cervical masses, a definitive assessment might only be possible during surgical exploration. In the authors' opinion, a CT scan likely offers the most cost-effective simultaneous evaluation of local invasiveness and metastatic spread in the preoperative evaluation of dogs with thyroid tumors (Fig. 28.2).

Evaluation of regional and distant metastases

Thyroid tumors metastasize primarily to the lungs and regional lymph nodes (retropharyngeal, mandibular, and cervical superficial), and up to 38% of dogs have evidence of pulmonary metastases at the time of diagnosis.

Thoracic radiographs provide a rapid and relatively inexpensive evaluation for pulmonary metastases and may allow the identification of ectopic thyroid neoplasia in the cranial mediastinum. However, CT is more sensitive for the detection of pulmonary metastases and also allows a thorough evaluation of regional lymph nodes and local invasiveness, making it arguably the most complete imaging modality for treatment planning in these patients.[22]

Planar thyroid scintigraphy, usually with technetium pertechnetate (99mTcO4), allows to confirm the thyroid origin of a cervical mass, to identify the presence of ectopic thyroid tissue (normal or neoplastic), and to detect thyroid cancer metastases if the metastatic tumor cells retain the ability to trap iodine, and also to give a rough indication about malignancy (Fig. 28.3). Although the pattern of radioiodine uptake does not correlate with tumor histology it can help predict the degree of capsular disruption and local invasiveness. Planar scintigraphy does not offer additional benefits for the detection of pulmonary metastases compared

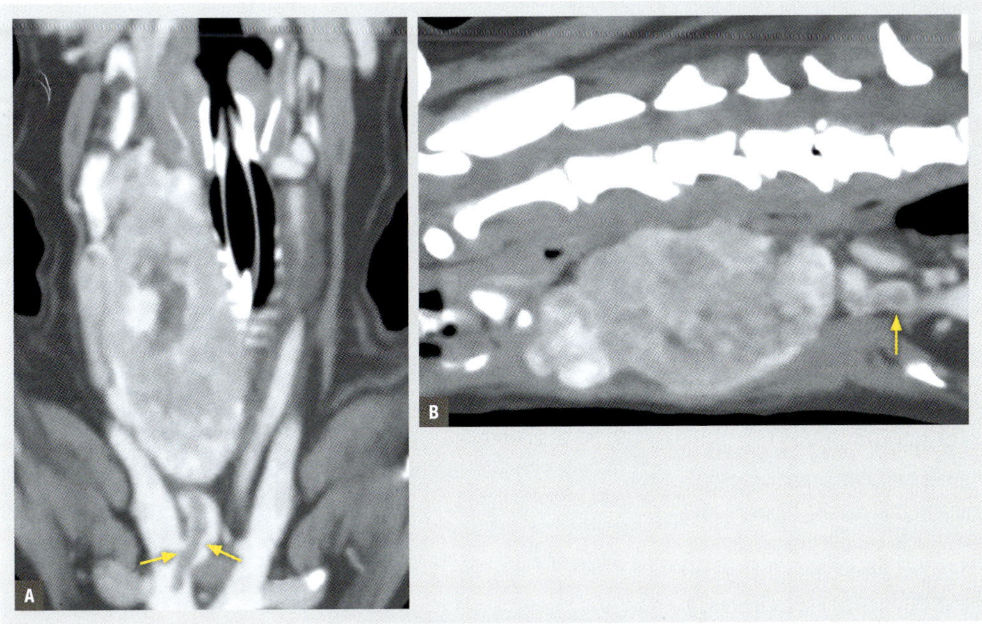

FIG. 28.2 Computed tomography image (A, coronal view; B, saggital view) of a right-sided follicular cell thyroid carcinoma in a dog showing gross vascular invasion. In the mid-thyroid vein, an irregular and centrally located linear filling defect that extends to the right internal jugular and right brachiocephalic veins is visible. Courtesy of the Radiology Department, AniCura Medisch Centrum voor Dieren.

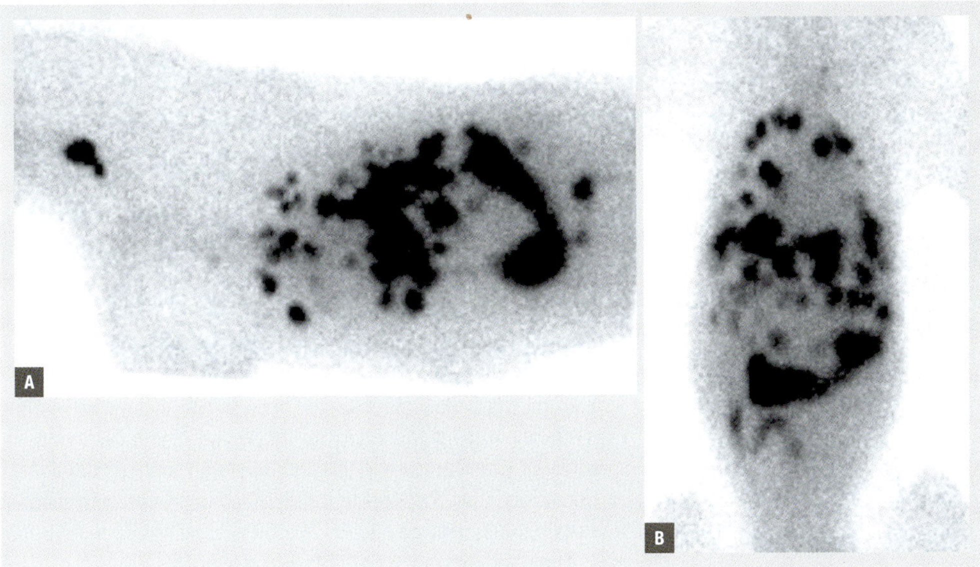

FIG. 28.3 Lateral and ventral views of a thyroid and thoracic planar technetium (99mTc) scintigraphy of a dog with left-sided thyroid carcinoma and multiple lung metastases exhibiting homogeneous uptake pattern. Courtesy of Gustavo Cobucci, Nuclear Medicine Department, Gamma Vet.

to thoracic radiographs. Thoracic SPECT provides higher sensitivity than radiographs to detect thoracic metastases; however, the technique is not widely available.[18]

Diagnosis

Next to thyroid tumors, the differentials of the ventral cervical mass include granuloma/hematoma with or without foreign body, carotid body tumors (especially in brachycephalic dogs), or lymphadenomegaly of the mandibular, medial retropharyngeal, or cervical lymph nodes. See Fig. 28.4 for a possible general clinical approach to a cervical mass in dogs.

Cytology

Fine-needle aspiration can be performed once a mass is detected, as cytology can provide information regarding the origin of the mass. Importantly, cytology cannot reliably distinguish benign from malignant disease, and thyroid tumors in dogs should be assumed to be malignant. A cytology sample contaminated with blood is highly suspicious of the presence of a thyroid tumor, as these tumors are highly vascularized.

Histopathology

Definitive diagnosis of thyroid gland neoplasia requires histopathology. Thyroid tumors are highly vascularized. Hence, an excisional biopsy is the safest way to obtain a definitive histopathological diagnosis. For unresectable tumors due to local invasiveness, a presumptive diagnosis based on cytology, scintigraphy, or even CT may be a preferable approach. Traditionally, incisional biopsies and large-bore needle biopsies are avoided because of an important risk of bleeding. However, a correct histopathologic diagnosis pretreatment could be helpful in defining an adequate treatment plan in dogs with a nonresectable thyroid mass. Recently, ultrasound-guided core needle biopsy (14G) was evaluated in a limited series of patients with canine thyroid tumors. This pilot study suggested it to be a safe biopsy technique that allows pretreatment histological diagnosis, including immunohistochemistry, but further investigation is warranted before this technique is recommended at large.[23]

TABLE 28.1 Clinical staging system of dogs with thyroid tumors based on the TNM system adapted from WHO (Owen et al., 1980).

Stage	Primary tumor (T)	Regional lymph nodes (N)	Distant metastases (M)
I	T_1a, b	N_0	M_0
II	T_0	N_1	M_0
	T_1a, b	N_1	
	T_2a, b	N_0 or N_1 a	
III	Any T_3	Any N	M_0
	Any T	Any N b	
IV	Any T	Any N	M_1

Staging

Staging of thyroid tumors is performed according to the World Health Organization staging system and is based on the size and mobility of the primary tumor and the presence of regional or distant metastases (Table 28.1).

Therapy

Thyroidectomy

Surgery is the preferred treatment for dogs with well-encapsulated thyroid tumors in the absence of distant metastases. The reported median survival time (MST) for unilateral or bilateral thyroid tumors is beyond 2.5-3 years.[24-27] When present, regional lymph node metastases should also be surgically removed, and surgery should still be considered in dogs with distant metastases (see prognosis).[28-32] After thyroidectomy, local recurrence is reported in 4-12% of dogs, and 8% develop metastases.[27]

Thyroidectomy typically allows marginal excision of the tumor. Wide resection of noninvasive tumors is not indicated because of high morbidity and low rate of local recurrence.[27] Radical resection of deeply invasive tumors is not recommended due to high morbidity and excellent prognosis with radiation therapy or radioactive iodine-131 (^{131}I).[28,33,34] Because thyroid tumors are highly vascularized, cytoreductive surgery is not recommended due to the risk of hemorrhage. If patients are selected adequately, complications of unilateral thyroidectomy are uncommon but include hemorrhage (8%), aspiration pneumonia (3%), and laryngeal paralysis (2%).[24,27,28] One exception to the preclusion of surgery to treat invasive thyroid tumors is ectopic sublingual thyroid tumors invading the hyoid bone. Partial hyoidectomy is well tolerated by most dogs and allows en bloc removal of the entire tumor without major complications.[9,19]

In dogs with well-encapsulated bilateral thyroid tumors, monitoring for postoperative iatrogenic hypoparathyroidism is critical as 70% of patients develop hypocalcemia, and about 50% require long-term treatment with calcitriol.[25]

Radiation therapy

Dogs with locally invasive thyroid tumors not amenable to complete surgical resection can be adequately treated and enjoy prolonged survival with radiation therapy.[33,35,36] Dogs typically receive 48 Gray (Gy) over 4 weeks on an alternate-day schedule of 4 Gy/fraction.[33,35] In dogs with no evidence of metastases, the reported progression-free survival (PFS) rate is 80% at 1 year and 72% at 3 years.[33] Reported time to maximum effect on tumor size is 8 to 22 months. Acute radiation reactions include mild dysphagia, hoarseness, and cough due to esophageal, tracheal, or laryngeal mucositis. Chronic radiation complications include skin fibrosis with permanent alopecia, dry cough due to chronic tracheitis, hypothyroidism, and hypoparathyroidism.[33,37]

Palliative hypofractionated radiation protocols have been reported in dogs with advanced disease.[38,39] In one study, dogs received 36 Gy divided into 4 weekly fractions; the tumor response rate was 77%, and the MST for the dogs with and without pulmonary metastases was 21 and 29 months, respectively.[38] In another retrospective study, dogs with nonresectable thyroid carcinoma and tumor-related clinical signs received 4 weekly fractions of 6.5 to 8 Gy. Tumor response rate was 25%, overall MST was 5.5 months, and MST of dogs with pulmonary metastases was 8 months.[39]

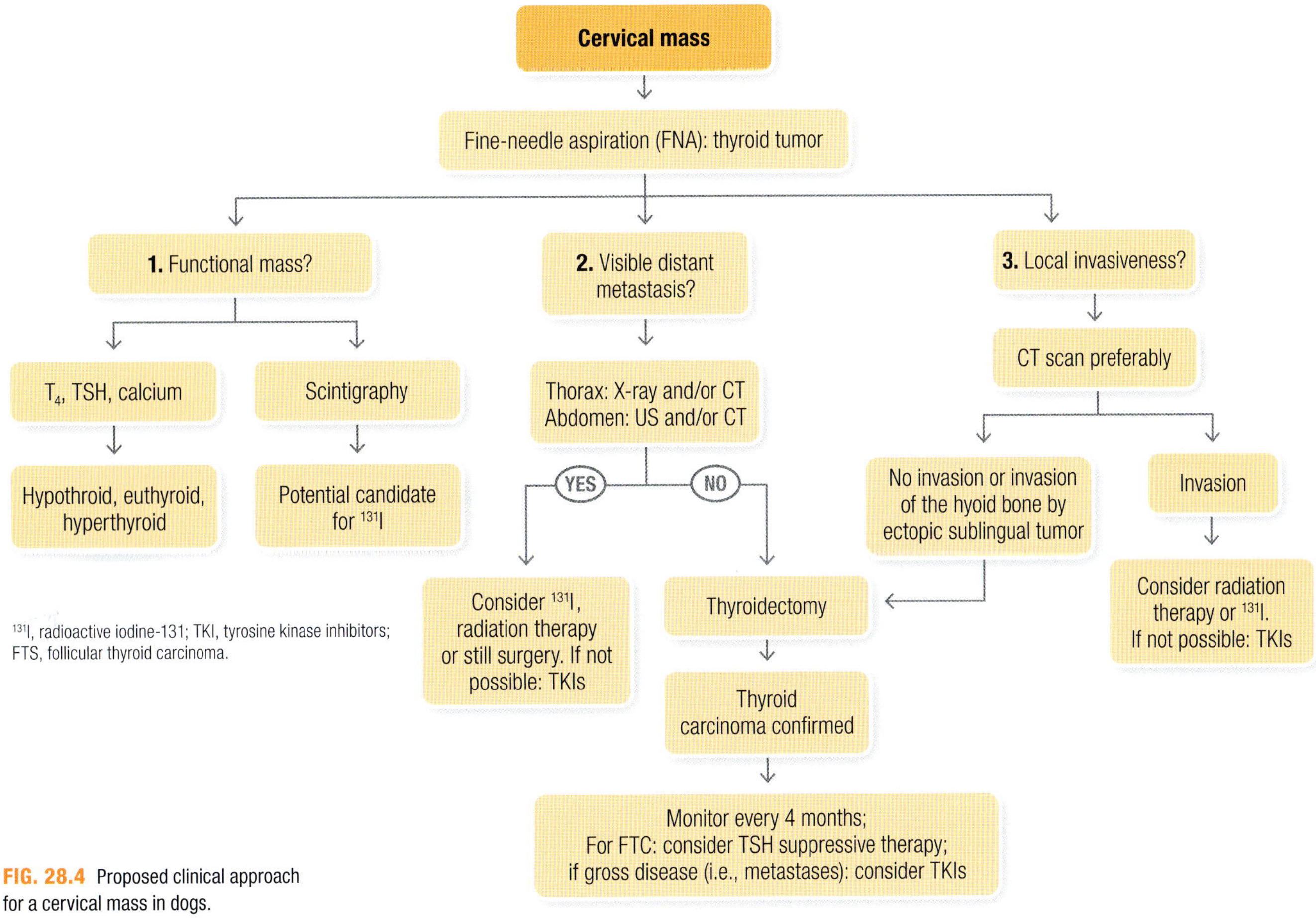

FIG. 28.4 Proposed clinical approach for a cervical mass in dogs.

Radioactive iodine ^{131}I

Locally invasive FTCs can also be treated with ^{131}I, which has the potential to target thyroid tissue regardless of its location.[21,34,40] For ^{131}I to deliver sufficient radiation to be effective, the tumor and possible metastases need to have adequate ^{131}I uptake (**Fig. 28.3**). Therefore, scintigraphy must be performed before treatment to select patients adequately. Tumors causing hyperthyroidism are expected to show high uptake of ^{131}I, and many euthyroid dogs with FTC are also good candidates. Overall, 70% of thyroid tumors (and 80% of FTCs) are reported to have normal to increased uptake on scintigraphy.[6,18] While uptake is homogeneous in 16% of tumors, 84% have heterogeneous or variable uptake.[18] This may be due to loss of cellular differentiation, necrosis, or hemorrhage in parts of the tumor and could limit treatment efficacy. In 13% to 28% of dogs, more than one ^{131}I treatment is needed for adequate tumor control.[21,34]

Other limitations of ^{131}I therapy in dogs include its limited availability and the need for high dosages of ^{131}I (11-191 mCi; 0.41-7.10 GBq). Depending on each country's regulations, this implies variable mandatory hospitalization periods.

The MST reported for dogs treated with ^{131}I as sole therapy is 30 months.[21] The survival time of dogs with stage II or III disease (MST 28 months) is significantly longer than for dogs with stage IV disease (MST 12 months).[34] In about 30% of dogs, the tumor can become resectable 3 to 6 weeks after ^{131}I therapy, but surgery does not seem to provide a significant survival benefit after ^{131}I treatment.[34] The administration of ^{131}I as an adjunct to surgery (MST 34 months) also does not seem to provide a survival benefit over surgery alone (MST not reached).[21] Thyroid function does not seem to be a prognostic factor.[21,34]

Myelosuppression is a potentially fatal complication described in 8% dogs[34] and is probably related to high ^{131}I dosages.

The efficacy of external beam radiation therapy versus ^{131}I in the treatment of unresectable thyroid tumors has never been directly compared. Even so, available studies show that external beam radiation likely provides a longer progression-free interval (PFS rate of 72% at 3 years) and may be more effective.[33] External beam radiotherapy is likely to deliver a more uniform radiation dosage to the whole tumor compared to ^{131}I, where radiation delivery is limited to tumor areas of functional FTC cells.[21] With ^{131}I, tumor heterogenicity could lead to areas of the tumor not being exposed to sufficient radiation levels to ensure cell death. Furthermore, only dogs with FTC are expected to be effectively treated with ^{131}I, but not dogs with MTC, which still represent one-third of all cases.

Chemotherapy

Chemotherapy with platinum compounds or doxorubicin can be considered in selected patients with thyroid carcinoma. Still, its efficacy as the sole treatment for inoperable thyroid tumors is disappointing compared to either radiation therapy or ^{131}I. Partial responses are reported in 44% to 54% of dogs and median survival times range from 3 to 8 months.[41] In dogs with distant metastases, the reported median survival time is only 4 months.

To date, no study has shown a clear benefit of adjuvant chemotherapy after thyroidectomy. In a retrospective study, the survival of dogs undergoing thyroidectomy alone (MST = 510 days; n = 28) was comparable to that of dogs also receiving adjuvant chemotherapy (MST = 518 days; n = 16).[28] Similar results have been reported in other studies.[29,42] However, the effect of chemotherapy has only been evaluated in retrospective studies with relatively low numbers of dogs, and it may be reasonable to consider it in dogs with negative prognostic factors, such as large tumor size, bilateral disease, metastases, evidence of microscopic or gross vascular invasion, high mitotic count, undifferentiated carcinoma and carcinosarcoma[6,27-30,33] (see prognosis).

Tyrosine kinase inhibitors

Toceranib phosphate is a tyrosine kinase inhibitor (TKI) that targets VEGFR (vascular endothelial growth factor receptor), PDGFR (platelet-derived growth factor receptor), Kit, CSF-1R (colony stimulating factor-1 receptor), and Flt-3. In line with earlier reports, a study in 42 dogs with thyroid carcinoma showed clinical benefit (complete remission, partial remission, or stable disease) in about 90% of dogs with naïve disease and 75% of dogs that had prior treatment.[43,44] Even though most dogs had presumed pulmonary metastases, the median survival time for treatment-naïve dogs and for dogs previously treated were 12 and 36 months, respectively. The objective responses of thyroid tumors to toceranib phosphate suggest that specific TKIs targeted by toceranib may be dysregulated and that this constitutes an effective treatment option for dogs where curative treatment is not pursued and dogs developing recurrent or metastatic disease after treatment. Reported adverse effects include diarrhea, anorexia, vomiting, and neutropenia.

TSH suppression, antithyroid drugs, and retinoic acid

In dogs, FTC cells conserve TSH receptors; thus, endogenous TSH may stimulate the growth of thyroid cancer cells and contribute to tumor progression. In people with high-risk differentiated FTC, TSH suppression with levothyroxine is associated with improved survival, and many clinicians (the authors included) use it routinely in adjunctive treatment of canine FTC.[45,46] To date, the efficacy of TSH suppression in dogs with thyroid carcinoma has not been adequately investigated. In a retrospective study, 13 of 28 dogs with differentiated FTC treated by thyroidectomy also received levothyroxine supplementation after surgery, but levothyroxine treatment did not affect patient survival.[6] In another study, 21 of 42 dogs with thyroid tumors undergoing different treatment modalities received levothyroxine with the aim of suppressing TSH, but no significant effect on survival was observed.[47] Although no studies support TSH suppression in dogs with FTC, given the evidence in human medicine, it should still be considered.

Antithyroid drugs are not routinely recommended in dogs with hyperthyroidism due to functional thyroid tumors, as this condition typically resolves by treating the underlying tumor. However, in untreated dogs with clinical signs of hyperthyroidism and dogs with tumor recurrence/progression following treatment, antithyroid drugs may be indicated to treat the hyperthyroid state. Methimazole can be started at dosages similar to those used in hyperthyroid cats (2.5 mg to 5 mg q12h) with subsequent increases as needed to control clinical signs and T_4.[48] If increasing dosages of methimazole or carbimazole are insufficient to control hyperthyroidism, prescribing an iodine-restricted diet has been shown to be successful in one dog.[49]

One study on a limited number of dogs suggested a longer disease-free interval when retinoic acid was used as an adjuvant therapy after thyroidectomy.[42]

Prognosis

Important negative prognostic factors reported in dogs with thyroid tumors include large tumor size, bilateral disease, presence of metastases at diagnosis, evidence of gross vascular invasion, high mitotic count, undifferentiated carcinoma, and carcinosarcoma.[6,27-30,33] Left untreated, median survival times for dogs with thyroid tumors range from 3 to 13 months.[21,29,47] As almost all clinically detected thyroid masses are malignant, the best prognosis is achieved in dogs with tumors amenable to surgery without gross vascular invasion or visible metastases at diagnosis.[43] However, with a selection of adequate treatment (thyroidectomy for dogs with removable tumors; external-beam radiation, ^{131}I or TKIs for dogs with invasive tumors), even dogs with unresectable tumors, gross vascular invasion (Fig. 28.5) or distant metastases can enjoy a long survival with good quality of life.

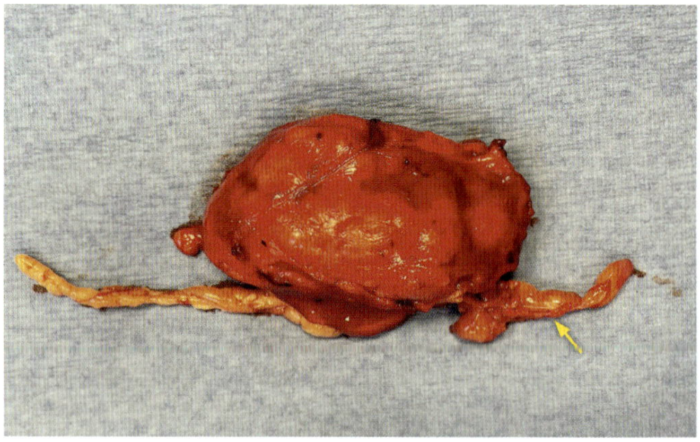

FIG. 28.5 Postoperative image of a well-encapsulated follicular cell thyroid carcinoma in a dog with gross evidence of vascular invasion of the thyroid vein. Courtesy of Nicolien van Klaveren, Soft Tissue Surgery Department, AniCura Medisch Centrum voor Dieren.

KEY POINTS

- In dogs, most clinically detected thyroid masses are carcinomas; therefore, all cervical masses should be investigated promptly.
- Cytology is needed to confirm diagnosis of a thyroid tumor, but cannot predict malignancy.
- Palpation of large thyroid masses that seem "fixed" can be misleading and can give the clinician the impression that the thyroid tumor is unresectable.
- Advanced medical imaging (mainly CT scan) is strongly recommended for appropriate staging and assessment of local invasion prior to treatment.
- Dogs without evidence of metastasis and amenable to thyroidectomy have the best prognosis.
- Many dogs with unresectable thyroid tumors and/or metastasis can also enjoy a long survival with a good quality of life with appropriate treatment such as radiation therapy, radioactive iodine ^{131}I, or tyrosine kinase inhibitors.

References

1. Ward RC. Canine hyperthyroidism. In Ettinger SJ, Feldman EC, Côté E (editors). Textbook of Veterinary Internal Medicine 8th edition. Elsevier, 2017, pp. 1757-1767.
2. Brodey RS, Kelly DF. Thyroid neoplasms in the dog. A clinicopathologic study of fifty-seven cases. *Cancer* 22:406-416, 1968.
3. Leav I, Schiller AL, Rijnberk A, et al. Adenomas and carcinomas of the canine and feline thyroid. *Am J Pathol* 83:61-122, 1976.
4. Wucherer KL, Wilke V. Thyroid cancer in dogs: An update based on 638 cases (1995-2005). *J Am Anim Hosp Assoc* 46:249-254, 2005.
5. Carver JR, Kapatkin A, Patnaik AK. A comparison of medullary thyroid carcinoma and thyroid adenocarcinoma in dogs: a retrospective study of 38 cases. *Vet Surg* 24:315-319, 1995.
6. Campos M, Ducatelle R, Rutteman G, et al. Clinical, pathologic, and immunohistochemical prognostic factors in dogs with thyroid carcinoma. *J Vet Intern Med* 28:1805-1813, 2014.
7. Campos M, Ducatelle R, Kooistra HS, et al. Immunohistochemical expression of potential therapeutic targets in canine thyroid carcinoma. *J Vet Intern Med* 28:564-570, 2014.
8. Liptak JM, Kamstock DA, Dernell WS, et al. Cranial mediastinal carcinomas in nine dogs. *Vet Comp Oncol* 6:19-30, 2008.
9. Broome MR, Peterson ME, Walker JR. Clinical Features and Treatment Outcomes of 41 Dogs with Sublingual Ectopic Thyroid Neoplasia. *J Vet Intern Med* 28:1560-1568, 2014.
10. Benjamin SA, Stephens LC, Hamilton BF, et al. Associations between lymphocytic thyroiditis, hypothyroidism, and thyroid neoplasia in beagles. *Vet Pathol* 33:486-494, 1996.
11. Benjamin SA, Saunders WJ, Lee AC, et al. Non-neoplastic and neoplastic thyroid disease in beagles irradiated during prenatal and postnatal development. *Radiat Res* 147:422-430, 1997.
12. Devilee P, Van Leeuwen IS, Voesten A, et al. The canine p53 gene is subject to somatic mutations in thypoid carcinoma. *Anticancer Res* 14:2039-2046, 1994.
13. Campos M, Kool MMJ, Daminet S, et al. Upregulation of the PI3K/Akt pathway in the tumorigenesis of canine thyroid carcinoma. *J Vet Intern Med* 28:1814-1823, 2014.
14. Urie BK, Russell DS, Kisseberth WC, et al. Evaluation of expression and function of vascular endothelial growth factor receptor 2, platelet-derived growth factor receptors-alpha and -beta, KIT, and RET in canine apocrine gland anal sac adenocarcinoma and thyroid carcinoma. *BMC Vet Res* 8:67, 2012.
15. Beatrice L, Boretti FS, Sieber-Ruckstuhl NS, et al. Concurrent endocrine neoplasias in dogs and cats: a retrospective study (2004-2014). *Vet Rec* 182:323, 2018.
16. Mooney CT. Canine hyperthyroidism. In Mooney CT, Peterson ME (editors). BSAVA manual of canine and feline endocrinology. Gloucestershire, British Small Animal Veterinary Association, 2012, pp. 86-91.
17. Köhler B, Stengel C, Neiger R. Dietary hyperthyroidism in dogs. *J Small Anim Pract* 53:182-184, 2012.
18. van den Berg MF, Daminet S, Stock E, et al. Planar and single-photon emission computed tomography imaging in dogs with thyroid tumors: 68 cases. *J Vet Intern Med* 1-9, 2020.
19. Milovancev M, Wilson DM, Monnet E, et al. Partial resection of the hyoid apparatus during surgical treatment of ectopic thyroid carcinomas in dogs: 5 cases (2011-2013). *J Am Vet Med Assoc* 245:1319-1324, 2014.
20. Taeymans O, Penninck DG, Peters RM. Comparison between clinical, ultrasound, CT, MRI, and pathology findings in dogs presented for suspected thyroid carcinoma. *Vet Radiol Ultrasound* 54:61-70, 2013.
21. Worth A, Zuber R, Hocking M. Radioiodide (131)I therapy for the treatment of canine thyroid carcinoma. *Aust Vet J* 83:208-214, 2005.
22. Armbrust LJ, Biller DS, Bamford A, et al. Comparison of three-view thoracic radiography and computed tomography for detection of pulmonary nodules in dogs with neoplasia. *J Am Vet Med Assoc* 240:1088-1094, 2012.
23. Scheemaeker S, Vandermeulen E, Ducatelle R, et al. Ultrasound-guided core needle biopsy in dogs with thyroid carcinoma. *Vet Comp Oncol* 21:349-356, 2023.
24. Klein MK, Powers BE, Withrow SJ, et al. Treatment of thyroid carcinoma in dogs by surgical resection alone: 20 cases (1981-1989). *J Am Vet Med Assoc* 206(7):1007-1009, 1995.
25. Tuohy JL, Worley DR, Withrow SJ. Outcome following simultaneous bilateral thyroid lobectomy for treatment of thyroid gland carcinoma in dogs: 15 cases (1994-2010). *J Am Vet Med Assoc* 241:95-103, 2012.
26. Frederick AN, Pardo AD, Schmiedt CW, et al. Outcomes for dogs with functional thyroid tumors treated by surgical excision alone. *J Am Vet Med Assoc* 256:444-448, 2020.
27. Reagan JK, Selmic LE, Fallon C, et al. Complications and outcomes associated with unilateral thyroidectomy in dogs with naturally occurring thyroid tumors: 156 cases (2003-2015). *J Am Vet Med Assoc* 255:926-932, 2019.
28. Nadeau ME, Kitchell BE. Evaluation of the use of chemotherapy and other prognostic variables for surgically excised canine thyroid carcinoma with and without metastasis. *Can Vet J* 52:994-998, 2011.
29. Giannasi C, Rushton S, Rook A, et al. Canine thyroid carcinoma prognosis following the utilisation of computed tomography assisted staging. *Vet Rec* 189:e55, 2021.
30. Enache D, Ferro L, Nicoli S, et al. Thyroidectomy in dogs with thyroid tumors: survival analysis in 144 cases (1994-2018). *J Vet Intern Med* 37:635-647, 2023.
31. Skinner OT, de M Souza CH, Kim DY. Metastasis to ipsilateral medial retropharyngeal and deep

cervical lymph nodes in 22 dogs with thyroid carcinoma. *Vet Surg* 50:150-157, 2021.
32. Latifi M, Skinner OT, Spoldi E, et al. Outcome and postoperative complications in 73 dogs with thyroid carcinoma with gross vascular invasion managed with thyroidectomy. *Vet Comp Oncol* 19:685-696, 2021.
33. Théon AP, Marks SL, Feldman ES, et al. Prognostic factors and patterns of treatment failure in dogs with unresectable differentiated thyroid carcinomas treated with megavoltage irradiation. *J Am Vet Med Assoc* 216:1775-1779, 2000.
34. Turrel JM, McEntee MC, Burke BP, et al. Sodium iodide I 131 treatment of dogs with nonresectable thyroid tumors: 39 cases (1990-2003). *J Am Vet Med Assoc* 229:542-548, 2006.
35. Pack L, Roberts RE, Dawson SD, et al. Definitive radiation therapy for infiltrative thyroid carcinoma in dogs. *Vet Radiol Ultrasound* 42:471-474, 2001.
36. Brearley MJ, Jeffery ND, Phillips SM, et al. Hypofractionated radiation therapy of brain masses in dogs: a retrospective analysis of survival of 83 cases (1991-1996). *J Vet Intern Med* 13:408-412, 1999.
37. Amores-Fuster I, Cripps P, Blackwood L. Post-radiotherapy hypothyroidism in dogs treated for thyroid carcinomas. *Vet Comp Oncol* 15:247-251, 2017.
38. Brearley MJ, Hayes AM, Murphy S. Hypofractionated radiation therapy for invasive thyroid carcinoma in dogs: a retrospective analysis of survival. *J Small Anim Pract* 40:206-210, 1999.
39. Tsimbas K, Turek M, Christensen N, et al. Short survival time following palliative-intent hypofractionated radiotherapy for non-resectable canine thyroid carcinoma: A retrospective analysis of 20 dogs. *Vet Radiol Ultrasound* 60:93-99, 2019.
40. Adams WH, Walker MA, Daniel GB, et al. Treatment of differentiated thyroid carcinoma in 7 dogs utilizing 131I. *Vet Radiol Ultrasound* 36:417-424, 1995.
41. Fineman LS, Hamilton T, de Gortari A, et al. Cisplatin chemotherapy for treatment of thyroid carcinoma in dogs: 13 cases. *J Am Anim Hosp Assoc* 34:109-112, 1998.
42. Castillo V, Pessina P, Hall P, et al. Post-surgical treatment of thyroid carcinoma in dogs with retinoic acid 9 cis improves patient outcome. *Open Vet J* 6:6-14, 2016.
43. Sheppard-Olivares S, Bello NM, Wood E, et al. Toceranib phosphate in the treatment of canine thyroid carcinoma: 42 cases (2009-2018). *Vet Comp Oncol* 7-13, 2020.
44. London C, Mathie T, Stingle N, et al. Preliminary evidence for biologic activity of toceranib phosphate (Palladia®) in solid tumours. *Vet Comp Oncol* 10:194-205, 2012.
45. Haugen BR, Alexander EK, Bible KC, et al. 2015 American thyroid association management guidelines for adult patients with thyroid nodules and differentiated thyroid cancer: the American Thyroid Association Guidelines Task Force on Thyroid Nodules and Differentiated Thyroid Cancer. *Thyroid* 26:1-133, 2016.
46. Jonklaas J, Sarlis NJ, Litofsky D, et al. Outcomes of patients with differentiated thyroid carcinoma following initial therapy. *Thyroid* 16:1229-1242, 2006.
47. Campos M. Pathogenesis and treatment of canine thyroid tumors. Faculty of Veterinary Medicine, Ghent University, 2014.
48. Scott-Moncrieff JC. Canine thyroid tumors and hyperthyroidism. In Feldman EC, Nelson RW, Reusch CR (editors). Canine and Feline Endocrinology. St Louis, Elsevier Saunders, 2015, pp. 196-212.
49. Looney A, Wakshlag J. Dietary management of hyperthyroidism in a dog. *J Am Anim Hosp Assoc* 53:111-118, 2017.

CHAPTER 29

Anatomy and physiology of parathyroid glands and calcium metabolism

Rodolfo Oliveira Leal
DVM, PhD, DECVIM-CA (Internal Medicine)

Anatomy of the canine parathyroid glands

Being one of the smallest endocrine organs, the parathyroid glands are pale, well-defined, ellipsoidal structures of 2-5 mm in diameter and 0.5-1 mm in width located in the cervical region adjacent to the thyroid glands.[1,2] Although their number may vary, dogs usually have four parathyroid glands (two cranial and two caudal). The two cranial, also known as external parathyroids, are located in the extrathyroidal fascia on the rostral end of the thyroid gland, while the two caudal ones are often embedded in the medial aspect of the thyroid parenchyma.[1,2] Their innervation, arteriolar blood supply, venous and lymphatic drainage are directly related to the corresponding thyroid tissues.[2]

Parathyroid physiology and its role in calcium homeostasis

Parathyroid glands are crucial in calcium metabolism, being responsible for parathyroid hormone (PTH) synthesis.[3-5] Calcium homeostasis involves the coordination and interaction of three hormones (PTH, calcitonin, and vitamin D) and their direct and indirect effect on three organs (intestine, bone, and kidney)[3-5] (Fig. 29.1 and Table 29.1).

Parathyroid hormone

Within the parenchyma in the parathyroid glands, the cells actively enrolled in the secretion of PTH are called chief cells.[3] PTH synthesis is similar to other protein hormones occurring within the rough endoplasmic reticulum and secreted by exocytosis in its active form, a single-chain 84 amino-acid polypeptide.[3,4] It has a short half-life in circulation (around 10 minutes) and is metabolized in the liver and kidneys.[3,4]

PTH secretion is mainly regulated by ionized calcium. Low iCa^{2+} levels stimulate its secretion, while high levels inhibit it. Phosphorus, 1,25-dihydroxycholecalciferol, magnesium, and epinephrine levels also affect PTH secretion. In detail, PTH is inhibited by high 1,25-dihydroxycholecalciferol levels and stimulated in case of hyperphosphatemia, hypomagnesemia or epinephrine release (through beta-adrenergenic receptors stimulation).[3,4] Although to a lesser extent, magnesium affects PTH in the same manner as calcium, being a cofactor for PTH synthesis and release.[3]

PTH has a direct effect in bones and kidneys and indirect action in the gastrointestinal tract. PTH induces bone resorption by inhibiting osteoblastic and enhancing osteoclastic activity, potentiating calcium and phosphorus release for the extracellular fluid. In kidneys, PTH potentiates calcium resorption in the distal convoluted tubule while it decreases phosphorus resorption in the proximal convoluted tubule.[4] Also, in kidneys, PTH stimulates the enzyme 1-alpha-hydroxilase that converts 25-hydroxycholecalciferol to 1,25-dihydroxycholecalciferol.[3,4] By itself, 1,25-dihydroxycholecalciferol stimulates calcium absorption in the gastrointestinal tract. Therefore, although PTH does not directly act in the gastrointestinal tract, it modulates calcium absorption due to this indirect effect on vitamin D metabolism.[3,4]

Vitamin D

In contrast to humans and other mammals in which the inactive form of vitamin D is mainly produced in the skin, dogs are less able to synthesize it, being mainly dependent on their dietary intake.[5] Inactive vitamin D is hydroxylated to 25-hydroxycholecalciferol (also inactive form) in the liver. In the kidneys, 25-hydroxycholecalciferol is hydroxylated by 1-alpha-hydroxylase to produce 1,25-hydroxycholecalciferol, the biologically active form of vitamin D. This is a relevant step for vitamin D production since 1-alpha-hydroxylase is positively regulated by hypocalcemia, increased PTH and, indirectly, by low phosphorus levels. Also in the kidneys, 25-hydroxycholecalciferol can be hydroxylated to 24,25-dihydroxycholecalciferol, an inactive metabolite, by 24-hydroxylase. This enzyme is inhibited by high PTH and positively regulated by high phosphorus levels.

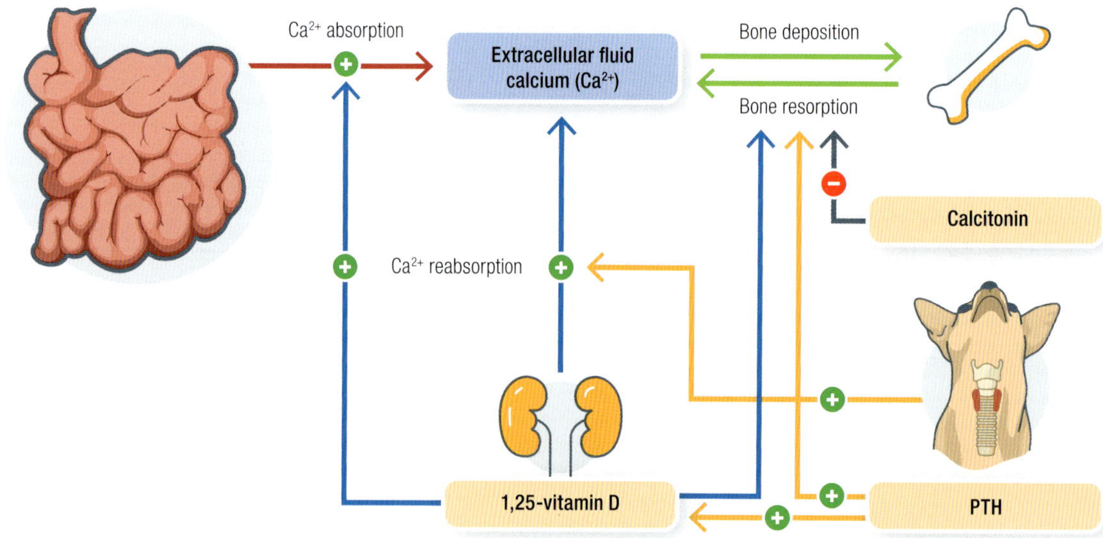

FIG. 29.1 Hormonal regulation of calcium homeostasis (original, adapted from Feldman 2015 and Costanzo, 2021).

Therefore, hyperphosphatemia indirectly induces a decrease in active vitamin D, shifting the pathway toward its inactive form[3-5] (Fig. 29.2). The most relevant action of vitamin D occurs in the small intestine, where it potentiates calcium (and phosphorus) absorption in a rate-limiting pathway by enterocytes.[3,4] Also, vitamin D increases calcium and phosphorus resorption in the kidneys.[3,5] In bone, vitamin D is responsible for remodeling and mineralization. Although it seems paradoxical, it stimulates bone resorption by osteoclasts to induce new bone mineralization by osteoblasts thereafter.[3,4] Overall, its main physiological action is coordinated to maintain high calcium and phosphorus levels (and consequently a high Ca × P product required for mineralization).[3,4]

Calcitonin

Calcitonin is a hormone produced by the parafollicular cells (C-cells) of the thyroid gland in response to hypercalcemia.[3,4] Among its physiological actions, calcitonin limits postprandial hypercalcemia in mammals.[5] This is achieved because gastrointestinal hormones such as gastrin, cholecystokinin, secretin, and glucagon stimulate calcitonin secretion.[3] By counterbalancing PTH action, calcitonin inhibits osteoclast activity and induces hypocalcemia.[3-5] The role of calcitonin in canine calcium physiology is discussable and considered less relevant than PTH and vitamin D.[3-5]

TABLE 29.1 Summary of the main stimulus and effect of hormones enrolled on calcium homeostasis.

		PTH	Vitamin D	Calcitonin
Stimulus for secretion		↓ Serum Ca^{2+}	↓ Serum Ca^{2+} ↑ PTH ↓ Serum phosphate	↑ Serum Ca^{2+}
Action on	Bone	↑ Resorption	↑ Remodeling	↓ Resorption
	Kidney	↓ P reabsorption ↑ Ca^{2+} reabsorption	↑ P reabsorption ↑ Ca^{2+} reabsorption	
	Intestine	↑ Ca^{2+} absorption (via activation of vitamin D)	↑ Ca^{2+} absorption ↑ P absorption	
Overall effect on	Serum Ca^{2+}	↑	↑	↓
	Serum phosphate	↓	↑	

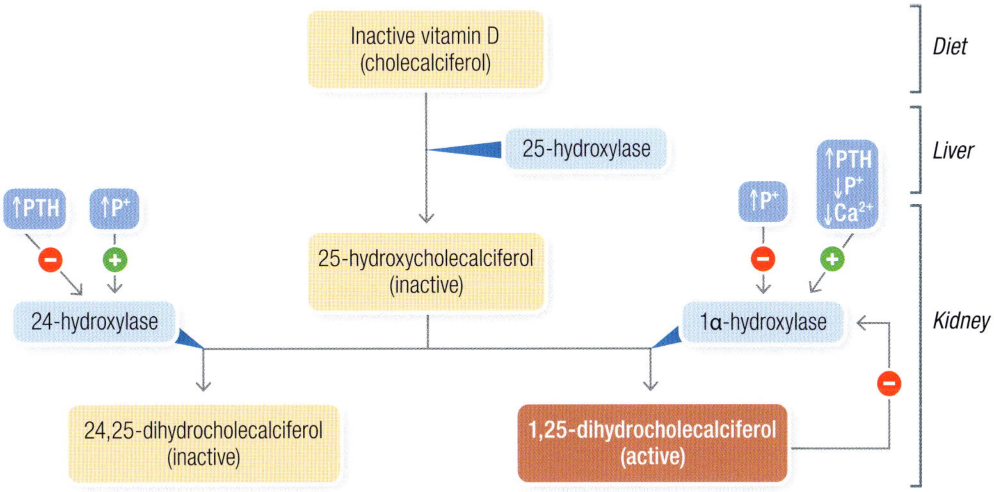

FIG. 29.2 Vitamin D hydroxylation pathways (original, adapted from Feldman 2015 and Costanzo, 2021).

KEY POINTS

- The parathyroid glands play a critical role in calcium metabolism, being responsible for parathyroid hormone (PTH) synthesis.
- PTH induces bone resorption by inhibiting osteoblastic and enhancing osteoclastic activity, potentiating calcium and phosphorus release for the extracellular fluid.
- Vitamin D is responsible for bone remodeling and mineralization.

References

1. Singh B (editor). Dyce, Sack and Wensing's Textbook of Veterinary Anatomy 5th edition. St. Louis, Elsevier, 2018.
2. Hermanson JW, de Lahunta A, Evans HE (editors). Miller and Evan's Anatomy of the Dog 5th edition. St Louis, Elsevier, 2019.
3. Klein BG (editor). Cunnigham's Textbook of Veterinary Physiology 6th edition. St.Louis, Elsevier, 2019.
4. Costanzo L (editor). Costanzo Physiology 7th edition. St.Louis, Elsevier, 2021.
5. Feldman E. Hypercalcemia and primary hyperparathyroidism. In Feldman EC, Nelson RW, Reusch C, Scott-Moncrieff JCR, Behrend E (editors). Canine and Feline Endocrinology. St. Louis, Elsevier, 2015, pp. 579-624.

CHAPTER 30

Primary hyperparathyroidism

Rodolfo Oliveira Leal
DVM, MSc, PhD
DECVIM-CA (Internal Medicine)

Etiology

Primary hyperparathyroidism (PHPTH) is an endocrine disorder characterized by an autonomous and inappropriate overproduction of parathyroid hormone (PTH), usually due to the presence of a solitary adenoma in one or more parathyroid glands.[1] The functional behavior of the disease results in hypercalcemia and low/low-normal phosphorus, both consequences of the autonomous secretion of PTH. Being the third most common disease associated with ionized hypercalcemia, PHPTH is infrequent in daily practice.[2]

Although out of the scope of this chapter, PHPTH is distinct from secondary hyperparathyroidism, which results from an overproduction of PTH induced by non-endocrine causes, namely chronic kidney disease or nutritional calcium imbalances.

PTH has a major impact on kidneys, bone, and, to a lesser degree, the gastrointestinal tract (see chapter 29). The consequences of inappropriate secretion of PTH in these organs are summarized in Fig. 30.1.

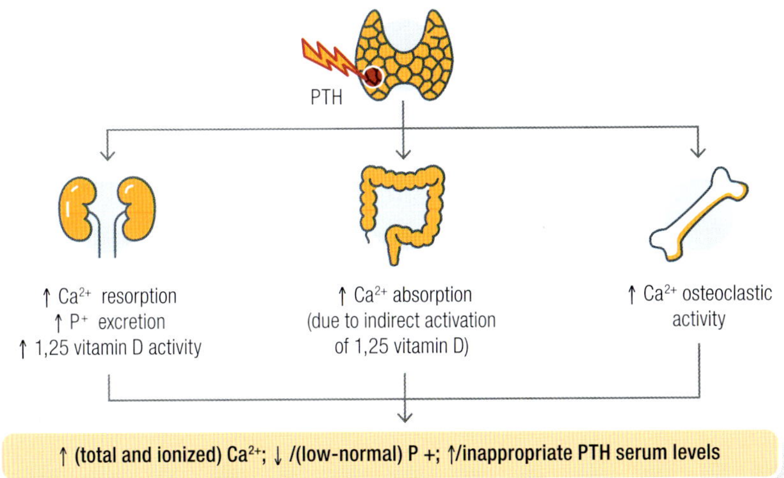

FIG. 30.1 Physiologic consequences of PTH overproduction in kidneys, bone, and gastrointestinal tract (original).

Clinical features

PHPTH mainly occurs in adult-geriatric dogs, most of them older than 7 years old, with a mean age of 11 (range 4-17) years.[1,3] There is no gender predisposition, and the reported mean body weight is 22 kg (range 2.6-60).[1,3] Although PHPTH can occur in every breed, Keeshonds, Labrador Retrievers, German Shepherds, Golden Retrievers, Poodles, Shih-Tzus, and Springer Spaniels are overrepresented.[1] Genetic studies have been conducted in Keeshonds, documenting PHPTH as an autosomal dominant disease in this breed.[4]

Clinical signs associated with PHPTH are often subtle and nonspecific, making it difficult for owners to have a proper perception of the disease. Consequently, PHPTH is often diagnosed not based on clinical signs but in the context of a fortuitous finding of hypercalcemia in a biochemistry panel conducted for another medical reason.[1,5]

The most frequent clinical features of PHPTH are urinary tract signs (stranguria, pollakiuria, and/or hematuria) and polyuria/polydipsia, both reported in about half of the cases.[3] Less frequent and nonspecific signs include weakness, decreased activity, or weight loss (Table 30.1).

Urinary signs directly result from hypercalciuria, subsequent urolithiasis, and eventual bacterial cystitis. Calcium cystic urolithiasis (calcium oxalate or mixed calcium phosphate and calcium oxalate) is present in 25-40% of dogs with PHPTH.[1,3] In opposition, ureterolithiasis or nephrocalcinosis are uncommon. Apart from hypercalciuria, suggested predisposing factors for urolithiasis include renal loss of phosphorus, increased urinary pH (secondary to bicarbonate loss, which potentiates calcium-phosphate precipitation), and unbalanced crystal aggregation inhibitors.[1] Bacterial cystitis is present in 20-30% of dogs with PHPTH and seems to be a consequence of urolithiasis and inappropriate urine concentration.[1,3] A decreased bladder tonus and inability to complete voiding secondary to muscle weakness and polyuria are also potential predisposing factors for bacterial cystitis in these cases.[1]

Polyuria/polydipsia develops in dogs with PHPTH since hypercalcemia activates calcium-sensing receptors in the collecting ducts, downregulating the expression of aquaporin-2 channels and consequently impairing correct vasopressin (AVP) action. Moreover, persistent

TABLE 30.1 Prevalence of main clinical signs in dogs with PHPTH (adapted from Feldman, et al., 2015).[1]

Clinical sign	% of dogs
Lower urinary tract signs	50
PU/PD	48
Weakness	46
Decreased activity	43
Decreased appetite	37
Weight loss/muscle wasting	18
Vomiting	13
Shivering/trembling	10

hypercalcemia also interacts with calcium-sensing receptors in the thick ascending limb, modulating the activity of $Na^+K^+2Cl^-$ channels and affecting the medullary osmotic gradient.[6]

Dogs with PHPTH may also show, less frequently, nonspecific signs such as lethargy, weakness, muscle atrophy, weight loss, shivering, and inappetence. Although physiopathology besides these findings is not completely understood, clinical signs may be justified by hyperpolarization of cell membranes induced by hypercalcemia and a consequent decrease in muscle excitability and gastrointestinal motility.[1] Although bone changes rarely have a significant clinical expression in PHPTH, skeletal pain, stiff gait, and fractures are reported in a minority of cases.[1]

Physical examination does not reveal significant changes in most cases of PHPTH, although a low body condition score, slight weakness, and generalized muscle atrophy may be present. Parathyroid nodules are usually undetectable on cervical palpation since they are small and often covered by cervical muscle layers.[1]

Clinicopathological findings

A complete blood count (CBC) and a routine biochemistry profile are one of the first complementary exams for the medical investigation of most systemic diseases, including PHPTH. In these cases, CBC is often unremarkable.

On the biochemistry profile, the identification of total hypercalcemia is one of the main relevant findings. When it is found, the ionized calcium concentration should be further evaluated (see chapter 18). In dogs with PHPTH, although it can slightly vary among analyzers and techniques, total (tCa^{2+}) and ionized calcium (iCa^{2+}) concentrations are usually above 13.6 mg/dL and 1.35 mmol/L, respectively.[1,3,7,8] Calcium should be assessed together with phosphorus, BUN, and creatinine concentrations. Because PTH inhibits phosphorus renal tubular resorption, it is usually low or low-normal in dogs with PHPTH (often <4 mg/dL with a median of about 2.8-2.9 mg/dL).[1,3,7,8] Therefore, PHPTH is a relevant differential diagnosis of hypophosphatemia, particularly in cases undergoing a well-balanced diet and without a history of phosphate binders medication.

TABLE 30.2 Comparison of the main laboratory findings observed in primary hyperparathyroidism and chronic kidney disease.

	PHPTH	Chronic kidney disease
Total calcium	High	High (10-15% of cases)
Ionized calcium	High	Usually normal to low
Phosphorus	Low-normal/low	Normal to high
Calcium × phosphorus product	<60	>60-80
PTH	High	High

Data concerning BUN in PHPTH is inconsistent. While in one study with 210 cases, about two-thirds of dogs had BUN below the reference range, another with 29 dogs reported an increase in about 45% of them.[3,7]

Serum/plasma creatinine is usually within the reference range, supporting the idea that dogs with PHPTH seem to have a low probability of developing azotemia.[1] However, diagnosis may be challenging to confirm when the uncommon combination of PHPTH and azotemia occurs since some clinicopathological changes may overlap (Table 30.2).

Liver enzymes are usually normal in dogs with PHPTH, apart from alkaline phosphatase, which may be mildly increased (about two to sixfold the reference range) in about 40% of cases.[1,3] This can be due to a reactive hepatopathy to systemic disease or secondary to bone resorption induced by PTH.[1]

On urine analysis, dogs with hypercalcemia show an inappropriate urine specific gravity (USG), regardless of its cause. About 60% of dogs with PHPTH have hyposthenuric or isosthenuric urine (mean USG of 1.012). In one-third of them, urine is classified as minimally concentrated (1.013-1.020), while less than 10% have USG higher than 1.021.[1,3] This inappropriate USG is due to the reversible nephrogenic diabetes insipidus, secondary to the effect of hypercalcemia on AVP action in the tubular renal tubules.[6] Urinary sediment may show hematuria, crystalluria, and bacteriuria, highlighting the presence of urolithiasis or bacterial cystitis, as already discussed.[1]

Endocrine tests

Parathyroid hormone

Parathyroid hormone (PTH) measurement is a cornerstone endocrine test for diagnosing PHPTH.

PTH is a single-chain 84-amino acid hormone produced by the chief cells of the parathyroid gland (see chapter 29). In the liver and within parathyroid secretory granules, the full-length 1-84PTH is degraded into carboxy-terminal peptides, 7-84PTH being the most described. Carboxy-terminal peptides have a higher half-life than 1-84PTH and are excreted in kidneys.[9] These metabolites are relevant to understand better the difference between "intact" and "whole" PTH assays. While intact PTH assays detect 1-84PTH and carboxy-terminal peptides (7-84PTH), the whole PTH assays only detect 1-84PTH. Over the years, several generations of assays have been developed to measure 1-84PTH, minimizing cross-reaction with the remaining fragments.[9] While the third-generation whole PTH assays seem accurate for this goal, they are still debatable if they are better.[9]

PTH amino acid sequence is conserved among several mammal species, with 88% homology between humans and dogs.[9] Over the years, several PTH human assays and different techniques have been used in dogs, namely immunoradiometric assays (IRMA),[10] immunoenzymatic methodologies,[11] chemiluminescence,[12,13] and ELISA.[14] IRMA was a pioneer in PTH measurement in dogs and cats and is considered a reliable technique. Data comparing different methodologies for PTH measurement is scarce. One study compared intact and whole PTH measured by IRMA with intact PTH assessed by chemiluminescence.[9] This study reinforced that IRMA is a more reliable method than chemiluminescence.[9] This study also showed an excellent correlation between whole versus intact PTH measured by IRMA, questioning the utility of this distinction in practice.

To date, not all assays are commercially available in every country, and some of the previous reliable and validated assays have been discontinued by manufacturers. Recognizing these practical issues, the author suggests that clinicians should ideally prioritize PTH dosage by IRMA. However, if this methodology is unavailable, immunoenzymatic, chemiluminescence or ELISA may be performed, being aware of the limitations of these alternative assays. Regardless of the methodology, results should always be correlated with the clinical context, and, in doubtful cases, PTH should be repeated in two distinct laboratories in order to assess consistency.

How should PTH measurement be interpreted?

PTH is usually high-normal or above the reference range in dogs with PHPTH. However, caution should be taken on its interpretation since it should never be performed as a single parameter and out of the clinical context. As a main rule, PTH results should always be interpreted in combination with calcium concentrations (either tCa^{2+} or, ideally, iCa^{2+}). In healthy dogs, PTH and calcium are inversely related. This means that in the case of hypercalcemia, it is expected to have a low PTH due to the negative physiological feedback induced by calcium on parathyroid glands. When a hypercalcemic dog presents with a concurrent PTH concentration within the reference range, that is considered inappropriate since it was expected to be low. This combination of results reinforces an autonomous PTH secretion regardless of the presence of hypercalcemia, supporting the diagnosis of a PHPTH. In case of doubtful or illogical results, calcium and PTH concentrations should be repeated to understand consistency and clarify potential hormone fluctuations.[1]

Parathyroid hormone-related protein

Several referral laboratories have specific "hypercalcemia panels", which often include not only the measurement of iCa^{2+} and PTH but also parathyroid hormone-related protein (PTHrp).

PTHrp is a hormone which is structurally and genetically similar to PTH. It has the same physiological action as PTH, with the difference that PTHrp neither stimulates calcitriol synthesis nor cross-reacts with conventional PTH assays.[1] In contrast to PTH, which is only produced in parathyroid glands, PTHrp is expressed in various normal fetal and adult tissues.[15] In daily practice, PTHrP is considered a useful biomarker of paraneoplastic hypercalcemia since it can be increased in dogs with various tumors; T-cell lymphoma and anal sac gland carcinoma are the most frequent ones.[16]

PTHrp can be measured using two-site IRMA or N-terminal radioimmunoassays (RIA), and the reference range in dogs is set as <1 pmol/L, with typical values usually below 0.5 pmol/L. Therefore, an increased PTHrp reinforces the suspicion of neoplasia. However, if PTHrp is within the reference range, hypercalcemia of malignancy cannot be excluded since there are other mechanisms through which tumors can induce hypercalcemia.[5,16]

Specifically concerning PTHrp in canine PHPTH, one study has documented that dogs with parathyroid solitary adenomas have PTHrp values within the reference range.[17]

Vitamin D metabolites

Vitamin D metabolites can sometimes be evaluated in the medical investigation of hypercalcemia, notably when hypervitaminosis D is suspected. These metabolites cannot be used to distinguish the different causes of hypercalcemia and are not routinely measured in the medical investigation of PHPTH. In case they are assessed, 1,25-dihydroxycholecalciferol (calcitriol) is expected to be normal to high, while 25-hydroxycholecalciferol is usually low-normal in dogs with PHPTH.[18]

Other complementary exams

Genetic tests (Keeshonds)

PHPTH has an autosomal dominant inheritance pattern in Keeshonds.[4] To the author's knowledge, a specific genetic test is currently available at the Animal Health Diagnostic Center at Cornell University, US (https://www.vet.cornell.edu/animal-health-diagnostic-center/testing/protocols/PHPT).

Diagnostic imaging

Thoracic and abdominal imaging

Diagnostic imaging is a key point in the medical investigation of hypercalcemia (chapter 18). In practice, thoracic radiographs, abdominal ultrasound, and/or advanced imaging (computed tomography) are routinely performed in dogs with hypercalcemia as a screening panel for direct/indirect signs of neoplasia.

In dogs with PHPTH, thoracic and abdominal imaging are usually unremarkable, apart from the possible identification of urolithiasis. Although rare, osteopenia may also be detected since these dogs may have mild bony changes.[1]

Cervical ultrasound

Cervical ultrasound is the most relevant imaging exam that supports the diagnosis of PHPTH.

Parathyroid glands on healthy dogs' cervical ultrasound are described as solitary, well-marginated, hypo to anechoic round structures of 1-3 mm of maximum diameter, surrounded by thyroid tissue. More than identifying masses within the parathyroid gland, this exam allows its characterization in terms of size and location in about 63-100% of cases.[1,7,8,13,19]

What is expected from a cervical ultrasound in dogs with PHPTH?

In 90% of dogs with PHPTH, a solitary nodule (usually adenoma) is identified in one of the parathyroids, with the remaining glands being small or atrophied (Fig. 30.2 and Fig. 30.3, Video 30.1). This nodule may be variable in diameter, with most measuring between 4 and 10 mm, with a median size of 6 mm (range 3 to 23 mm).[3] A recent study has documented that parathyroid lesions larger than 8 mm are more likely to be malignant (carcinoma), highlighting the potential role of cervical ultrasound in predicting malignancy.[20]

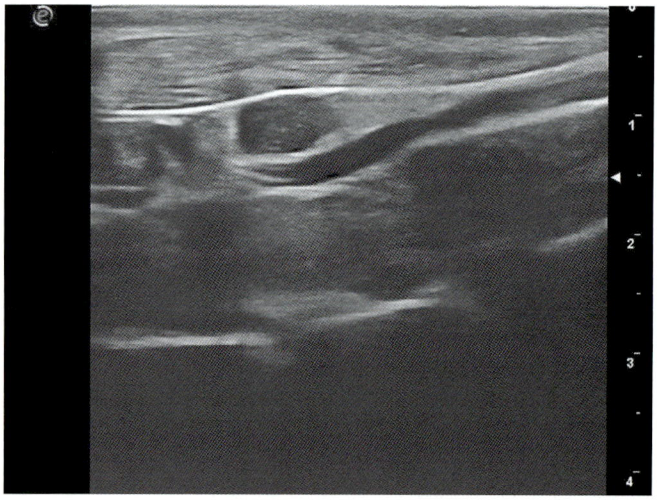

FIG. 30.2 Left thyroid and parathyroid gland of a dog with hypercalcemia. A well-marginated and hypoechoic parathyroid nodule is identified in this cervical ultrasound image. Credits: Rui Lemos Ferreira, Hospital Escolar Veterinário – Faculdade de Medicina Veterinária, Universidade de Lisboa, Lisbon, Portugal.

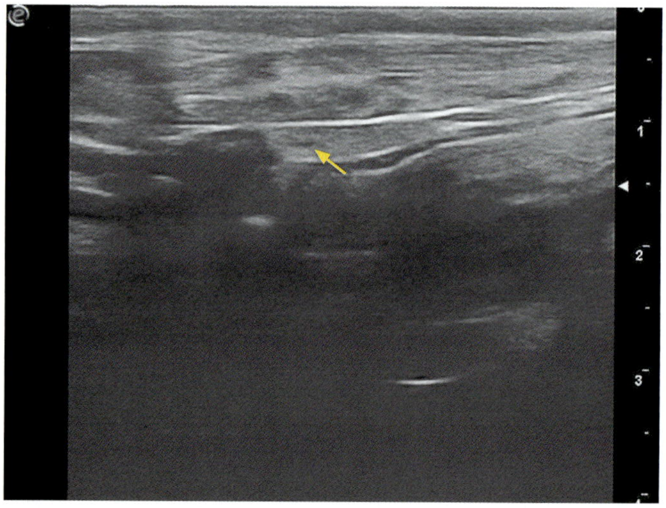

FIG. 30.3 Right thyroid gland from the same dog as Fig. 30.1, showing a small ill-defined hypoechoic structure (arrow) compatible with an atrophied parathyroid gland. Credits: Rui Lemos Ferreira, Hospital Escolar Veterinário – Faculdade de Medicina Veterinária, Universidade de Lisboa, Lisbon, Portugal.

In about 10% of cases, dogs can have more than one nodule, usually two distinct lesions, each in a different parathyroid gland.[1,3] Some dogs can even show a diffuse enlargement of all the parathyroid glands, compatible with hyperplastic disease. Although adenomatous hyperplasia is more commonly identified in secondary hyperparathyroidism, this has also been sparsely described in dogs with PHPTH.[21,22]

In some cases, it may be challenging to identify if a cervical nodule is of thyroid or parathyroid origin, and imaging features may overlap. Moreover, thyroid and parathyroid masses can coexist in the same dog. In fact, a study has shown that about 15% of hypercalcemic dogs undergoing a cervical ultrasound have an identified thyroid nodule.[23] This was described as an incidental finding since they were neither palpable cervical masses nor clinical signs of thyroid disease. However, although the association between thyroid nodules and hyperparathyroidism is unclear if a thyroid nodule is identified, further investigation with subsequent cytology and biopsy is recommended.[23]

Similarly to humans, there are some described cases of ectopic parathyroid tumors in dogs.[24] In cases in which clinicopathological findings and PTH measurement are in agreement with PHPTH and parathyroid glands are small in size or not visible, an ectopic parathyroid tumor should be suspected and explored. When present, ectopic parathyroid tumors tend to be located near the thyroid lobes, cranial to the thoracic inlet, and in the mediastinum.[24]

Video 30.1

Ultrasound capture of a well-marginated and hypoechoic parathyroid nodule in a dog with hypercalcemia. Credits: Rui Lemos Ferreira, Hospital Escolar Veterinário – Faculdade de Medicina Veterinária, Universidade de Lisboa, Lisbon, Portugal.

Regardless of the main findings identified on cervical ultrasound, it is worthwhile to mention that its accuracy is highly dependent on the available equipment as well as the expertise of the radiologist.

Computed tomography and magnetic resonance

Previous studies have shown that parathyroid glands are difficult to identify on CT and MRI.[25,26] Specifically, concerning dogs with PHPTH, data focusing on CT and MRI features is scarce. A recent study described CT findings in parathyroid adenomas, adenocarcinomas, and hyperplasia.[24] This study highlighted that CT can be relevant for the identification of parathyroid changes and presurgical planning. The same study also opened new insights on contrast-enhanced CT, highlighting its potential utility in the identification of parathyroid malignancy.

Scintigraphy

The utility of double-phase parathyroid scintigraphy using technetium-99m-sestamibi was briefly evaluated in dogs with PHPTH.[27] Due to its poor sensitivity and specificity, it is not recommended for routine use in daily practice.

Diagnosis

Diagnosis of PHPTH results from a combination of compatible clinical signs (if present), a persistent total and (ideally) ionized hypercalcemia with concurrent low/low-normal phosphorus, inappropriately high PTH concentrations, and the evidence of a solitary nodule in one of the parathyroid glands. Even if other forms of the disease are possible (such as diffuse hyperplasia or two distinct parathyroid nodules), those are uncommon in daily practice.

Therapy

The definitive treatment for PHPTH requires the ablation or removal of the parathyroid nodule(s). This can be achieved by surgery (classic parathyroidectomy or minimally invasive technique), ultrasound-guided percutaneous heat ablation, or ethanol ablation.[1,28]

Rare cases in which dogs with suspected PHPTH have a diffuse enlargement of all parathyroid glands are a therapeutic dilemma. Up to three out of the four glands can be removed without the risk of iatrogenic hypoparathyroidism.[29] However, the causes of secondary hyperparathyroidism should be scrutinized before an eventual surgical approach.

Parathyroidectomy

Surgery is one of the current preferred techniques for PHPTH treatment, particularly in cases showing larger nodules (>10 mm). After a cervical ventral midline approach, the solitary nodule is easily identified and removed (Fig. 30.4). Although delicate, the surgical technique is not considered difficult. If the nodule is located in the external parathyroids, it is easily removed. If it is in the internal ones, surgeons may need to resect adjacent thyroid tissue (partial thyroidectomy), or, in case of apparent invasion or carcinoma suspicion, a concurrent total thyroidectomy may be required.

With the current advances in diagnostic imaging, there is a high confidence in diagnosis prior to surgery concerning dimensions and location, allowing a good procedure plan. A recent study has shown that agreement between ultrasound and surgery was 66% for the number of affected glands.[20] Concerning laterality, studies point to an agreement of around 70-75%.[8,20] From a perioperative perspective, one study evaluated systemic and local PTH concentration (measured in venous blood from saphenous and each of the jugular veins, respectively). This study aimed to help the surgeon precise the nodule's location and confirm the success of the procedure by measuring PTH before and after parathyroid tissue removal. Although a systemic decrease of >50% of PTH confirmed the removal of the autonomous functional tissue, the assessment of laterality was inconsistent and unreliable.[13]

With the development of minimally invasive interventions in dogs, video-assisted parathyroidectomy was recently described and is considered a potential and promising alternative for conventional surgery in the near future.[30]

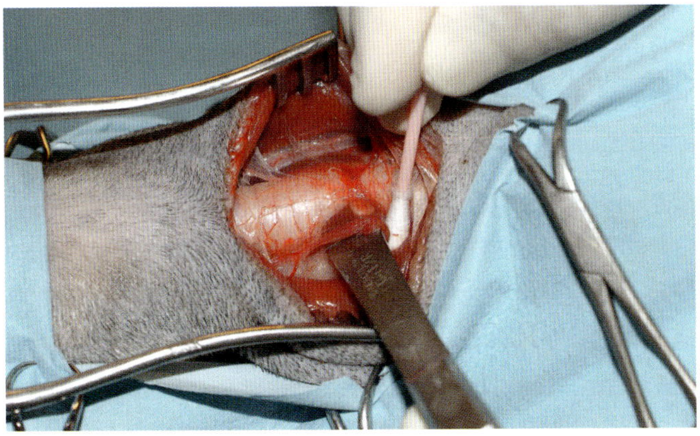

FIG. 30.4 Parathyroid nodule identified during a parathyroidectomy procedure in a dog with PHPTH. Credits: Juan Hernandez/Cyrill Poncet, Centre Hospitalier Vétérinaire Fregis, Paris, France.

Percutaneous heat ablation

This ultrasound-guided procedure uses radiofrequency waves converted into heat and allows the thermic necrosis of the parathyroid lesion.[31] An 18 to 20-gauge tip needle (or similar catheter) is placed into the mass. Using a radiofrequency unit, energy discharges of 5-10 seconds are applied, and wattage is progressively increased until echogenic bubbles are seen on the ultrasound and the tissue becomes hyperechoic (Video 30.2). The needle can be redirected when necessary in order to cover the entire mass. The detailed protocol can be consulted in the specific literature.[31,32] Caution should be taken in large masses and/or in dogs with concurrent hypothyroidism since both factors were associated with treatment failure using this technique.[33] The success rate of heat ablation is overall high and similar to surgery (90 vs. 94%, respectively).[34] However, it is also worth mentioning that a learning curve is required, which may impact the individual success rate in daily practice.

Ethanol ablation

Ethanol induces vascular thrombosis and tissue necrosis. Being an ultra sound-guided procedure, a specific volume of ethanol is slowly instilled within the parathyroid nodule. This technique has been considered a cheaper and more effective alternative to conventional surgery. Its success is variable among studies but considered inferior to the remaining techniques overall.[34,35]

Medical treatment

Since phosphorus is low/low-normal in these dogs, the calcium-phosphorus product (Ca × P) is usually below 60-80.[1] Consequently, the risk of tissue mineralization is low in PHPTH when compared to the remaining causes of hypercalcemia, which requires rapid stabilization, such as hypervitaminosis D or kidney disease. Therefore, medical management of PHPTH is neither an emergency nor an essential step before definitive treatment.

Accordingly, symptomatic support mainly consists of offering water *ad libitum* to dogs. Although not essential, in cases in which owners decline definitive treatment, the medical management of hypercalcemia may be judged in an individual-based approach. This may include parenteral fluid therapy (which corrects dehydration and optimizes diuresis); furosemide (that acts as calciuretic); glucocorticoids (which decrease bone resorption, are calciuretic and decrease calcium intestinal absorption) or bisphosphonates (e.g., pamidronate or alendronate, which reduce the number and action of osteoclasts, minimizing bone resorption).[1] These latter ones can be used in the chronic management of hypercalcemia, but their accessibility may change among countries. Due to their low bioavailability when given PO, parenteral options should be prioritized. For drug dosages, see Table 18.2 in chapter 18. Cinacalcet, a calcium sensing-receptor modulator that increases the sensitivity of parathyroid cells to calcium and decreases PTH secretion, is currently used in the medical management of primary hyperparathyroidism in humans, particularly if

Video 30.2

Ultrasound-guided radiofrequency heat ablation. During the procedure, a heat discharge is applied, and it is visible on the video that the hypoechoic lesion turns hyperechoic. Credits: Juan Hernandez, Oniris, Nantes-Atlantic College of Veterinary Medicine and Foond Sciences, Nantes, France.

parathyroidectomy is not an option.[36] Although data is scarce in dogs, this compound seems effective in canine PHPTH (0.5 mg/kg PO once daily as the initial dose but individually titrated according to side effects and ionized calcium decrease, with a final dose range between 1.0 mg/kg q4 days and 9.4 mg/kg q12h).[37] However, due to its side effects (lethargy, anorexia, vomiting, and non-hypocalcemic shaking episodes), the interindividual dose variation, and duration of action, further studies are needed for a robust recommendation of its use.

Post-treatment management

With the presence of a parathyroid single nodule, the remaining glands are often atrophied. Consequently, transient hypocalcemia is expected when the autonomous functional nodule is removed until the remaining glands recover their physiological activity. Several studies have been conducted to explore potential pretreatment predictors of post-treatment hypocalcemia.[1,7,8,20,38-40] However, results are conflicting and inconsistent, stressing the unpredictability of calcium fluctuation after definitive therapeutic options. It is generally agreed that PTH concentration rapidly decreases within the first 24h and that iCa^{2+} reaches the respective nadir in the first 48h after the procedure. Therefore, close monitoring of tCa^{2+} and/or, ideally, iCa^{2+} concentrations (at least once q12h for a minimum of 72h after the procedure) is essential to anticipate potential complications.[39-40]

It is also debatable whether a medical treatment with calcitriol should be started prior to definitive therapy. While some internists defend a prophylactic administration of calcitriol, others consider it necessary to document a calcium decrease before beginning treatment.

In line with historical recommendations and based on personal experience, the author considers a safe decision to administer calcitriol (20-30 ng/kg PO) in the morning of the procedure for all dogs undergoing a definitive PHPHT treatment.

After the first administration, it is usually suggested to continue calcitriol treatment with half dosage (10-15 ng/kg PO q12h), starting the evening after the procedure and continuing for at least 48h, followed by slow decreases in 10% intervals.[1] Although calcitriol does not seem to prevent a decrease in calcium concentrations immediately after the procedure, it reduces the severity of clinical and biochemical hypocalcemia.[1] According to its pharmacokinetics, calcitriol takes several days to induce a therapeutic effect, and individual variation is expected. Also, caution should be taken to avoid vitamin-D-induced hyperphosphatemia.[40] Calcitriol should be adjusted in accordance with calcium concentrations: if tCa^{2+} and iCa^{2+} are below 8.5 mg/dL (2.1 mmol/L) or 3.8 mg/dL (0.9 mmol/L), respectively, the dose should be increased; in case of hypercalcemia, calcitriol must be stopped, and if values are in the upper reference range, it should be decreased. The medical goal is to keep calcium in the lower range (tCa and iCa^{2+} within 8.0-9.5 mg/dL [2.0-2.4 mmol/L] and 3.6-4.8 mg/dL [0.9-1.2 mmol/L], respectively), optimizing the functional recovery of the remaining atrophied parathyroids and avoiding clinical signs, not expected to occur at this level of slight hypocalcemia.[1]

In opposition to this historical protocol, a recent study has failed to support calcitriol administration in the postoperative period after parathyroidectomy, stressing the need for further prospective investigation on this subject.[40]

The author does not routinely continue calcitriol supplementation after definitive PHPHT treatment since most dogs tolerate the procedure well without developing postoperative clinical hypocalcemia. However, regardless of the decision, dogs should be kept hospitalized and ideally at rest (since physical activity may worsen and potentiate clinical signs of hypocalcemia), with regular calcium monitoring for at least 3-5 days.[1] If hypocalcemia becomes evident during hospitalization, calcitriol treatment should then be prolonged. Recommendations about the length of hospitalization are inconsistent since previous data has shown that postsurgical hypocalcemia can occur as early as in the first 12 hours after definitive PHPTH treatment to about 20 days later.[1] Recognizing this later scenario is extremely rare, and most dogs stabilize calcemia over the first week; hospitalization is adapted on a case-by-case basis, often depending on financial concerns and calcium monitoring results. However, a minimum of 3 days of hospitalization after the procedure is recommended, with ionized calcium (or total, if ionized is not available) monitored q8-12h. If calcium continues to decrease on the day of discharge, hospitalization should be prolonged for two more days until calcium stabilization is reached. When hospitalization for more than 3 days is not affordable, as an alternative, dogs may be discharged with recommendations of reduced activity at home and daily calcium controls at the assistant veterinarian.

Histopathology

On histopathology, parathyroid gland features can be classified as adenoma, carcinoma, or hyperplasia, accounting for 87%, 8%, and 5% of the reported cases, respectively.[1] Regardless of the histological classification, their biological behavior and overall long-term prognosis are similar. It is worthwhile to mention that the distinction between adenoma and hyperplasia is not clinically relevant since both have functional autonomy, being debatable whether hyperplasia is a multiple form of parathyroid adenoma.[21]

A large recent study on parathyroid carcinoma has shown a good long-term outcome after surgical excision, with a median survival time of 2 years.[19]

Prognosis

The overall prognosis of PHPHT is excellent, with a recurrence rate estimated in 5-10% of cases.[1] In these, a single parathyroid mass identified in one of the remaining parathyroid glands is the most frequent scenario. Since recurrence is possible, regular monitoring of calcium concentrations in dogs already treated is strongly advised.

Data is scarce for non-treated dogs or those only receiving medical management. However, there are two published cases showing acute hypocalcemia in a previous context of untreated PHPTH.[1,41] In these cases, an acute auto-infarction or parathyroid necrosis was documented, which led to hypocalcemia secondary to the concurrent atrophy of the remaining parathyroid glands.[41] Although it is a rare scenario, clinicians should be aware of this unusual presentation in dogs with untreated PHPTH.

Parathyroids and concurrent endocrine diseases

Although only briefly reported in dogs, parathyroid glands may also be involved in cases of concurrent endocrine neoplasia, namely multiple endocrine neoplasia (MEN)[1] (enteropancreatic endocrine, pituitary, and parathyroid gland neoplasia) or MEN-2a (medullary thyroid carcinoma, unilateral or bilateral pheochromocytoma, and parathyroid hyperplasia or adenoma).[1]

It is also known that hypercortisolism may induce calcium dysregulation, and a combination of this endocrine disease with hyperparathyroidism has been advoked.[1] Most dogs with hypercortisolism have an increased PTH, although no changes in total and ionized calcium were observed.[42] Furthermore, treatment of hypercortisolism is associated with a decline of intact PTH.[43] A recent study assessed calcium metabolism and bone turnover in dogs with hypercortisolism, concluding that this PTH increase does not seem to be associated with decreased bone formation or increased bone resorption.[44] Another recent study also reported that hyperphosphatemia and high urine calcium excretion may contribute to calcium metabolism disruption in dogs with hypercortisolism.[45] All in all, the term adrenal secondary hyperparathyroidism is suggested as a broad definition to summarize these changes in dogs with hypercortisolism.

KEY POINTS

- Primary hyperparathyroidism (PHPHT) results from an inappropriate production of PTH by one or more parathyroid glands.
- It mainly occurs in adult-geriatric dogs, and Keeshonds are genetically predisposed to the disease.
- Clinical signs are frequently imperceptible to owners, and hypercalcemia is often fortuitously discovered on routine bloodwork.
- Diagnosis results from a combination of persistent hypercalcemia, low/low-normal phosphorus, inappropriate PTH concentrations, and the evidence of a solitary parathyroid nodule, which is present in about 90% of cases.
- Treatment requires the ablation or removal of the parathyroid nodule either by conventional or minimally invasive parathyroidectomy, ultrasound-guided percutaneous heat ablation, or ethanol ablation.
- Post-treatment hypocalcemia is likely regardless of the therapeutic modality, and data concerning its prediction is inconsistent.
- Prophylactic calcitriol administration is debatable and should be based on individual cases and clinician preferences.
- Biological behavior of parathyroid adenomas, carcinomas, or hyperplasia is similar, and the overall prognosis of PHPTH is excellent.

References

1. Feldman EC. Hypercalcemia and primary hyperparathyroidism (PHP) in dogs. In Feldman EC, Nelson RW, Reusch CE (editors). Canine and Feline Endocrinology. Missouri, Elsevier, 2015, pp. 579-624.
2. Messinger JS, Windham WR, Ward CR. Ionized hypercalcemia in dogs: A retrospective study of 109 Cases (1998-2003). *J Vet Intern Med* 23:514-519, 2009.
3. Feldman EC, Hoar B, Pollard R, et al. Pretreatment clinical and laboratory findings in dogs with primary hyperparathyroidism: 210 cases (1987-2004). *J Am Vet Med Assoc* 227:756-761, 2005.
4. Goldstein RE, Atwater DZ, Cazolli DM, et al. Inheritance, mode of inheritance, and candidate genes for primary hyperparathyroidism in Keeshonden. *J Vet Intern Med* 21:199-203, 2007.
5. Skelly BJ. Primary hyperparathyroidism. In Ettinger SJ, Feldman EC, Côté E (editors). Textbook of Veterinary Internal Medicine. Missouri, Elsevier, 2017, pp. 1715-1727.
6. Jepson R. Polyuria and Polydipsia. In Elliott J, Grauer GF, Westropp JL (editors). BSAVA Manual of Canine and Feline Nephrology and Urology. Gloucester, BSAVA, 2017, pp. 8-23.
7. Gear RNA, Neiger R, Skelly BJS, et al. Primary hyperparathyroidism in 29 dogs: diagnosis, treatment, outcome and associated renal failure. *J Small Anim Pract* 46:10-16, 2005.
8. Milovancev M, Schmiedt CW. Preoperative factors associated with postoperative hypocalcemia in dogs with primary hyperparathyroidism that underwent parathyroidectomy: 62 cases (2004-2009). *J Am Vet Med Assoc* 242:507-515, 2013.
9. Mooney CT, Shiel RE, Fawcett K, et al. A comparison of canine whole and intact parathyroid hormone concentrations as measured by different assays. *J Small Anim Pract* 60:507-513, 2019.
10. Parker VJ, Harjes LM, Dembek K, et al. Association of vitamin D metabolites with parathyroid hormone, fibroblast growth Factor-23, calcium, and phosphorus in dogs with various stages of chronic kidney disease. *J Vet Intern Med* 31:791-798, 2017.
11. Zambarbieri J, Tagliasacchi F, Moretti P, et al. Analytical and clinical validation of a new immunoenzymatic method for the measurement of canine parathyroid hormone. *Animals* 10:2411, 2020.
12. Graham K, Wilkinson M, Culvenor J, et al. Intraoperative parathyroid hormone concentration to confirm removal of hypersecretory parathyroid tissue and time to postoperative normocalcaemia in nine dogs with primary hyperparathyroidism. *Aust Vet J* 90: 203-209, 2012.
13. Ham K, Greenfield CL, Barger A, et al. Validation of a rapid parathyroid hormone assay and intraoperative measurement of parathyroid hormone in dogs with benign naturally occurring Primary hyperparathyroidism. *Vet Surg* 38:122-132, 2009.
14. Warland J, Skelly B, Knudsen C, et al. Apparent resolution of canine primary hypoparathyroidism with immunosuppressive treatment. *J Vet Intern Med* 29:400-404, 2015.
15. Epstein FH, Strewler GJ. The physiology of parathyroid hormone-related protein. *N Engl J Med* 342:177-185, 2000.
16. Bailey DB. Paraneoplastic syndromes. In Vail DM, Thamm HD, Liptak JM (editors). Withrow & MacEwen's Small Animal Clinical Oncology. Missouri, Elsevier, 2020, pp. 98-112.
17. Mellanby RJ, Craig R, Evans H, et al. Plasma concentrations of parathyroid hormone-related protein in dogs with potential disorders of calcium metabolism. *Vet Rec* 159:833, 2006.

18. Gerber B, Hauser B, Reusch CE. Serum levels of 25-hydroxycholecalciferol and 1,25-dihydroxycholecalciferol in dogs with hypercalcaemia. *Vet Res Commun* 28:669-680, 2004.
19. Erickson AK, Regier PJ, Watt MM, et al. Incidence, survival time, and surgical treatment of parathyroid carcinomas in dogs: 100 cases (2010-2019). *J Am Vet Med Assoc* 259:1-9, 2021.
20. Burkhardt SJ, Sumner JP, Mann S. Ambidirectional cohort study on the agreement of ultrasonography and surgery in the identification of parathyroid pathology, and predictors of postoperative hypocalcemia in 47 dogs undergoing parathyroidectomy due to primary hyperparathyroidism. *Vet Surg* 50:1379-1388, 2021.
21. Vonderen IK van, Kooistra HS, Peeters ME, et al. Parathyroid hormone immunohistochemistry in dogs with primary and secondary hyperparathyroidism: the question of adenoma and primary hyperplasia. *J Comp Pathol* 129:61-69, 2003.
22. Vessieres F, Selgas AG, Rasotto R, et al. Primary hyperparathyroidism associated with hyperplasia of multiple parathyroid glands in a dog. *Vet Rec Case Rep* 3:e000191, 2015.
23. Pollard RE, Bohannon LK, Feldman EC. Prevalence of incidental thyroid nodules in ultrasound studies of dogs with hypercalcemia (2008-2013). *Vet Radiol Ultrasound* 56:63-67. 2015.
24. Cordella A, Bertaccini J, Rondena M, et al. Multidetector-row CT findings in dogs with different primary parathyroid gland diseases. *Vet Sci* 9:273, 2022.
25. Taeymans O, Dennis R, Saunders JH. Magnetic resonance imaging of the normal canine thyroid gland. *Vet Radiol Ultrasound* 49:238-242, 2008.
26. Lautscham E, von Klopmann C, Schaub S, et al. CT imaging features of the normal parathyroid gland in the dog. *Tierärztliche Prax Ausg K: Kleintiere Heimtiere* 48:313-320, 2020.
27. Matwichuk CL, Taylor SM, Daniel GB, et al. Double-phase parathyroid scintigraphy in dogs using technetium-99M-sestamibi. *Vet Radiol Ultrasound* 41:461-469, 2000.
28. Townsend KL, Ham KM. Current concepts in parathyroid/thyroid surgery. *Vet Clin North Am Small Animal Pract* 52:455-471, 2022.
29. Lunn KF, Boston SE. Tumors of the endocrine system. In Vail DM, Thamm DH, Liptak JM (editors). Withrow & MacEwen's Small Animal Clinical Oncology. Missouri, Elsevier, 2020, pp. 565-596.
30. Young KM, Degner DA. Surgical description and outcome of ultrasound-guided minimally invasive parathyroidectomy in 50 dogs with primary hyperparathyroidism. *Vet Surg* 52:18-25, 2023.
31. Leal RO, Pascual LF, Hernandez J. The use of percutaneous ultrasound-guided radiofrequency heat ablation for treatment of primary hyperparathyroidism in eight dogs: outcome and complications. *Vet Sci* 5:91, 2018.
32. Pollard RE, Long CD, Nelson RW, et al. Percutaneous ultrasonographically guided radiofrequency heat ablation for treatment of primary hyperparathyroidism in dogs. *J Am Vet Med Assoc* 218:1106-1110, 2001.
33. Bucy D, Pollard R, Nelson R. Analysis of factors affecting outcome of ultrasound-guided radiofrequency heat ablation for treatment of primary hyperparathyroidism in dogs. *Vet Radiol Ultrasound* 58:83-89, 2017.
34. Rasor L, Pollard R, Feldman EC. Retrospective evaluation of three treatment methods for primary hyperparathyroidism in dogs. *J Am Anim Hosp Assoc* 43:70-77, 2007.
35. Guttin T, Knox VW, Diroff JS. Outcomes for dogs with primary hyperparathyroidism following treatment with percutaneous ultrasound-guided ethanol ablation of presumed functional parathyroid nodules: 27 cases (2008-2011). *J Am Vet Med Assoc* 247:771-777, 2015.
36. Chandran M, Bilezikian JP, Lau J, et al. The efficacy and safety of cinacalcet in primary hyperparathyroidism: a systematic review and meta-analysis of randomized controlled trials and cohort studies. *Rev Endocr Metab Disord* 23:485-501, 2022.
37. Ward H, Schenck P, Lupo M, et al. Abstract EN17: efficacy and tolerability of generic cinacalcet in dogs with primary hyperparathyroidism. In 2022 ACVIM Forum Proceedings. Austin, 2022, p. 694.
38. Dear JD, Kass PH, Maggiore AMD, et al. Association of hypercalcemia before treatment with hypocalcemia after treatment in dogs with primary hyperparathyroidism. *J Vet Intern Med* 31:349-354, 2017.
39. Arbaugh M, Smeak D, Monnet E. Evaluation of preoperative serum concentrations of ionized calcium and parathyroid hormone as predictors of hypocalcemia following parathyroidectomy in dogs with primary hyperparathyroidism: 17 cases (2001-2009). *J Am Vet Med Assoc* 241:233-236, 2012.
40. Armstrong AJ, Hauptman JG, Stanley BJ, et al. Effect of prophylactic calcitriol administration on serum ionized calcium concentrations after parathyroidectomy: 78 cases (2005-2015). *J Vet Intern Med* 32:99-106, 2018.
41. Rosol TJ, Chew DJ, Capen CC, et al. Acute hypocalcemia associated with infarction of parathyroid gland adenomas in two dogs. *J Am Vet Med Assoc* 192:212-214, 1988.
42. Ramsey IK, Tebb A, Harris E, et al. Hyperparathyroidism in dogs with hyperadrenocorticism. *J Small Anim Pract* 46:531-536, 2005.
43. Tebb AJ, Arteaga A, Evans H, et al. Canine hyperadrenocorticism: effects of trilostane on parathyroid hormone, calcium and phosphate concentrations. *J Small Anim Pract* 46:537-542, 2005.
44. Mooney CT, Shiel RE, Sekiya M, et al. A preliminary study of the effect of hyperadrenocorticism on calcium and phosphate concentrations, parathyroid hormone and markers of bone turnover in dogs. *Front Vet Sci* 7:311, 2020.
45. Corsini A, Dondi F, Serio DG, et al. Calcium and phosphate homeostasis in dogs with newly diagnosed naturally occurring hypercortisolism. *J Vet Intern Med* 35:1265-1273, 2021.

CHAPTER 31

Hypoparathyroidism: naturally occurring and iatrogenic

Barbara J Skelly
MA, VetMB, PhD, DACVIM, DECVIM-CA (Internal Medicine), AFHEA, MRCVS

Hypoparathyroidism describes a condition in which parathyroid tissue has been excised or damaged iatrogenically or endogenously through an immune-mediated mechanism, leaving the animal with no means of synthesizing parathyroid hormone (PTH). This is a rare condition in people and dogs and extremely uncommon in cats, with very few case reports. The pattern of endocrine gland destruction or loss and management with hormone replacement therapy is a common one across all species in many different endocrine diseases, but hypoparathyroidism is unusual in that hormone replacement with PTH was first approved in the USA for people only as far back as 2015[1] and it is yet to be used in small animals. Instead, as veterinarians, we attempt to approximate the function of PTH in other ways, and disease control is, therefore, more challenging and crude.

This chapter describes the pathophysiology of hypoparathyroidism, its features and diagnosis, and current management strategies for small animals.

Pathogenesis of PTH deficiency

PTH can be deficient for a number of different reasons (Table 31.1). Firstly, and most simply, surgery (typically thyroid surgery) or damage to the ventral neck through injury[2] can mean that parathyroid glands are removed, have their blood supplies compromised, or fail to survive transplantation techniques. Recovery is possible, but support of serum calcium concentration is necessary over the short to medium term. One specific cause of hypocalcemia occurs in dogs with hyperparathyroidism postparathyroidectomy or ablation (see chapter 30). Autonomously functioning parathyroid glands suppress the remaining normal glands, which may be chronically inactive and atrophied. Support for calcium homeostasis is frequently required over the short to medium term. This phenomenon has been debated; some publications show that calcium/vitamin D supplementation is usually ineffective,[3] and some support its use.[4]

Secondly, immune-mediated parathyroid gland destruction can reduce functional gland capacity, making PTH production inadequate. This process is a direct parallel of the proposed etiology of canine hypoadrenocorticism and also, in some cases, of type 1 diabetes mellitus. Triggers are infrequently recognized, and we are rarely able to recognize and stop the process before end-stage destruction has occurred.[5]

Thirdly, functional hypoparathyroidism is apparent in cases where there is concurrent magnesium imbalance, either with hyper- or hypomagnesemia. Magnesium, as a divalent cation, is able to activate the calcium-sensing receptor (CaSR) and turn off PTH synthesis. Conversely, magnesium is essential as a mediator of PTH synthesis and release, so a magnesium-deficient state can also lead to relative hypoparathyroidism. Either way, it is clear that magnesium status should be considered when diagnosing absolute PTH deficiency, but also that interpretation of magnesium measurements is challenging in small animals. Oral magnesium supplementation and repeated PTH measurement may be used to confirm hypoparathyroid status.

TABLE 31.1 The mechanisms through which parathyroid-dependent hypocalcemia develops.

Type of hypoparathyroidism	Disease/syndrome
Naturally-occurring (due to irreversible loss of functional parathyroid tissue)	■ **Primary** (idiopathic, immune-mediated destruction) ■ Iatrogenic following surgical removal
Acquired (may be reversible)	■ Following treatment for hyperparathyroidism ■ Spontaneous infarction of parathyroid adenoma ■ **Secondary** to trauma or surgery that disrupts blood supply
Functional (reversible)	■ Magnesium dysregulation/deficiency

Signalment of animals with hypoparathyroidism

Hypoparathyroidism most commonly affects middle-aged female dogs. In a series of 735 dogs with hypoparathyroidism, 62% were female and 38% male.[6] Terrier breeds, Schnauzers, Dachshunds, and Poodles may be more commonly affected, and in Australia and New Zealand, Saint Bernard appears to be predisposed.[7,8,6,10] However, these publications are all historical, and there are no recent publications or case series documenting the current breed predispositions of this disease, which probably vary geographically.

History and clinical manifestation of hypoparathyroidism

Owners commonly recognize muscle twitching, depression, reluctance to exercise, and stiffness on exercise as key features of hypoparathyroidism (Table 31.2). Severe, more rapidly developing hypocalcemia (iCa <0.8 mmol/L, 3.2 mg/dL, tCa <1.8 mmol/L, 7.2 mg/dL) produces more pronounced clinical signs such as muscle cramps, tetany, laryngospasm, and tetanic seizures. The likelihood of clinical signs occurring is easier to predict when iCa is measured compared to when tCa is measured since this is unaffected by other changes in the blood, e.g., hypoalbuminemia. Clinical signs are made worse by stress, excitement, and exercise. The reason for this is twofold: panting and tachypnea, which result in increased carbon dioxide loss, and a progressive respiratory alkalosis, which reduces the ionized calcium fraction. Meanwhile, exercise triggers neuromuscular conduction, and the low extracellular calcium concentration means that sodium conductance and therefore depolarization is enhanced to the point that repetitive depolarization and tetany results. Other rarer reported neuromuscular clinical signs include synchronous diaphragmatic flutter (hiccups).[9]

Hypocalcemic cataracts are reported in people and small animals. They are described as posterior and punctate or linear in appearance (Fig. 31.1).

Cardiac changes are not commonly clinically significant in dogs and range between ECG changes and fulminant myocardial failure.

Inappetence, anorexia, vomiting, and diarrhea are common. Anorexia in people may be due to hyperphosphatemia, and the same may be true in dogs, though this is more difficult to assess on an individual case basis. Hypocalcemia-induced steatorrhea is caused by a deficiency of cholecystokinin, leading to exocrine pancreatic deficiency.[11] This is in contrast

TABLE 31.2 Clinical manifestations of hypoparathyroidism.

Neuromuscular excitability	Behavioral changes	Cardiac changes	Ocular changes	Gastrointestinal problems
Muscle fasciculations or tremors	Agitation	Tachycardia/bradycardia	Cataracts	Anorexia
Face rubbing	Anxiety	Lengthening of ST segment and QT interval on ECG		Vomiting
Biting or licking at paws or body	Vocalization	Myocardial failure	Blepharospasm	Diarrhea
Hypersensitivity to external stimuli	Aggression	Hypotension	Blepharitis	
Stiff, stilted gait	Pacing			
Ataxia	Panting*			
Tetanic seizures				
Respiratory arrest				
Weakness				
Hyperthermia related to muscle activity				
Panting*				
Circling				

*Panting probably has multifactorial causes, both neuromuscular and also induced by anxiety.

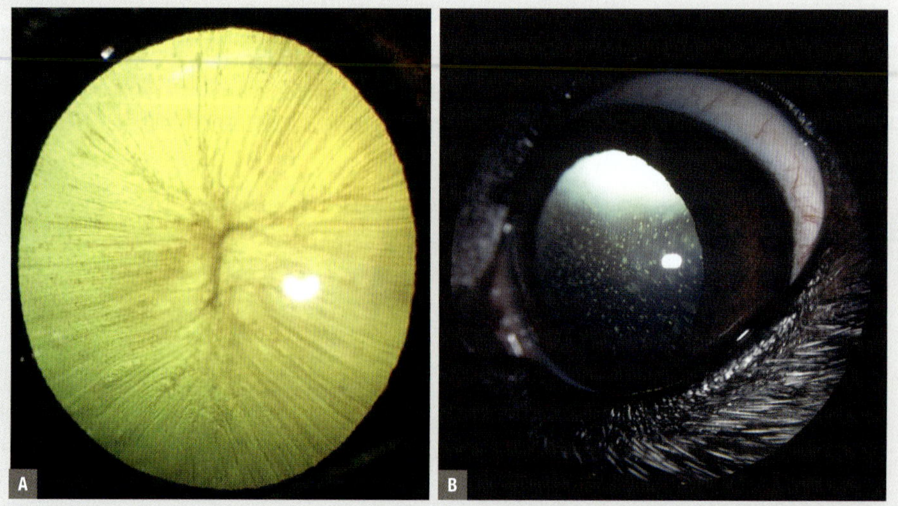

FIG. 31.1 (A) Photograph of the lens of a Border Collie with hypoparathyroidism. There are marked linear opacities in the anterior and posterior subcapsular cortex as well as anterior and posterior suture lines. Visual acuity would be expected to be affected, though this dog was still able to negotiate obstacles. Photograph courtesy of David Williams (with permission). (B) Photograph of punctate opacities in the lens of a dog with hypoparathyroidism. Photograph courtesy of David Gould (with permission). Reproduced with permission from BSAVA Manual of Canine and Feline Endocrinology 5th edition. ©BSAVA.

with protein-losing enteropathy (PLE), which is a differential diagnosis as a cause of hypocalcemia; in cases of PLE, PTH would be measured as high or high normal.

Diagnostic procedures and endocrine testing

Biochemistry

Features of hypoparathyroidism include total and ionized hypocalcemia coupled with low or undetectable PTH concentrations. Phosphate concentrations are high-normal, or high. Other biochemical parameters that may be abnormal include the markers of muscle damage, aspartate aminotransferase (AST), alanine aminotransferase (ALT), and creatine kinase (CK).

Urinalysis

There are no specific urinalysis changes, although in the human literature, the documentation of hypercalciuria by showing an increased fractional excretion of calcium or increased urinary calcium:creatinine ratio is a useful diagnostic test. We have yet to adopt this approach in small animals mainly due to the lack of useful and accepted appropriate reference ranges and the difficulty of doing the recommended 24-hour urine collection.

Endocrine tests

PTH measurement is offered at many diagnostic laboratories. PTH is labile, and EDTA-separated plasma should be frozen quickly to avoid misdiagnosis through hormone degradation. If the laboratory reports that they received thawed plasma, a low to undetectable hormone concentration is not a reliable measurement, and it is recommended that this be repeated. For more details on PTH measurement, see chapter 30.

Vitamin D metabolites (1,25-dihydroxycholecalciferol, 25-hydroxycholecalciferol, and 24,25-dihydroxycholecalciferol) should support a failure of activation of 25-hydroxycholecalciferol by 1-alpha-hydroxylase as this is a PTH-enabled reaction. Although 25-hydroxycholecalciferol is synthesized in the liver independently of PTH, the second hydroxylation to 1,25-dihydroxycholecalciferol is catalyzed by 1-alpha-hydroxylase, the production of which PTH directly stimulates in the cells of the proximal convoluted tubule. In a hypoparathyroid animal 25-hydroxycholecalciferol and 24,25-dihydroxycholecalciferol (the first stage on the catabolic pathway of vitamin D) would be predicted to be normal or above normal range, whilst 1,25-dihydroxycholecalciferol may be low or low normal. A lack of PTH will, therefore, lead to a decreased activation rate of vitamin D and a subsequent reduction in intestinal calcium and phosphate absorption.

The diagnostic algorithm is represented in Fig. 31.2. Imaging is rarely informative in cases of hypoparathyroidism. Ultrasonographic evaluation of the thyroid gland and associated parathyroid tissue may show parathyroid gland atrophy but is not often included in a diagnostic workup. Survey radiographs and abdominal ultrasound may be carried out to

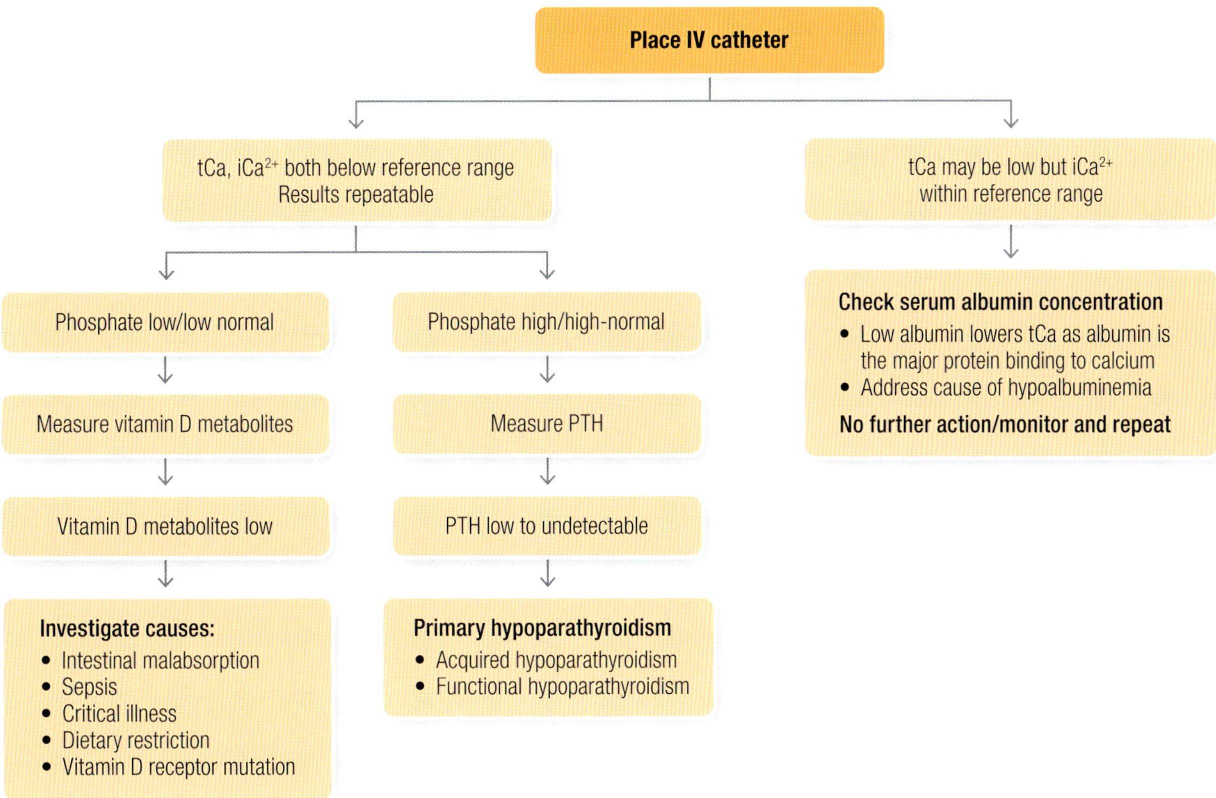

FIG. 31.2 Algorithm for the investigation of hypocalcemia.

rule out triggers for immune-mediated disease but would be expected to be unremarkable.

Treatment

The treatment of hypocalcemia is depicted in **Fig. 31.3**. Vitamin D and, at least initially, calcium supplementation is used to maintain calcium homeostasis. This approach has drawbacks; vitamin D enhances calcium and phosphate uptake through the gastrointestinal tract, whilst PTH increases urinary phosphate loss. A hypoparathyroid animal will be both hypocalcemic and hyperphosphatemic and this latter is worsened via the action of exogenous vitamin D, which will increase gut phosphate as well as calcium absorption. In people, this is a significant problem, whereas in animals, we rarely have to manage the negative effects of hyperphosphatemia, although inappetence may be persistent. Frequent monitoring of serum iCa is necessary from the outset, and target calcium concentrations should be maintained at a low normal or just below the normal reference interval to avoid excessive calciuria and hypercalcemia. Hypercalcemia is recognized by owners usually because the animal develops polyuria and polydipsia, whilst prolonged periods of hypercalciuria are detrimental to renal function.

When calcium intake is high, oral calcium is absorbed passively through the gut, which can be advantageous when waiting for vitamin D concentrations to rise. Conversely, when calcium intake is low, vitamin D is required for absorption.[12] Calcium carbonate is most commonly used (40% elemental calcium) and has the added benefit of being a phosphate binder so that hyperphosphatemia is not worsened.

Two forms of vitamin D are most commonly employed; calcitriol in the US and Europe (1,25- dihydroxycholecalciferol) and alfacalcidol in Europe (1-hydroxycholecalciferol). Both are available as capsules and also as liquid formulations, so they can be titrated to effect in dogs of all sizes. Calcitriol is the biologically active form of vitamin D but alfacalcidol needs to be hydroxylated by the liver, a non-rate-limiting step, meaning that the onset of action is similar to calcitriol. Alternatively, dihydrotachysterol is a vitamin D analog that only requires hydroxylation by the liver. Non-biologically active vitamin D (ergosterol (D_2) from plant sources or cholecalciferol (D_3) found in oily fish and other animal sources) has a longer lag time to maximum effect, and when dose adjustment is required, so these products are more difficult to get to acceptable therapeutic steady-state concentrations. Furthermore, these products require both hepatic and renal hydroxylation, the latter of which is disabled through the absence of PTH. The standard doses of calcium preparations and active forms of vitamin D are listed in **Table 31.3**. As in other endocrine diseases, some cases may be difficult to stabilize, and doses higher than those cited may be required. This is particularly true with long-standing hyperparathyroid dogs post-parathyroidectomy. Human literature suggests that cholecalciferol may replenish stores of 25-hydroxycholecalciferol and that intermediates of vitamin D metabolism may have functions that make therapy more holistic; this approach is not regularly recommended in small animals.[13]

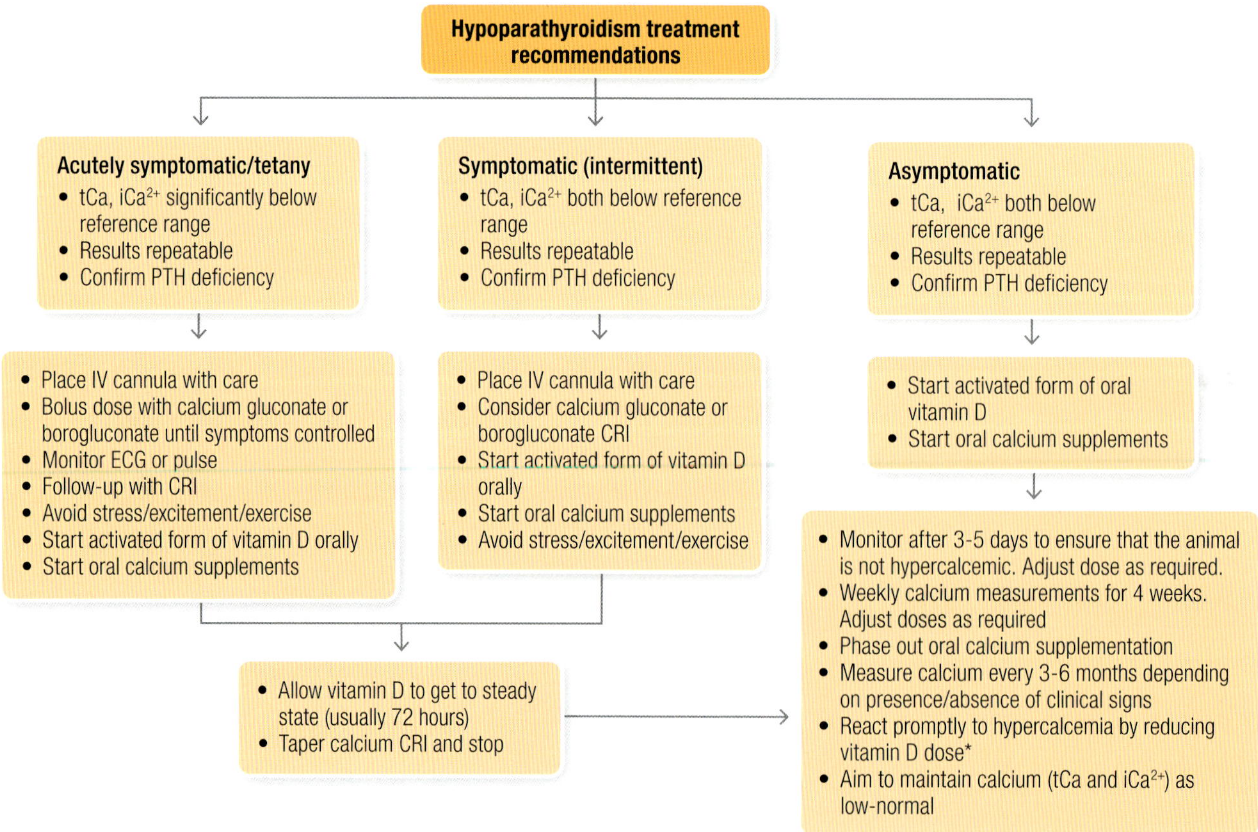

FIG. 31.3 Algorithm illustrating decision-making for dogs with hypoparathyroidism.

*Regular monitoring is essential to avoid prolonged hypercalcemia, particularly in cases where reversible hypoparathyroidism is suspected, e.g., post-parathyroidectomy for primary hyperparathyroidism. Vitamin D must be reduced with care and with the appreciation of possible significant delays between dose reduction and a reduction of tCa and iCa^{2+}.

TABLE 31.3 The treatment of acute, subacute, and chronic hypocalcemia.

	Drug	Dose	Precautions
Acute	■ 10% Calcium gluconate	0.5-1.5 mL/kg slow IV over 20-30 minutes	Monitor heart by auscultation, pulse palpation, or ECG for bradycardia, shortened QT interval, and ST segment elevation
	■ 10% Calcium borogluconate	0.5-1.0 mL/kg slow IV over 20-30 minutes	
	■ 10% Calcium chloride†	0.16-0.5 mL/kg slow IV over 20-30 minutes	
Subacute	■ 10% Calcium gluconate	10-15 mL/kg IV over 24 hours in 0.9% NaCl	Do not give subcutaneously
	■ 10% Calcium borogluconate	6-9 mL/kg IV over 24 hours in 0.9% NaCl	
	■ 10% Calcium chloride†	3-5 mL/kg IV over 24 hours in 0.9% NaCl	
Chronic	■ Calcium carbonate ■ Calcium gluconate ■ Calcium lactate	25-50 mg/kg of elemental calcium*	Can be stopped once vitamin D dose is appropriate
	■ Calcitriol	0.02-0.06 µg/kg/day PO once or divided twice** a day. The recommended starting dose is 0.02-0.03 µg/kg/day	Time to maximum effect <4 days
	■ Alfacalcidol	0.02-0.06 µg/kg once or divided twice** daily. The recommended starting dose is 0.02-0.03 µg/kg/day	Time to maximum effect <4 days
	■ Dihydrotachysterol	0.02-0.03 mg/kg daily, reducing to 0.01-0.02 mg/kg every 24-48 hours as required	Time to maximum effect <7 days

*1 mg calcium = 11.2 mg calcium gluconate = 7.7 mg calcium lactate = 2.5 mg calcium carbonate. *IV*, intravenous. †Calcium chloride is extremely irritant compared to calcium gluconate and calcium borogluconate. It is recommended that calcium chloride is not used except when there is no alternative in a life-threatening situation and, when used, that it is diluted >1:2. All forms of calcium are irritant both intravascularly and when extravasated. **Due to the turnover time for intestinal crypt cells that absorb calcium, twice daily dosing is optimum.

Does hungry bone syndrome exist in dogs?

Hungry bone syndrome describes hypocalcemia alongside normal or elevated PTH and is seen especially in people postparathyroidectomy for hyperparathyroidism where there has been long-standing disease and loss of bone density.[14] The extreme calcium requirements post-parathyroidectomy of dogs that have been hyperparathyroid for months to years may provide a parallel clinical presentation, but more investigation is needed to confirm this hypothesis.

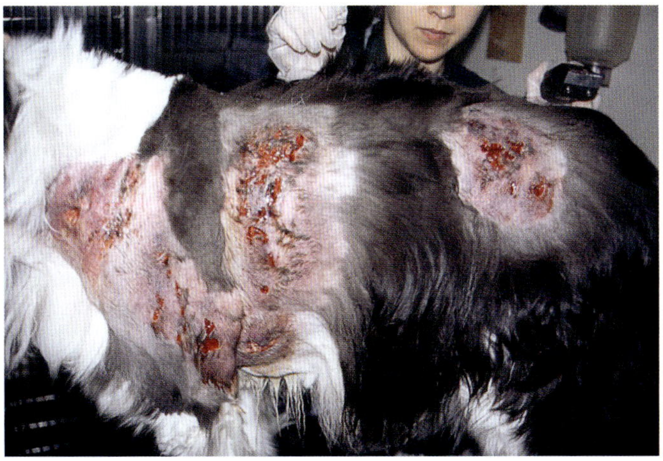

FIG. 31.4 A Border Collie with hypoparathyroidism that had received multiple subcutaneous injections of diluted 10% calcium gluconate in several sites. Photograph courtesy of Andria Cauvin (with permission). Reproduced with permission from BSAVA Manual of Canine and Feline Endocrinology 5th edition. ©BSAVA.

Acute management of symptomatic hypocalcemia

Acute management relies on bolus intravenous calcium supplementation followed by constant rate infusion (CRI). Stability is often not achieved quickly, so boluses are always better followed up with CRI treatment until oral vitamin D supplements begin to work, usually for a period of 2-4 days. **Table 31.3** details methods of calcium supplementation. Calculations for dose vary depending on which calcium salt is used; calcium gluconate or borogluconate are the best tolerated, although they can still cause significant phlebitis and are highly irritant when extravasated. Even when diluted, subcutaneous calcium solutions can cause significant problems, including tissue sloughing (**Fig. 31.4**) and the development of crystalline calcium deposits in the skin.[15]

Concurrent conditions complicating the management of primary idiopathic hypoparathyroidism

Common immune-mediated conditions, including immune-mediated hemolytic anemia (IMHA) and immune-mediated thrombocytopenia (ITP), can occur alongside primary hypoparathyroidism. Management includes immunosuppressive prednisolone/prednisone and/or additional drugs, including cyclosporine, azathioprine, chlorambucil, and mycophenolate mofetil. Glucocorticoids induce calciuria and make calcium homeostasis challenging.[16] The relationship between glucocorticoids and refractory hypocalcemia is described in people and is recognized clinically, however, it is an under-reported complication in dogs, which, in this author's experience, can have a devastating effect on disease stability.

The combination of primary hypoparathyroidism with ITP is described in a case report detailing recovery from primary hypoparathyroidism.[5] The inclusion of hypoparathyroidism necessitates adjunctive therapy for immunosuppression so that treatment is not reliant on glucocorticoids. Patients receiving glucocorticoids may remain dependent on intravenous calcium preparations, and tissue necrosis and skin sloughing can result, as was reported in the poodle who went on to recover parathyroid function[5] and also in the Pomeranian dog reported by Jaffey.[16] This latter publication suggests that the recovery shown by the Poodle could be because the immune-mediated antibody response was to the calcium-sensing receptor (CaSR) blocking function rather than against the gland itself.[17] The minority of cases with primary hypoparathyroidism will have parathyroid gland biopsy, so it is difficult to know how many have gland destruction and fibrosis, but historically in the literature, there are reports of non-supportive parathyroid histology in dogs with presumed parathyroid gland immune-mediated destruction so this possibility may justify further investigation.[2,17]

Long-term treatment and prognosis

Long-term treatment relies on chronic administration of active vitamin D (calcitriol or alfacalcidol). Extra oral calcium is rarely needed because commercial food contains sufficient. Regular monitoring of calcium concentration is required to avoid sustained hypercalcemia and possible renal damage. Concurrent conditions can significantly impact disease stability, particularly other immune-mediated diseases, as discussed, but also malabsorptive gastrointestinal conditions that impair fat-soluble vitamin (vitamin D) and, therefore, calcium uptake. The prognosis in uncomplicated, monitored cases is good.

KEY POINTS

- Hypoparathyroidism results from damage, dysfunction or removal of the parathyroid glands.
- Primary hypoparathyroidism without known surgery or trauma is due to immune-mediated damage or functional impairment of the parathyroid glands.
- Loss of parathyroid tissue leads to a deficiency of parathyroid hormone (PTH).

References

1. Zavatta G, Clarke BL. Challenges in the management of chronic hypoparathyroidism. *Endocr Connect* (10):R229-R240, 2020.
2. Wolf J, Vigani A, Schaer M. Trauma-induced primary hypoparathyroidism following severe bite wound injury to the neck in a dog. *J Vet Emerg Crit Care* 30(3):331-335, 2020.
3. Armstrong AJ, Hauptman JG, Stanley BJ, Klocke E, Burneko M, Holt DE, et al. Effect of prophylactic calcitriol administration on serum ionized calcium concentrations after parathyroidectomy: 78 Cases (2005-2015). *J Vet Intern Med* 32(1):99-106, 2018.
4. Dear JD, Kass PH, Della Maggiore AM, Feldman EC. Association of hypercalcemia before treatment with hypocalcemia after treatment in dogs with primary hyperparathyroidism. *J Vet Intern Med* 31(2):349-354, 2017.
5. Warland J, Skelly B, Knudsen C, Herrtage M. Apparent resolution of canine primary hypoparathyroidism with immunosuppressive treatment. *J Vet Intern Med* 29(1):400-404, 2015.
6. Refsal K, Provencher-Bollinger, A, Graham P, Nachreiner R. Update on the diagnosis and treatment of disorders of calcium regulation. *Vet Clin North Am Small Anim Pract* 31(5):1043-1062, 2001.
7. Kornegay JN, Greene CE, Martin C, Gorgacz EJ, Melcon DK. Primary hypoparathyroidism in dogs. *J Am Anim Hosp Assoc* 16(5):723-734, 1980.
8. Jones BR, Alley MR. Primary idiopathic hypoparathyroidism in St Bernard dogs. *N Z Vet J* 33(6):94-97, 1985.
9. Vrabelova D, Gilor C, Habing A, Schober KE, Johnson S. Synchronous diaphragmatic flutter secondary to primary hypoparathyroidism in a dog. *J Am Anim Hosp Assoc* 51(6):392-395, 2015.
10. Russell NJ, Bond KA, Robertson ID, Parry BW, Irwin PJ. Primary hypoparathyroidism in dogs: a retrospective study of 17 cases. *Aust Vet J* 84(8):285-290, 2006.
11. Abboud B, Daher R, Boujaoude J. Digestive manifestations of parathyroid disorders. *World J Gastroenterol* 17(36):4063-4066, 2011.
12. De Brito Galvao JF, Chew DJ, Nagode LA, Schenck PA. Treatment of hypoparathyroidism. In Bonagura JF (editor). Kirk's Current Veterinary Therapy XV. St. Louis, Elsevier Saunders, 2014, p. e122.
13. Bilezikian JP. Hypoparathyroidism. *J Clin Endocrinol Metab* 105(6):1722-1736, 2020.
14. Jakubauskas M, Beiša V, Strupas K. Risk factors of developing the hungry bone syndrome after parathyroidectomy for primary hyperparathyroidism. *Acta Medica Litu* 25(1):45-51, 2018.
15. Schaer M, Ginn PE, Fox LE, Leon J, Ramirez FM. Severe calcinosis cutis associated with treatment of hypoparathyroidism in a dog. *J Am Anim Hosp Assoc* 37(4):364-369, 2001.
16. Jaffey J, DeClue A, Cannon A, Tocci L, Hyland J. Presumptive glucocorticoid-induced refractory hypocalcemia in a dog with idiopathic immune-mediated hypoparathyroidism, thrombocytopenia, and hemolytic anemia. *J Am Anim Hosp Assoc* 55(1):e551-e604, 2019.
17. Kifor O, McElduff A, LeBoff MS, Moore FD, Butters R, Gao P, et al. Activating antibodies to the calcium-sensing receptor in two patients with autoimmune hypoparathyroidism. *J Clin Endocrinol Metab* 89(2):548-56, 2004.

CHAPTER 32

Anatomy and physiology of the adrenal glands

Darja Pavlin
DVM, PhD

Anatomy

The paired adrenal glands are located in the retroperitoneal space near the craniomedial border of the corresponding kidneys. Beneath a prominent fibrous capsule are two structurally and functionally distinct parts, each with a different developmental origin. The central part, the medulla, is enveloped by the outer layer, the cortex.[1] The adrenal medulla is composed of polygonal chromaffin cells named due to their ability to stain dark brown with chromium-containing fixatives. Chromaffin cells are modified postganglionic sympathetic neurons that synthesize catecholamines (epinephrine, norepinephrine, dopamine) and other molecules (chromogranin A, serotonin). About 80% of chromaffin cells in dogs produce epinephrine, and the remaining 20% produce norepinephrine. The adrenal cortex is divided into three main zones based on their structure, function, and regulation (Fig. 32.1). The outermost layer, the zona glomerulosa, produces mineralocorticoids. The middle layer, the zona fasciculata, is the largest of the three cortical zones and functions with the innermost zona reticularis as a unit to produce glucocorticoids. The zona reticularis additionally produces adrenal androgens. The adrenocortical cells contain abundant cytoplasmic lipids.[2]

Physiology

Adrenal medulla

Catecholamines are essential for the response to acute stress by mediating the so-called "fight-or-flight" response and the regulation of intermediary metabolism. After release into the systemic circulation, they bind to adrenergic receptors. There are two main groups, α- and β-adrenergic receptors. These G protein-coupled receptors differ in their affinity for the specific types of catecholamines. α-adrenergic receptors (α1 and α2) have the same affinity for epinephrine and norepinephrine. β-adrenergic receptors (β1 and β2) have a higher affinity for epinephrine. The effects of catecholamines in different tissues depend on the type and number of receptors. The effects on metabolism are mediated mainly by epinephrine. They include stimulation of lipolysis in adipose tissue, increase in glucose concentration by activation of glycogenolysis and gluconeogenesis, inhibition of insulin secretion, and increase in basal metabolic rate. Non-metabolic effects, e.g., effects on cardiac function, smooth muscle tension, and acclimatization to cold, are mediated by both epinephrine and norepinephrine.[3]

Adrenal cortex

Each adrenocortical steroid hormone is synthesized from a common precursor, cholesterol. During steroidogenesis, cholesterol is converted to the different steroid hormones by multiple intermediate steps, which are catalyzed by steroidogenic enzymes. Each zone expresses a different set of steroidogenic enzymes to ensure that each adrenocortical zone produces a different end product. The crucial enzyme for functional zonation of the canine adrenal cortex is 17α-hydroxylase/17,20-lyase (CYP17), which is expressed only in the zona fasciculata and zona reticularis. This results in zone-specific production of

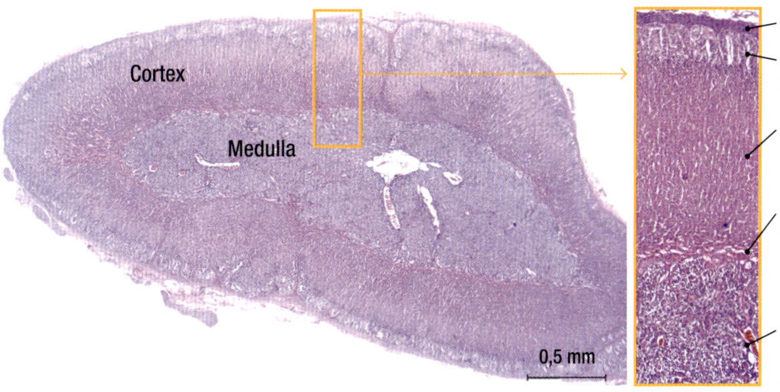

FIG. 32.1 Histological structure of the canine adrenal gland including main secretory hormones. (Photos courtesy of Prof. Dr. Valentina Kubale Dvojmoč, Veterinary Faculty of Ljubljana, Slovenia).

cortisol and androgens in these zones and restriction of aldosterone synthesis to the zona glomerulosa.[4]

Adrenocortical hormones are not stored but are immediately secreted into the blood by simple diffusion across the cell membrane. Because of their lipophilic structure, transport in the blood depends on transport proteins, although about 10% of circulating cortisol and 40% of aldosterone are in an unbound state. The primary transport proteins are albumin for aldosterone and transcortin for cortisol.[5]

Mineralocorticoid regulation and function

Aldosterone is responsible for metabolizing sodium, potassium, and chloride ions and maintaining blood pressure. The two main regulatory mechanisms for mineralocorticoid production are extracellular potassium concentration and angiotensin, although other factors, such as adrenocorticotropic hormone (ACTH) and natriuretic factors, also play a role. Hypotension or decreased renal perfusion activate the renin-angiotensin-aldosterone system, ultimately leading to the production of angiotensin II, which stimulates aldosterone secretion. In addition, plasma potassium concentration has an independent effect on aldosterone secretion.[3]

The main target tissues for the action of mineralocorticoids are epithelial tissues such as kidneys, colon, salivary, and sweat glands. Aldosterone binds to cytoplasmic mineralocorticoid receptors (MR), which have a similar affinity to aldosterone and cortisol. In epithelial cells and vascular smooth muscle cells, the enzyme 11β-hydroxysteroid dehydrogenase type 2 (11β-HSD2) converts cortisol to the inactive metabolite cortisone. This prevents glucocorticoids, which are present in higher concentrations, from outcompeting mineralocorticoids for the MR. In other non-epithelial cells, e.g., cardiomyocytes and neurons, glucocorticoids can antagonize the action of aldosterone since 11β-HSD2 is present to a lesser extent.[5]

Glucocorticoid regulation and function

The major glucocorticoid produced in the adrenal glands of dogs is cortisol. Its secretion is strictly controlled by the hypothalamic-pituitary-adrenal axis, with ACTH serving as a principal stimulator of cortisol synthesis and release.[2]

As a response to stress, immune response, and inflammation, neurons in the hypothalamus produce corticotropin-releasing hormone (CRH). CRH enters the hypothalamo-hypophyseal portal system and stimulates corticotropic cells in the anterior lobe of the pituitary gland (adenohypophysis) to secrete ACTH. Binding of the ACTH to its receptor (ACTHR, MC2R-melanocortin type 2 receptor) on the surface of the zona fasciculata cells subsequently initiates steroidogenesis. Increased circulating cortisol, in turn, has a negative feedback effect on the hypothalamus and pituitary gland and inhibits the secretion of ACTH and CRH. ACTH also has a direct short-loop feedback effect on the secretion of CRH.[3]

Glucocorticoids have a variety of effects in different tissues. They play an important role in intermediary metabolism, especially in gluconeogenesis and glycogenolysis, effectively increasing blood glucose concentrations. Other effects on metabolism include stimulation of lipolysis and catabolism of proteins. They also have immunosuppressive and anti-inflammatory effects by inhibiting phagocytosis, suppressing antibody production, and inhibiting the synthesis of inflammatory mediators, e.g., prostaglandins, thromboxanes, and leukotrienes.

KEY POINTS

- The adrenal glands consist of two structurally, functionally, and developmentally distinct parts: the inner medulla and the outer cortex.
- The medulla consists of chromaffin cells that synthesize the catecholamines epinephrine, norepinephrine, and dopamine.
- The cortex is divided into three zones extending from the capsule toward the medulla: zona glomerulosa, zona fasciculata, and zona reticularis.
- Aldosterone from the zona glomerulosa is the major mineralocorticoid and is regulated by the renin-angiotensin system and potassium concentration.
- The zona fasciculata and zona reticularis function as a unit to produce glucocorticoids. Cortisol is the main glucocorticoid in dogs, and its secretion is regulated by the hypothalamic-pituitary-adrenal axis.
- The zona reticularis additionally produces androgens.

References

1. Hermanson JW, de Lahunta, Evans HE. The endocrine system. In Hermanson JW, de Lahunta A (editors). Miller and Evan's Anatomy of the Dog 5th edition. St. Louis, Elsevier Saunders, 2018, pp. 469-581.
2. Hullinger R, Andrisani OM. Endocrine system. In Eurell JO, Frappier BL (editors). Dellman's Textbook of Veterinary Histology 6th edition. Ames, Iowa, Blackwell Publishing, 2006, pp. 298-319.
3. Greco DS, Stabenfeldt GH. Endocrine glands and their function. In Klein BG (editor). Cunningham's Textbook of Veterinary Physiology 5th edition. St. Louis, Elsevier Saunders, 2013, pp. 374-407.
4. Sanders K, Mol JA, Kooistra HS, et al. New insights in the functional zonation of the canine adrenal cortex. *J Vet Intern Med* 30(3):741-750, 2016. doi:10.1111/jvim.13946.
5. Goff JP. The endocrine system. In Reece WO, Erickson HH, Goff JP, Uemura EE (editors). Duke's Physiology of Domestic Animals 13th edition. Ames, Iowa, John Wiley & Sons, 2015, pp. 617-653.

CHAPTER 33

Hypoadrenocorticism

Nadja S. Sieber-Ruckstuhl
Prof., Dr. med. vet., DACVIM, DECVIM-CA (Internal Medicine)

Felicitas S. Boretti
Prof., Dr. med. vet., FVH, DACVIM, DECVIM-CA (Internal Medicine)

Hypoadrenocorticism is caused by reduced adrenal cortex function. Diagnosis requires a high level of suspicion due to vague and intermittent clinical signs. Failure to recognize the disease can result in life-threatening complications and significant mortality. It is crucial to consider hypoadrenocorticism before administering glucocorticoids, as they can interfere with diagnostic testing.

Etiology

The adrenal cortex comprises three distinct zones, each with unique functions and morphological characteristics. The outermost layer, the zona glomerulosa, is responsible for synthesizing mineralocorticoids, predominantly aldosterone. The middle and inner layers, zona fasciculata and zona reticularis, function together to produce glucocorticoids, primarily cortisol, as well as androgens.

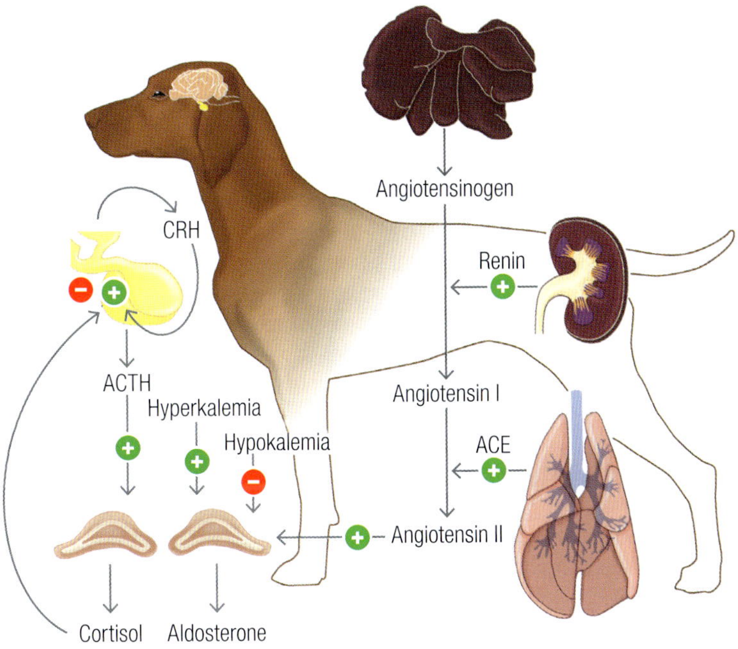

FIG 33.1 Schematic illustration of cortisol and aldosterone production from the adrenal glands. ©Vetsuisse Faculty Zurich, UZH / J. Peter, Vetcom.

A comprehensive understanding of the various forms of hypoadrenocorticism necessitates an understanding of the physiological regulation of adrenal cortex hormone production (Fig. 33.1). The renin-angiotensin system and extracellular potassium concentration are the main regulators of aldosterone secretion. In contrast, cortisol secretion is regulated by the hypothalamus-pituitary-adrenal axis, with adrenocorticotropic hormone (ACTH) serving as the principal stimulator of cortisol synthesis and release.

There are two main forms of hypoadrenocorticism based on the underlying disease process: (1) primary hypoadrenocorticism, which arises from dysfunction within the adrenal cortices, and (2) secondary hypoadrenocorticism, which occurs due to inadequate ACTH production by the pituitary gland. It is possible that a third form, tertiary hypoadrenocorticism, exists, of which the cause is the deficient secretion of corticotropin-releasing hormone (CRH) by the hypothalamus. This results in decreased ACTH and cortisol production. However, distinguishing between secondary and tertiary disease poses challenges, and this particular form has not yet been documented in veterinary medicine.

The primary form of hypoadrenocorticism most commonly arises from progressive immune-mediated destruction of the adrenal cortices, leading to adrenal atrophy. This condition, often called Addison's disease, has a significant genetic component in certain breeds.[1] An autoimmune-mediated origin is suspected, as antibodies against the cytochrome P450 side-chain cleavage enzyme (P450scc) are detectable in some affected dogs.[2] The destruction typically involves all layers of the adrenal cortex, leading to deficiency in both glucocorticoids and mineralocorticoids. As a consequence, negative feedback to the pituitary and hypothalamus is lost, resulting in increased concentrations of ACTH.

In rare instances, the destructive process within the adrenal glands may be limited to the middle and inner zone of the adrenal cortex, resulting in isolated glucocorticoid deficiency. This form of primary hypoadrenocorticism, characterized by normal electrolyte concentrations, is referred to as eunatremic, eukalemic primary hypoadrenocorticism according to the Agreeing Language in Veterinary Endocrinology (ALIVE) project of the European

Society of Veterinary Endocrinology (ESVE). Even more uncommonly, isolated cases have been reported where the destruction is confined solely to the outer zone of the adrenal cortex (zona glomerulosa), leading to isolated hyperreninemic hypoaldosteronism.

Adrenal cortex destruction, leading to primary hypoadrenocorticism, can also be caused by other factors such as granulomatous or neoplastic infiltration, hemorrhagic infarction, amyloidosis, and trauma. Additionally, iatrogenic primary hypoadrenocorticism resulting from adrenal necrosis can be induced by drugs like mitotane (o,p'-DDD) or trilostane.

Secondary hypoadrenocorticism, characterized by ACTH deficiency, primarily leads to isolated cortisol deficiency, as only the middle and inner zones of the adrenal cortices undergo atrophy. Secondary hypoadrenocorticism is rare (<5%) and can arise from various pituitary diseases (post-traumatic, neoplastic, inflammatory, infectious, vascular, congenital). Surgical hypophysectomy can also result in secondary hypoadrenocorticism.

The most common cause of secondary hypoadrenocorticism, specifically referred to as iatrogenic hypoadrenocorticism, arises from the exogenous administration of glucocorticoids or progestins followed by the sudden withdrawal of the medication. Hence, accurately measuring endogenous ACTH is crucial to substantiate the diagnosis.

TABLE 33.1 **Possible clinical signs and physical examination findings typically observed in dogs with hypoadrenocorticism.**

Clinical signs	Physical examination findings
■ Loss of appetite or hyporexia* ■ Vomiting* ■ Diarrhea* ■ Weight loss ■ Hematemesis ■ Melena ■ Polyuria/polydipsia ■ Shivering ■ Collapse	■ Lethargy* ■ Dehydration ■ Hypovolemia ■ Weakness* ■ Hypotension ■ Poor body condition score ■ Abdominal pain ■ Bradycardia ■ Signs of hypovolemic shock

*Common clinical signs and physical examination findings (seen in >50% of dogs)

Clinical features

Although hypoadrenocorticism can occur at any age (reported age range: 2 months to 14 years), the most typically affected dogs fall within the young to middle-aged range (reported median age of onset: 3.2-4.8 years). Any breed can be affected, but hereditary factors have been identified in certain breeds, such as the Standard Poodle, Portuguese Water dog, Nova Scotia Duck Tolling Retriever, Soft-coated Wheaten Terrier, and Bearded Collie.[3,4] Furthermore, an increased prevalence of the disease has been reported in certain family lines of Leonbergers and Pomeranians.[3,4] Even though inheritance is proven in some breeds, providing generalized breeding advice is challenging as a complex inheritance pattern seems more likely than the often-postulated autosomal recessive trait.[3] Inbreeding, however, should be viewed critically, as it has been shown that inbreeding increases the susceptibility to hypoadrenocorticism.[5]

In general, females seem to be more affected than males.[3,4] However, in some breed-specific studies, a gender predisposition could not be clearly demonstrated.

The clinical signs of dogs with hypoadrenocorticism can be acute or insidious, vague or intermittent, and waxing and waning. A history of intermittent gastrointestinal signs that improve with fluid therapy and other supportive measures (e.g., glucocorticoid therapy) or a history of signs occurring especially after stressful situations should raise suspicion of hypoadrenocorticism. Typical clinical signs of dogs with hypoadrenocorticism are listed in Table 33.1.

Among the most common signs are lethargy, loss of appetite, vomiting, diarrhea, and weight loss. Less frequent gastrointestinal signs include hematemesis and melena. Gastrointestinal signs are attributed to the physiological role of glucocorticoids in maintaining the integrity of the gastrointestinal tract. Regurgitation due to the presence of megaesophagus has been reported in some cases; however, the precise underlying mechanism remains unknown. Electrolyte disturbances (hyponatremia and hyperkalemia) are discussed as impacting membrane potential and neuromuscular function, but muscle weakness resulting from cortisol deficiency has been suggested as an alternative explanation, as megaesophagus has also been observed in dogs suspected to have eunatremic, eukalemic primary hypoadrenocorticism (isolated glucocorticoid deficiency).

Other reported clinical signs are polyuria and polydipsia. Polyuria primarily arises from aldosterone deficiency, leading to hyponatremia, which then decreases renal medullary hypertonicity and the concentration gradient, impairing water reabsorption. Additionally, hyponatremia compromises the release of arginine vasopressin (AVP) by reducing serum osmolality.[4] If ionized hypercalcemia is present, it can also cause altered responsiveness to AVP. Compensatory polydipsia, an increased water intake, is commonly observed in the early stages of the disease. As the illness progresses, however, water intake can be compromised, contributing to dehydration and hypovolemia. Less commonly described symptoms include seizures caused by hypoglycemia and muscle cramping.[3,4]

Physical examination findings are often vague and nonspecific and include lethargy, dehydration, hypovolemia, weakness, hypotension, poor body condition, abdominal pain, bradycardia, and, in severe cases, hypovolemic shock (e.g., weak pulse, hypothermia, decreased capillary refill time).[3] The absence of compensatory tachycardia in a dog with hypovolemic shock or the presence of bradycardia in this scenario should raise suspicion of hypoadrenocorticism.

Dogs with eunatremic, eukalemic primary hypoadrenocorticism (isolated glucocorticoid deficiency) often go undiagnosed for longer periods since their symptoms are similar to those seen in primary gastrointestinal diseases. Additionally, as they do not suffer from mineralocorticoid deficiency, the specific clinical and clinicopathological manifestations of aldosterone shortage are absent, which is why hypoadrenocorticism should be considered in dogs with chronic, recurrent gastrointestinal signs. Although the reported frequency of hypoadrenocorticism in this population is low (between 0.35 and 4%), recognition of the disease is important as further progress could finally lead to a life-threatening crisis.[6,7,8]

Clinicopathological findings

The most important laboratory findings in dogs with hypoadrenocorticism include hyponatremia, hyperkalemia, azotemia, mild non-regenerative anemia, and absence of a stress leukogram (Table 33.2). However, these clinicopathologic abnormalities do not have to be present in all cases and are not pathognomonic for hypoadrenocorticism as they can also be seen with other diseases (e.g., acute kidney injury and renal failure, hepatic failure, chronic effusions). Therefore, it is of utmost importance

TABLE 33.2 Possible clinicopathological findings typically observed in dogs with hypoadrenocorticism.

Hematology	Biochemistry	Urinalysis
■ Anemia ■ Relative erythrocytosis ■ Eosinophilia ■ Neutrophilia ■ Lymphocytosis	■ Hyponatremia* ■ Hyperkalemia* ■ Hypochloremia ■ Increased urea* ■ Increase creatinine* ■ Hyperphosphatemia* ■ Hypercalcemia ■ Hypoglycemia ■ Hypocholesterolemia ■ Hypoalbuminemia ■ Increased liver enzymes ■ Increased TSH	■ Specific gravity <1.030 in combination with azotemia*

*Common clinicopathological findings (seen in > 50% of dogs)

that clinicians consider hypoadrenocorticism as a differential for any dog with vague and unclear clinical signs. Hypoadrenocorticism can usually be easily ruled out but can lead to death if unrecognized.

Hematology

Various hematological abnormalities have been described. These include normocytic, normochromic non-regenerative anemia, relative erythrocytosis, eosinophilia, neutrophilia, and lymphocytosis.[3]

Anemia can be attributed to a lack of stimulation of erythropoiesis due to glucocorticoid deficiency or gastrointestinal bleeding.[3] In some cases, anemia is only apparent after rehydration therapy because it can be masked by concurrent dehydration. Furthermore, it has been observed that dogs with isolated glucocorticoid deficiency suffer from anemia more frequently than those with concurrent mineralocorticoid deficiency.[9] The cause could be the longer duration of illness in this subgroup of dogs, as well as the less severe dehydration.[4]

A common finding in dogs with hypoadrenocorticism is the absence of a stress leukogram. This is somehow unexpected as the systemic illness represents a major stress to the body.[4] A characteristic stress leukogram manifests as lymphopenia, neutrophilia, and eosinopenia. Dogs with hypoadrenocorticism may demonstrate lymphocytosis and eosinophilia or may have neutrophils and lymphocyte counts within the reference range, which should be considered abnormal in this setting. Therefore, the presence of such a leukogram in a severely ill dog should raise suspicion of hypoadrenocorticism.

Biochemistry

The predominant biochemical abnormalities, occurring in over 80% of dogs with hypoadrenocorticism, are a consequence of aldosterone deficiency and manifest as hyponatremia and hyperkalemia. When evaluating such electrolyte changes, it is important to consider several other diseases as differential diagnoses, including acute kidney injury, urinary tract obstruction, uroabdomen, acute gastroenteritis due to intestinal parasitism or perforation, liver failure, acute pancreatitis, pleural or abdominal effusion, and congestive heart failure.

Elevated concentrations of urea (seen in more than 80% of cases), creatinine (more than 60% of cases), and phosphate (up to almost 60% of cases) are other biochemical deviations often observed in dogs with hypoadrenocorticism. These elevations can be attributed to the decreased glomerular filtration rate resulting from dehydration and hypovolemia. It is important to note that the azotemia associated with hypoadrenocorticism typically represents prerenal azotemia. However, differentiating it from renal causes can be challenging due to the frequent reduction in urine specific gravity (see below).

Gastrointestinal hemorrhage can be another cause of increased urea concentrations and may even lead to proportionally higher urea concentrations than creatinine concentrations. This is a consequence of absorbed intestinal blood, its metabolized ammonia in the colon, subsequent absorption into the portal system, and final metabolism to urea in the liver.

Hypercalcemia has also been observed in cases of hypoadrenocorticism. Total calcium elevation, occurring in approximately 30% of cases, is more commonly reported than ionized calcium elevation, observed in about 18% of cases.[3,4] The precise underlying mechanism is not well understood, but several factors have been proposed. These include volume contraction, reduced glomerular filtration rate leading to decreased calciuresis, enhanced intestinal calcium absorption, and metabolic acidosis, which primarily contributes to ionized hypercalcemia.[10]

Dogs with hypoadrenocorticism may exhibit other biochemical abnormalities, including hypoglycemia, hypocholesterolemia, and hypoalbuminemia. Hypoglycemia, observed in up to 30% of cases, results from decreased hepatic gluconeogenesis and increased peripheral insulin sensitivity. Although hypoglycemia is typically mild, it can be severe and even lead to seizure activity.

Hypocholesterolemia and hypoalbuminemia are frequently seen, particularly in cases of eunatremic, eukalemic primary hypoadrenocorticism (isolated glucocorticoid deficiency).[9,11] Decreased cholesterol concentrations are attributed to reduced fat absorption or concurrent hepatopathy, while hypoalbuminemia is primarily associated with gastrointestinal losses (protein loss or blood loss), decreased hepatic production due to hepatopathy, and reduced oral intake.[11] Dogs with isolated glucocorticoid deficiency are more likely to exhibit hypocholesterolemia and hypoalbuminemia, which in turn is probably due to the longer duration of the disease, as they do not experience aldosterone deficiency, thus reducing the likelihood of developing hypovolemia and shock.

Mild-to-moderate elevations in liver enzymes can be observed in up to 30% of dogs with hypoadrenocorticism. In most cases, these changes can be attributed to decreased hepatic perfusion. However, some authors have discussed the possibility of decreased hepatic function accompanied by abnormal liver function tests, although this appears to resolve spontaneously without requiring specific treatment.[12]

In some commercial laboratories, a complete chemistry panel often includes the measurement of total thyroxine. However, it is important to note that total thyroxine (and free thyroxine) concentrations can be reduced in dogs with nonthyroidal illnesses, a condition formerly known as euthyroid sick syndrome. Additionally, TSH (thyroid-stimulating hormone) concentrations have been shown to be increased in up to 30% of dogs with newly diagnosed and untreated hypoadrenocorticism.[13] Thyroid-stimulating hormone usually normalizes without thyroxine supplementation after glucocorticoid treatment has been started and given for several weeks. This phenomenon has to be clearly differentiated from another condition: Schmidt's syndrome, also known as polyglandular autoimmune syndrome type 2, a rare autoimmune disorder that affects multiple endocrine glands in dogs. It is characterized by the combination of hypoadrenocorticism together with hypothyroidism. On the basis of clinical signs, it cannot be differentiated whether a dog is suffering from hypoadrenocorticism alone or hypoadrenocorticism and concurrent hypothyroidism. Testing of autoimmune markers is not available; therefore, the evaluation of thyroid status is best postponed until after several weeks of long-term treatment with glucocorticoids, as postponing diagnosis and potential treatment of hypothyroidism is not life-threatening.[13]

Urinalysis

Ideally, a urine sample should be collected prior to initiating fluid therapy in dogs with hypoadrenocorticism. Despite experiencing hypovolemia, dehydration, and prerenal azotemia, the majority of dogs with hypoadrenocorticism exhibit diluted urine with a specific gravity below 1.030. This impaired ability to concentrate urine is attributed to the low sodium concentration and the loss of the normal medullary concentration gradient. As a result, differentiating hypoadrenocorticism from kidney disease, particularly acute kidney injury, can be challenging in certain cases.

Endocrine testing

ACTH stimulation test

The ACTH stimulation test is the test of choice for confirming the diagnosis of hypoadrenocorticism. In unstable patients, proceeding directly to this test without initially measuring baseline cortisol concentrations is recommended.

Test performance

A synthetic form of ACTH (cosyntropin or tetracosactrin) is administered at a supraphysiological dosage of 5 µg/kg. Blood should be sampled to determine the cortisol concentration before and one hour after intravenous ACTH administration. While intramuscular administration is possible, it is advisable to avoid it in dehydrated and hypovolemic dogs due to potential delays in absorption, which may impact the interpretation of the test results. Since intravenous fluid therapy is necessary for hypovolemic and dehydrated animals, the catheter required for fluid administration can also be utilized for the administration of ACTH.

Interpretation

In dogs with normal adrenal gland function, the administration of ACTH leads to a significant increase in cortisol concentration, typically surpassing 138 nmol/L (5 µg/dL). However, in dogs with hypoadrenocorticism, the post-stimulation cortisol concentrations are below 55 nmol/L (2 µg/dL) or even below the detection limit of the assay.[4] In very rare cases, post-stimulation cortisol concentrations may range between 55 and 83 nmol/L (2-3 µg/dL) (personal observation). When the post-ACTH cortisol concentration falls between the threshold of 55 nmol/L (2 µg/dL) and the level indicating sufficient adrenal reserve (>138 nmol/L or >5 µg/dL), it is considered borderline or within the gray zone. In this case, the measurement of endogenous ACTH is recommended.

Various factors can contribute to an inadequate response to ACTH stimulation besides hypoadrenocorticism. The administration of glucocorticoids (topically or systemically) or progestins prior to the test is a significant factor. Depending on the glucocorticoid product and duration of use, post-stimulation cortisol concentrations often range from 55-138 nmol/L (2-5 µg/dL).[14] In some cases, cortisol concentrations may be even lower, dropping below the detection limit of the cortisol assay due to suppression of the hypothalamic-pituitary-adrenal axis. Other reasons for a borderline or inadequate response include treatment with trilostane or ketoconazole, non-cortisol-secreting adrenal tumors, loss of potency of the administered ACTH product due to improper or prolonged storage, use of an incorrect ACTH dosage, and errors in administration or timing of sample collection.

Additionally, synthetic glucocorticoids (e.g., prednisolone, methylprednisolone) given on the same day as the test can directly interfere with cortisol measurement and lead to falsely elevated cortisol values. However, this interference does not occur when using dexamethasone. Therefore, dexamethasone can be a suitable option for providing glucocorticoid support to critically ill patients when needed. Like other glucocorticoids, dexamethasone inhibits endogenous cortisol production directly, but this effect typically takes several hours to manifest. To avoid artificially decreased post-ACTH cortisol concentrations, it is crucial to ensure that the ACTH stimulation test is conducted within a few hours after administering dexamethasone. By doing this, correct interpretation and exclusion of hypoadrenocorticism should still be possible after a single dose of dexamethasone.[15]

The ACTH stimulation test alone cannot distinguish between different forms of adrenal insufficiency in animals. These include primary hypoadrenocorticism, eunatremic, eukalemic primary hypoadrenocorticism, secondary adrenal insufficiency resulting from chronic pituitary dysfunction, or secondary adrenal insufficiency due to recently discontinued long-term glucocorticoid administration. Therefore, in cases in which electrolyte concentrations are within the reference range, it is crucial to thoroughly exclude any prior administration of glucocorticoids (topically or systemically). Additionally, measuring endogenous ACTH concentration can help differentiate between these various forms (see below).

Baseline serum cortisol

In stable patients suspected of having hypoadrenocorticism, measuring a baseline cortisol concentration is possible. A baseline cortisol level exceeding 55 nmol/L (>2 µg/dL) can effectively rule out hypoadrenocorticism. This cut-off value remains valid regardless of the specific cortisol assay used for measurement.[3,4]

A baseline cortisol level of ≤55 nmol/L (≤2 µg/dL) exhibits a sensitivity ranging between 99% and 100% for diagnosing hypoadrenocorticism. Due to the relatively low specificity, ranging between 63% and 78%, an ACTH stimulation test must be conducted in these cases to confirm the diagnosis.

Endogenous ACTH

Dogs with primary hypoadrenocorticism typically exhibit increased or very high ACTH concentrations (above the reference range, and most of the time much higher), and dogs with secondary hypoadrenocorticism have subnormal or undetectable values.[3,4]

Determination of the endogenous ACTH concentration can be especially beneficial in cases in which the ACTH stimulation test results are in the gray zone and in which serum electrolyte concentrations are within the reference range. Elevated ACTH concentrations indicate primary hypoadrenocorticism and close monitoring of electrolyte concentrations is crucial, as the condition may progress from isolated glucocorticoid deficiency to combined glucocorticoid and mineralocorticoid deficiency. Lastly, it is crucial to emphasize that endogenous ACTH concentration alone should not be relied upon as the sole parameter in confirming a diagnosis. It is important to take into account that the administration of glucocorticoids can lead to decreased ACTH concentration, with them occasionally falling below the detection limit of the assay.

Sample processing is of utmost importance as endogenous ACTH is highly unstable, and improper handling can lead to erroneously low results. Chilled EDTA plasma should be collected and promptly separated and frozen within 30 minutes of collection to ensure accuracy. Furthermore, it is essential to avoid contact with glass and use plastic tubes instead, as ACTH can adhere to glass. Once separated, the plasma can be stored at −20°C for an extended period. It is important to note that specific sample collection and handling procedures may vary depending on the assay utilized. Therefore, it is advisable to consult the laboratory concerned for their recommended guidelines regarding sample handling. Additionally, it is crucial to inquire whether the assay has been validated for use in dogs and if reference ranges are available.

Cortisol-to-ACTH ratio

The determination of the cortisol-to-ACTH ratio (CAR) has been suggested as a potential alternative to the ACTH stimulation test, particularly in regions where obtaining synthetic ACTH is challenging or cost-prohibitive. In dogs with primary hypoadrenocorticism, there is typically a decrease in cortisol concentrations and an increase in ACTH concentrations due to the absence of negative feedback on the pituitary gland. As a result, the CAR is expected to be significantly lower in dogs with hypoadrenocorticism compared with healthy dogs or dogs with non-adrenal illnesses, as supported by findings from several studies.[16-18]

Based on these findings, the calculation of the CAR can be considered a valuable screening test for the diagnosis of primary hypoadrenocorticism. However, it is important to acknowledge that some overlap has been observed between the groups (healthy, hypoadrenocorticism, non-adrenal illness), which introduces the possibility of misdiagnosis. Also, the diagnostic reliability of CAR in dogs with secondary hypoadrenocorticism has not been evaluated in a larger population of dogs. Further research is necessary to assess its usefulness in this specific context.

In one study, a CAR threshold of >0.01 demonstrated a diagnostic sensitivity of 100% and specificity of 99% in excluding hypoadrenocorticism.[18] However, it is important to note that despite employing the same assay for cortisol and endogenous ACTH measurement, variations in CAR cut-off values were observed between two different studies.[17,18] Therefore, although CAR shows promising sensitivity and specificity, it should not be used as a stand-alone test for definitive diagnosis. Further research of CAR cut-off values are warranted to establish its optimal utility in diagnosing hypoadrenocorticism.

Aldosterone

In dogs with primary hypoadrenocorticism, serum aldosterone concentrations have been shown to be markedly lower compared with those of healthy dogs and dogs with non-adrenal diseases.[16,19] However, even when measuring aldosterone concentrations after ACTH stimulation, overlapping values have been observed among the groups.[19] Consequently, the determination of aldosterone has limited diagnostic value in identifying hypoadrenocorticism. Interestingly, aldosterone concentrations have been found to fall below the detection limit of the assay, even in dogs with eunatremic, eukalemic primary hypoadrenocorticism where serum sodium and potassium concentrations remain unaffected.[19] Therefore, the aldosterone level alone is not a fully reliable parameter for distinguishing between eunatremic, eukalemic primary hypoadrenocorticism and secondary hypoadrenocorticism.

Plasma renin activity and aldosterone-to-renin ratio

Aldosterone deficiency physiologically leads to reduced sodium resorption, hypovolemia, and, consequently, an increase in renin activity. In primary hypoadrenocorticism, there is a deficiency of aldosterone accompanied by elevated plasma renin activity, and compared with healthy dogs, those with hypoadrenocorticism showed a significantly lower aldosterone-to-renin ratio.[16] Unlike single measurements of aldosterone and renin, there is less overlap in the aldosterone-to-renin ratio between dogs with and without hypoadrenocorticism.[16] Currently, the measurement of renin activity is not routinely available as a diagnostic test. In summary, while these hormone measurements show promise, they cannot yet be recommended as a definitive diagnostic tool for diagnosing hypoadrenocorticism.

Utility of changes in serum blood chemistry, CBC, and urine parameters in the diagnosis of hypoadrenocorticism

Sodium to potassium ratio

The calculation of the sodium to potassium (Na^+/K^+) ratio has been suggested by several authors as a potential diagnostic tool for hypoadrenocorticism. According to this approach, a lower ratio, resulting from lower sodium and higher potassium concentrations, could indicate the presence of hypoadrenocorticism, while a higher ratio may potentially exclude the condition.

However, it is important to acknowledge that both scenarios are possible, as a higher ratio can still be observed in dogs with hypoadrenocorticism, and a low ratio can occur in dogs without the condition. Therefore, relying solely on the Na^+/K^+ ratio for diagnosis is not recommended.

In cases where a dog presents with hyponatremia and/or hyperkalemia, along with clinical signs consistent with hypoadrenocorticism, it is crucial to consider it as a candidate for hypoadrenocorticism, regardless of the Na^+/K^+ ratio. More reliable diagnostic tests, such as the ACTH stimulation test, should be employed to confirm or rule out hypoadrenocorticism.

Leukogram: eosinophilia, lymphocytosis

It has been shown that dogs with hypoadrenocorticism display a significantly higher eosinophil count (≥570/μL) than dogs without the condition. Moreover, in dogs with clinical suspicion of hypoadrenocorticism, a lymphocyte count ≥750/μL has been reported to show 100% sensitivity in detecting the presence of hypoadrenocorticism, although its specificity is low (35%). Furthermore, dogs with hypoadrenocorticism exhibit a significantly lower neutrophil-to-lymphocyte ratio than dogs without the disease. In cases where hypoadrenocorticism is suspected, a neutrophil-to-lymphocyte ratio ≤2.3 predicts the presence of hypoadrenocorticism with a sensitivity of 67% and a specificity of 82%.[20] However, the most reliable diagnostic performance has been achieved by combining a neutrophil-to-lymphocyte ratio ≤2.3 and a sodium-to-potassium ratio ≤22. This combination revealed a specificity of 100% for the disease and could identify the disease in 68% of cases correctly.[20]

In summary, a leukogram can help raise suspicion of hypoadrenocorticism or aid in the interpretation of an inconclusive ACTH stimulation test. However, it cannot be used to confirm or exclude the diagnosis definitively.

Urine electrolyte concentrations

Urine electrolyte concentrations have also been evaluated as potential diagnostic parameters for the determination of hypoadrenocorticism.[21,22]

However, due to the significant overlap between results from dogs with hypoadrenocorticism and those without the disease, the measurement of urine electrolyte concentrations cannot currently be recommended as a reliable method for confirming the diagnosis of hypoadrenocorticism.

Urinary cortisol-creatinine ratio

The urine cortisol-to-creatinine ratio (UCCR) has been shown to be significantly reduced in dogs with hypoadrenocorticism compared to that of both healthy dogs and dogs with non-adrenal illnesses.[23] This suggests that UCCR could potentially serve as a valuable screening test for excluding hypoadrenocorticism, similar to the determination of baseline cortisol concentration. Further investigation is, however, necessary to establish an optimal cut-off value and assess the robustness and reliability of UCCR as a diagnostic tool in clinical practice.

Diagnostic imaging

Ultrasonography

Dogs affected by primary hypoadrenocorticism display significantly thinner adrenal glands compared with healthy dogs and dogs with diseases that mimic hypoadrenocorticism.

A left adrenal gland thickness of less than 3.2 mm has been proposed as a strong indicator of the disease.[24] Taking a measurement of the left adrenal gland width of <3.9 mm resulted in a sensitivity of 80% and a specificity of 82.4% specific for the diagnosis of glucocorticoid-deficient hypoadrenocorticism.[25] Based on these numbers, which indicate a considerable overlap in adrenal gland size between dogs with and without hypoadrenocorticism, ultrasound findings alone are insufficient to establish a diagnosis of hypoadrenocorticism. As shown in healthy dogs and dogs with non-adrenal illness, adrenal gland thickness is affected by body weight, age, and sex. However, the finding of small adrenal glands on ultrasonographic examination in a dog with appropriate clinical symptoms is a strong indicator of the presence of hypoadrenocorticism and warrants further endocrinological testing.

It should also be emphasized that the administration of exogenous glucocorticoids can lead to a significant reduction in adrenal gland size (Fig. 33.2). Therefore, obtaining a thorough history and consulting with the owner or referring veterinarian is crucial before initiating diagnostic procedures.

Studies have demonstrated slight variations in measurements when the dorsal and lateral recumbency positions of the dog during the ultrasound examination are compared. However, minimal differences were observed in the caudal pole thickness when measured from the longitudinal plane. As a result, measuring the maximal thickness of the adrenal glands at this caudal pole has been recommended.[26] This approach helps minimize any variation attributable to the dog's position. Furthermore, the caudal pole thickness is widely regarded as the preferred dimension for assessing adrenal gland size due to its low variability, ease of measurement, and high reliability.[26]

Treatment

The treatment of hypoadrenocorticism can be divided into two phases: treatment during the adrenal crisis and long-term treatment.

Treatment during the adrenal crisis

Acute Addisonian crisis represents a life-threatening emergency situation. Therefore, immediate initiation of therapy is required for every patient with strong clinical evidence of adrenal insufficiency. The initial emergency treatment aims to restore fluid volume, correct electrolyte imbalances, and administer rapid-acting glucocorticoids. Simultaneously with emergency care, further diagnostic evaluation should be conducted, e.g., an ACTH stimulation test. Confirming the diagnosis before starting glucocorticoid treatment is important, as glucocorticoids can complicate the diagnostic workup (Fig. 33.3).

While long-term treatment for dogs with primary hypoadrenocorticism involves both glucocorticoid and mineralocorticoid therapy, mineralocorticoid treatment is not necessary during the acute phase of treatment but should only be started after the dog has been stabilized.

Fluid therapy

Initial fluid therapy should be tailored to address hypovolemia and dehydration. In cases of hypovolemic shock, boluses of 20-30 mL/kg of crystalloids are administered over 10-20 minutes until the patient achieves hemodynamic stability. The response should be evaluated by assessing heart rate, pulse quality, capillary refill time, mental status, and blood pressure. Subsequently, fluid therapy should be continued as deemed necessary based on these parameters, which, in most cases, is at a rate of approximately 1.5 to 2 times the maintenance rate.

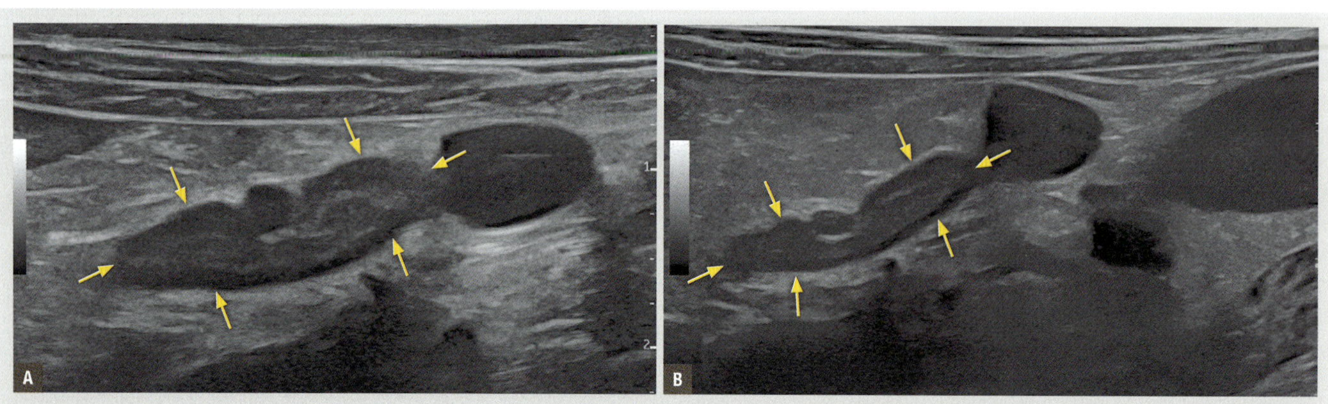

FIG. 33.2 Left adrenal gland of a healthy beagle dog before (A) and after (B) prednisolone therapy for 20 weeks. Dimensions: (A) cranial pole 4.9 mm, caudal pole 5.3 mm; (B) cranial pole 3.5 mm, caudal pole 4.2 mm. ©Vetsuisse Faculty Zurich, UZH/M. Dennler.

Isotonic crystalloid solutions with low potassium concentrations, such as Plasmalyte A, Normosol-R, or Ringer's solution, are recommended as the preferred fluids. These solutions effectively dilute potassium, enhance renal perfusion, and mitigate metabolic acidosis due to their alkalizing properties. Despite their minimal potassium content, these crystalloid solutions are favored over 0.9% saline, which was previously advocated. Using 0.9% saline may seem justified due to its lack of potassium and higher sodium content compared to the fluids mentioned above. However, it is associated with disadvantages, including its acidifying tendency and the potential risk of excessively rapid sodium concentration elevation.

In cases of severe hyponatremia (<125 mmol/L), it is crucial to avoid rapid increases in sodium concentrations to prevent neurological damage, such as osmotic demyelination syndrome characterized by the loss of neuronal myelin sheath in neuronal tissues, particularly the pons and other brain regions. This condition can manifest as neurological symptoms such as ataxia, postural deficits, dysphagia, and altered mental status, which may appear hours or days after initiating treatment.[4] Therefore, for patients with severe hyponatremia, using isotonic crystalloid solutions is mandatory, and the rate of sodium concentration increase should not exceed 10-12 mmol/L/day (or <0.5 mmol/L/h). Close monitoring is essential to ensure appropriate and controlled elevation of sodium concentrations.

Dogs with mild to moderate increases in potassium usually do not require additional treatment for hyperkalemia, as they respond to fluid therapy alone. However, in patients with severe hyperkalemia (>8 mmol/L) and possible accompanying ECG alterations (e.g., loss of P waves, prolonged P-R interval, bradycardia), additional emergency management is necessary and can be life-saving. A 5-10 mL/kg bolus of 50% dextrose over 20 minutes should be administered intravenously. If given through a peripheral vein, it should be diluted to a 25% concentration in an isotonic crystalloid solution to prevent venous irritation caused by the high glucose concentration. This approach utilizes the physiological glucose-potassium cotransport mechanism to decrease

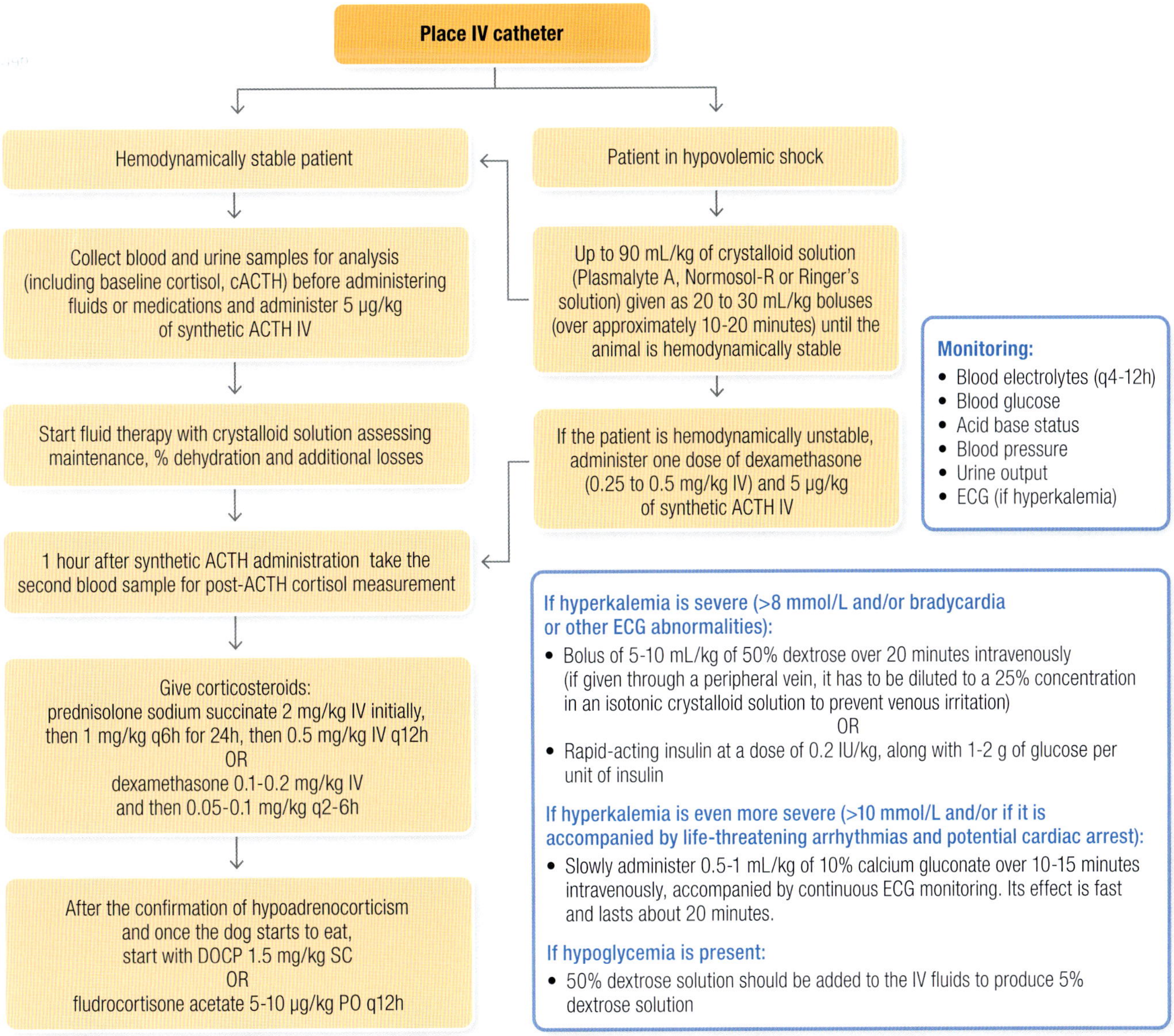

FIG. 33.3 Treatment during the adrenal crisis.

extracellular potassium concentration. Additionally, the glucose infusion can be combined with a rapid-acting insulin at a dose of 0.2 IU/kg, along with 1-2 grams of glucose per unit of insulin administered. This combination accelerates the decrease in potassium concentrations. The combined effect of insulin and dextrose is rapid and lasts approximately 15-30 minutes. Because of the potential development of hypoglycemia, regular monitoring of glucose concentrations is essential during this treatment. The use of 5% dextrose should be avoided, as it can become hypotonic and enter the interstitial space once the dextrose is metabolized.

In cases of even more severe hyperkalemia (>10 mmol/L) and/or if it is accompanied by life-threatening arrhythmias and potential cardiac arrest, administration of 0.5-1 mL/kg of 10% calcium gluconate over 10-15 minutes intravenously should be considered, accompanied by continuous ECG monitoring. Its effect is fast and lasts about 20 minutes. Rapid administration should be avoided, as it may lead to the development of additional arrhythmias and more severe bradycardia. It is important to note that calcium gluconate does not decrease serum potassium concentrations but counteracts the negative effects of potassium on cardiac myocytes. To decrease the potassium concentration, the above-described methods must be used simultaneously. Further, calcium chloride should not be used due to the potential for venous irritation.

Glucocorticoid replacement

Whenever feasible, the administration of glucocorticoids should be postponed until diagnostic tests for hypoadrenocorticism (ACTH stimulation test; endogenous ACTH measurement) have been completed. Delaying the initiation of glucocorticoid therapy is usually not problematic as long as adequate intravenous fluid therapy has been implemented.

However, in cases in which a patient appears to be hemodynamically unstable (e.g., persistent hypotension) and glucocorticoid administration cannot be delayed, treatment with intravenous dexamethasone (0.25-0.5 mg/kg) can be started concurrently while starting the ACTH stimulation test. As dexamethasone is a synthetic glucocorticoid, it does not cross-react with most cortisol assays. The ACTH stimulation test should be started in parallel, as dexamethasone can lead to a diminished cortisol response (approximately 35%) within several hours for up to three days.

After the ACTH stimulation test is terminated, replacement therapy for hypoadrenocorticism can be achieved using various other rapid-acting glucocorticoids (e.g., prednisolone sodium succinate or hydrocortisone sodium succinate). Prednisolone exhibits a relative glucocorticoid activity that is approximately four times greater than that of hydrocortisone, while its mineralocorticoid activity is approximately 0.8 times that of hydrocortisone.[27] A commonly used treatment protocol recommended by our clinic is prednisolone sodium succinate at a starting dose of 2 mg/kg IV; then 1 mg/kg IV every 6 hours for the next 24 hours; the dose can subsequently be reduced to 0.5 mg/kg twice daily until the patient is stable, at which point oral treatment can be started. At discharge from the hospital, the dose can be lowered to 0.5 mg/kg once daily to avoid overt side effects of glucocorticoid therapy. Further lowering and adaptation of the therapy should be tried as soon as possible (see the long-term treatment section below).

Other protocols have been described and recommended.[28,29] However, the choice of a glucocorticoid product and dosing regimen are primarily based on the clinician's experience and preference rather than on the results of randomized controlled trials. In a retrospective study, it was shown that hydrocortisone (a synthetic analog of cortisol with equipotent mineralocorticoid and glucocorticoid activity) at a dose of 0.5 or 0.625 mg/kg/h, together with IV fluids, led to a rapid resolution of hyperkalemia, was well tolerated and reduced the need for extensive fluid resuscitation in certain patients.[28] In a recent and retrospective study comparing hydrocortisone with the conventional protocol of dexamethasone and prednisolone, no clear benefit of hydrocortisone could be shown.[29] Moreover, it seemed as if the use of intravenous hydrocortisone may necessitate longer hospital stays and more intensive monitoring compared to conventional glucocorticoid therapy. In conclusion, while intravenous hydrocortisone is considered safe, there is currently insufficient evidence to support its routine use as an alternative. Prospective studies would be needed to determine its potential advantages and disadvantages compared to those of standard glucocorticoid treatment.

Additional supportive therapy during hospitalization

In dogs with gastrointestinal signs, administering gastroprotectants or antiemetics can help improve general conditions more quickly. The prophylactic use of antibiotics is no longer recommended; instead, its prescription should be based on individual needs. The danger of gastrointestinal translocation leading to sepsis or aspiration pneumonia in cases with megaesophagus are examples of when its use is justified.

In patients with severe anemia, blood transfusions should be considered. Regular reassessment of patients is essential after the initial stabilization phase. Fluid rates should be adjusted to address dehydration and azotemia. Electrolyte concentrations should undergo re-evaluation following the initial stabilization phase and subsequently at regular intervals of 6 to 12 hours to ensure that optimal electrolyte balance is achieved and maintained.

Continuous electrocardiogram (ECG) monitoring is recommended until any arrhythmias are resolved.

If a diagnosis of Addisonian crisis is suspected and emergency treatment is promptly initiated, the majority of patients typically show a rapid response to treatment, with noticeable improvements observed within hours. Discharge from the hospital is usually possible after 2-5 days.

Long-term treatment

Long-term therapy for primary hypoadrenocorticism involves lifelong replacement of both mineralocorticoids and glucocorticoids. Mineralocorticoid treatment should be started during hospitalization as soon as the dog is clinically stable and the danger of a too-rapid increase in serum sodium has passed. Two formulations of mineralocorticoids are available, one long-acting (desoxycortone pivalate) and the other short-acting (fludrocortisone). The most commonly used medication for substituting glucocorticoids is prednisolone.

It is important to emphasize that in the beginning, frequent follow-up evaluations will be required to determine the optimal doses (mineralocorticoid and glucocorticoid medication) for each individual dog. Thereafter, regular lifelong check-ups are also essential, as dosages may need to be adjusted over time.

Mineralocorticoid treatment

Desoxycorticosterone pivalate

Desoxycorticosterone pivalate (DOCP) is a long-acting synthetic mineralocorticoid. Due to the absence of both 11β- and 17α-hydroxylation, it is theoretically expected that it possesses minimal to no glucocorticoid activity. It is available as a prolonged-release suspension in two registered products for treating dogs with hypoadrenocorticism. In the European Union, only desoxycorton pivalate is registered.

The recommended starting dose of DOCP, as indicated in the package insert, is 2.2 mg/kg administered at approximately 25-day intervals.

The products are approved for intramuscular or subcutaneous administration and were shown to be equally potent. Therefore, the choice should be based on the registration of the product in the country in which it is used.

It has been shown that substantially lower doses than those recommended by the manufacturer are sufficient for most dogs with hypoadrenocorticism, independent of the product used.[30-33] Doses as low as 0.4 mg/kg were effective in controlling clinical signs and stabilizing electrolytes within the reference range.[30] Dogs treated with lower doses were not at higher risk of developing an adrenal crisis. This was also demonstrated in more recent studies using DOCP at a starting dose of 1.1 and 1.5 mg/kg, respectively.[31-33] Median maintenance dose during the course of therapy can be anticipated to be around 1.3 mg/kg.[31,32] When the lower dose protocol (1.1 mg/kg) was compared with the standard dose of 2.2 mg/kg, it could be shown that it was just as safe and effective in treatment outcome.[33] In fact, dogs treated with the higher dose had lower urine specific gravity and, on the basis of their overly suppressed plasma renin activity, were more likely to have been overtreated.[33]

Our standard treatment protocol includes a starting dose of 1.5 mg/kg every 28 days for adult dogs, while dogs under 1 year of age receive a higher starting dose of 2.2 mg/kg every 28 days.

After the initial DOCP injection, electrolyte concentrations should be rechecked at 14 and 28 days, aiming to maintain serum sodium and potassium concentrations within the reference range. Adjustments of the DOCP dose can be made according to **Table 33.3**. The authors consistently rely on absolute electrolyte concentrations and advise against using the Na^+/K^+ ratio, as it may be potentially misleading. Subsequent rechecks are typically done after 28 days unless the DOCP dose requires adjustment, in which case **Table 33.3** should be consulted again. The 14-day follow-up examination enables the assessment of treatment response and dictates the dose adjustments to be made for the next injection. Similarly, the 28-day follow-up visit allows for precise modulation of the frequency of DOCP administration based on individual patient requirements.

We recommend taking care if the maintenance dose is lowered below 0.5 mg/kg. The lower the maintenance dose, the higher the potential risk of a crisis if the owner does not strictly adhere to the prescribed dosing schedule.

Extending the dosing interval of DOCP beyond one month has been suggested as an alternative approach in order to reduce treatment costs.[34] While some clinicians recommend this approach, we caution against it: increasing the interval between injections raises the risk of owners forgetting the next administration, which can potentially lead to a life-threatening adrenal crisis. Owner compliance can probably improve if they adhere to a once-monthly injection regimen. Therefore, we prefer to adjust the DOCP dose as described above and summarized in **Table 33.3**.

Once the appropriate DOCP dose has been determined, regular rechecks are recommended every 4-6 months, aligned with the scheduled DOCP injections. A well-controlled dog should exhibit an active and happy demeanor, have a healthy appetite, and show no signs of overtreatment, such as excessive urination, increased thirst, muscle wasting, a dull hair coat, or hair loss. Serum potassium and sodium concentrations should be within the reference interval.

One drawback of using DOCP is that it has to be injected (**Video 33.1**). Additionally, pain at the injection site may occur with DOCP administration. However, following the proper manufacturer's instructions can help minimize discomfort. Prior to drawing the suspension into the syringe, it should be thoroughly resuspended by gently rolling and shaking the vial. The injection should be given immediately, ensuring the suspension remains well-mixed. A needle with a large diameter (at least 22G) should be used to facilitate swift injection of the entire volume (**Video 33.1**). Most owners can be instructed in this procedure so that they are able to inject the dog on their own.

TABLE 33.3 Adjustment of DOCP dose according to the potassium concentrations on days 14 and 28 after DOCP injection.

Day 0	Day 14*/**	Day 28*/**	Recommended dose adaption	Special comment
Adult dogs: DOCP 1.5 mg/kg SC **Dogs <1 year and cats:** DOCP 2.2 mg/kg SC	K^+ normal	K^+ normal	Inject DOCP at the same dose.	Recheck after 28 days, if this was after the first DOCP injection. Recheck after 3 months, if this was after the second DOCP injection.
	K^+ normal	K^+ low	No DOCP injection. Recheck electrolytes every 7 days until K^+ is within the reference range. At that time, inject DOCP, but reduce the dose by 10% for every 7-day delay.***	Recheck after 28 days.
	K^+ normal	K^+ high	Inject DOCP and increase dose by 10%.	Recheck after 28 days.
	K^+ low	K^+ normal	Inject DOCP and decrease dose by 10%.***	Recheck after 28 days.
	K^+ low	K^+ low	No DOCP injection. Recheck electrolytes every 7 days until K^+ is normal. At that time inject DOCP but reduce the dose by 10% for every 7-day delay.***	Recheck after 28 days.
	K^+ low	K^+ high	Inject DOCP and increase dose by 10%.	Recheck after 14 and 28 days.
	K^+ high	K^+ high	Inject DOCP and increase dose by 10-20%.	Recheck after 14 and 28 days.

*At each recheck, sodium and potassium should be measured. Measuring the electrolytes in the same material (serum, heparin-plasma) is always important. Otherwise, the values cannot be compared. **Sodium alone is less suitable for dose control than potassium. Ideally, sodium should be in the upper half of the reference range on day 14 and in the lower half of the reference range on day 28. ***If potassium is within the reference range and sodium shows significant deviations, the dose adjustment on day 28 must also be based on the sodium concentration (e.g., if sodium is below the reference range, there is no decrease in the DOCP dose).

Video 33.1

Video showing the material needed for a DOCP injection and the important points of the procedure. ©Vetsuisse Faculty Zurich, UZH. Film director: Prof. Dr. med. Nadja Sieber-Ruckstuhl; date: 4.10.2023; title: DOCP injection.

Fludrocortisone acetate

Fludrocortisone acetate, a short-acting mineralocorticoid, not only demonstrates significant mineralocorticoid activity but also possesses notable glucocorticoid activity, estimated to be approximately 10 times that of cortisol. It is available in two oral formulations (both human products) and can serve as an alternative to DOCP for supplementing mineralocorticoids. While therapy with short-acting formulations may be more cost-effective in certain countries, it is crucial to adhere to national regulations, considering that these formulations are not licensed for use in dogs.

The recommended starting dose is 0.01-0.02 mg/kg/day administered orally, divided into two daily doses. The effectiveness of fludrocortisone acetate treatment is regularly evaluated by monitoring clinical manifestations, renal function (blood urea nitrogen and serum creatinine concentration), and serum electrolyte concentrations (sodium and potassium). Adjustments of the fludrocortisone acetate dosage primarily depend on the serum potassium concentrations. Dose modifications are typically made in increments of 0.025-0.1 mg per dog, considering the individual dog's size. The main drawback of fludrocortisone acetate is its significant glucocorticoid activity. In many dogs, especially large breed dogs, the fludrocortisone dose must be increased to reach sufficient mineralocorticoid effect (to get the potassium concentration into the normal range). With the higher fludrocortisone dose, however, many dogs experience significant glucocorticoid side effects (Fig. 33.4 and Fig. 33.5). One study showed that fludrocortisone acetate is inferior to DOCP in its overall mineralocorticoid efficacy, as it is less effective in suppressing the increased plasma renin activity.[35] Another advantage of DOCP is that it lacks glucocorticoid effects, allowing for separate management of mineralocorticoid and glucocorticoid needs, thereby reducing the risk of glucocorticoid-related side effects through overdosing. The results of an online survey conducted among Western European veterinarians revealed that almost 80% preferred prescribing DOCP over fludrocortisone as a first-line treatment for mineralocorticoid supplementation.[36]

Glucocorticoid treatment

Dogs with DOCP

In dogs undergoing DOCP treatment, a daily administration of glucocorticoids is an absolute requirement. Upon discharge, dogs are typically prescribed an initial dose of 0.5 mg/kg/day of prednisolone, which can subsequently be reduced to 0.25 mg/kg/day after three days. At the first recheck, scheduled 14 days after DOCP injection (see above), a gradual reduction in prednisolone dosage is initiated, with an approximate 50% decrease every seven days. The aim is to achieve a final dosage of about 0.05-0.1 mg/kg/day. However, it should be noted that certain dogs, particularly those of larger breeds, may exhibit increased sensitivity to glucocorticoid side effects. Therefore, in such cases, it is advisable to individualize the final glucocorticoid dosage towards the lower end of the recommended range or even below it.

Dogs with fludrocortisone

Fludrocortisone acetate possesses some glucocorticoid activity, which may eliminate the need for additional glucocorticoid therapy in certain dogs, especially those requiring higher doses of fludrocortisone. Our approach involves initiating dogs on 0.5 mg/kg/day of prednisolone upon discharge, with the dose reduced to 0.25 mg/kg/day after three days. At the first recheck, scheduled 14 days after discharge, a gradual reduction in prednisolone dosage is initiated, with an approximate 50% decrease every seven days. The aim is to achieve a final dosage of about 0.05 mg/kg/day.

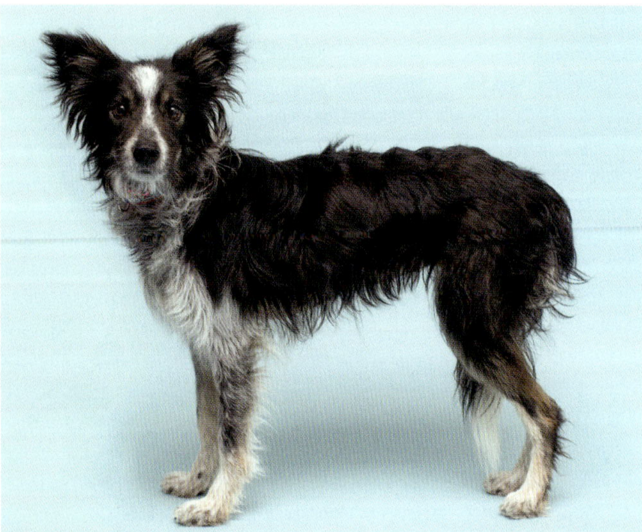

FIG. 33.4 A 5-year-old Border Collie with hypoadrenocorticism, treated with fludrocortisone and prednisolone and showing clear signs of iatrogenic hyperadrenocorticism (polyuria, polydipsia, thin skin, hair coat changes). ©Vetsuisse Faculty Zurich, UZH/M.A. Oesch.

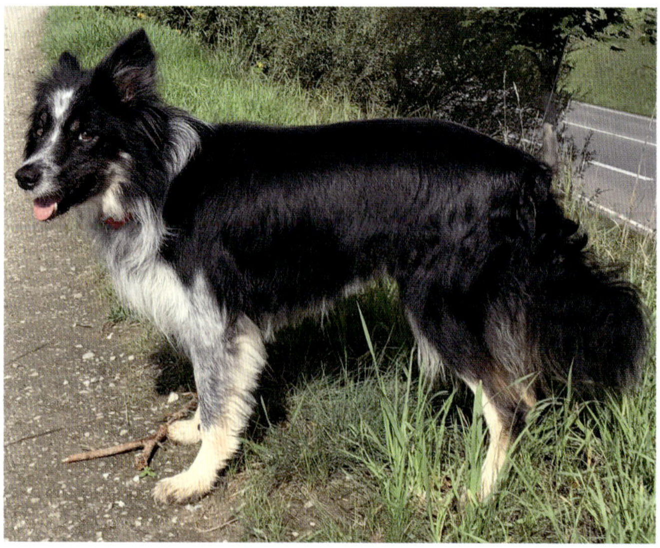

FIG. 33.5 The same Border Collie as in Fig. 33.4, 3 years after changing the therapy to DOCP and prednisolone. Picture taken by the dog's owner.

In cases where glucocorticoid side effects manifest, an attempt should be made to gradually withdraw the dog from additional glucocorticoid treatment entirely. Approximately 50% of dogs treated with fludrocortisone acetate will not require glucocorticoid therapy in the long run. Generally, the dosage of glucocorticoids in dogs with hypoadrenocorticism is adjusted on the basis of their clinical condition. The aim is to ensure the dogs are stable in their daily lives without manifesting signs of glucocorticoid overtreatment. One study investigated the utility of monitoring endogenous ACTH concentrations as a means of optimizing glucocorticoid dose during replacement therapy.[37] The findings showed the potential benefits of this approach. However, due to the limited sample size, further investigations are warranted to establish the validity and applicability of ACTH measurement during long-term treatment.

Glucocorticoid requirements during stressful situations

The demand for glucocorticoids increases during periods of stress. However, the need for dosage adjustments depends on several factors, including the daily long-term glucocorticoid dose, individual stress perception, and the dog's temperament.

Initially, basic training is provided to dog owners during the first rechecks, and general guidelines are offered. However, it is crucial for them to promptly seek veterinary assistance, especially in acute episodes.

Following our guidelines for a glucocorticoid boost:

- Mild to moderate stressors, such as long car or train journeys or an influx of visitors during holidays, may require doubling or tripling the daily glucocorticoid dose. This recommendation, however, depends on the individual response and needs to be adjusted accordingly.
- In the case of an acute event, such as sudden illness or an accident, the dose should be increased to 0.5-2 mg/kg/day, depending on the severity of the incident.
- For planned surgical procedures, a dose escalation to 0.5-2 mg/kg/day (based on the procedure's severity) is advised two days prior, as well as maintaining this dosage until discharge or one day thereafter.

While adjusting the glucocorticoid dose during stressful situations is important, caution should be exercised to avoid excessive and frequent dose increases due to owner anxiety. Long-term excessive dosing can lead to chronic glucocorticoid overdosing and the iatrogenic induction of hyperadrenocorticism, characterized by typical clinical symptoms such as polyuria, polydipsia, panting, hair loss, and muscle wasting.

Prognosis

With proper treatment and diligent monitoring, the prognosis for dogs diagnosed with naturally occurring hypoadrenocorticism is very good. Reported survival time was shown to be approximately 5 years, and the majority of deaths were attributed to causes unrelated to hypoadrenocorticism.[38,39] It is crucial to emphasize to owners the importance of lifelong, consistent medication administration and regular veterinary monitoring of the dog. Deviation from the prescribed DOCP medication schedule, including skipping doses or extending the treatment interval without veterinary authorization, can significantly elevate the risk of a crisis. It is of utmost importance to strictly adhere to the recommended treatment protocol and seek professional guidance to prevent such complications. Consequently, a high level of commitment is required of the owner, and it can be anticipated that the disease will have an impact on the daily routine of both the owner and the dog. According to an online survey conducted among owners of dogs with hypoadrenocorticism, the majority of owners reported that their own quality of life was not affected by their dog's disease; however, only about one-third of the owners reported no discernible effect on their dog's quality of life resulting from the disease.[38,39] The primary concerns highlighted by owners included the apprehension of their dog experiencing an adrenal crisis (49%) and feeling hesitant to leave their dog unattended (37%). About two-thirds perceived a strengthened bond between themselves and their canine companion following the diagnosis.

References

1. Boag AM, Catchpole B. A review of the genetics of hypoadrenocorticism. *Top Companion Anim Med* 29(4):96-101, 2014. doi:10.1053/j.tcam.2015.01.001.
2. Boag AM, Christie MR, McLaughlin KA, et al. A longitudinal study of autoantibodies against cytochrome P450 side-chain cleavage enzyme in dogs (*Canis lupus familiaris*) affected with hypoadrenocorticism (Addison's disease). *Vet Immunol Immunopathol* 202:41-45, 2018. doi:10.1016/j.vetimm.2018.05.013.
3. Guzmán Ramos PJ, Bennaim M, Shiel RE, et al. Diagnosis of canine spontaneous hypoadrenocorticism. *Canine Med Genet* 9(1):6, 2022. doi:10.1186/s40575-022-00119-4.
4. Scott-Moncrieff JC. Hypoadrenocorticism. In Feldman EC, Nelson RW, Reusch C, Scott-Moncrieff JC (editors). Canine and Feline Endocrinology and Reproduction 4th edition. St. Louis, Elsevier, 2015, pp. 485-520.
5. Oberbauer AM, Bell JS, Belanger JM, et al. Genetic evaluation of Addison's disease in the Portuguese Water Dog. *BMC Vet Res* 2:15, 2006. doi:10.1186/1746-6148-2-15.
6. Tardo AM, Del Baldo F, Leal RO, Galiazzo G, Pietra M, Gaspardo A, Fracassi F. Prevalence of eunatremic, eukalemic hypoadrenocorticism in dogs with signs of chronic gastrointestinal disease and risk of misdiagnosis after previous glucocorticoid administration. *J Vet Intern Med*, 2023 doi:10.1111/jvim.16921. Epub ahead of print.
7. Gallego AF, Gow AG, Boag AM. Evaluation of resting cortisol concentration testing in dogs with chronic gastrointestinal signs. *J Vet Intern Med* 36(2):525-531, 2022. doi:10.1111/jvim.16365.
8. Hauck C, Schmitz SS, Burgener IA, et al. Prevalence and characterization of hypoadrenocorticism in dogs with signs of chronic gastrointestinal disease: A multicenter study. *J Vet Intern Med* 34(4):1399-1405, 2020. doi:10.1111/jvim.15752.
9. Thompson AL, Scott-Moncrieff JC, Anderson JD. Comparison of classic hypoadrenocorticism with glucocorticoid-deficient hypoadrenocorticism in dogs: 46 cases (1985-2005). *J Am Vet Med Assoc* 230(8):1190-1194, 2007. doi:10.2460/javma.230.8.1190.
10. Adler JA, Drobatz KJ, Hess RS. Abnormalities of serum electrolyte concentrations in dogs with hypoadrenocorticism. *J Vet Intern Med* 21(6):1168-73, 2007. doi:10.1892/06-270.1.
11. Langlais-Burgess L, Lumsden JH, Mackin A. Concurrent hypoadrenocorticism and hypoalbuminemia in dogs: a retrospective study. *J Am Anim Hosp Assoc* 31(4):307-311, 1995. doi:10.5326/15473317-31-4-307.
12. Feldman EC, Nelson RW. Hypoadrenocorticism (Addison's disease). In Feldman EC, Nelson RW (editors). Canine and Feline Endocrinology and Reproduction 3rd edition. St. Louis, Saunders/Elsevier, 2004, pp. 394-439.

13. Reusch CE, Fracassi F, Sieber-Ruckstuhl NS, et al. Altered serum thyrotropin concentrations in dogs with primary hypoadrenocorticism before and during treatment. *J Vet Intern Med* 31(6):1643-1648, 2017. doi:10.1111/jvim.14840.
14. Lathan P, Thompson AL. Management of hypoadrenocorticism (Addison's disease) in dogs. *Vet Med (Auckl)* 9:1-10, 2018. doi:10.2147/VMRR.S125617.
15. Kemppainen RJ, Sartin JL, Peterson ME. Effects of single intravenously administered doses of dexamethasone on response to the adrenocorticotropic hormone stimulation test in dogs. *Am J Vet Res* 50(11):1914-1917, 1989.
16. Javadi S, Galac S, Boer P, et al. Aldosterone-to-renin and cortisol-to-adrenocorticotropic hormone ratios in healthy dogs and dogs with primary hypoadrenocorticism. *J Vet Intern Med* 20(3):556-61, 2006. doi:10.1892/0891-6640(2006)20[556:aachri]2.0.co;2.
17. Lathan P, Scott-Moncrieff JC, Wills RW. Use of the cortisol-to-ACTH ratio for diagnosis of primary hypoadrenocorticism in dogs. *J Vet Intern Med* 28(5):1546-1550, 2014. doi:10.1111/jvim.12392.
18. Boretti FS, Meyer F, Burkhardt WA, et al. Evaluation of the cortisol-to-ACTH ratio in dogs with hypoadrenocorticism, dogs with diseases mimicking hypoadrenocorticism and in healthy dogs. *J Vet Intern Med* 29(5):1335-1341, 2015. doi:10.1111/jvim.13593.
19. Baumstark ME, Sieber-Ruckstuhl NS, Müller C, et al. Evaluation of aldosterone concentrations in dogs with hypoadrenocorticism. *J Vet Intern Med* 28(1):154-159, 2014. doi:10.1111/jvim.12243.
20. Zeugswetter FK, Schwendenwein I. Diagnostic efficacy of the leukogram and the chemiluminometric ACTH measurement to diagnose canine hypoadrenocorticism. *Tierarztl Prax Ausg K Kleintiere Heimtiere* 42(4):223-230, 2014.
21. Lennon EM, Hummel JB, Vaden SL. Urine sodium concentrations are predictive of hypoadrenocorticism in hyponatraemic dogs: a retrospective pilot study. *J Small Anim Pract* 59(4):228-231, 2018. doi:10.1111/jsap.12792. Erratum in *J Small Anim Pract* 59(7):450, 2018.
22. Dropkin CA, Kruger JM, Langlois DK. Evaluation of urine electrolytes for the diagnosis of hypoadrenocorticism in dogs. *Vet Clin Pathol* 50(4):507-514, 2021. doi:10.1111/vcp.13018.
23. Del Baldo F, Gerou Ferriani M, Bertazzolo W, et al. Urinary cortisol-creatinine ratio in dogs with hypoadrenocorticism. *J Vet Intern Med* 36(2):482-487, 2022. doi: 10.1111/jvim.16358. Erratum in *J Vet Intern Med* 37(3):1287, 2023.
24. Wenger M, Mueller C, Kook PH, et al. Ultrasonographic evaluation of adrenal glands in dogs with primary hypoadrenocorticism or mimicking diseases. *Vet Rec* 167(6):207-210, 2010. doi:10.1136/vr.c4235.
25. Reagan KL, McLarty E, Marks SL, et al. Characterization of clinicopathologic and abdominal ultrasound findings in dogs with glucocorticoid deficient hypoadrenocorticism. *J Vet Intern Med* 36(6):1947-1957, 2022. doi:10.1111/jvim.16564.
26. Seiler GS, Cohen EB, d'Anjou MA, et al. ACVR and ECVDI consensus statement for the standardization of the abdominal ultrasound examination. *Vet Radiol Ultrasound* 63(6):661-674, 2022. doi:10.1111/vru.13151.
27. Sieber-Ruckstuhl NS, Reusch CE. Glucocorticoid therapy. In Feldman EC; Fracassi F, Peterson ME (editors). Feline Endocrinology. Milano, Edra Publishing, 2019, pp. 422-430.
28. Gunn E, Shiel RE, Mooney CT. Hydrocortisone in the management of acute hypoadrenocorticism in dogs: a retrospective series of 30 cases. *J Small Anim Pract* 57(5):227-33, 2016. doi:10.1111/jsap.12473.
29. Mitropoulou A, Häuser MK, Lehmann H, et al. Comparison of hydrocortisone continuous rate infusion and prednisolone or dexamethasone administration for treatment of acute hypoadrenocortical (Addisonian) crisis in dogs. *Front Vet Sci* 8:818515, 2022. doi:10.3389/fvets.2021.818515.
30. Bates JA, Shott S, Schall WD. Lower initial dose of desoxycorticosterone pivalate for treatment of canine primary hypoadrenocorticism. *Aust Vet J* 91(3):77-82, 2013. doi:10.1111/avj.12019.
31. Sieber-Ruckstuhl NS, Reusch CE, Hofer-Inteeworn N, et al. Evaluation of a low-dose desoxycorticosterone pivalate treatment protocol for long-term management of dogs with primary hypoadrenocorticism. *J Vet Intern Med* 33(3):1266-1271, 2019. doi:10.1111/jvim.15475.
32. Münch L, Münch M, Paul H, et al. Therapie des primären Hypoadrenokortizismus beim Hund mit niedrig dosiertem Desoxycorticosteronpivalat [Therapy of primary hypoadrenocorticism in dogs with low dose desoxycorticosterone pivalate]. *Tierarztl Prax Ausg K Kleintiere Heimtiere* 48(3):171-175, 2020. doi:10.1055/a-1166-8800.
33. Vincent AM, Okonkowski LK, Brudvig JM, et al. Low-dose desoxycorticosterone pivalate treatment of hypoadrenocorticism in dogs: A randomized controlled clinical trial. *J Vet Intern Med* 35(4):1720-1728, 2021. doi: 10.1111/jvim.16195.
34. Jaffey JA, Nurre P, Cannon AB, et al. Desoxycorticosterone pivalate duration of action and individualized dosing intervals in dogs with primary hypoadrenocorticism. *J Vet Intern Med* 31(6):1649-1657, 2017. doi:10.1111/jvim.14828.
35. Baumstark ME, Nussberger J, Boretti FS, et al. Use of plasma renin activity to monitor mineralocorticoid treatment in dogs with primary hypoadrenocorticism: desoxycorticosterone versus fludrocortisone. *J Vet Intern Med* 28(5):1471-1478, 2014. doi:10.1111/jvim.12426.
36. Rebocho R, Domínguez-Ruiz M, Englar RE, et al. Use of deoxycorticosterone pivalate by veterinarians: A Western European survey. *Vet Sci* 8(11):271, 2021. doi:10.3390/vetsci8110271.
37. Zeugswetter FK, Haninger T. Prednisolone dosages in Addisonian dogs after integration of ACTH measurement into treatment surveillance. *Tierarztl Prax Ausg K Kleintiere Heimtiere* 46(2):90-96, 2018. doi:10.15654/TPK-170668.
38. Hupfeld J, Dölle M, Volk H, et al. Effect of long-term management of hypoadrenocorticism on the quality of life of affected dogs and their owners. *Vet Rec* 191(10):e1977, 2022. doi:10.1002/vetr.1977.
39. Hazuchova K. Optimising the long-term management of dogs with hypoadrenocorticism. *Vet Rec* 191(10):414-416, 2022. doi:10.1002/vetr.2458.

CHAPTER 34

Cushing's syndrome

Carolina Arenas
DVM, PhD, DECVIM-CA (Internal Medicine)

Carlos Melián
DVM, PhD

Sara Galac
DVM, PhD

Henk van den Broek
DVM, PhD, DECVDI

Stefanie Veraa
DVM, PhD, DECVDI

Stefania Golinelli
DVM, PhD

Björn Meij
DVM, PhD, DECVS

Sara Del Magno
DVM, PhD, DECVS

Sebastiaan A. van Nimwegen
DVM, PhD, DECVS

Maurice Zandvliet
DVM, PhD, DECVIM-CA (Medicine and Oncology)

Jérôme Benoit
DVM, DACVR (Radiation Oncology), DECVDI (Radiation Oncology)

Pathogenesis and clinical manifestations

Carolina Arenas, Carlos Melián

Cushing's syndrome, or hypercortisolism (HC), is a common endocrine disorder in dogs resulting from chronic exposure to an excess of glucocorticoid activity. Canine HC can occur as a naturally-occurring condition or from the administration of exogenous glucocorticoids, and it may represent a challenge in veterinary practice due to its diverse clinical manifestations and potential complications. This chapter aims to provide a comprehensive overview of the pathogenesis and clinical manifestation and endocrine diagnosis of naturally-occurring HC.

Pathogenesis

Cortisol is secreted by the adrenal cortex, and its production and release are regulated by the adrenocorticotropic hormone (ACTH), which is produced and secreted in the pars distalis and pars intermedia of the pituitary gland.[1,2] HC can be broadly classified into two categories based on its underlying cause: ACTH-dependent and ACTH-independent hypercortisolism.[3] Pituitary-dependent hypercortisolism (PDH) is the most common form of ACTH-dependent HC, while most cases of ACTH-independent hypercortisolism are caused by an autonomous cortisol secretion by the adrenal cortex.[1-3] Less common types of ACTH-dependent HC include ectopic ACTH syndrome, and ACTH-independent HC as a result of aberrant adrenocortical receptor expression.

ACTH-dependent hypercortisolism

In 80% to 85% of cases, spontaneous canine HC is pituitary-dependent and caused by a dysregulation of ACTH secretion by the pituitary gland due to a pituitary corticotroph tumor or hyperplasia, resulting in autonomous secretion of ACTH, bilateral adrenocortical hyperplasia and chronic hypercortisolism[1,3] (Fig. 34.1). In approximately 70% of dogs with PDH, the pituitary tumor arises from the pars distalis and the remaining 30% from the pars intermedia. Most pituitary tumors are adenomas, while invasive adenomas and carcinomas are considered rare. Advanced imaging methods can be helpful in identifying invasive adenomas by detecting their growth into surrounding brain tissue or nearby structures and carcinomas when there is metastatic disease.[3]

Ectopic ACTH syndrome is a rare cause of ACTH-dependent HC in dogs caused by an uncontrolled secretion of ACTH from a nonpituitary site, usually a carcinoid (a malignant tumor of neuroendocrine origin).[3] Isolated case reports of canine HC due to ectopic ACTH secretion have been described in dogs with several types of neuroendocrine tumors, including metastatic neuroendocrine tumors involving pancreatic lymph nodes and liver, mesenteric neuroendocrine tumors, liver carcinoids, and pheochromocytoma.[4-7]

ACTH-independent hypercortisolism

In approximately 15-20% of dogs with Cushing's syndrome, HC originated in the adrenal cortex (adrenal-dependent hypercortisolism or ADHC), generally associated with adrenal neoplasia (adenoma or adenocarcinoma) or, less commonly, with primary adrenal hyperplasia.[3,5] Excessive circulating cortisol concentration results in negative feedback on the hypothalamus and pituitary gland, leading to suppressed endogenous ACTH concentration, which tends to cause atrophy of the contralateral adrenal gland and the remaining non-neoplastic cortisol-secreting cells of the affected gland[1] (Fig. 34.1). Most functional adrenal tumors are unilateral, although bilateral tumors can occur.

A less common form of ACTH-independent HC has been reported and is caused by an aberrant expression of receptors in the adrenal cortex.[6,7] Food-responsive hypercortisolism due to receptors for the gastrointestinal hormone gastric inhibitory polypeptide (GIP) is considered a subtype of aberrant adrenal expression. In this form of HC, food ingestion induces GIP release from the small intestine that binds to its receptor in the adrenal gland, causing excess cortisol secretion.[6] Recently, luteinizing

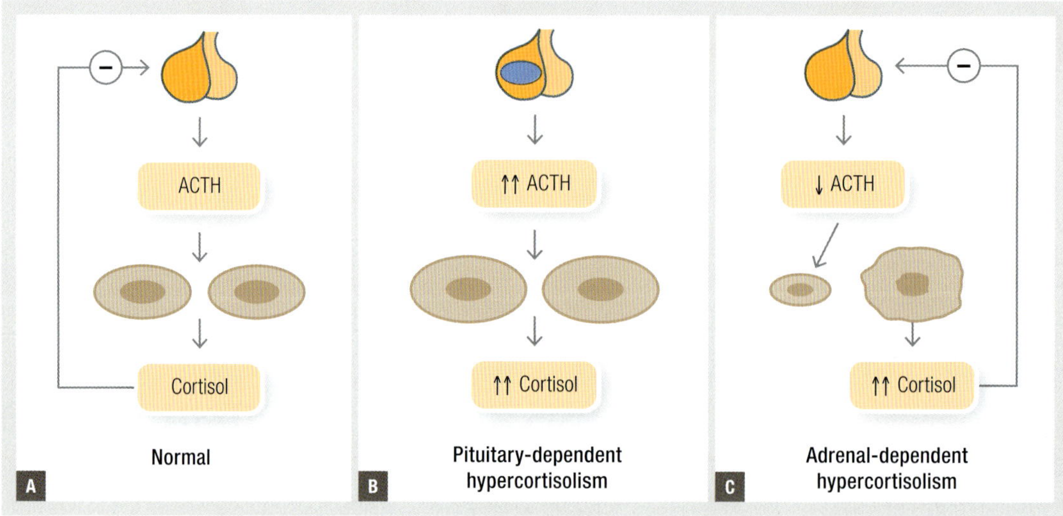

FIG. 34.1 Simplified scheme of the pituitary-adrenal gland axis in normal dogs (**A**), in dogs with pituitary-dependent hypercortisolism (**B**), and dogs with adrenal-dependent hypercortisolism (**C**).

hormone (LH)-dependent HC has been proposed to occur in spayed female dogs. The elevated circulating LH concentrations after spaying could be responsible for aberrant LH receptor activation in the adrenal cortex resulting in hypercortisolemia.[7]

Epidemiology

Hypercortisolism is a very common endocrine disease, with a recently reported prevalence between 0.2- 0.28%.[8,9] It occurs in middle-aged to older dogs. The mean age at diagnosis in several studies ranges from 10 to 11 years. Although the majority of dogs with HC are >6 years of age, dogs younger than 2 years have also been reported presenting growth retardation alongside the classical clinical signs.[1,2,8-10] Sex association is still questionable as female dogs have been over-represented in some studies, whereas others have not shown major sex association with HC.[1,8-10] Some breeds have been reported to be at risk for HC, including Bichon Frisé, Border Terrier, Jack Russell Terrier, Yorkshire Terrier, Miniature Schnauzer, Miniature Poodle, Boxer, and Dachshund.[9-11] The proportion of dogs >20 kg is significantly higher in dogs with functional adrenal tumors compared to those with PDH.[2]

Clinical features

Clinical signs, irrespective of the etiology, are caused by excess serum cortisol secretion. These signs may develop over months, and many owners consider early signs as part of the normal aging process and may not seek veterinary attention until the signs are more advanced. Clinical signs of iatrogenic HC are identical to those with naturally-occurring HC. The most common clinical findings at presentation (Table 34.1) are polyuria, polydipsia (PU/PD), polyphagia, abdominal distension, alopecia, panting, and muscle weakness. Polyuria-polydipsia is observed in around 80-90% of dogs. There are multiple factors that may contribute to PU/PD in dogs with HC, which include increased renal glomerular filtration rate, a direct effect of glucocorticoid on renal responsiveness to vasopressin, impaired osmoregulation of vasopressin release and osmotic diuresis secondary to glycosuria in dogs with concurrent diabetes mellitus.[1-3] Some dogs develop a degree of bladder atonicity, which can lead to overflow incontinence.[2] Urinary tract infection (UTI) is also common in dogs, with HC being *E. coli* the most frequent pathogen identified. However, UTI might be subclinical in a great proportion of dogs due to the anti-inflammatory effects of glucocorticoids.[12] Urolithiasis has been reported in 2.8% of dogs with HC and may also contribute to UTI.[11] Calcium-containing stones are the most frequently reported as glucocorticoids increase urinary calcium excretion.

Polyphagia is also frequent (46-84%), and it is assumed to be a direct effect of glucocorticoids on appetite and can be exacerbated in dogs with concurrent diabetes mellitus.[2] In some cases, hyporexia or even anorexia can occur, which is frequently associated with the presence of a concurrent disease and/or a severely enlarged pituitary tumor.[2,13]

Abdominal distension is a classical clinical sign and frequent in these dogs, occurring in up to 73% of dogs with HC. This "potbellied" appearance develops as a result of abdominal muscular weakness (due to cortisol-induced protein catabolism), fat accumulation within the abdomen, and increased abdominal contents (due to hepatomegaly resulting from glycogen deposition and a large urinary bladder due to polyuria).[1-3]

Muscular weakness and lethargy are also frequently reported due to muscular wasting secondary to the catabolic effects of glucocorticoids.[2] Infrequently, some dogs may have difficulty standing up. Panting

TABLE 34.1 Clinical signs and comorbidities of canine hypercortisolism.

Most common	Less common	Uncommon
Polyuria/polydipsia	Lethargy	Calcinosis cutis
Polyphagia	Hyperpigmentation/comedones/pyoderma	Mucocele
Abdominal distension	Facial nerve paralysis	Thromboembolism
Panting	Anestrus/testicular atrophy	Ligament rupture
Alopecia	Urinary tract infection	Urinary calculi
Thin skin	Neurological signs	Anorexia
Muscle weakness	Diabetes mellitus	Pseudomyotonia
Systemic hypertension		

Modified from Behrend EN, et al., 2013.[22]

(Fig. 34.2) is common and can be due to respiratory muscle weakness; however, other factors such as increased diaphragmatic pressure due to abdominal distension, pulmonary hypertension, pulmonary and bronchial mineralization leading to decreased lung compliance, and, less commonly, pulmonary thromboembolism, may contribute.[1,14]

Dermatological signs are also frequent and a common owner concern. These include bilateral symmetric alopecia (Fig. 34.3A and Fig. 34.4), thin skin (Fig. 34.3B), hyperpigmentation (Fig. 34.5), pyoderma, comedones, and poor hair regrowth. Less common dermatological manifestations include calcinosis cutis and bruising. Calcinosis cutis occurs (Fig. 34.6) due to dystrophic calcium dermal deposition, but the pathogenesis is not completely understood; abnormal collagen fibrils as a direct effect of glucocorticoids and/or secondary hyperparathyroidism may play a role in its development.[15,16] Bruising (Fig. 34.3B) may occur secondary to venipuncture, minor trauma and/or after surgery, as well as poor wound healing. Cortisol-induced inhibition of collagen synthesis, leading to weaker and fragile blood vessel walls and atrophy of subcutaneous tissue may predispose to it.[2]

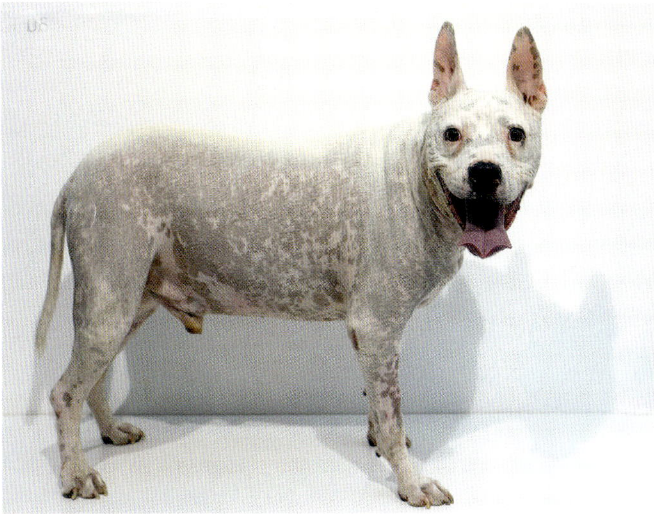

FIG. 34.2 A 10-year-old castrated male mixed breed dog with pituitary-dependent hypercortisolism with continuous panting, hair thinning, and distended abdomen.

Neurological signs may develop in 10-30% of dogs with PDH; these might include inappetence, anorexia, dullness, altered mentation, stupor, behavioral changes, circling, head pressing, aimless wandering, ataxia, and seizures.[1,17] In some studies, these neurological signs have been reported even in a higher proportion of dogs, probably reflecting the fact that nonspecific clinical signs (e.g., mental dullness, lethargy, and inappetence) were also included.[13] Neurological signs may develop secondary to an enlarged pituitary tumor, which is compressing and invading the hypothalamus and other suprasellar structures, but also due to pituitary apoplexy, a syndrome characterized by acute neurological signs that result from hemorrhage or infarction within the pituitary gland.[13,18,19]

Hypertension is also common, affecting as much as 82% of dogs with HC, and its pathogenesis is likely multifactorial.[20] Nearly half of the dogs that develop systemic hypertension are severely hypertensive (systolic blood pressure >180 mmHg). Risk factors associated with its development are thrombocytosis, hypokalemia, and proteinuria.[20] Both dogs with PDH and ADHC are at risk of developing systemic hypertension. While some studies have found no difference in the prevalence and the severity of systemic hypertension between dogs with PDH and ADHC,[20] some others have reported a higher frequency of systemic hypertension in dogs with functional adrenal tumors.[2,20] Systemic hypertension does not always improve despite adequate medical treatment in dogs with PDH, and some dogs may even develop systemic hypertension during treatment with trilostane.[21]

Thromboembolism is a complication associated with HC with a reported frequency of 6.1% in a recent study;[11] particularly, pulmonary thromboembolism has been identified in 2.7% of dogs with HC on necropsy.[3]

Less common clinical presentations include anestrus, testicular atrophy, facial palsy, ligament laxicity that may lead to tearing and lameness and pseudomyotonia.[1,11,22] Severe muscle stiffness, also known as pseudomyotonia or Cushing's myotonia, is a myopathy characterized by persistent, active muscle contraction of the thoracic legs, all four legs or more frequently just affecting the pelvic legs (Video 34.1). It is a condition that most commonly affects dogs with PDH, although it has also been described in dogs with iatrogenic HC.[23,24] The condition is nonpainful and results in an extremely stiff and stilted gait and, in more advanced cases, an inability to ambulate.[2,23] Electromyography shows myotonic, bizarre, and high-frequency discharges. Histopathology

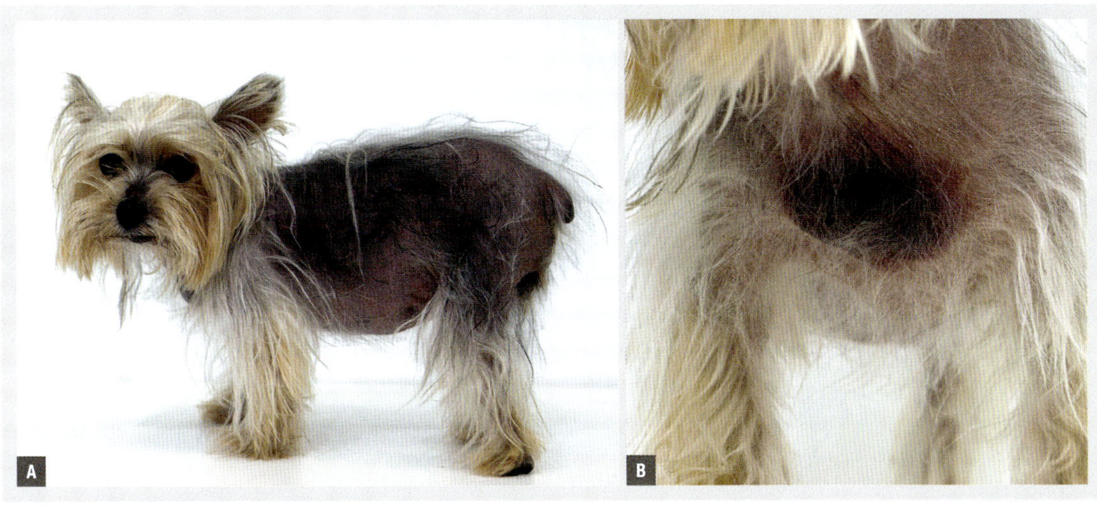

FIG. 34.3 A 9-year-old intact female Yorkshire Terrier with pituitary-dependent hypercortisolism with a 6-month history of polyuria and polydipsia. (A) Distended abdomen and truncal alopecia. (B) Thin skin and bruising at the jugular venipuncture site.

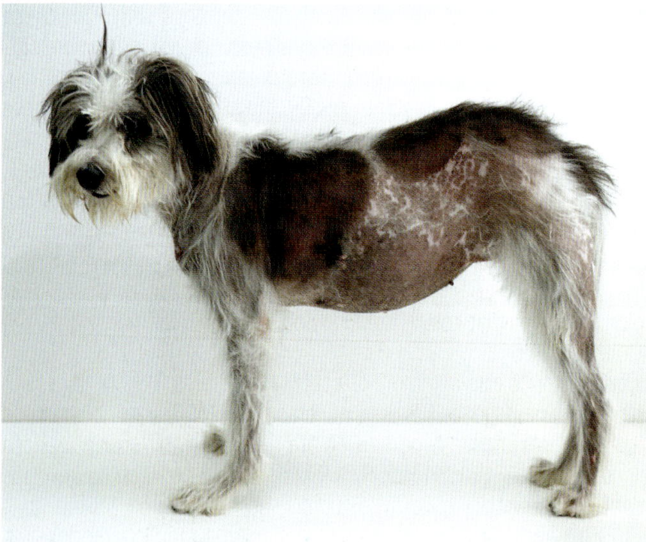

FIG. 34.4 A 10-year-old female spayed mixed breed with pituitary-dependent hypercortisolism with a distended abdomen and truncal alopecia.

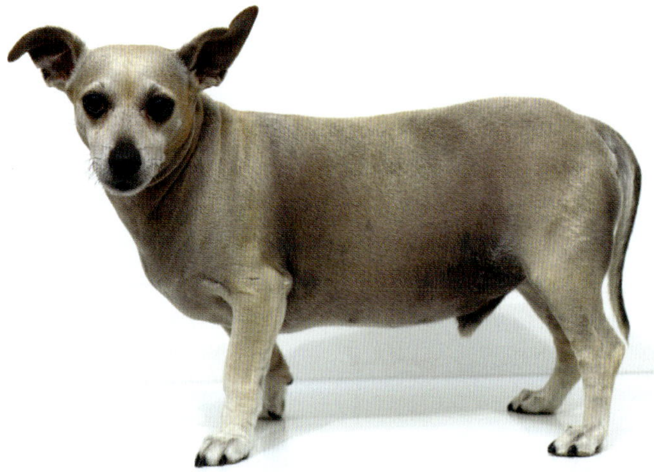

FIG. 34.5 An 8-year-old male, mixed breed, with adrenal-dependent hypercortisolism and diabetes mellitus with a 7-month history of weight gain, weakness, polydipsia, increased appetite, and hyperpigmentation.

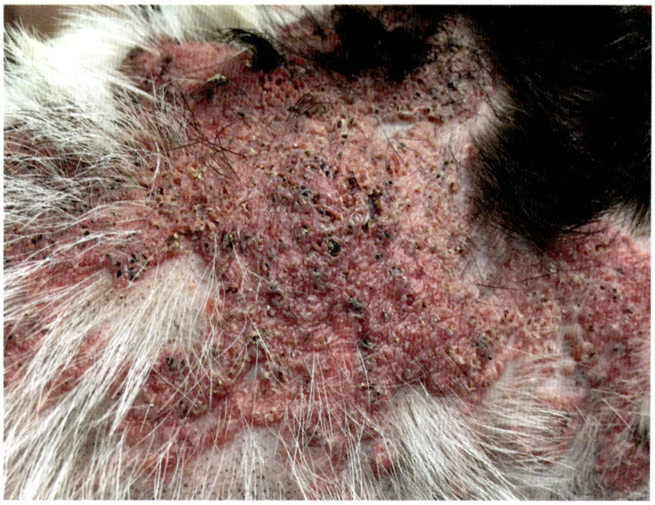

FIG. 34.6 Close-up of a calcinosis cutis lesion in the neck of a 10-year-old female spayed French Bulldog with pituitary-dependent hypercortisolism.

Video 34.1

Same dog as Fig. 34.3 showing muscle stiffness in the rear limbs.

includes fiber size variation, focal necrosis, fiber splitting, and fatty infiltration, although it may also be relatively unremarkable.[2,23] In a study including 36 dogs with pseudomyotonia, two dogs developed progressive difficulty eating and drinking because of masticatory muscle involvement.[23] In the majority of reported dogs with spontaneous HC, despite successful treatment, pseudomyotonia does not seem to resolve completely (although mild or partial improvement can be seen);[23,24] substantial improvement might be seen in cases of iatrogenic HC once corticosteroid administration is stopped.[24]

In dogs with ADHC, tumor-related signs, such as abdominal pain due to abdominal or retroperitoneal hemorrhage, ascites, or rear limb paresis, can also occur, but the prevalence of these signs is unknown.[1]

The association between HC and pancreatitis is controversial; biochemical markers commonly used to assess pancreatitis (canine pancreatic lipase [cPL] and/or DGR lipase 1,2-o-dilauryl-rac-glycero-3-glutaric acid-(60-methylresorufin) ester [DGGR]) might be abnormal in dogs without clinical signs of pancreatitis and changes on pancreas echogenicity assed by ultrasound are also more frequent in dogs with HC than controls.[3]

Dogs with HC have an odds ratio 29 times higher for gallbladder mucocele formation than dogs without HC, and it has been identified in up to 23% of dogs with HC.[3,11] Having HC was associated with nearly a two-fold increase in odds of death in a study including 1,194 dogs with gallbladder mucocele.[25]

Clinicopathological findings

The most common clinicopathological abnormalities are listed in Table 34.2. However, these findings should not be used on their own to screen dogs for HC; these clinicopathological abnormalities must always be interpreted together with the dog's clinical signs, as the absence of common clinical signs previously described should decrease the suspicion of HC.[22]

Complete blood count

At the complete blood count (CBC), the most common finding is the presence of a stress leukogram, which includes an elevated white blood cell (WBC) count with neutrophilia, monocytosis, lymphopenia, and/

TABLE 34.2 Clinicopathological abnormalities observed in dogs with hypercortisolism.

Complete blood count	Most common	■ Neutrophilia ■ Lymphopenia ■ Eosinopenia
	Less common	■ Erythrocytosis ■ Thrombocytosis
Biochemistry	Most common	■ Increased ALP ■ Increased ALT ■ Hypercholesterolemia ■ Hypertriglyceridemia ■ Hyperglycemia
	Less common	■ Low urea ■ Hyper/hypophosphatemia ■ Increased bile acids
Urinalysis	Most common	■ Low USG (<1.015) ■ Proteinuria
	Less common	■ Glycosuria
Coagulation parameters		■ Decreased prothrombin time (PT) ■ Increased fibrinogen ■ Increased maximum angle (TEG) ■ Elevated alpha angle (TEG) ■ Short K value (TEG)

ALP: alkaline phosphatase; ALT: alanine aminotransferase; USG: urine specific gravity; TEG: thromboelastography.

or eosinopenia. Neutrophilia and monocytosis are due to steroid-enhanced capillary demargination, lymphopenia is most likely due to steroid-induced lympholysis, and eosinopenia is caused by bone marrow sequestration. Other frequent findings are mild erythrocytosis, which is related to direct bone marrow stimulation and/or ventilatory problems frequently found in these dogs, and thrombocytosis, which is also due to bone marrow stimulation.[1,2]

Biochemistry

The most common findings include increased alkaline phosphatase (ALP) and alanine aminotransferase (ALT) activities, hypercholesterolemia, decreased urea concentration, and hyperglycemia. Increased ALP is related to steroid-induced hepatic isoenzyme activity in the dog, but vacuolar hepatopathy may also contribute to some degree. There is no correlation between ALP activity and the severity of the disease or prognosis. Vacuolar hepatopathy is also the cause of increased ALT activity. Elevation in ALP activity is greater than that of ALT activity. Steroid-induced lipolysis causes hypercholesterolemia and hypertriglyceridemia, and low urea is likely secondary to increased renal clearance from polyuria.[1,2]

Another common laboratory finding is fasting hyperglycemia, but concurrent diabetes mellitus and HC only occur in 10-13.6% of dogs.[11] Glucocorticoids antagonize the effects of insulin, leading to increased hepatic gluconeogenesis and decreased peripheral glucose utilization.

Hyperphosphatemia is a common finding in dogs with PDH, and serum parathyroid hormone (PTH) concentrations are also increased in dogs with HC, a condition sometimes named adrenal secondary hyperparathyroidism; however, hypophosphatemia may also occur in dogs with HC due to increased urinary excretion of phosphate.[2,16]

Bile acid tests may show a mild increase in as many as 30% of dogs with HC.[2]

Urinalysis

Urinalysis usually reveals low specific gravity, i.e., <1.015, as 90% of patients with HC have PU/PD. Glycosuria is generally absent unless overt diabetes mellitus develops. Proteinuria is also common, with protein to creatinine ratio ranging from 1 to 6 in most cases.[1] Dogs with HC are predisposed to UTIs, secondary to chronic immunosuppression, loss of urinary concentration, and persistent bladder overdistention.

Coagulation parameters

At the time of diagnosis, up to 89% of dogs will show coagulation abnormalities consistent with a hypercoagulable state, which is probably multifactorial.

Endocrine testing

Sara Galac

Based on patient history, clinical manifestations, and clinicopathological findings, the suspicion of hypercortisolism (HC) necessitates confirmation by endocrine testing. The unexpected finding of an adrenal mass discovered on imaging in a dog primarily not suspected of HC or the identification of a large pituitary mass during evaluation for neurological symptoms also warrants testing for HC.[22]

The diagnosis of HC depends on the demonstration of two key features: increased cortisol production and reduced sensitivity of the hypothalamic-pituitary-adrenal axis to negative glucocorticoid feedback.[1] The diagnosis of HC is a two-step procedure that relies on a screening test that distinguishes dogs with HC from dogs without HC and discrimination tests that differentiate between pituitary-dependent hypercortisolism (PDH) and adrenal-dependent hypercortisolism (ADHC). Differentiation between PDH and ADHC is essential to choosing the most optimal treatment.

The low-dose dexamethasone suppression test (LDDST) is primarily a screening test, but the results may also indicate the presence of PDH due to an anterior lobe tumor, so it also serves as a differentiation test. A test that combines screening and differentiation is the urinary cortisol-to-creatinine ratio (UCCR) when combined with an oral high-dose dexamethasone suppression test (oHDDST). The ACTH stimulation test (ACTHst) is a screening test only.[26] None of the tests is 100% accurate, and each has its advantages and disadvantages. Testing for HC should be avoided if the patient is seriously ill, and postponing testing until concurrent illness is resolved or controlled is recommended. Recent administration of glucocorticoids and progestogens may suppress the hypothalamic-pituitary-adrenal axis and consequently affect endocrine testing.[27]

The laboratory method used to measure the cortisol concentration, either in plasma, serum, or urine, is of utmost importance in interpreting endocrine tests, and the reference ranges cannot be used interchangeably. Various methods of cortisol measurement generate variations in cortisol concentrations, and ideally, reference ranges for each method should be established and periodically re-evaluated.[22]

Low-dose dexamethasone suppression test

The LDDST is the most recommended test for confirming the diagnosis of HC. This test relies on assessing the response of the hypothalamic-pituitary-adrenal axis to negative glucocorticoid feedback. In healthy dogs, administration of exogenous dexamethasone will rapidly suppress ACTH secretion and subsequently result in prolonged suppression of cortisol secretion, while dogs with HC are abnormally resistant to dexamethasone suppression.[1]

Serum or plasma samples for cortisol concentration are collected before, 4h, and 8h after IV administration of 0.01 mg/kg dexamethasone. The test can be performed at any time of the day. Feeding should be avoided because lipemic serum can influence cortisol measurements. In dogs without HC, cortisol concentrations at 4h and 8h after dexamethasone are below or very close to the detection limit of current assays. The laboratory cutoff for plasma cortisol concentrations varies between 27.6 nmol/L (1,0 µg/dL) and 39 nmol/L (1,4 µg/dL) and depends on the methodology as well as the material (plasma vs. serum) used.[28–30] Therefore, laboratory-specific references should be considered for the interpretation.

The LDDST is the oldest test used to diagnose HC in dogs. Basal and 8h post-dexamethasone cortisol results are used for the screening portion of the interpretation. Meanwhile, the 4h sample and the percentage of suppression in 4h and/or 8h post dexamethasone cortisol may be valuable for distinguishing between the PDH and ADHC (Fig. 34.8B). Recently, several studies reevaluated the performance of the LDDST (Fig. 34.7B).[29,30,31] Furthermore, several new patterns have been recognized, and their diagnostic value has been reported (Fig. 34.7). A cortisol concentration above the laboratory cutoff 8h after dexamethasone administration has historically been considered consistent with HC irrespective of the patterns observed.[28] Failure to suppress dexamethasone (post dexamethasone cortisol at 4h and 8h higher than the diagnostic cutoff and >50% of basal cortisol concentration) confirms the diagnosis of HC. This "lack of suppression pattern" is not helpful in discriminating between PDH and ADHC, and further differentiation with diagnostic imaging and endogenous ACTH measurements is warranted. A suppression of >50%, compared to the basal cortisol concentration, at 8h or 4h in dogs with confirmed HC, is indicative of PDH and is termed a "partial suppression pattern". The "escape pattern" is defined as post dexamethasone cortisol at 4h falls below and at 8h rises above the laboratory cutoff. An "inverse pattern" is diagnosed when post dexamethasone cortisol concentration at 8h is below the laboratory cutoff, but at 4h, it exceeds it. While highly suspicious, an inverse pattern is nondiagnostic for HC, and further testing for HC should be pursued when there is a strong clinical indication.[28,29]

The reported sensitivity and specificity of the LDDST range from 85 to 100% and from 67 to 80%, respectively. A "lack of suppression pattern" exhibits the highest positive predictive value for diagnosing HC (range from 94 to 100%), followed by a "partial suppression pattern" (range 73 to 94%). The positive predictive values of "escape pattern" and "inverse pattern" are based on a low number of dogs and vary from 37 to 86% and from 27 to 40%, respectively.[28,29]

Urinary cortisol-to-creatinine ratio

The UCCR represents an integrated measure of corticoid production over an interval (usually one night), smoothing the effects of short-term fluctuations in plasma cortisol levels. Determination of basal UCCRs can be performed in tandem with an oHDDST. The combination has the advantage of potentially demonstrating both increased cortisol production and decreased sensitivity to glucocorticoid feedback, i.e., to differentiate between PDH and ADHC. The reported sensitivity and specificity of the UCCR for diagnosis of HC range from 75-100% and 20-25%, respectively.[22]

The UCCR should always be performed at home to minimize stress influence and at least two days after a visit to a veterinary clinic to prevent false positive results. The owner collects urine samples on two consecutive mornings for baseline UCCRs. After collecting the second urine sample, dexamethasone is administered PO in a dosage of 0.1 mg/kg

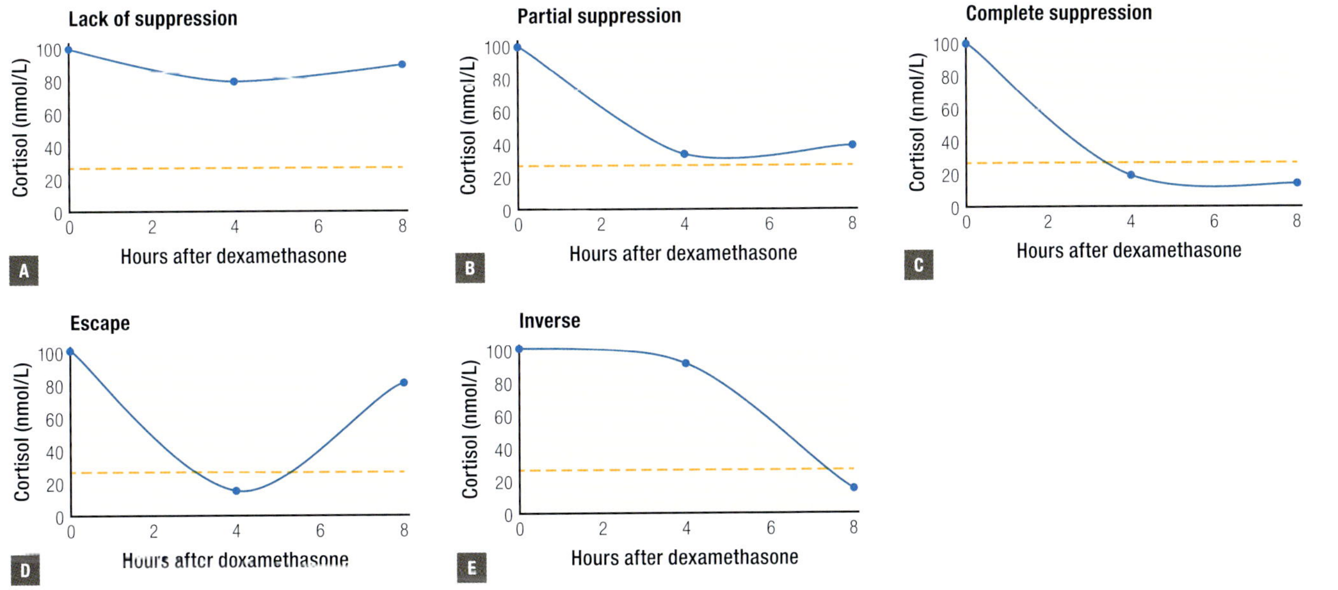

FIG. 34.7 Suppression patterns of the low-dose dexamethasone suppression test, including lack of suppression (t4 and t8 ≥27.6 nmol/L*, and >50% of t0 cortisol concentration); partial suppression (t4 and t8 ≥27.6 nmol/L, but either one or both <50% of t0 cortisol concentration); complete suppression (t4 and t8 <27.6 nmol/L); escape (t4 <27.6 nmol/L and t8 ≥27.6 nmol/L); and inverse patterns (t4 ≥27.6 nmol/L and t8 <27.6 nmol/L). Traditionally, a cortisol concentration ≥27.6 nmol/L at t8 is considered a positive test irrespective of the suppression pattern observed. *27.6 nmol/L = 1 µg/dL. Adapted from: Zeugswetter FK, Carranza Valencia A, Glavassevich K, Schwendenwein I. Patterns of the low-dose dexamethasone suppression test in canine hyperadrenocorticism revisited. *Vet Clin Pathol* 50:62-70, 2021.

at 12:00, 18:00, and 24:00 hours. The next morning, about 8 hours after administration of dexamethasone, the third urine sample is collected (Table 34.3).

In dogs with severe polyuria that also present with nocturia, the test is less reliable, as the morning sample will not reflect the accumulation of glucocorticoids in the urine for several hours. The reliability of the UCCR test also depends on the availability of a trustworthy assay and the method-specific reference ranges and diagnostic cutoffs.[32] There are considerable differences between the laboratories providing the UCCR measurements, and the UCCR cutoffs vary from 10×10^{-6} to even 60×10^{-6}.[33] The differences are due to various assays and antibodies used and the urinary extraction methods. Traditionally, UCCR measurements were based on radioimmunoassay (RIA), and the diagnostic thresholds were well established.[34] Nowadays, chemiluminescent immunoassay (CLIA) and tandem mass spectrometry (LC-MSMS) are being applied with each method having its own diagnostic thresholds and cutoff values.[33]

Interpretation of the UCCR combined with oHDDST is provided in Fig. 34.8A.

Various factors can influence the performance of the UCCR, including the recent administration of glucocorticoids or progestagens. Some glucocorticoids, like prednisolone, may cross-react in cortisol assays, potentially affecting UCCR results. Therefore, just like in other endocrine tests for HC, when interpreting UCCR results, it is important to consider any recent administration of medications and their potential effects on cortisol levels.[27]

TABLE 34.3 Test protocol for urinary cortisol-to-creatinine ratio (UCCR) combined with the oral high-dose dexamethasone suppression test (oHDDST).

- The owner is asked to collect the first urine sample at home on three consecutive days.
- On the second day, dexamethasone tablets are administered orally in a dose of 0.1 mg/kg three times (at 12:00, 18:00, and 24:00).
- On the third day, approximately 8 hours after the last dexamethasone administration, the third urine sample is collected.

Day 1	Collect morning urine sample	UCCR 1
Day 2	Collect morning urine sample	UCCR 2
	12:00 dexamethasone, 0.1 mg/kg; first dose	
	18:00 dexamethasone, 0.1 mg/kg; second dose	
	24:00 dexamethasone, 0.1 mg/kg; third dose	
Day 3	Collect morning urine sample	UCCR 3

ACTH stimulation test

The ACTH stimulation test assesses adrenocortical reserve and is the gold standard for diagnosing iatrogenic HC. This test does not involve assessing decreased sensitivity of the hypothalamic-pituitary-adrenal axis to negative glucocorticoid feedback and does not allow differentiation between PDH and ADHC.[22]

The ACTH stimulation test is a quick test and can be performed at any time of the day. Plasma cortisol is measured twice. After IV or IM administration of synthetic ACTH, peak cortisol secretion occurs at 60-90 minutes.[35] Synthetic ACTH is commercially available in liquid, lyophilized, or depot forms. The current dose recommendation is to use 5 µg/kg body weight of synthetic ACTH instead of the total dose of 250 µg/dog. The use of 1 µg/kg of synthetic ACTH resulted in a different clinical interpretation in approximately 25% of cases suspected of HC and is not recommended.[36]

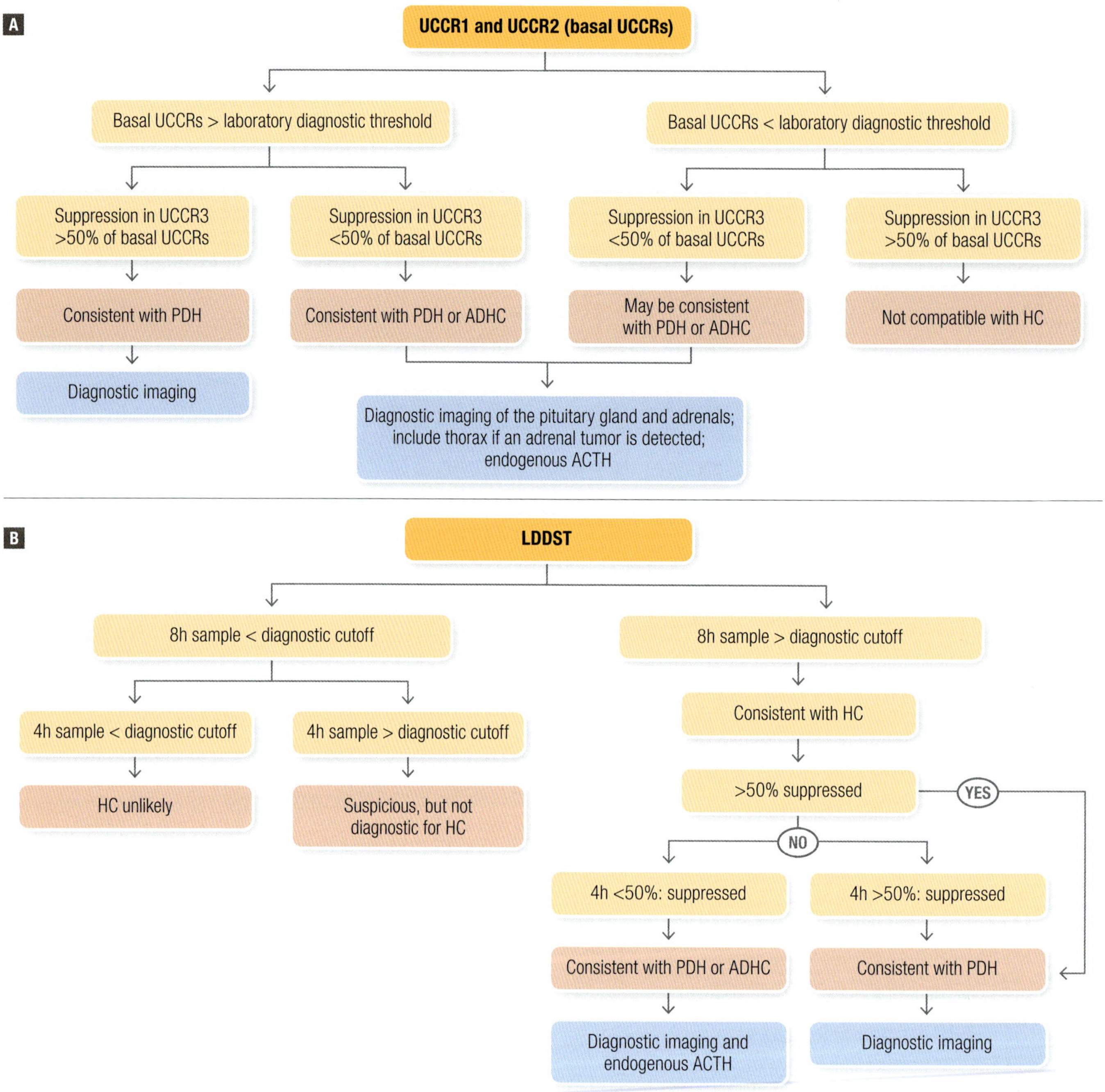

FIG. 34.8 (A) Interpretation of the urinary cortisol to creatinine ratio (UCCR) combined with the oral high-dose dexamethasone suppression test (oHDDST). (B) Interpretation of low-dose dexamethasone suppression test (LDDST).

C

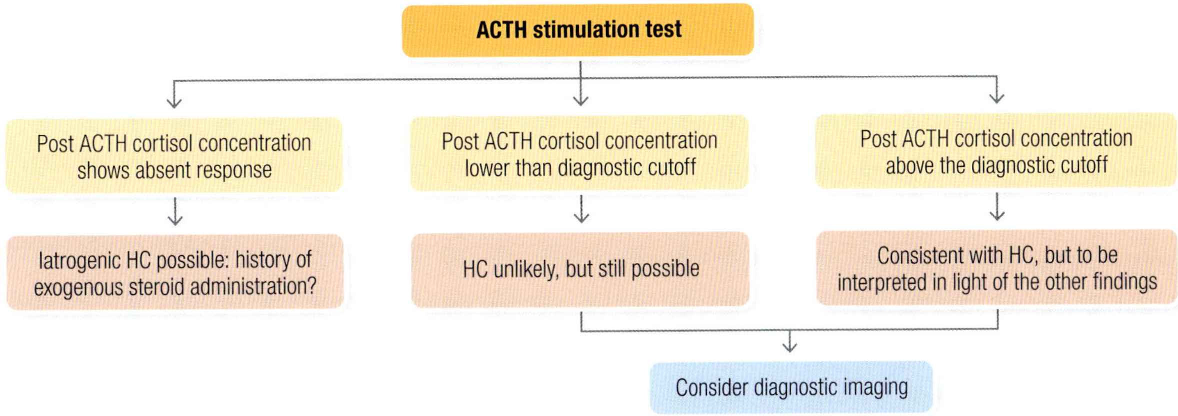

FIG. 34.8 *Continued.* (C) Interpretation of the ACTH stimulation test. HC, hypercortisolism; PDH, pituitary-dependent hypercortisolism; ADHC, adrenal-dependent hypercortisolism.

The sensitivity of the ACTH stimulation test for spontaneous HC ranges between 80-83% for PDH and from 57-63 % for ADHC. The low sensitivity of the ACTH stimulation test in ADHC is most likely associated with the downregulation of the ACTH receptor (MC2 receptor) in adrenocortical carcinomas. The specificity ranges between 59 and 93%.[26] Because of its low sensitivity for ADHC and the inability to differentiate between PDH and ADHC, the diagnostic usefulness of the ACTH stimulation test is inferior to the LDDST (Fig. 34.7C).

Endogenous ACTH

Endogenous ACTH (eACTH) is secreted from the pituitary gland in an episodic, pulsatile fashion. Circulating concentrations of eACTH overlap considerably between healthy dogs and those with PDH. Consequently, its measurement is not useful to screen for HC. In dogs with ADHC, the eACTH is expected to be low or undetectable. Endogenous ACTH is the most accurate stand-alone biochemical test for differentiating PDH from ADHC in dogs with proven HC.[26] A low circulating eACTH concentration is also a characteristic of other forms of ACTH-independent HC, such as food-induced HC.

The accuracy of differentiating PDH from ADHC depends on analytical sensitivity, the working range of the ACTH assay, and proper sample handling. Dogs' endogenous ACTH is collected into chilled, silicon-coated glass or plastic tubes containing EDTA, centrifuged within 15 minutes (ideally in a cooled centrifuge), and the plasma transferred to plastic tubes and frozen immediately.[22]

High-dose dexamethasone suppression test

The indication for the IV-HDDST is to differentiate between PDH and ADHC when the LDDST is nonsuppressible. The HDDST should be performed as the LDDST, except that the dosage is 0.1 mg/kg IV. When suppression of >50% on an HDDST occurs, the diagnosis of PDH can be made. If there is no suppression in the LDDST (at 8h sample and/or 4h sample), the HDDST will provide differentiation in only 12% additional cases. Therefore, this test is not recommended anymore. Instead, diagnostic imaging and eACTH measurements are advised to differentiate between PDH and ADHC in dogs with nonsuppressible LDDST.[22]

Conclusion

Several endocrine tests exist to confirm the diagnosis of HC. While their diagnostic accuracy is influenced by various analytical factors, assessment of the patient's signalment, history, and clinical presentation should always be encountered alongside test results.

Diagnostic imaging

Henk van den Broek and Stefanie Veraa

Diagnostic imaging of preferentially both pituitary and adrenal glands should be included in the diagnostic evaluation of every dog with spontaneous hypercortisolism (HC) when the diagnosis has been confirmed with an endocrine test. Diagnostic imaging allows clinicians to differentiate between pituitary-dependent hypercortisolism (PDH) and adrenal-dependent hypercortisolism (ADHC), to choose the most optimal treatment, and to estimate prognosis. Finding normal pituitary and normal adrenal glands on diagnostic imaging does not rule out HC.

Abdominal ultrasonography

Ultrasonography is a relatively inexpensive and noninvasive technique to image the adrenal glands. Adrenal gland thickness increases with body weight in dogs, and different reference intervals have been proposed for the left and right adrenal glands in different body weight categories (Table 34.4; Fig. 34.9; Video 34.2 and Video 34.3).[37] B-mode ultrasound is used to help distinguish between PDH and ADHC, but also to support a clinical suspicion of HC by findings such as hepatomegaly, gallbladder sludge or mucocele, speckled spleen, thrombosis, and a hyperechoic pancreas.

In PDH, bilateral adrenomegaly is expected as excessive secretion of ACTH will stimulate the proliferation of both adrenal glands. In unilateral cortisol-secreting adrenal tumors, an enlargement of one adrenal gland is observed, while the contralateral gland is expected to decrease in size (Fig. 34.10; Video 34.4). A maximal dorsoventral thickness of ≤5 mm suggests an atrophic adrenal gland.[38] Bilateral cortisol-secreting tumors causing ADHC are possible and complicate the differentiation between PDH and ADHC. In addition, equivocal adrenal asymmetry is observed in a large proportion of dogs with HC, representing a biological variation or caused by nodular hyperplasia.[38] Malignant adrenal masses are associated with size exceeding 2 cm, irregular margination, thromboembolism, and metastasis to the liver, pancreas, and kidneys. Contrast-enhanced ultrasound (CEUS) has been described in dogs with PDH and dogs with

TABLE 34.4 Ultrasonographic upper limits for dorsoventral adrenal gland thickness (height) measured on the sagittal plane in clinically healthy dogs according to Melián et al., 2021.[37]

Body weight	Maximal left adrenal gland height	Maximal right adrenal gland height
≥2.5-5 kg	5.1 mm	5.3 mm
>5-10 kg	5.5 mm	6.8 mm
>10-20 kg	6.4 mm	7.5 mm
>20-40 kg	7.3 mm	8.7 mm

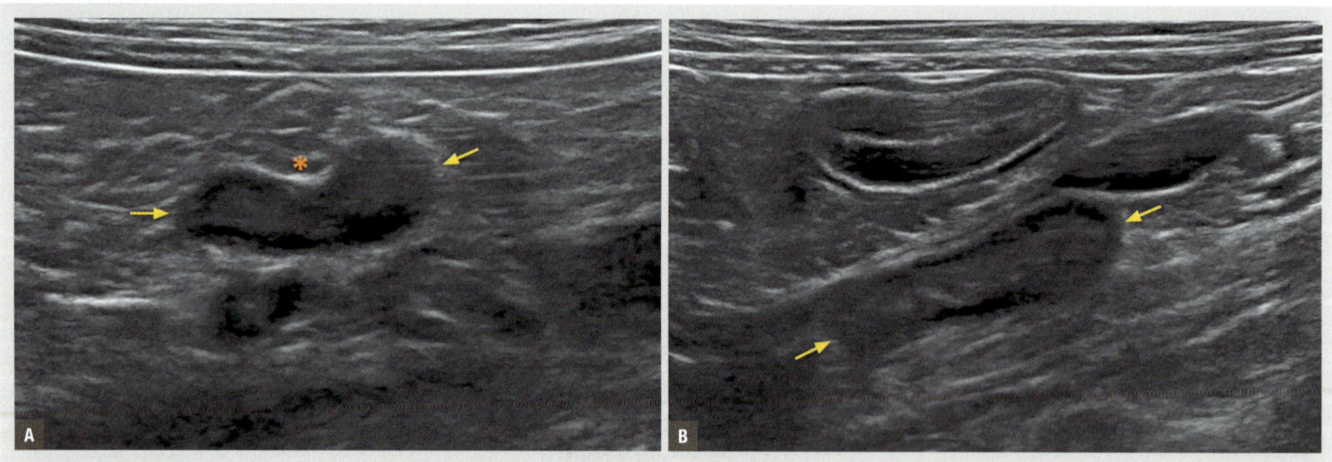

FIG. 34.9 (A) Ultrasonographic image of a normal left adrenal gland in the long axis (cranial on the left side of the image). Note the bean-shaped adrenal gland, consisting of a cranial and caudal pole with the presence of a central indentation and phrenicoabdominal vein on the ventral aspect (asterix). (B) Ultrasonographic image of a normal right adrenal gland in the long axis (cranial on the left side of the image). Note the visible corticomedullary distinction in this dog.

Video 34.2

Ultrasonography of a normal left adrenal gland; long-axis view with movement of the transducer from the aorta at the location of the celiac and cranial mesenteric artery towards the more laterally positioned adrenal gland.

Video 34.3

Ultrasonography of a normal right adrenal gland; long-axis view with movement of the transducer from the right kidney area towards the caudal vena cava.

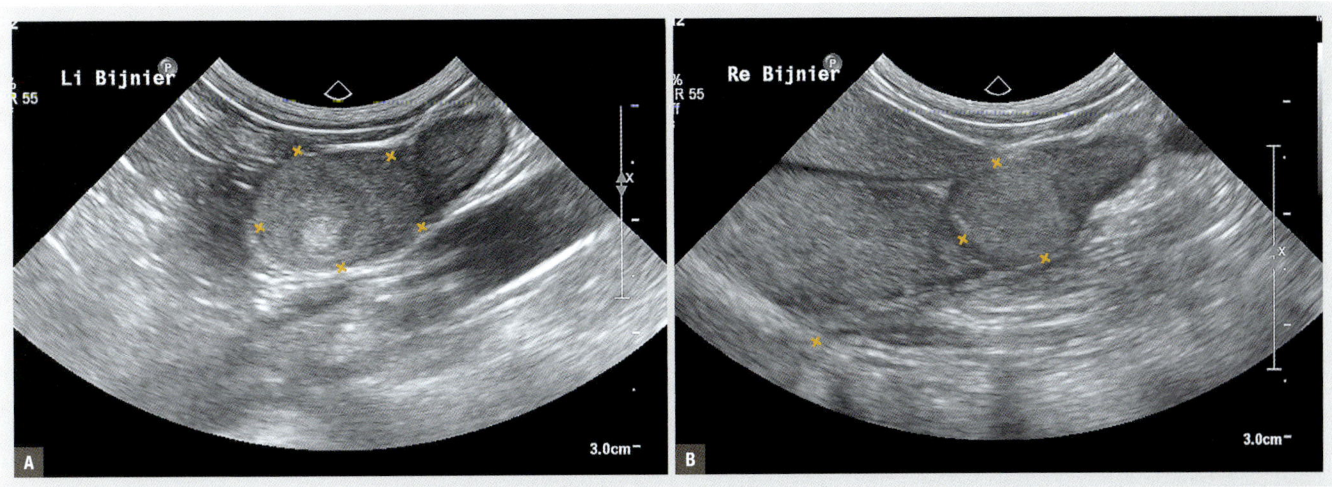

FIG. 34.10 (A) Ultrasonographic image of an enlarged left adrenal gland in the long axis (cranial on the left side of the image). A well-defined echogenic mass lesion is visible in the cranial pole, deforming the outer contours of the adrenal gland. (B) Ultrasonographic image of an enlarged right adrenal gland in the long axis (cranial on the left side of the image). A well-defined echogenic mass lesion is visible in the medulla of the cranial pole, deforming the outer contours of the adrenal gland.

Video 34.4

Ultrasonography of a normal left adrenal gland; long-axis with movement of the transducer from the aorta at the location of the celiac and cranial mesenteric artery towards the more laterally positioned adrenal gland.

adrenal neoplasia and aids in further differentiation and characterization of different types of adrenal tumors.[39-41] Dogs with PDH showed increased and chaotic contrast enhancement in both the medulla and cortex. Adrenocortical adenomas were characterized as homogeneous lesions during CEUS examination, whereas adrenocortical carcinomas were characterized as non-homogeneous lesions with the presence of both hypoperfused areas and intralesional disordered microcirculation. Combining enhancement degree and vascularity, CEUS can discriminate malignant versus benign adrenal lesions with a sensitivity of 100%, a specificity of 80%, and an accuracy of 92%.[39]

Computed tomography

Computed tomography (CT) is the preferred imaging modality for canine HC in the authors' institution because it allows simultaneous assessment of both the pituitary and adrenal glands. In the case of an adrenal tumor, a screening of the thorax for metastasis can be included. Furthermore, CT aids surgical and radiotherapy planning in patients with PDH.

The basic scanning protocol for the pituitary gland consists of pre- and postcontrast series. The normal canine pituitary CT dimensions (length × width × height) are approximately 5 × 6 × 4.5 mm.[42] The pituitary gland is considered enlarged when it protrudes dorsal to the suprasellar extensions of the intercrural cistern, and calculation of the pituitary height/brain area (P/B value) has a high discriminative index to distinguish enlarged (P/B >0.31) from nonenlarged (P/B ≤ 0.31) pituitary glands. To measure the P/B value, the height of the pituitary is measured on the image with the largest cross-section of the gland, and adjustments are made for variations in dog size by tracing the brain edges on this image and calculating the enclosed area. The P/B value is calculated by dividing the height of the pituitary (mm × 100) by the calculated brain area (mm^2) (Fig. 34.11A).

The localization of microadenomas that do not alter the size and shape of the pituitary gland, can be visualized indirectly by the displacement of the neurohypophysis. The centrally located neurohypophysis has a direct arterial blood supply and shows early enhancement in a dynamic CT study, the so-called neurohypophyseal flush.[43] The presence of an otherwise inconspicuous small adenoma in the surrounding adenohypophysis could be detected by distortion or displacement of the neurohypophyseal flush.[43,44] Still, an unremarkable CT study of the pituitary gland does not rule out the presence of a microadenoma. In a study involving 55 dogs with PDH, 10 dogs exhibited unremarkable size and contrast-enhancement of the pituitary gland, and even empty sella has been described[43] (Fig. 34.11B; Video 34.5, Video 34.6, and Video 34.7). Traditionally, pituitary masses are arbitrarily divided into macrotumor (>10 mm in height) (Fig. 34.11C) and microtumor (<10 mm in height) (Fig. 34.11B). This classification was adapted from human medicine but should be avoided in dogs. Because of the large variability in body and skull size in dogs, the classification between enlarged and nonenlarged pituitary glands based on the 10 mm cutoff value is not correct. In small breeds, for instance, pituitary adenomas between 6 and 10 mm in height enlarge the pituitary gland to such an extent, that they may induce neurological signs and therefore should not be classified as microadenomas. The highest discriminatory power in distinguishing enlarged from nonenlarged pituitaries is the P/B value, with 0.31 as the cutoff value. The P/B value can be measured both on CT and MRI images.

Pituitary tumors are usually adenomas and are round with homogenous contrast enhancement, whilst invasive adenomas tend to become more oval or irregular in shape, could show mineralization, and have a markedly increased P/B value.[45] Sphenoid bone resorption can be found in more aggressive types of tumors, such as adenocarcinoma. Intratumoral hemorrhage (i.e., pituitary apoplexy) may occur in large pituitary tumors and is characterized by precontrast heterogeneity, hyperattenuation, and heterogeneous contrast enhancement.[46]

For imaging of the adrenal glands, dynamic CT is not required, and pre- and postcontrast series suffice. In healthy dogs, the mean volume

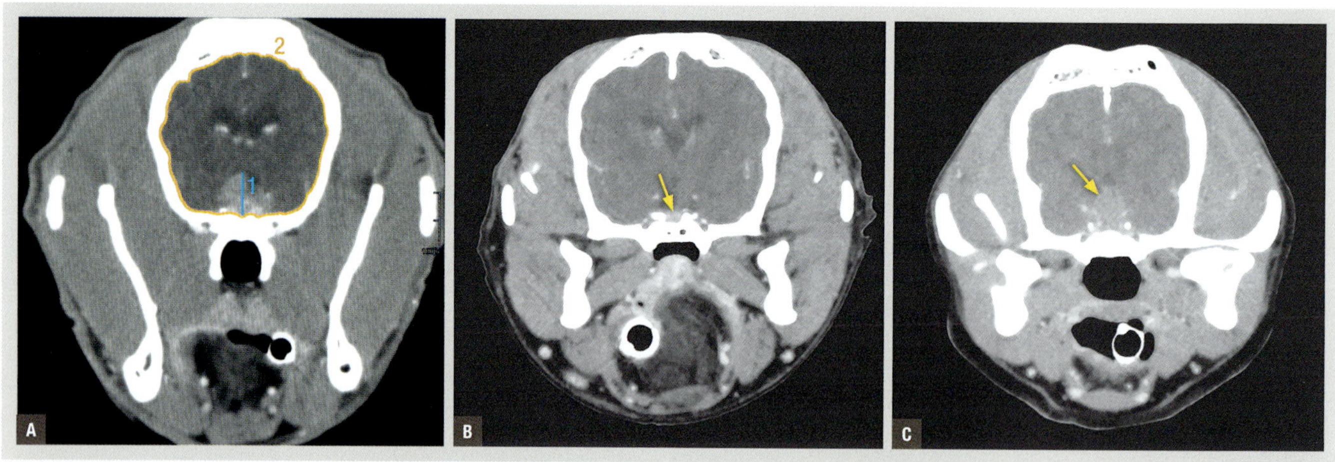

FIG. 34.11 (**A**) Transverse CT contrast-enhanced image of the head at the level of the pituitary gland demonstrating the pituitary/brain value (P/B). The pituitary height (P, marked as 1) is measured on the image with the largest cross-section of the gland. The orange line represents the brain edges and the enclosed area is calculated (B, marked as 2). The P/B is calculated by dividing the P (mm x 100) by the calculated B (mm^2). The P in this case is 1250 (12.5 mm x 100) and the B is 2000 mm^2. P/B value is (1250/2000) =0.62. (**B**) Transverse CT contrast-enhanced image of the head of a dog at the level of the pituitary gland (left is to the right of the image). A normal-sized pituitary gland (arrow) is visible that is retained within the sellar boundaries, P/B <0.31. (**C**) Transverse CT contrast-enhanced image of the head of a dog at the level of the pituitary gland (left is to the right of the image). A severely enlarged, mildly asymmetric, and diffuse enhancing pituitary gland (arrow) is visible (P/B >0.31) that is reaching the ventral boundary of the hypoattenuating third ventricle. No bone lysis was noted.

of the left adrenal gland was determined to be 0.60 cm^3 and of the right adrenal gland 0.55 cm^3, with a mean nonenhanced attenuation value of 35 HU and contrast-enhanced attenuation value of 100 HU[47] (Fig. 34.12A). Considerable overlap in adrenal gland size measurements exists between dogs with PDH and ADHC. However, the maximum adrenal gland diameter ratio, reflecting adrenal gland size asymmetry, is useful in discriminating between PDH and ADHC, with a ratio ≤ 2.08 on reformatted images suggestive of ADHC (Fig. 34.12A). Vascular invasion and adrenal calcification were also more common in ADHC.[48] When an adrenal mass is identified, thoracic CT must be performed to screen for pulmonary metastasis. In 5% of dogs with dexamethasone-resistant HC, concurrent pituitary and adrenal lesions were identified, underlining the need to image both organs for proper diagnostic workup and treatment planning.[49]

Video 34.5

Transverse dynamic CT at the level of the pituitary gland (left is to the left in the video). A normal centrally located contrast flush is noted in the neurohypophysis.

Video 34.6

Transverse dynamic CT at the level of the pituitary gland (left is to the right in the video). An eccentric right-sided contrast flush is noted in neurohypophysis, indicative of a microadenoma.

Video 34.7

Transverse dynamic CT at the level of the pituitary gland (left is to the left in the video). An empty sella is visible without any signs of pituitary gland enhancement, and increased fluid attenuation is noted in this region.

Magnetic resonance imaging

Magnetic resonance imaging (MRI) has superior contrast resolution compared to CT. Intravenous contrast medium administration is not necessary to assess the pituitary gland, although the dorsal border is better delineated. The neurohypophysis is hyperintense on T1W images, named the pituitary bright spot (Fig. 34.13A). Analogous to the neurohypophyseal flush on dynamic CT, displacement of the bright spot on MRI could indicate the presence of a microadenoma, whereas a diffuse enhancement of the adenohypophysis is otherwise visible (Fig. 34.13B). The bright spot is best seen on the precontrast T1W sequence, and dorsal displacement is associated with PDH caused by a microtumor.[50] In T2W images, the pituitary gland is equal to brain intensity and outlined by the bright cavernous sinuses (Fig. 34.14A). The diagnostic performance of 0.2 Tesla MRI was equal to dynamic CT in dogs with PDH.[51] In general, size measurements of the pituitary gland are larger, and the thickness of the sphenoid bone is smaller on MRI compared to CT, but the P/B value does not differ.[51] Severely enlarged pituitary tumors are typically T1W isointense and mildly T2W hyperintense with marked diffuse enhancement (Fig. 34.14B). Pituitary microtumors are usually not identified, but secondary changes such as increased convexity of the dorsal border of the pituitary gland and displacement of the neurohypophysis suggest their presence.[50] Like CT, MRI cannot distinguish between tumor types, but larger size, irregular shape and margination, and sphenoid bone lysis suggest invasive adenoma or adenocarcinoma. Metastases are usually not identified on MRI.

Advanced imaging with a CT/MRI scan in dogs with HC is indicated not only in dogs intended to be treated by surgery or radiation but also before starting medical treatment to provide additional information on the prognosis and quality of life of dogs with HC by screening for concommitant diseases.

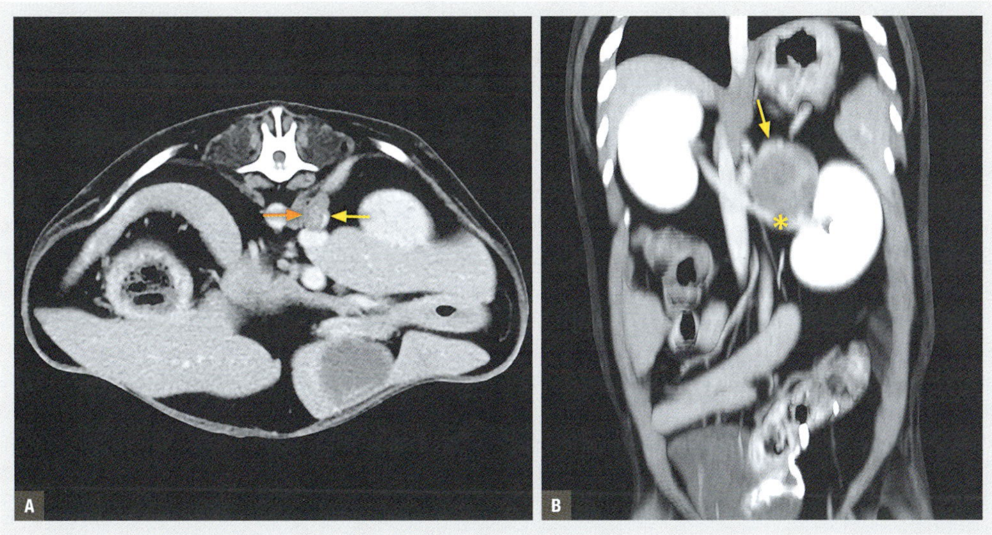

FIG. 34.12 (**A**) Transverse CT contrast-enhanced image of the abdomen of a dog at the level of the left adrenal gland (left is to the right of the image). A diffuse enhancing left adrenal gland (orange arrow) can be noted dorsal to the caudal vena cava and axial to the left cranial pole of the kidney. Note the small phrenicoabdominal vein along the lateral surface of the adrenal gland (yellow arrow). (**B**) Dorsal multiplanar reconstruction (MPR) CT contrast-enhanced image of the dorsal abdomen of a dog at the level of the left adrenal and kidneys. A severely enlarged, patchy left adrenal gland (arrow) can be noted wedged between the caudal vena cava and left kidney, displacing the left renal vein slightly caudally (asterix). No invasion in the adjacent vasculature was seen.

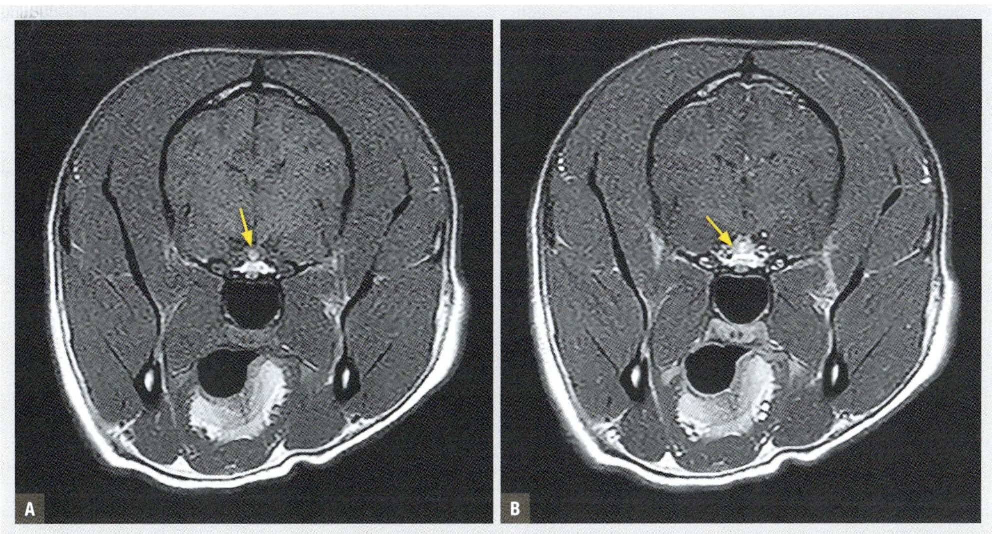

FIG. 34.13 (**A**) Transverse MRI T1-weighted image of the head of a dog at the level of the pituitary gland (left is to the right of the image). Note the bright spot in the middle of the pituitary gland (arrow). (**B**) Transverse MRI T1-weighted contrast-enhanced image of the head of the same dog at the level of the pituitary gland (left is to the right of the image). Note the diffuse contrast enhancement (arrow).

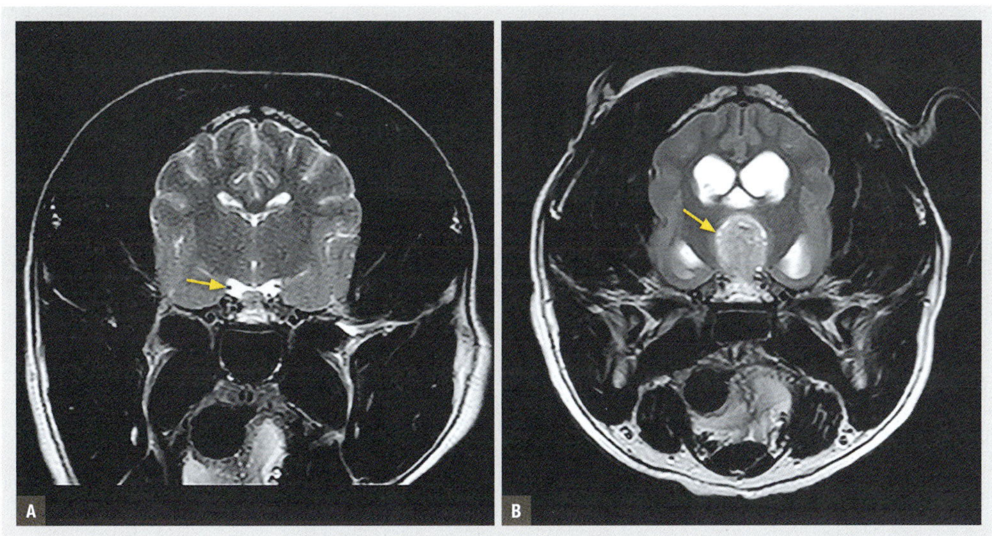

FIG. 34.14 (**A**) Transverse MRI T2-weighted image of the head of the same dog at the level of the pituitary gland (left is to the right of the image). Note the hyperintense signal of the cavernous sinuses outlining the pituitary gland (arrow). (**B**) Transverse MRI T2-weighted image of the head of a dog at the level of the pituitary gland (left is to the right of the image). The irregular hyperintense pituitary gland is severely enlarged, displacing the surrounding brain and ventricular structures (arrow). Osteolysis of the underlying sphenoid bone surface is suspected.

General treatment considerations

Sara Galac

The goals of treating canine hypercortisolism (HC) would optimally be to eliminate the source of either ACTH or autonomous cortisol excess, to achieve normocortisolism, to eliminate the clinical signs, to reduce long-term complications and mortality, and to improve the quality of life.[52] Treatment strategies depend on whether HC is pituitary-dependent (PDH) or adrenal-dependent (ADHC) (Fig. 34.15). Therefore, diagnostic imaging is essential in the decision-making process.[49] Additionally, the severity of the condition, the existence of HC-related complications or concurrent conditions, such as diabetes mellitus, hypertension, calcinosis cutis, and the general health of the patient aid the decision.

Both PDH and ADHC can be treated either surgically[53,54] or medically,[55,56] and pituitary tumors can also be treated with radiotherapy.[57] The medical treatment of HC aims to suppress cortisol secretion and control the clinical signs. Trilostane is the most commonly used drug to treat HC in dogs. It has been shown to be safe and effective, but its dosage needs to be monitored regularly, and its long-term effects are not yet fully known.[58]

A PHD caused by a pituitary microadenoma can be treated with the adrenocorticostatic drug trilostane. Hypophysectomy or radiation therapy is not necessary, since in dogs with a pituitary microadenoma, the main problem is cortisol excess rather than the pituitary mass itself. In relatively young patients, a follow-up CT scan is recommended after 12 months of trilostane therapy to reassess the size of the pituitary tumor. If the tumor has significantly increased in size, surgical intervention or radiotherapy is advised.[53,57] In PDH dogs with an enlarged pituitary tumor, treatment targeting the pituitary level is preferred over medical treatment (targeting the adrenal level). While trilostane therapy effectively controls the clinical signs of HC, it does not inhibit pituitary tumor growth, which can potentially lead to neurological signs. In patients with severely enlarged pituitary tumors, radiotherapy or surgical debulking are possible options. In both cases, medical treatment with trilostane is usually required to control the clinical signs of HC.

Cortisol-secreting adrenocortical tumor(s) (AT) causing ADHC can be malignant, and therefore, adrenalectomy is the best treatment option.[54] In cases of unilateral ATs, supplementation with glucocorticoids is required following surgery because the contralateral adrenal cortex is atrophic due to feedback suppression of pituitary ACTH secretion, but this reverses within 2 months. After bilateral adrenalectomy, lifelong supplementation with both glucocorticoids and mineralocorticoids is needed. Adrenalectomy, like hypophysectomy, requires special facilities and a team consisting of an experienced surgeon, endocrinologist, radiologist, anesthesiologist, and critical care specialist. While the major indication for medical treatment with trilostane is PDH, it can also be used in ADHC when surgery is not possible due to the presence of metastasis or for other reasons. Mitotane is still available for use in dogs with PDH resistant to trilostane and in dogs with inoperable and/or metastatized cortisol-secreting ATs.[52]

A detailed description of treatment options is provided in the following subchapters.

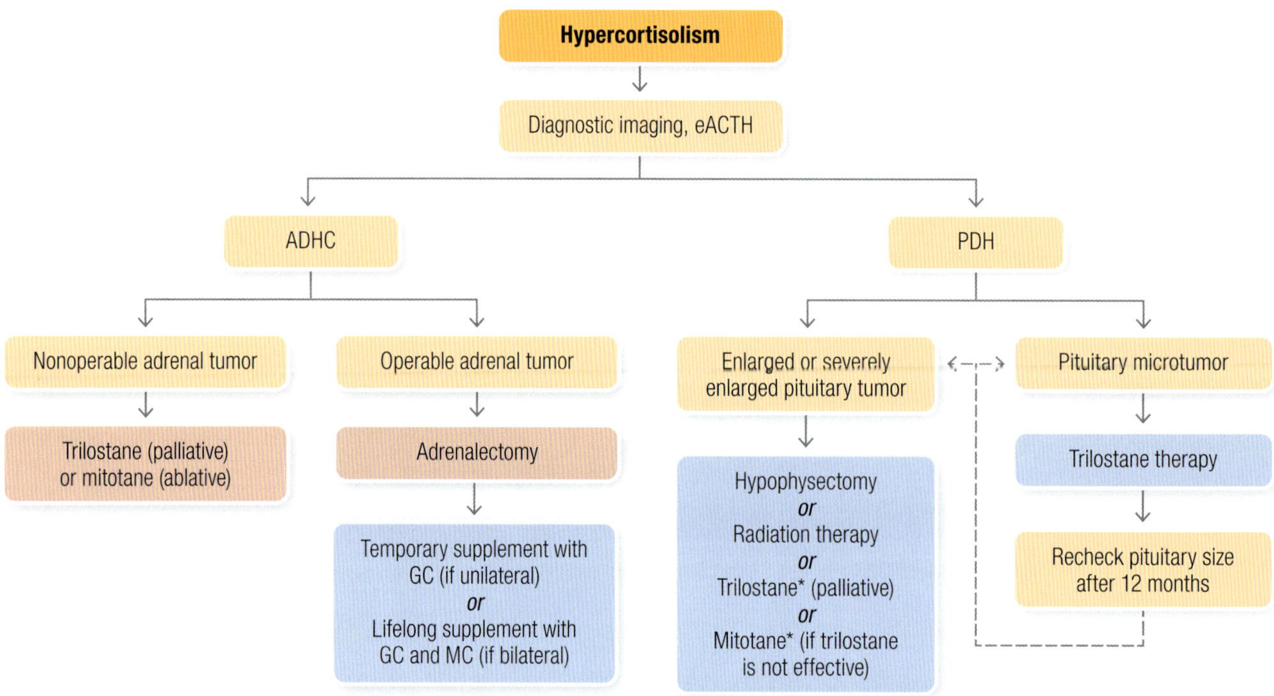

FIG. 34.15 Treatment strategies for canine hypercortisolism. *Only in patients with good appetite and no serious comorbidities. PDH, pituitary-dependent hypercortisolism; ADHC, adrenal-dependent hypercortisolism; eACTH, endogenous adrenocorticotropic hormone; GC, glucocorticoids; MC, mineralocorticoids.

Medical treatment

Stefania Golinelli

Medical treatment is the most common approach to canine hypercortisolism (HC). It mainly involves adrenal-targeting drugs, while novel medical treatments aimed at modulating both adrenal and pituitary function are still under investigation. This chapter will address the current medical strategies with trilostane and mitotane and briefly discuss future strategies.

Adrenal-directed drugs (traditional options)

Adrenal-directed drugs are designed to act upon the adrenal gland, leading to a decrease in cortisol secretion by inhibiting the process of steroidogenesis. Due to their mechanism of action, these drugs are categorized as "inhibitors of steroidogenesis". Among them, trilostane is widely employed, with mitotane used to a lesser extent.[52]

Trilostane

History, mechanism of action, and pharmacology

Trilostane, a synthetic steroid analog, emerges as a pivotal therapeutic agent in the medical management of canine HC. Trilostane exerts its effects through competitive inhibition of the steroidogenic enzyme 3-beta-hydroxysteroid dehydrogenase (3βHSD), a key player in the biosynthesis of all adrenocortical hormones[59] (**Fig. 34.16**). By targeting 3βHSD, trilostane disrupts the production of cortisol and aldosterone, inducing a cascade of hormonal responses. This includes a surge in plasma ACTH levels due to cortisol suppression, leading to a loss of negative feedback and a compensatory increase of plasma renin activity due to reduced aldosterone production.[55,56,60]

Trilostane suppression of 3βHSD is substantiated through the observed reduction in plasma cortisol levels coupled with simultaneous elevations in 17-alpha-hydroxy-pregnenolone concentrations. Notably, the concentrations of 17-alpha-hydroxy-progesterone remain unchanged, while cortisol concentrations markedly decreased, implying the possibility of

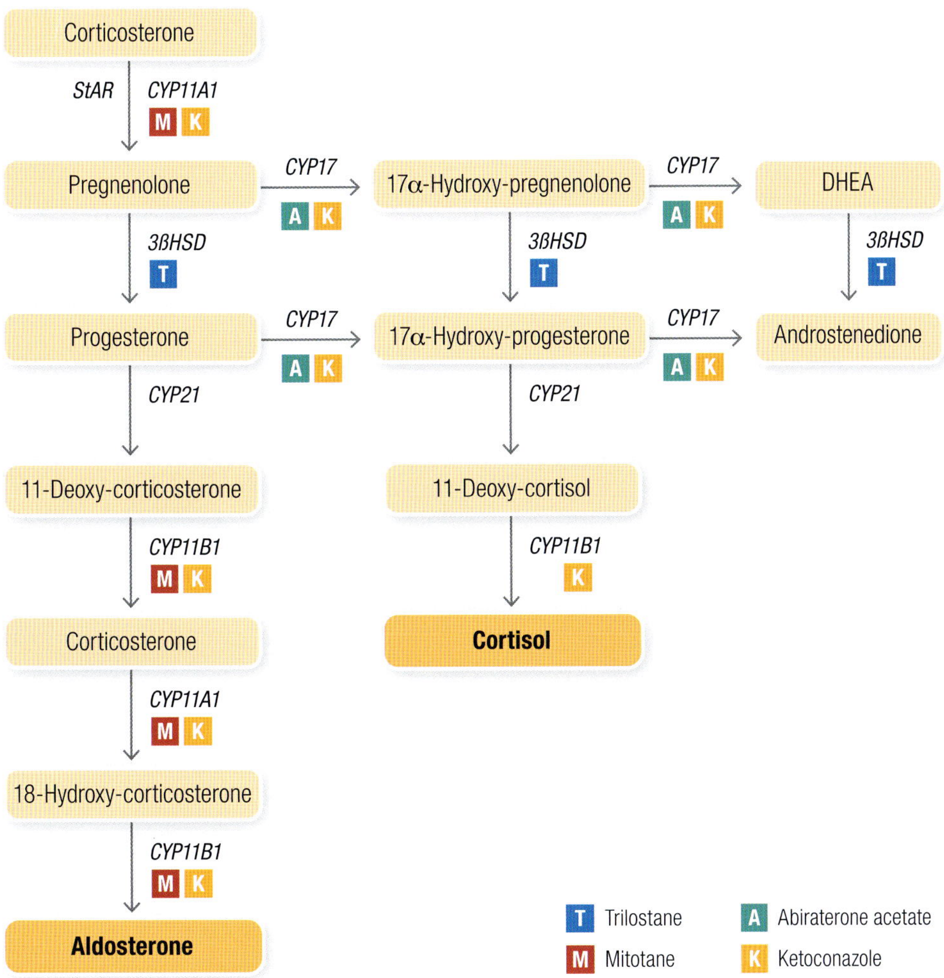

FIG. 34.16 Schematic overview of the site of action of steroidogenesis inhibitors. StAR, steroidogenic acute regulatory protein; CYP11A1, cholesterol side-chain cleavage enzyme; 3βHSD, 3β-hydroxysteroid dehydrogenase; CYP17, 17α-hydroxylase/17,20-lyase; CYP21, 21-hydroxylase; CYP11B1, 11β-hydroxylase. Adapted from: Sanders K, Kooistra HS, Galac S. Treating canine Cushing's syndrome: current options and future prospects. *Vet J* 241:42-51, 2018.

trilostane's additional inhibition of enzymes of the hormone cascade, like 11-beta-hydroxylase and possibly 11-beta-hydroxysteroid dehydrogenase (11βHSD).[61]

The peak of trilostane concentrations is achieved approximately 1.5 hours post administration, followed by a decline to initial levels within an approximate span of 18 hours.[62] The variation in systemic trilostane levels following oral dosing may be due to suboptimal absorption resulting from its limited aqueous solubility. It has been established that administering trilostane with food enhances its absorption.[63] Therefore, trilostane should be always administered with food.

Indication for PDH and ADHC treatment

Since 1998 trilostane has been approved for the medical treatment of both canine pituitary-dependent hypercortisolism (PDH) and adrenal-dependent hypercortisolism (ADHC). However, most investigations regarding trilostane utilization have been conducted in dogs affected by PDH.[64-66] In contrast, comprehensive investigations on the treatment of ADHC with trilostane remain lacking.[67,68] The therapeutic effect of trilostane on cortisol-secreting adrenocortical tumors (AT) is limited to mitigating clinical signs and does not exert influence or potential metastatic progression. Nevertheless, trilostane-based palliative intervention in dogs with AT has demonstrated efficacy in effectively managing clinical signs.[69,70]

Dosing and frequency of administration

Dosage regimens, administration frequencies, and monitoring protocols for trilostane remain subjects of ongoing evaluation.

For initial treatment, trilostane should be administered at the dose of 0.5-1 mg/kg PO q12h, with a maximum initial dose of 30 mg/dog for dogs >30 kg. When using lower initial dosages, it might take a longer time to achieve control of clinical signs, but this regime frequently proves sufficient while simultaneously minimizing overdose risk.[71,72] Although q12h administration suffices for effective HC management, some cases are well controlled only when trilostane is administered q8h. Irrespective of the chosen starting dose and administration frequency, treatment mandates tailoring to meet the patient's and owner's unique requirements. Moreover, as body weight increases, the requisite trilostane dosage tends to decrease.[73]

Presently, the prescribed dosage for ADHC is identical to that recommended for PDH. Clinical observations suggest that dogs with ADHC may exhibit heightened sensitivity to trilostane therapy, indicating the initiation of treatment with a relatively conservative initial dosage of 0.5 mg/kg q12h. Trilostane is commercially available in capsule formulations of 5, 10, 30, 60 and 120 mg. Compounded doses, if required, should exclusively employ the licensed trilostane product and must be prepared by skilled pharmacists.[74]

Efficacy

Approximately 7-10 days after commencing trilostane, owners should observe heightened activity and reduced polyuria/polydipsia.[64-66] Among these, polyphagia might exhibit a gradual decline over several weeks. The resolution of dermatological issues may extend over several months (Fig. 34.17). Initially, some dogs might experience a perceived deterioration in their hair coat due to the shedding of dead hair and dry skin, resulting in exacerbated alopecia and pronounced flaking. Calcinosis cutis can show complete resolutions in some patients with trilostane therapy, although it usually takes from months to years to occur.

Typical laboratory anomalies associated with HC, such as elevated alkaline phosphatase, show improvement with trilostane treatment.[64,75] Proteinuria, detected by the urinary protein-to-creatinine ratio, tends to improve with trilostane treatment over time, yet some dogs remain proteinuric even after a year of therapy.[76] Hypercortisolism correlates with calcium imbalance, leading to the formation of calcium-oxalate uroliths, soft tissue mineralization like calcinosis cutis, or perihilar bronchial mineralization.[77] The effectiveness of trilostane ranges from 67% to 100% in resolving different clinical signs of HC over a period of 3 to 6 months in both PDH and ADHC.[65-67]

Monitoring

Regular and frequent monitoring is imperative for the effective management of HC with trilostane. Over the past decade, significant efforts have been directed toward identifying the optimal approach for monitoring trilostane therapy.[58,78-88] Regardless of the chosen method, the evaluation of clinical signs stands as the initial step (Table 34.5).

Among the available monitoring methods, the frequently employed approach entails the utilization of the ACTH-stimulation test (ACTHst). This test is used to assess the adrenal glands' capacity to secrete cortisol in response to stimulation and is regarded as an indicator of cortisol reserve.[78]

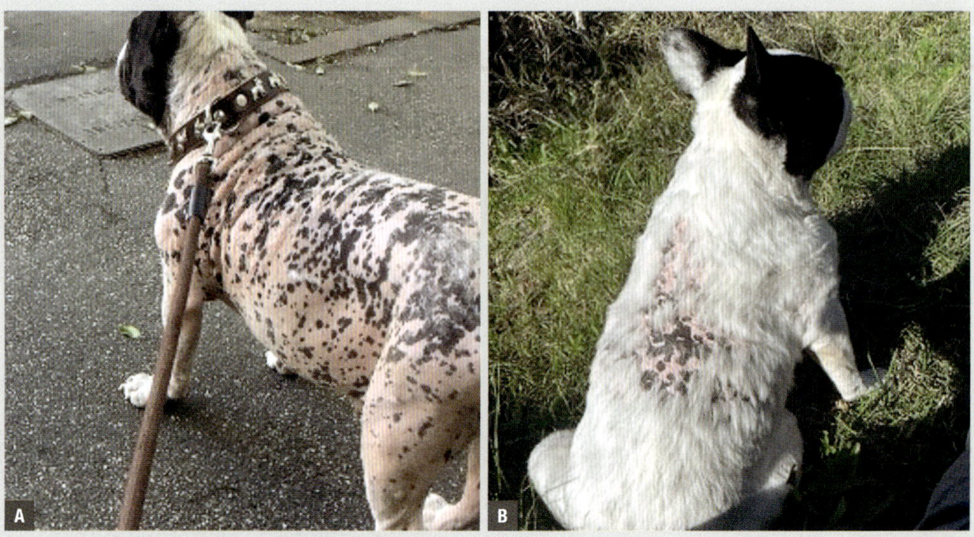

FIG. 34.17 An 11-year-old neutered female French Bulldog with pituitary-dependent hypercortisolism. (**A**) Generalized alopecia at diagnosis. (**B**) Coat improvement after 4 months of trilostane treatment.

As such, an ACTHst evaluates the safety of trilostane dosages. The timing of the ACTHst to monitor trilostane therapy is of paramount importance, as it can substantially influence the test results.[89] It is recommended to schedule the test in close alignment with the peak action of trilostane, which is approximately 2-3 hours post trilostane administration, to ensure accurate assessment.[62] Given that trilostane absorption is influenced by food intake, the medication is typically administered with a meal, and the patient should not fast on the morning of the test.

An alternative method involves measuring the pre-trilostane administration cortisol (prepill) and correlating it with clinical signs reported by owners.[80] This approach proposes that cortisol concentration, measured after the effects of trilostane have diminished, could provide objective insights into optimal dosage and frequency for the dog. Among the various monitoring tests investigated, the prepill appeared to exhibit the strongest correlation with clinical assessment. However, it still has limitations. For instance, when two prepill cortisol measurements were taken at one-hour intervals, conflicting information regarding therapeutic control was achieved. In 30% of dogs with paired results, each of which would have led to entirely different treatment decisions.[87] Moreover, the prepill measurement does not provide insights into adrenal reserve and the risk of overdosing.

A recent study aimed to compare various monitoring methods that have been proposed over the years to determine the most effective one. Despite haptoglobin, γ-glutamyl transferase, and ALT seemed to best correlate with the clinical picture, none of the proposed methods was able to identify overdosed dogs. The study failed to pinpoint a single test that could serve as a replacement for clinical assessment.[58]

TABLE 34.5 Compilation from 10 studies of possible trilostane monitoring methods in dogs with hypercortisolism.

Study referenced	Total number of dogs (PDH) (ADH)	Monitoring methods evaluated	Gold standard for the treatment control	Conclusion
McGrotty et al., 2015[88]	12 (/) (/)	Haptoglobin	Clinical evaluation	Clinical control of HC did not closely correlate to haptoglobin
Galac et al., 2009[82]	18 (18) (0)	UCCR	ACTHst	UCCR cannot be used as an alternative to ACTHst
Arteaga et al., 2010[83]	13 (/) (/)	Acute phase proteins, ALP, prepill	ACTHst	No additional info in comparison with ACTHst
Cook and Bond, 2010[84]	103 (/) (/)	Basal cortisol (4-6h post-trilostane)	ACTHst	Basal cortisol provided clinically useful information
Burkhardt et al., 2013[85]	40 (/) (/)	Pre-ACTH	ACTHst	ACTHst cannot be replaced
Boretti et al., 2016[81]	97 (/) (/)	Pre-ACTH, Post-ACTH, eACTH	Clinical evaluation	Clinical signs matched poorly with cortisol and eACTH
Macfarlane et al., 2016[80]	67 (23) (4) (40 unknown)	Prepill, 2h post-trilostane, 3h post-trilostane, post-ACTH	Clinical evaluation	Prepill and 3h post-trilostane are potentially better monitoring methods than ACTHst
Woolcock et al., 2016[86]	22 (/) (/)	Pre-ACTH	ACTHst	Pre-ACTH cannot be used as a sole monitoring method
Arenas Bermejo et al., 2020[75]	22 (22) (/)	Pre-ACTH, prepill, USG, UCCR	Clinical evaluation	No variable discriminates between adequate controlled and uncontrolled dogs
Golinelli et al., 2021[58]	45 (44) (1)	Pre-ACTH, post-ACTH, prepill, eACTH, prepill/eACTH, haptoglobin, USG, UCCR, ALT, GGT, ALP	Clinical evaluation	No monitoring methods can substitute clinical evaluation
Wehner et al., 2021[78]	49 (40) (4) (3 PDH + ADH) (2 unknown)	ACTHst	Clinical evaluation	Clinical signs of hypercortisolism were not predicted from ACTHst

UCCR, urine cortisol creatinine ratio; ALP, alkaline phosphatase activity; prepill, pretrilostane administration cortisol concentration; pre-ACTH, pre-ACTH stimulation cortisol concentration; post-ACTH, post-ACTH stimulation cortisol concentration; eACTH, endogenous ACTH; USG, urinary specific gravity; ALT serum alanine aminotransferase; GGT; γ-glutamyl transferase.

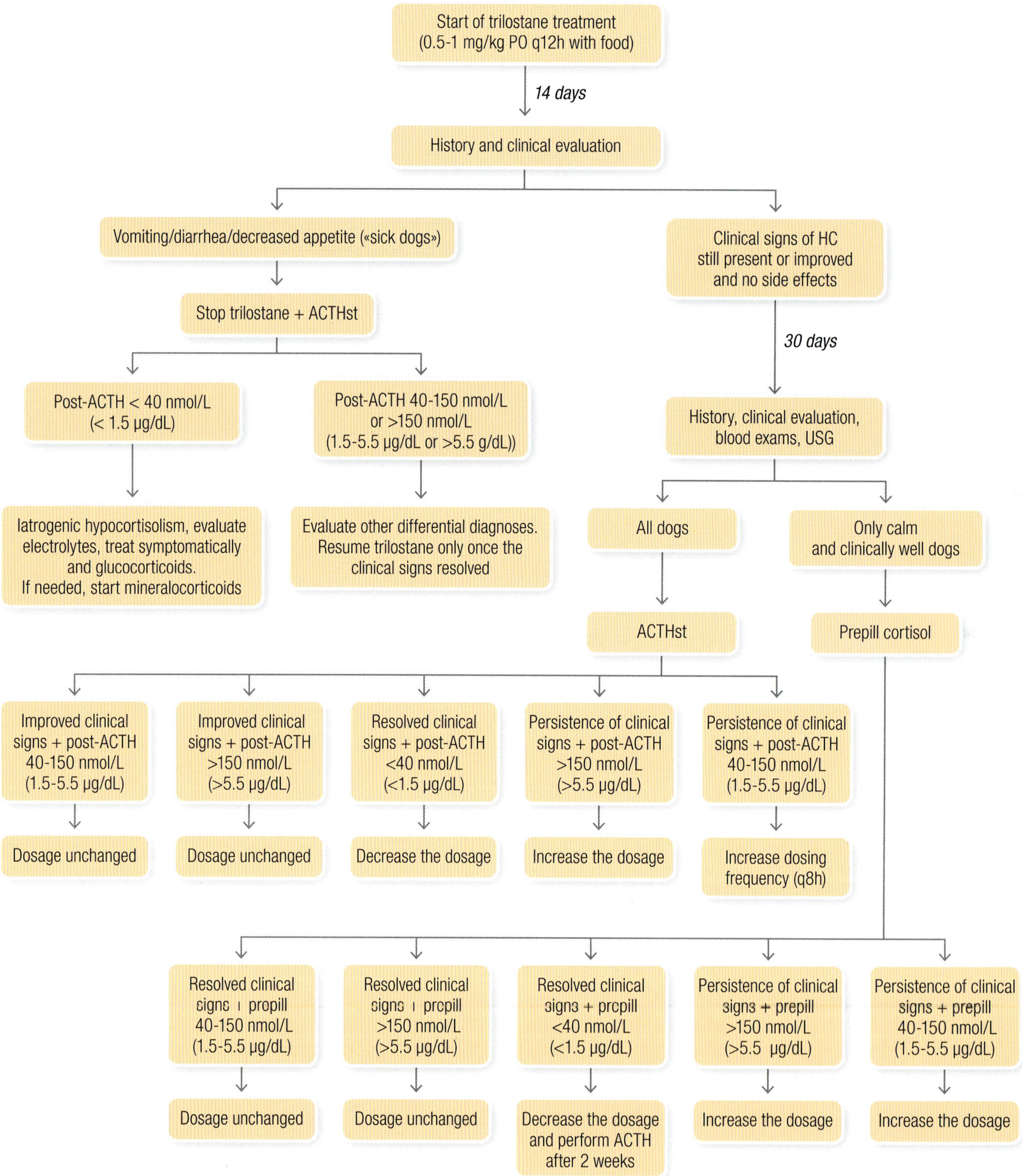

FIG. 34.18 Protocol for the use and monitoring of trilostane treatment in dogs with hypercortisolism. USG, urinary specific gravity; ACTHst, ACTH stimulation test; post-ACTH, post-ACTH stimulation cortisol concentration; prepill, pretrilostane administration cortisol concentration. The suggested cortisol values refer to measurements with the chemiluminescence.

At present, therapeutic monitoring relies on clinical assessment combined with comprehensive blood and urine examination. Depending on the patient (susceptibility to stress, cooperative or noncooperative behavior) and the treatment progress (persistence or resolution of signs related to HC, suspected overdosing), either prepill or the ACTHst can be employed (**Fig. 34.18**).[58,80]

The optimal cortisol concentrations for a dog undergoing trilostane therapy are generally within 40 to 150 nmol/L (1.5 to 5.5 µg/dL) both for post-ACTH and prepill. However, when evaluating the post-ACTH cortisol concentration, consideration must be given to the pre-ACTH value as well. In a dog with a pre-ACTH cortisol concentration of 30 nmol/L (1.4 µg/dL) and a post-ACTH of 40 nmol/L (1.5 µg/dL), the adrenal stimulation is insufficient, despite the post-ACTH concentration being within the reference range. Attention must be paid to signs of overdosed treatment.

In the past, the recommended protocol involved conducting the first assessment within 10 to 14 days after initiating trilostane or adjusting doses, followed by endocrine tests at 1, 3, and subsequently every 3 to 6 months once the trilostane dosage stabilizes. It is generally acknowledged that in some dogs, both clinical symptoms and cortisol concentrations continue to ameliorate within the initial month of commencing trilostane therapy. Consequently, apart from the onset of symptoms indicative of overdosage (e.g., vomiting, diarrhea, anorexia, lethargy), the first check-up is recommended 1 month after the start of therapy.

It is recommended to conduct an assessment within 1 month following any dose modification. Once the dog's clinical status and dose are stable, subsequent check-ups should be carried out at 30 and 90 days after trilostane' start, followed by every 3 months for the first year of treatment. For well-controlled dogs, check-ups should be planned 1 to 2 times for years. The extent of dosage adjustment, whether upward or downward, is often influenced by available capsule sizes, generally hovering around 25-50%.

Side effects and potential risks

Trilostane is generally well-tolerated. The main adverse effects include transient hypocortisolism (deficiency of glucocorticoids), possibly combined or followed by complete hypoadrenocorticism (deficiency of both glucocorticoids and mineralocorticoids). Around 15% of dogs on trilostane therapy experience clinical hypocortisolism within the first two years.[90]

Mild side effects of trilostane include lethargy and reduced appetite, while severe effects encompass depression, anorexia, vomiting, diarrhea, and more.[55,56] If concerning clinical signs appear, trilostane should be discontinued first. Most adverse effects resolve upon discontinuation, with possible continuation of trilostane treatment at a lower dose only when clinical signs of HC reoccur.

While theoretically reversible within 1 to 2 days, trilostane suppression effect can last weeks to years.[91,92] The role of trilostane in causing adrenal necrosis as the reason for permanent hypoadrenocorticism is debatable, with some studies implicating increased ACTH production as responsible.[56,93]

Caution is needed when administering trilostane with ACE inhibitors or aldosterone antagonists due to cumulative suppression of aldosterone concentration. As trilostane diminishes adrenal reserve, it is imperative to discontinue the medication during periods of stress, such as concurrent illnesses or surgical procedures. Given these potential complications, careful monitoring and recommended evaluations are crucial for dogs on trilostane, even if they appear clinically stable.

Dogs with HC display higher parathyroid hormone and phosphate concentrations compared to healthy dogs, and these irregularities tend to improve during trilostane treatment.[77]

Consequences of HC, like hypertension, present in over 50% of HC patients, often persist even after a year of trilostane treatment.[94]

Limited information exists regarding trilostane use in dogs with concurrent HC and diabetes mellitus. Excessive cortisol levels induce insulin resistance, complicating the management of diabetes in dogs with concurrent uncontrolled HC. Insulin resistance is expected to partially improve with trilostane treatment, necessitating vigilant blood glucose monitoring for dogs with both conditions.

Prognosis

Median survival times for PDH dogs undergoing trilostane treatment range from 662 to 852 days.[95-97] Dogs with PDH dogs under q12h trilostane administration have notably higher median survival times (900 days) compared to PDH dogs treated q24h (662 days). Median survival times for dogs with ADHC on trilostane therapy range from 353 to 427 days.[69,70] In dogs with PDH, trilostane effectively mitigates the clinical manifestations of glucocorticoid excess, but it does not affect the growth of the pituitary tumor. While this seems less relevant for dogs initially presented with nonenlarged pituitary glands (characterized by a pituitary brain value (P/B) of ≤0.31), the pituitary tumor may exhibit growth over time (**Fig. 34.19**). It is noteworthy that in healthy dogs, the P/B value has been

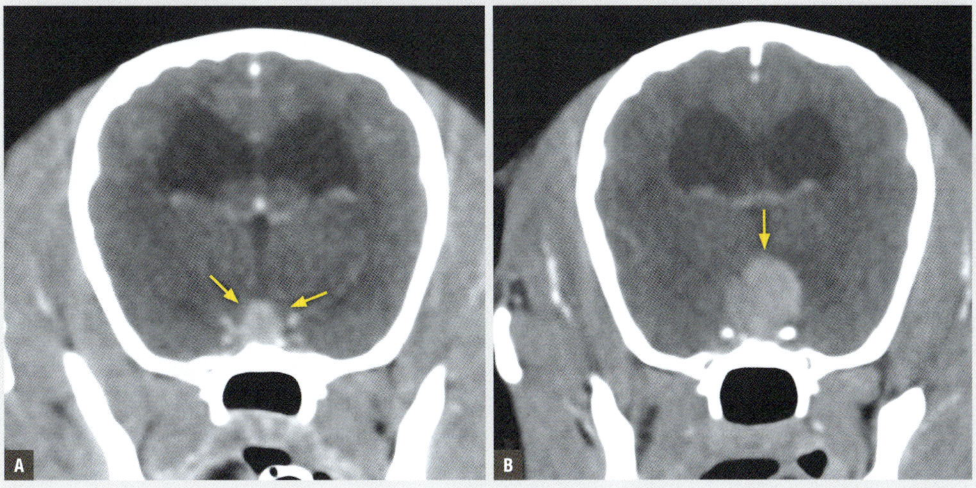

FIG. 34.19 Postcontrast cross-sectional images of the cranial region involving the pituitary fossa in a mixed-breed dog with pituitary-dependent hypercortisolism. (**A**) Pituitary tumor prior to the star of trilostane treatment (0.7 cm in height × 0.5 cm in width × 0.6 cm in length). (**B**) The same pituitary tumor after one year of trilostane treatment (1.2 cm in height × 1.3 in weight × 2.6 cm in lenght).

shown to notably increase subsequent to trilostane therapy; however, this phenomenon remains unexplored in dogs with PDH.[98] Notwithstanding, particularly in younger dogs with PDH, the consideration of a follow-up computed tomography (CT) or magnetic resonance imaging (MRI) scan after one year of treatment is advisable to re-evaluate pituitary size and reevaluate the treatment choice.

Mitotane

History, mechanism of action, and pharmacology

Mitotane (o,p'-DDD) is an adrenocorticolytic agent derived from the insecticide DDT.[99] It hinders the production of cortisol-inhibiting steroidogenic enzymes, including CYP11A1 and CYP11B1, and induces additional cytochrome P450 enzymes that alter glucocorticoid clearance[52] (**Fig. 34.16**). The exact mechanism underlying mitotane actions has not been fully elucidated. Recent research has revealed a mechanism involving the inhibition of sterol-O-acyl-transferase 1 (SOAT1), an enzyme catalyzing the conversion of free cholesterol to cholesterol esters. This inhibition elevates intracellular free cholesterol levels, triggering endoplasmic reticulum stress and subsequent cell apoptosis.

Although largely replaced by trilostane due to its efficacy and safety profile, mitotane offers several advantages, including notably high efficacy, particularly in cases of PDH non-responsive to trilostane and non-surgical ADHC (**Fig. 34.20**).

Mitotane can be employed to induce partial degradation of the adrenal cortex, preserving the zona glomerulosa (standard protocol or selective protocol), or to cause the necrosis of the entire adrenal cortex (non-selective or ablative protocol). Despite the zona glomerulosa's relative resistance to mitotane effects, in a subset of dogs receiving mitotane with standard protocol complete adrenocortical insufficiency can arise.[100] Aldosterone deficiency resulting from this can pose life-threatening implications, and this was one of the main reasons for introducing selective protocol.

Standard protocol

The initial induction phase involves administering mitotane tablets at 30 to 50 mg/kg/day for 8-10 days or until signs of hypocortisolism emerge. Owners should vigilantly monitor their dogs' behavior, appetite, and water intake to assess the need for drug discontinuation or ACTHst. An early and commonly observed adverse sign is a decrease in appetite, which typically precedes the development of other adverse clinical signs like vomiting, weakness, and complete anorexia. Due to this, the dog's owner should carefully observe the dog's appetite before administering the daily dosage of mitotane. Mitotane should be administered with food to enhance gastrointestinal absorption due to its fat-soluble nature. The duration of the loading phase cannot be predicted based on the severity of the disease or initial cortisol levels (**Fig. 34.21**).[100]

The efficacy and safety of mitotane therapy are mainly assessed through ACTHst, aiming for post-ACTH cortisol concentrations between 27 and 135 nmol/L (1 to 5 µg/dL). Each dog's response to mitotane during the induction phase varies. The typical duration required to achieve effective control is around 11 days, but due to individual sensitivity, it can span from 5 days to 2 months.

Approximately 10% to 15% of dogs exhibit an exacerbated response to exogenous ACTH after the induction phase and an insufficient clinical response. For these dogs, it is advised to maintain the daily mitotane administration and conduct the ACTHst again on a weekly basis until either adverse clinical signs emerge or the circulating cortisol concentration aligns with the targeted range.

Roughly 33% of dogs may exhibit a serum cortisol concentration below the optimal level (e.g., post-ACTH cortisol concentration <30 nmol/L (<1 µg/dL) after induction; in such cases, mitotane therapy should be halted, and an ACTHst should be performed after 2 weeks to evaluate adrenal function. During this period, prednisone can be administered at physiological doses (0.2 mg/kg q24h).[100] If prednisone or prednisolone is administered, it is crucial to wait at least 12 hours before conducting an ACTHst, as prednisone can cross-react in cortisol assays.

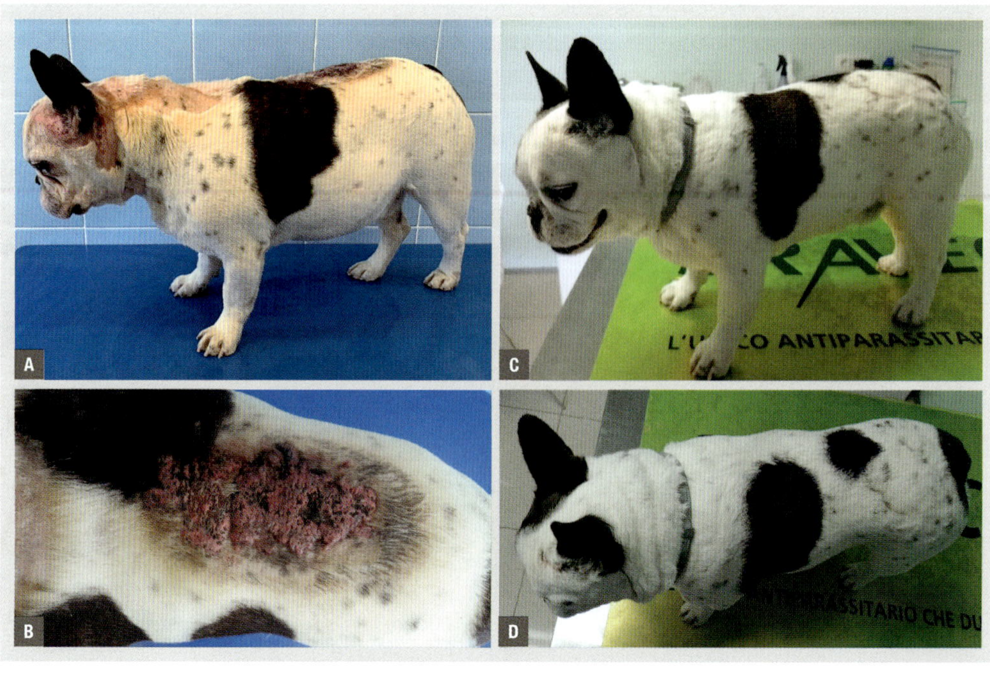

FIG. 34.20 A 7-year-old intact male French Bulldog with pituitary-dependent hypercortisolism. (A) and (B) Alopecia, abdominal enlargement, calcinosis cutis after 1 year of trilostane treatment. (C) and (D) A visible improvement 6 months after transitioning to mitotane treatment.

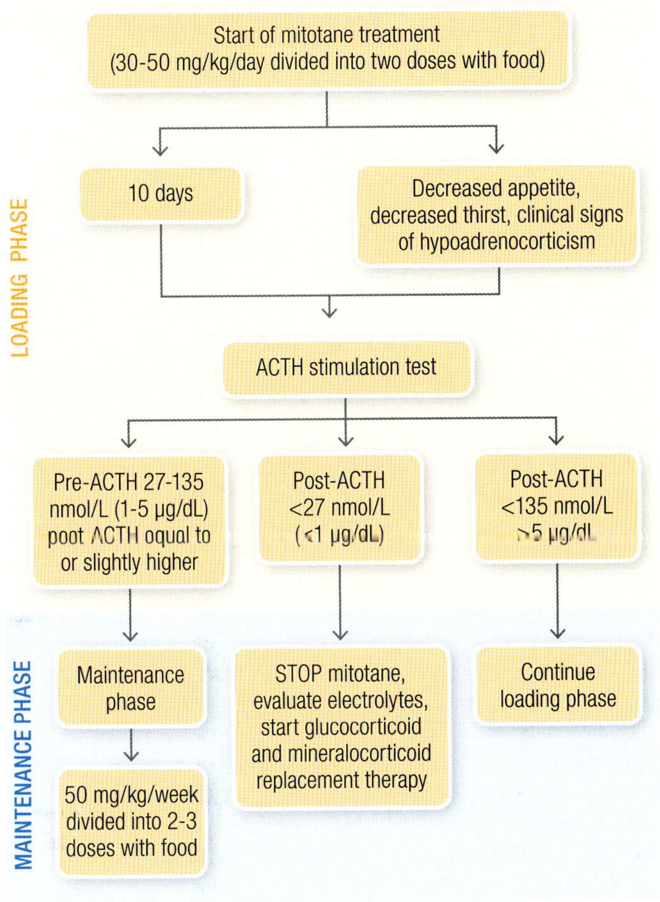

FIG. 34.21 Scheme for the use and monitoring of the selective mitotane protocol. Pre-ACTH, pre-ACTH stimulation cortisol concentration; post-ACTH, post-ACTH stimulation cortisol concentration.

Once documentation of cortisol secretion recovery is confirmed and the concentrations fall within the desired range, the maintenance phase can commence. Maintenance involves a weekly mitotane dosage of about 50 mg/kg divided into three administrations, along with periodic ACTHst to ensure appropriate control.

Nonselective protocol

The nonselective protocol aims to achieve complete destruction of the adrenal cortex layers. The treatment regimen involves administering mitotane at a dose of 50 to 75 mg/kg per day. Initially, mitotane is given daily for 5 days, followed by every other day dosing over a span of 40 days (25 doses of mitotane in total). For smaller dog breeds, a higher dosage of up to 100 mg/kg might be necessary. It is recommended to divide each daily dose into three or four portions.[101]

Substitution therapy commences on the third day, involving daily administration of glucocorticoids (e.g., 2 mg/kg cortisone acetate) and mineralocorticoids (e.g., 0.0125 mg/kg fludrocortisone acetate) divided into at least two portions. Following the initial mitotane course, the glucocorticoid dose is reduced (e.g., 0.5-1 mg/kg cortisone acetate). To prevent relapse, mitotane should be administered at the initial daily dose once weekly for at least 6 months or potentially throughout the dog's lifetime, which is usually the case for dogs with ADHC.

To assess the complete destruction of the adrenal cortex, the urinary cortisol-to-creatinine ratio ([UCCR] assessed by radioimmunoassay) can be measured in morning urine after the initial mitotane course (i.e., after day 45), and subsequently every 6 months. Before collecting morning urine for UCCR measurement, evening doses of glucocorticoids and mineralocorticoids should be withheld. Effective destruction of the adrenal cortex results in very low or undetectable UCCRs. This approach is only possible when cortisone acetate is used as a supplement for glucocorticoids. Additionally, regular measurements of blood sodium and potassium are essential to regulate the dosage of administered mineralocorticoids.[52]

Throughout both mitotane protocols, side effects such as lethargy, anorexia, vomiting, and diarrhea are common, largely due to direct drug intolerance rather than being attributed to absolute or relative hypoadrenocorticism.

If a dog undergoing mitotane treatment experiences any form of stress (such as illness, trauma, surgery, or others), the initiation of stress dosage of glucocorticoids is recommended. While a dog with HC generally possesses adequate adrenal reserve for routine daily activities, this reserve might be insufficient to cope with significant instances of stress.

Prognosis

In general, dogs treated with a selective mitotane protocol exhibit median survival times of 102 to 476 days.[95,97] The survival times of dogs treated with a nonselective mitotane protocol are unknown.

Ketoconazole

Ketoconazole, an imidazole antifungal drug, exerts its pharmacological influence by not only combatting fungal infections but also impeding the biosynthesis of glucocorticoids and androgens.[52] It inhibits various cytochrome P450 enzymes, including CYP11A1 and CYP11B1 (**Table 34.16**), thereby reducing cortisol synthesis. Its impact on cortisol levels within circulation is noteworthy, while its impact on mineralocorticoid production remains relatively inconspicuous.[102] Ketoconazole is no longer used due to its limited effectiveness and high incidence of adverse effects.

Adrenal-directed drugs (future options)

Emerging pharmaceutical options show promise in refining treatment strategies for HC. These include melanocortin 2 receptor antagonists, CYP17 inhibitors like abiraterone acetate, steroidogenic factor-1 (SF-1) inverse agonists, SOAT1 inhibitors, and some other potential drugs that have emerged only in humans in the last years (**Box 34.1**).[52]

Pituitary-directed drugs

The optimal approach to managing PDH involves specifically addressing the pituitary tumor. Due to their inhibitory functions within the pituitary gland, dopamine (DA) and somatostatin (SST) have gained significant attention.

The focus on pituitary-directed drugs centers around three primary receptor subtypes: dopamine receptor subtype 2 (DRD2), somatostatin receptor subtype 2 (SSTR2), and somatostatin receptor subtype 5 (SSTR5). In canine corticotroph adenomas, the predominant receptor subtype expressed is SSTR2, whereas DRD2 and, particularly, SSTR5 are expressed at considerably lower levels.[103] It is noteworthy that when comparing treatment approaches between dogs and humans, the

Box 34.1 Medical treatment of hypercortisolism: future perspectives.

Melanocortin 2 receptor (MC2R) antagonist

The MC2R receptor is a member of a cluster of five melanocortin receptors referred to as MC1R through MC5R. These receptors are triggered by melanocortin peptides derived from the precursor molecule pro-opiomelanocortin (POMC). What sets MC2R apart is its unique affinity for specific ligands. While various melanocortin peptides can interact with the other MC receptors, MC2R exclusively binds to ACTH.[108] Consequently, the development of a potent MC2R antagonist holds considerable promise for innovative treatments by selectively impeding ACTH-dependent hypercortisolism.

In the realm of human research, CRN04894, a potent and orally bioavailable nonpeptide, has demonstrated significant *in vitro* efficacy as a highly selective antagonist for the melanocortin type 2 receptor (MC2R). Currently, it is undergoing evaluation in a phase 1 clinical trial to thoroughly assess its safety, pharmacokinetics, pharmacodynamics, and tolerability in healthy individuals.[109,110]

Additionally, in a recent study, two MC2R antagonist peptide compounds, namely BIM-22776 (#776) and BIM-22A299 (#299), were assessed using primary adrenocortical cell cultures from normal canine adrenal glands. This study indicated efficacy, particularly in the case of #299.[111] However, to establish their effectiveness *in vivo*, further investigations are warranted.

Abiraterone acetate

Abiraterone acetate (AA) serves as an irreversible inhibitor of the 17α-hydroxylase/17, 20-lyase enzyme (CYP17) and is utilized in human patients with prostate cancer. In this context, AA plays a pivotal role in the suppression of cortisol and androgen levels in humans. Recent investigations involving adult patients afflicted with adrenocortical carcinomas have underscored AA efficacy in promptly limiting cortisol excess.[112]

Notably, research has established that while the CYP17 enzyme is indispensable for cortisol production in dogs, it is not essential for aldosterone synthesis.[113] Moreover, a more contemporary study has elucidated the proficiency of AA in specifically inhibiting cortisol production without exerting any impact on aldosterone production within canine adrenocortical cell cultures.[114]

As we look to the future, *in vivo* investigations are needed to ascertain whether AA holds promise as a valuable addition to the existing array of treatment choices for canine hypercortisolism.

Steroidogenic factor-1 (SF-1) inverse agonists

SF-1, an orphan nuclear receptor, orchestrates adrenal development, growth, and steroidogenesis.[115] The transcriptional activity of SF-1 is activated by ACTH, thereby increasing the expression of genes encoding steroidogenic enzymes. Elevated SF-1 activity stands as a notable feature in dogs afflicted by pituitary-dependent hypercortisolism (PDH). Furthermore, research has indicated that the expression of SF-1 mRNA was markedly higher in adrenocortical tumors (ATs) of dogs experiencing hypercortisolism recurrence within 2.5 years following adrenalectomy, compared to ATs of dogs without recurrence.[116]

Recent advancements have unveiled a promising avenue with the identification of a specific SF-1 inverse agonist compound, denoted as compound #31. This compound effectively inhibits cortisol production and suppresses the expression of SF-1 target genes within canine adrenocortical cells *in vitro*.[116] The inhibition of SF-1 activity demonstrates considerable potential as a prospective treatment strategy in both PDH and cortisol-secreting ATs.

Sterol-o-acyltransferase 1 (SOAT1) inhibitors

ATR-101, a selective sterol-o-acyltransferase 1 (SOAT1) inhibitor, is an innovative oral adrenal-targeted medication that is presently undergoing clinical assessment as a potential treatment for Cushing's syndrome, adrenal cortical carcinoma, and congenital adrenal hyperplasia in humans. Distinguishing itself from existing adrenal-targeted drugs that affect steroidogenesis enzymes, such as mitotane, ATR-101 operates on SOAT1a transmembrane enzyme pivotal in cholesterol metabolism.[117]

A study on 18 healthy Beagle dogs demonstrated that ATR-101 induced degeneration and necrosis in the adrenal zona fasciculate and reticularis, leading to adrenal insufficiency. Interestingly, adrenocortical degeneration manifested across all dose levels, while adrenal insufficiency signs and symptoms showed a dose-dependent correlation.[118]

In canine adrenocortical cell cultures, ATR-101 was found to impair mitochondrial respiration and impede adrenal cholesterol efflux, suggesting a potential role in the cytotoxic elevation of intracellular free cholesterol.[119]

Other two studies involving dog models have examined the impact of ATR-1 on cortisol secretion.[118,120] One study with three female dogs demonstrated that ATR-101 treatment at 3 mg/kg/day and 30 mg/kg/day resulted in reductions of 62% and 71% in ACTH-stimulated cortisol levels, respectively. Similarly, ATR-101 treatment led to decreased ACTH-stimulated levels of cortisol precursors and androgens.[120]

In another study involving 10 dogs with hypercortisolism, ATR-101 treatment reduced ACTH-stimulated cortisol levels in 90% of cases. Overall, the cohort observed a significant decrease in ACTH-stimulated cortisol levels within the first week of treatment, which was maintained throughout the four-week study period. Improvement was seen in 70% of cases, 20% remained stable, and 10% experienced worsening symptoms. Adverse events included a slight decline in hematocrit and serum albumin (within the normal range), along with increased alanine aminotransferase levels, mildly elevated alkaline phosphatase levels, and isolated episodes of vomiting and diarrhea.[121]

Considering the notably pronounced effect of ATR-101 in dogs, this strategy shows considerable potential as a promising pathway for treating dogs dealing with ATs.

Other potential drugs

Ongoing research is dedicated to exploring potential new adrenal-directed agents for treating Cushing's syndrome, both in humans and dogs.

Recently, cytochrome P450 Family 26 Subfamily B Member 1 (CYP26B1) has emerged as a novel prognostic marker and a promising therapeutic target for both canine and human corticotroph adenomas. Future investigations encompassing *in vitro* and *in vivo* studies could shed light on whether CYP26B1 inhibitors have the capability to impede tumor growth in both dogs and humans affected by ACTs.[122]

Among adrenal-directed agents in humans, metyrapone stands as the sole historical agent currently undergoing evaluation within a prospective, multicenter, international clinical trial. This trial holds the potential to provide crucial insights into the efficacy and safety of metyrapone across a substantial patient population afflicted with Cushing's syndrome.[123]

Additionally, osilodrostat, a small molecule inhibitor of 11β-hydroxylase available in oral form, shares a mechanism of action akin to metyrapone. Recently approved in the European Union for the treatment of endogenous Cushing's syndrome in humans, osilodrostat is presently undergoing regulatory review in the USA for treating Cushing's disease.[124]

Furthermore, levoketoconazole, a distinct chemical formulation of the historical agent ketoconazole, remains under scrutiny within clinical trials. Initial evidence suggests that it effectively and safely manages Cushing's syndrome.[123]

Cabergoline

Cabergoline functions as a dopamine agonist, binding to the dopamine receptor D2 (DRD2). Corresponding to the moderate expression of DRD2 in corticotroph adenomas of canines, the response of canine corticotroph cells to cabergoline was relatively modest when examined *in vitro*.[103]

However, *in vivo* experiments revealed a notable outcome: 43% of dogs afflicted with PDH exhibited positive responses to cabergoline treatment. These positive responses were characterized by a reduction in clinical manifestations, diminished pituitary adenoma sizes, and lower urinary cortisol creatinine ratios (UCCRs).[104] Notably, the variance in effectiveness observed could potentially be attributed to differences in the durations of the treatment periods.

The authors treated two groups of PDH dogs: one group received cabergoline in addition to trilostane, while the other group received trilostane alone. In the dogs treated with cabergoline, pituitary height and pituitary-to-brain value (P/B) were decreased in 4 out of 12 (30%) cases. This percentage corresponds to findings observed in humans and indicates that the effectiveness of cabergoline in reducing the size of pituitary tumors is evident only in a limited fraction of treated dogs.[105]

Pasireotide

Pasireotide (SOM230) is categorized as a multiligand somatostatin analog that effectively binds to four different somatostatin (SST) receptors (SSTR): SSTR 1, SSTR 2, SSTR 3, and SSTR 5.[125] In a study involving 20 dogs diagnosed with PDH, pasireotide demonstrated a notable reduction in plasma ACTH concentration along with improvements in clinical signs. Importantly, this response was achieved without the manifestation of severe adverse effects.[106] Another recent study focused on administering pasireotide to dogs afflicted with macroadenomas that were simultaneously undergoing trilostane or mitotane treatment. Among these cases, six out of nine dogs experienced a reduction in pituitary tumor volume, while the remaining three displayed an increase. Remarkably, no overt neurological signs or substantial adverse effects were observed.[125]

In the context of human application, pasireotide efficacy has been validated, leading to its approval in both Europe and the USA as a second-line treatment for PDH patients when surgical interventions have proven unsuccessful or unfeasible.[126] Notably, due to the distinct expression patterns of specific receptors, there is potential for an SST analog with a higher affinity for SST2 than pasireotide to yield enhanced efficacy in canines, as corroborated by *in vitro* experiments.[103]

Octreotide

Octreotide, an SST analog, exhibits high affinity binding to SSTR2 and moderate affinity binding to SSTR3 and SSTR5.[103] In concordance with the substantial expression of SSTR2 in corticotroph adenomas of canines, octreotide exerted a significant inhibitory effect on ACTH release in canine corticotroph cells when evaluated *in vitro*. This inhibitory effect was found to be more potent compared to the effects of pasireotide or cabergoline.[103]

While octreotide can induce gastrointestinal side effects in humans, its impact on dogs in this regard is less extensively documented. In other medical contexts, such as insulinoma, octreotide is occasionally employed as adjunctive treatment to mitigate insulin secretion. Nonetheless, its limited duration of action following subcutaneous injection restricts its applicability.[127]

Recently, a novel technology has emerged that enhances drug molecule absorption by transiently opening the tight junctions of the intestinal epithelium. This innovation has enabled the attainment of therapeutic levels of octreotide after oral administration in humans.[128] The potential advantage of orally administered octreotide lies in its avoidance of injection-related side effects. However, its usage would necessitate a rigorously adhered to twice-daily fasting dosing regimen in humans.[128] Given the substantial expression of SSTR2 in corticotroph tumors of canines, the introduction of oral octreotide treatment holds promise as an intriguing therapeutic avenue for dogs afflicted with PDH.

Retinoic acid

For the production of ACTH, the precursor molecule pro-opiomelanocortin (POMC) undergoes cleavage to yield multiple peptide hormones. The gene expression of POMC is regulated by various factors, including the transcription factors AP-1 and Nur77. Retinoic acid, functioning as a regulatory agent governing multiple cellular processes, influences these transcription factors' binding to their respective DNA binding sites. Consequently, ACTH secretion is inhibited.

A study involving 22 dogs treated with retinoic acid reported a decrease in plasma ACTH concentration, a reduction in UCCRs, resolution of clinical symptoms, and a diminishment in pituitary size.[129] In human application, retinoic acid has been associated with adverse effects such as teratogenicity, mucocutaneous toxicity, impaired liver function, and heightened photosensitivity. Strategies like minimizing light exposure have been explored to mitigate these effects.[130]

Notably, recent research indicated that 9-cis retinoic acid, an active isomer of retinoic acid, triggers activation of the DRD2 promoter, thereby rendering pituitary adenomas more responsive to dopaminergic treatments.[131] Furthermore, a synthetic retinoid analog named bexarotene has shown the potential to induce hypopituitarism. Consequently, a phase I and II clinical trial has been initiated in humans.

These comprehensive findings and ongoing investigations offer a broad spectrum of potential treatment avenues and hold promise for advancing our understanding and management of PDH.

distribution of these receptor subtypes differs to some extent. In human corticotroph adenomas, the main receptors are SSTR5 and DRD2. Cabergoline, a DRD2 agonist, along with pasireotide and octreotide, both somatostatin analogs, has been evaluated in canine studies. Cabergoline has demonstrated efficacy in 43% of dogs with PDH, reducing pituitary tumor size and UCCR and improving clinical signs of HC.[104] Recently, cabergoline combined with trilostane resulted in a reduction of pituitary size in 30% of treated dogs.[105] Pasireotide has also been used in dogs with PDH, either alone or in combination with trilostane, showing reductions in pituitary size and eACTH, and enhancing clinical signs of HC.[106] Lastly, octreotide has been shown to reduce eACTH levels *in vitro* more effectively than cabergoline and pasireotide, likely due to its higher affinity for SSTR2.[107] As of now, none of these drugs are approved for addressing PDH in dogs, and their use is off-label (**Box 34.1**)

Surgical treatment: trans-sphenoidal hypophysectomy

Björn Meij and Sara Del Magno

Trans-sphenoidal hypophysectomy is the treatment of choice for dogs with pituitary-dependent hypercortisolism (PDH) because it addresses both pituitary hormonal hypersecretion and the mass effect. It is superior to medical treatment with trilostane, which only addresses hormonal hypersecretion at the adrenal level, and radiation therapy, aiming to shrink the tumor mass over time (months) but is unable to address hormonal hypersecretion in the short-term.[52]

In humans with Cushing's disease, surgery aims to selectively remove the microadenoma (selective adenomectomy) while preserving the unaffected pituitary tissue. In dogs, the goal of surgery remains the complete removal of the pituitary mass since it is difficult to distinguish between the normal pituitary tissue and the pituitary tumor tissue pre- and intraoperatively.[53]

Hypophysectomy in patients with multiple hormonal and metabolic issues requires a multidisciplinary team approach before, during, and after surgery to prevent, monitor, and treat potential complications.[132] The team includes dedicated surgeons, endocrinologists, anesthesiologists, radiologists, and intensivists. The (surgical) learning curve and absence of expert team members may be the primary reason why this technique, although successful, is not widely available and performed.[53]

The technique can also be applied to treat other pituitary masses, such as somatotroph pituitary adenoma causing hypersomatotropism (see chapter 24) or non-hormonally functional adenomas (NFA). Corticotroph pituitary tumors are mostly adenomas; less frequently, they invade the surrounding tissues (invasive adenomas) and rarely show intracranial or extracranial metastasis (adenocarcinomas). Due to their growth, pituitary masses may cause compression of normal pituitary gland tissue or surrounding brain structures with secondary hormonal effects like diabetes insipidus, pituitary insufficiency, and/or mass effects like loss of appetite, dullness, hypothalamic disturbance, and cranial nerve deficits.[18]

Pituitary apoplexy in dogs, which is defined as hemorrhage and/or infarction of pre-existent sellar tumor (silent or endocrinologically active tumor), causes sudden onset of severe neurological signs like stupor/coma.[19,46] In humans, pituitary apoplexy may lead to sudden onset of loss of vision, which requires immediate trans-sphenoidal surgery. In dogs, information regarding the medical, surgical, or radiation treatment for pituitary apoplexy is still scarce. However, surgery may be considered when patients are stable enough to undergo anesthesia. Trans-sphenoidal hypophysectomy has been reported in one case with pituitary apoplexy, and the tumor was incompletely removed due to adhesions.[133]

Preoperative evaluation

Patients with PDH considered for hypophysectomy must have a thorough workup to ensure they are good surgical candidates. Preoperative evaluation entails comprehensive clinical and neurological examination, endocrine testing, and complete blood and urinalyses. Surgical planning necessitates an assessment of the dog's skull type, such as mesocephalic, dolichocephalic, or brachycephalic. Dolicho- and brachycephalic skull types increase surgical difficulty.

High owner compliance is mandatory for successfully managing the hormonal balance after surgery, and expectations should be clearly communicated with the owner during the patient-selection phase.

Surgical anatomy and diagnostic imaging

The pituitary gland is located at the base of the skull in the hypophyseal fossa of the sphenoid bone (sella turcica). The fossa is limited rostrally by the tuberculum sellae and caudally by the dorsum sellae (Fig. 34.22). The pituitary gland is located ventrally to the diencephalon and is largely outside the blood-brain barrier and covered ventrally by the dura mater. The pituitary gland is surrounded by vessels, laterally on both sides by the cavernous sinus that contains the internal carotid artery and dorsally by the arterial cerebral circle. The optic chiasm is located rostrally to the gland, which is not affected by dorsal enlargement of pituitary masses in dogs. The hypothalamus and third ventricle connect and extend to the pituitary gland by way of the infundibulum. All these structures are depicted in Fig. 34.22.

Pituitary imaging in dogs can be performed with CT or high-field MRI. Full-body CT allows imaging of the skull, thorax, and abdomen and is an essential step in evaluating the size and shape of the pituitary gland. It may also exclude the presence of concomitant adrenal tumors, other comorbidities, and metastasis (rare).

CT (or high-field MRI) is crucial for preoperative planning. The traditional approach to the pituitary fossa is based on the individual anatomy of the landmarks that can be best visualized on CT and then identified during surgery. The position of the hamular processes of the pterygoid bone and the shape of the outer surface of the sphenoid bone are considered landmarks for locating the fossa hypophysealis. The hamular processes

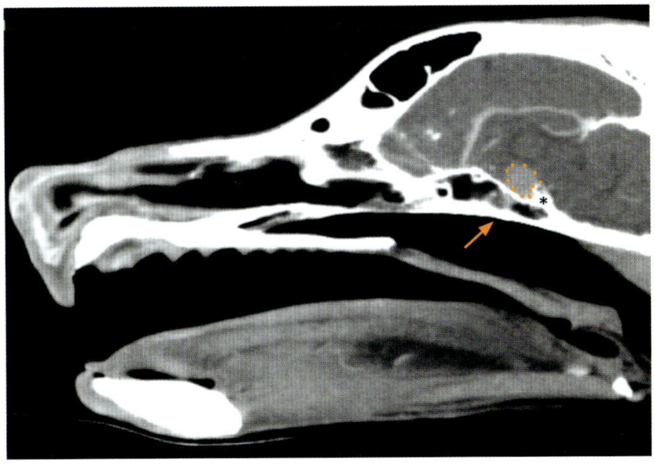

FIG. 34.22 Sagittal multiplanar reconstruction of contrast-enhanced CT in a mesocephalic dog with pituitary-dependent hypercortisolism. The enlarged pituitary gland shows typical suprasellar extension (orange dots). Other important anatomic features for the pituitary surgeon are the pituitary fossa, the double cortical layered sphenoid bone (arrow), the relation of the tumor to the dorsum sellae (*), and tuberculum sellae, the soft palate, and the extension of the hard palate.

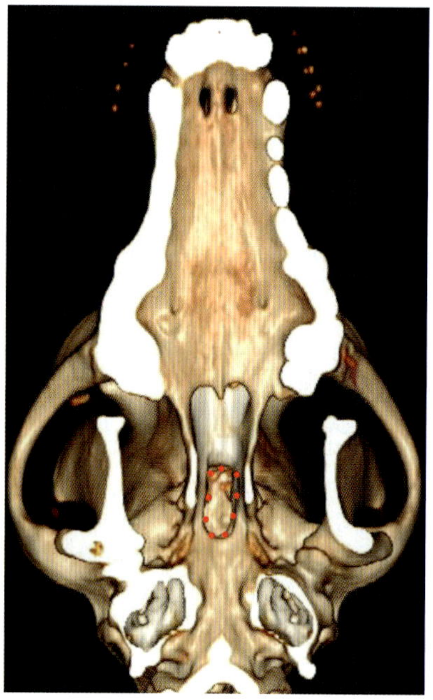

FIG. 34.23 Ventral view of a 3D skull reconstruction in a dog with pituitary-dependent hypercortisolism that underwent trans-sphenoidal hypophysectomy (same dog as depicted in Fig. 34.22). The round pituitary adenoma with a diameter of 12 mm was extracted through a burr hole (8 × 15 mm, red dots) and performed by careful preoperative assessment of anatomic CT bone landmarks only. In silico digital bone-cutting surface markings are shown in white.

are easily palpable through the soft palate, before and after the access to the nasopharynx during surgery; the outer cortex of the basisphenoid frequently has a ridge-to-groove transition from rostrocaudal as can be seen on spatial CT and palpated during surgery and linked to the pituitary enhancement on CT. All landmarks help in the exact positioning of the burr hole underlying the hypophyseal fossa. The thickness of the sphenoid bone to access the fossa can also be measured preoperatively to guide intraoperative access (Fig. 34.23).

However, experience is required to identify the correct location for access to the pituitary fossa, especially in dogs with more complex skull conformations like dolichocephalic and brachycephalic dogs. Recently, different modifications to the technique described in 1997 by Meij, et al.[134] have been proposed to facilitate pituitary localization before the burring of the bone, including:

- 3D printed custom guides based on CT images.[135,136]
- Neuronavigation system to intraoperatively locate the pituitary gland.[137]
- Intraoperative CT after drilling two initial pilot holes to relate to the position of the fossa.[138]
- In silico 3D skull reconstruction in brachycephalic dogs, to preoperatively dry-practice the surgical approach with ostectomy of the caudal portion of the hard palate.[139]

High-field MRI is an excellent diagnostic imaging technique to diagnose pituitary tumors.[140] However, microadenomas may also be difficult to visualize, and bony landmarks are less identifiable on MRI than on CT. Recently an MRI classification scheme has been developed to correlate the extension of the pituitary tumors and the indications for surgery. The classification is mainly based on the involvement of the vessels surrounding the pituitary tumor (circle of Willis or cavernous sinus) and the rostrocaudal and dorsal extension of the tumor. When there is no or minimal involvement of the blood vessels, with mild-moderate extension over the dorsum sellae and dorsal extension to the maximum of the third ventricle or the mammillary bodies, the tumor can be considered surgically removable. In more extreme cases, the surgery becomes challenging with an unpredictable outcome.[140]

Preoperative management and surgical technique

In patients pretreated with trilostane, it is advised to stop treatment three to four days before surgery.[52] During preoperative preparation, the application of a central venous catheter, an arterial catheter, and an indwelling urinary catheter is essential to allow precise monitoring of the fluid balance, hemodynamics, and electrolytes during and after surgery. The anesthesia protocol varies based on each patient's clinical condition.

The surgical approach in dogs with PDH is trans-oral and trans-sphenoidal. Magnification using an operating loupe, videoexoscope (VITOM), or freely moveable operating microscope is essential for pituitary surgery.

The dog is placed in a supinate position with the head elevated, and the table is usually tilted at around 40° angle. Traditionally, the maxilla is fixed to a support structure (e.g., metal bar behind canines) or halo frame, and the mandible is kept open without severe traction (**Fig. 34.24A**). This position allows direct access to the oral cavity, a midline approach, and facilitates the removal of the pituitary gland tissue added by gravity, and at the same time, allows a good flow in the jugular veins to avoid an increase of intracranial pressure.

A full-thickness incision of the soft palate is performed on the midline in the region where the hamular processes are palpable. The mucoperiosteum that covers the sphenoid bone is incised and elevated with a periosteal elevator. The shape and position of the hamular processes and of the outer cortex of the sphenoid bone are palpated and correlated to the CT images to precisely locate the fossa hypophysealis and the pituitary gland. Generally, the location for burring is at the basisphenoid bone.

The normal pituitary gland in dogs usually appears as white-to-pinkish tissue, and using a ball-tipped neural probe, the margins of the gland are palpated, and gentle traction is used to remove the gland. In the case of adenomas, the tissue may appear more greyish, dark blue, brown, or greenish due to hemorrhages, necrosis, and cholesterol crystals, and the structure may become more mucoid to fluid-like. In the case of large tumors, debulking is performed by first centrally removing pituitary tumor fragments, followed by circumferential traction of the remnant adenoma capsule (**Fig. 34.24B**). The neurohypophysis, which is usually removed at the end, can be recognized due to its posterior localization against the dorsum sellae. Following its removal, hemorrhage usually occurs due to its direct arterial supply from the caudal hypophyseal artery, which can easily be stopped using bipolar electrocautery.

After the complete pituitary gland is removed, the ventral portion of the hypothalamus is visible together with the entrance to the third ventricle. CSF can freely flow out at this point. To improve the vision, the VITOM exoscope or rigid endoscope can be introduced close to or in the fossa

Video 34.8

Video showing surgical planning on CT, trans-sphenoidal hypophysectomy, and recovery on intensive care in a 9-year-old female castrated Australian Shepherd dog diagnosed with pituitary-dependent hypercortisolism due to enlarged pituitary tumor measuring 12 × 10 × 11 mm and a P/B of 0.70.

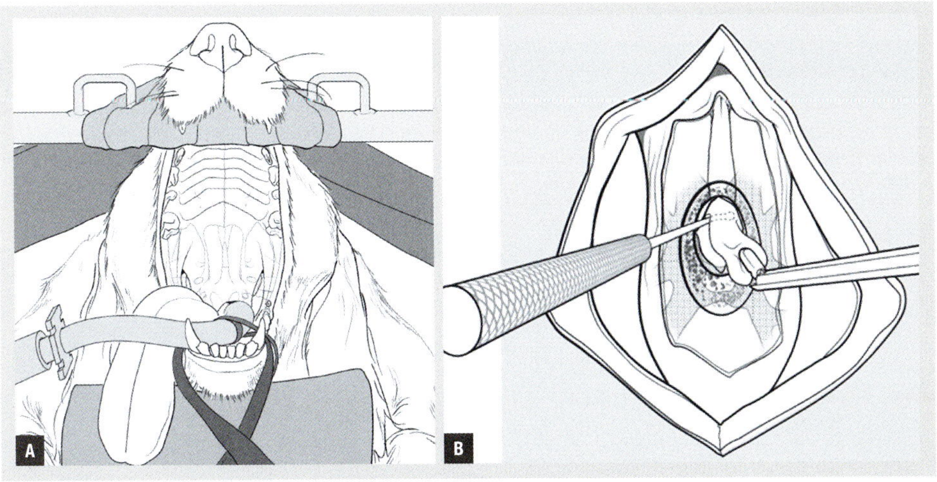

FIG. 34.24 (A) Schematic presentation of the positioning and surgical field in pituitary surgery. The surgeon faces the dog from the frontal side for the transoral, transnasal, and trans-sphenoidal approach to the pituitary fossa at the skull base. The maxilla is firmly attached to a support structure, whereas the mandibula is only loosely retracted ventrally. (B) The pituitary gland is carefully detached laterally, rostrally, dorsally, and caudally from its surroundings with a ball-tipped neural probe and grasped and extracted with neurosurgical biopsy forceps. Gentle traction is applied with simultaneous detachment by the probe (drawing courtesy of Remko van Deijk).

to check for remnants in the lateral, rostral, and caudal portions of the fossa. Once the removal of the mass is completed, the fossa is filled with a round portion of gelatin sponge, the hole in the bone is closed with bone wax, and the mucoperiosteum is partially sutured. The soft palate is sutured in two layers. A good inspection and removal of fluid from the oral cavity is important to avoid aspiration pneumonia during the recovery period (Video 38.8).

Postoperative care

In the postoperative period, professional intensive care support is essential to manage the complications that can occur after surgery (Table 34.6). Usually, dogs resume oral water and food intake the first days after surgery. Replacement therapy after hypophysectomy consists of the life-long administration of glucocorticoids (preferably cortisone acetate) and levothyroxine. Desmopressin, a synthetic vasopressin analog, is needed, at least temporarily, because removal of the pituitary adenoma by hypophysectomy also implies removal of the neurohypophysis, via which vasopressin, secreted by the hypothalamic paraventricular and supraoptic nuclei, reaches the systemic circulation.[136] Hypophysectomy results in transient central diabetes insipidus for up to 2 months, after which desmopressin can be gradually withdrawn. However, in about 22% of cases, the central diabetes insipidus remains permanent especially in case of large tumors (Table 34.7).

After hypophysectomy, high owner compliance in close cooperation with a well-informed local veterinary professional is mandatory for successful hormonal balance management. The owner needs to follow the medication scheme tightly and learn how to anticipate extreme stress situations.

Prognosis

Perioperative mortality (within 4 weeks after surgery) varies between 8-19%; while the intraoperative mortality is very low.[138,141,142]

Increased risk of death and shorter survival are related to elevated preoperative endogenous ACTH (eACTH) values, older age, and larger tumors.[142] The best outcome may be achieved when hypophysectomy is installed as the primary treatment for dogs with nonenlarged or moderately enlarged pituitaries following early diagnosis of PDH. Although a high pituitary brain (P/B) value is a negative prognosticator, hypophysectomy remains a good treatment option also for large pituitary tumors.[142] Brachycephalic dogs create a surgical challenge due to their skull conformation complicating the surgical approach and due to concurrent brachycephalic obstructive airway syndrome in varying degrees. However, even with an increased complication rate, postoperative survival remains good in the hands of an experienced surgeon.[139]

In large pituitary tumors and NFA, it is advised to perform immediate postoperative CT imaging with contrast to check for possible remnant tumors (Fig. 34.25). In dogs with PDH, the postoperative 5-hour trend of eACTH levels helps to predict remission of hypercortisolism in the short-term.[143] In the long-term, hormonal remission is evaluated by the absence of clinical signs and periodic measurement of urinary cortisol to creatinine ratios (UCCR) in urine samples collected at home, starting at 2 and 10 weeks after surgery. Monitoring in the long-term is advised with UCCR measurement every 6-12 months after surgery. The owner is instructed to omit the evening cortisone acetate dose and to collect the first morning urine sample. This monitoring is only possible when cortisone acetate is used because its short halftime does not interfere with urinary cortisol measurement and allows the measurement of endogenous glucocorticoids only. After complete hypophysectomy and full remission, the UCCR is very low ($<1\times10^{-6}$), often even under the detection level of the hormone assay.

Persistence of the disease can occur in cases of incomplete removal of the pituitary tumor, and recurrences are more frequent in cases of large pituitary tumors and thicker sphenoid bones, as these create more difficulties in visualization of the tumor and its complete removal.

In cases of very large pituitary tumors or recurrences, surgery can be followed with adjuvant radiation therapy to obtain a longer survival time. A second surgery, if feasible, can also be considered in case of recurrence. The long-term reported survival in dogs treated with hypophysectomy for PDH was 86% at 1 year, 79% at 2 years, 74% at 3 years, and 72% at 4 years. Estimated 1-year, 2-year, 3-year, and 4-year disease-free fractions were 89%, 79%, 74%, and 64%, respectively (Fig. 34.26). A recurrence rate of 27% is reported after a median of 555 days, more frequently in dogs with large tumors.[142,143,144]

TABLE 34.6 Postoperative complications after trans-sphenoidal hypophysectomy in dogs.

Postoperative complications	Frequency	Cause	Treatment	Prognosis
Hypernatremia (>160 mmol/L)	In the past, almost all dogs experienced hypernatremia, nowadays around 46% of dogs	Diabetes insipidus causes loss of free water through polyuria, dehydration	Adequate fluid therapy, stimulate oral water intake, and desmopressin administration	No influence on outcome
Hyponatremia (<135 mmol/L)	8.6%	Not known, in humans due to syndrome of inappropriate antidiuretic hormone secretion (SIADH), possibly due to hypothalamic trauma	Fluid therapy with higher sodium levels and immediate cessation of desmopressin administration	No influence on outcome
Transient diabetes insipidus	All dogs, where complete hypophysectomy is achieved	Temporary lack of vasopressin due to the removal of the neurohypophysis, restoration when neovascularization is complete	Administration of desmopressin for a minimum of 3 weeks after surgery, then gradually taper off and stop according to clinical effect	No influence on outcome
Persistent diabetes insipidus	Mainly in case of large pituitary tumors; 35% prolonged 22% lifelong	Prolonged or delayed dysfunction of hypothalamic nuclei that produce vasopressin, incomplete neovascularization and insufficient release of vasopressin into the systemic circulation	Prolonged or life-long administration of desmopressin	No influence on outcome, increased incidence in severely enlarged pituitary tumors
Neurogenic hyperthermia (>40°C)	Mainly in case of large pituitary tumor or traumatic surgery	Trauma or inflammation of the hypothalamic thermoregulation center	Active cooling, sedation	Fatal if severe (>41°C) and not addressed adequately
Keratoconjunctivitis sicca (KCS)	Breed predisposition (brachycephalic breeds), anesthesia (no eyelid function), endocrine disease (suppression of tear production), excessive and long duration open mouth	Subclinical minimal tear production preoperatively becomes clinical postoperatively. Traumatic or ischemic damage of the major petrosal nerves, resulting in deficit in tear production of the lacrimal glands	Administration of artificial tears every 6h and full KCS medication protocol (corneal protectants, antibiotics, anti-inflammatory agents, cyclosporine)	Usually transient
Exophthalmos	Excessive and long duration of open mouth	Excessive compression of the mandibular coronoid process in retrobulbar area region induces inflammation	Analgesia, anti-inflammatory drugs, topical eye lubricant	Usually transient, management of discomfort
Edema of the upper airways	Infrequent, brachycephalic dogs predisposed	Linked to the incision of the soft palate and brachycephalic skull conformation, edema at the base of the tongue	In severe cases, intubation may be required or temporary tracheostomy while the swelling decreases	Variable, can be life-threatening when obstruction of the upper airways is severe
Neurologic deterioration	Low frequency, mainly in large tumors	Hemorrhage, hematoma formation, cerebral edema or neural tissue damage, and necrosis	Symptomatic treatment with mannitol and dexamethasone. In case of signs of increased intracranial pressure, supplementation of oxygen, anticonvulsants	Variable, minimal central neurological signs may resolve within days, severe signs may require long rehabilitation
Rhinitis	Low frequency	Bacterial infection of the nasopharynx	Systemic antibiotic treatment	Good
Aspiration pneumonia	Low frequency	Leakage of lavage fluids alongside the cuff, long anesthesia, and surgery, possible gastroesophageal reflux that causes esophagitis and regurgitation	Supplementation of oxygen if required, large spectrum intravenous antibiotic treatment, nebulization	Variable
Pulmonary thromboembolism	Rare	Predisposition by cushingoid status	Pulmonary and cardiovascular monitoring and treatment	Typically peracute onset and sudden death, unpredictable
Dehiscence of the soft palate incision	Low frequency in dogs, higher frequency in cats, especially when starting with hypophysectomy (learning curve)	Long retraction during surgery, excessive use of electrocautery, ischemic soft tissue damage	Revision by debridement of the margins and suture in two layers. In case of a lack of tissue, tension-relieving techniques are required	Possible rhinitis, middle ear infection, or aspiration pneumonia when oronasal fistula is not treated
Hypocortisolism	Rare	Low cortisol blood level results in dullness, reduced activity, decreased appetite	Increase cortisone acetate dosage and monitor according to clinical signs	Good
Hypothyroidism	Rare	Low total T_4 concentrations results in dullness, excessive sleeping, reduced activity	Increase levothyroxine dosage and monitor with T_4 measurements	Good

TABLE 34.7 Postoperative medication for trans-sphenoidal hypophysectomy in dogs.

Postoperative medications	Type	Route of administration	Duration of treatment	Dosage/actions
Intravenous fluid therapy	Low-sodium maintenance fluid (0.45% NaCl + 0.5% glucose solution + 10 mEq KCl/500 mL) + isotonic balanced fluid	Intravenous	Until normal oral intake of food and water	Fluid input is regulated, matching fluid output
Intravenous fluid therapy in case of hypernatremia*	Hypotonic solution with low sodium (NaCl 0.45% + 2.5% glucose) or no sodium (0.5% glucose) added to maintenance	Intravenous	Until normonatremia is reached	Depending on the severity of hypernatremia and output; consider increasing frequency of desmopressin
Intravenous fluid therapy in case of hyponatremia*	NaCl 0.9% with K^+ supplementation or isotonic balanced fluid	Intravenous	Until normonatremia is reached	Depending on the cause, severity of hyponatremia, and urinary output; consider discontinuation of desmopressin
Hydrocortisone	100 mg/2 mL	Intravenous	On ICU until oral intake of cortisone	1 mg/kg q6h
Cortisone acetate	Cortisone acetate 5 mg tablet	Oral	Lifelong	1 mg/kg q12h, taper gradually to 0.33 mg/kg q12h
Desmopressin	Nasal solution (0.1 mg/mL, drops) or desmopressin tablet (0.1 mg)	Drops: in the conjunctival sac, intermittent left and right eye. Tablet: orally	Try to stop 3 weeks after surgery, taper dose gradually, and monitor drinking/urination	1 drop q8h, or 0.5 tablet q8h; adjust according to urinary output, starting immediately after surgery
Levothyroxine	200 or 400 µg tablet	Oral	Lifelong	Start with 15 µg/kg q12h, adjust according to T_4 measurement
Amoxicillin and clavulanic acid	50, 250, or 500 mg tablet	Oral	7-10 days	20 mg/kg q12h
Methadone	Solution (10 mg/mL)	Intravenous	First days	0.1 mg/kg q4-6h
Buprenorphine	Solution (0.3 mg/mL)	Intravenous	First days after methadone	0.015 mg/kg q6-8h
Paracetamol	250 or 500 mg tablet	Oral	3-5 days	15 mg/kg q8h

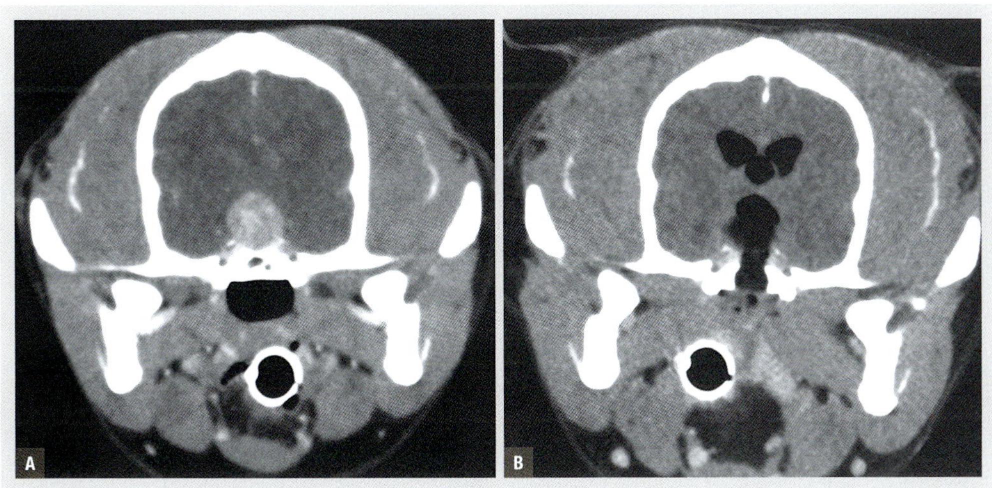

FIG. 34.25 Transverse contrast-enhanced CT scan images in a mesocephalic dog with pituitary-dependent hypercortisolism before (A) and immediately after (B) successful hypophysectomy. The width of the burr hole (8 mm) allowed complete extraction of the 12 mm round pituitary adenoma. The pneumoencephalograph (B), together with the absence of pituitary contrast enhancement, confirmed the completeness of hypophysectomy. The dog recovered uneventfully and was discharged from the hospital after 3 days.

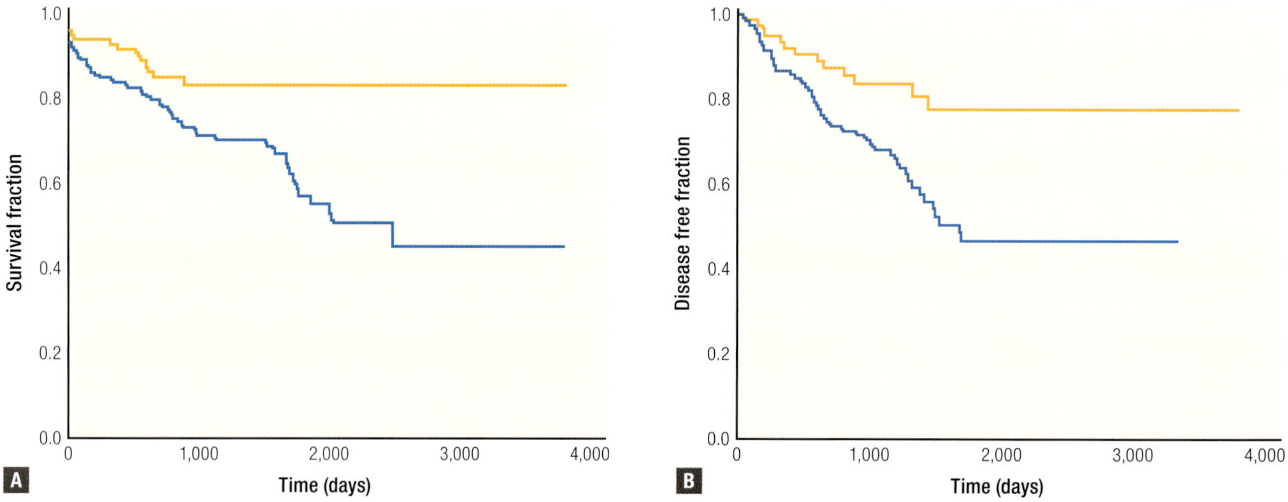

FIG. 34.26 (**A**) Survival curves for dogs with pituitary-dependent hypercortisolism (PDH) and enlarged pituitary (n = 197, pituitary/brain value (P/B) >0.31; blue line) and nonenlarged pituitary (n = 99, P/B ≤0.31; orange line). Censored cases (i.e., dogs that died from unrelated causes or were still alive at the last follow-up) are represented with vertical bars. p = 0.003. (**B**) Disease-free fraction curves for dogs with PDH with an enlarged pituitary (n = 169, P/B > 0.31; blue line) and nonenlarged (n = 86, P/B ≤0.31; orange line). Censored cases (i.e., dogs that died from unrelated causes or were still alive at the last follow-up) are represented with vertical bars. p = 0.002. Adapted from: Van Rijn SJ, Galac S, Tryfonidou MA, et al. The influence of pituitary size on outcome after trans-sphenoidal hypophysectomy in a large cohort of dogs with pituitary-dependent hypercortisolism. *J Vet Intern Med* 30(4):989- 995, 2016.

Surgical treatment: adrenalectomy

Sebastiaan A. van Nimwegen

Adrenalectomy is the preferred treatment for dogs with cortisol-secreting adrenal tumors (ATs) underlying adrenal-dependent hypercortisolism (ADHC). Treatment has two objectives: removal of AT and potential malignancy and establishment of normocortisolism. After successful adrenalectomy, there is no need for lifelong medication, which contrasts with the need for ongoing medical treatment with trilostane or mitotane.[52]

Surgical anatomy and disease staging

The adrenal glands are located retroperitoneally craniomedially to the kidneys. The right adrenal gland lies dorsolateral to the caudal vena cava (CVC), adhered to the CVC adventitia, covered by the caudate process of the liver and the cranial pole of the right kidney (Fig. 34.27). The left adrenal gland lies lateral to the aorta, caudolaterally of the cranial mesenteric artery, and is less attached and easier accessible than the right adrenal gland (Fig. 34.28). The numerous adrenal capsular arterioles arise from all neighboring arteries. Venous drainage is through a short adrenal vein directly entering the phrenicoabdominal vein (PAV), which runs over the lateroventral surface of both adrenal glands before entering the CVC in the area of adherence of the right adrenal gland and near the left renal vein for the left adrenal gland. The left adrenal vein can also connect to the left renal vein.

With increasing AT size, capsular arterioles increase in size and number, and the risk of adhesion to the renal vein and artery caudally and the CVC (right adrenal), aorta, and cranial mesenteric artery (left adrenal) medially increases, rendering surgical excision more challenging. Larger ATs that show infiltrative growth beyond the adrenal capsule may encase important blood vessels and invade adjacent organs, severely complicating surgical intervention. In addition, large ATs tend to form intravenous

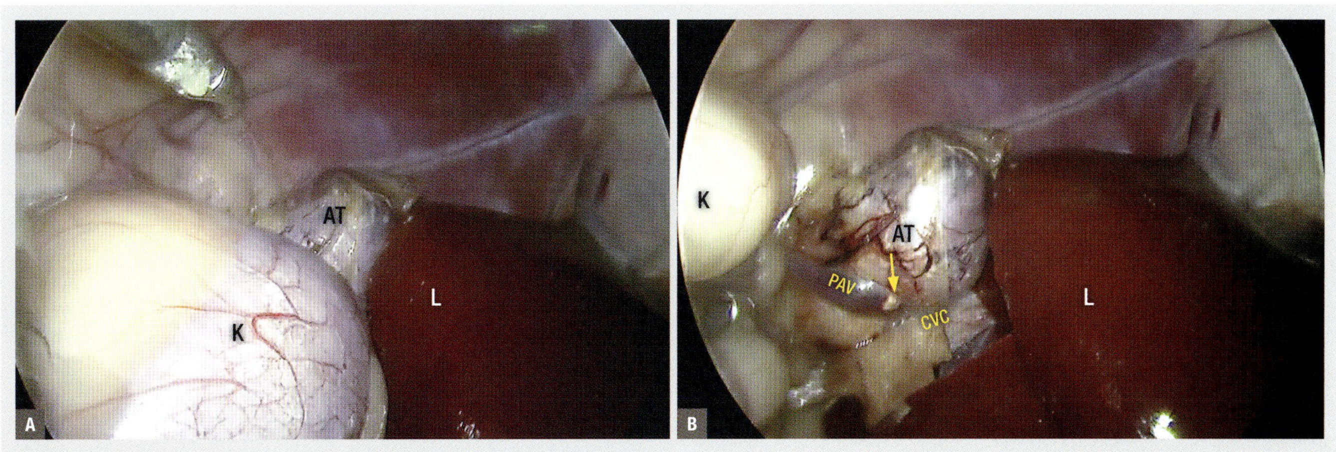

FIG. 34.27 (A) Laparoscopic view of a right-sided adrenocortical carcinoma (AT) in situ and (B) with the kidney (K) retracted, showing the AT situated dorsal of the caudal vena cava (CVC), with small intravascular tumor thrombus (arrow) in the phrenicoabdominal vein (PAV); L, liver.

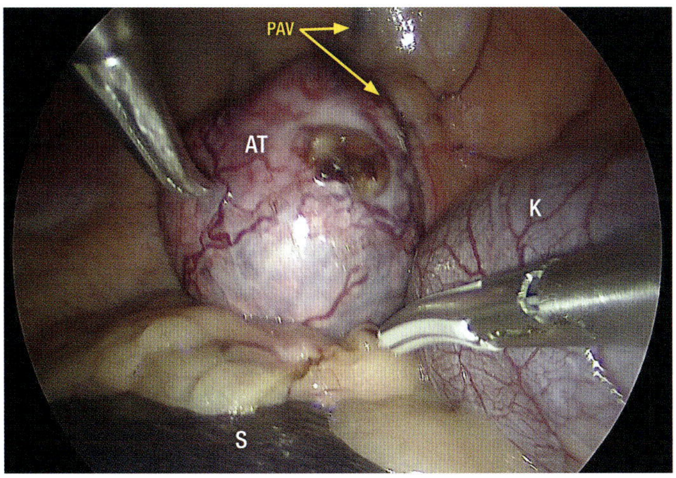

FIG. 34.28 Laparoscopic view of a left-sided adrenocortical tumor (AT) in situ, patient in sternal recumbency. The phrenicoabdominal vein (PAV) and caudal pole of the adrenal gland are covered by retroperitoneal fat and the left kidney (K). S, spleen.

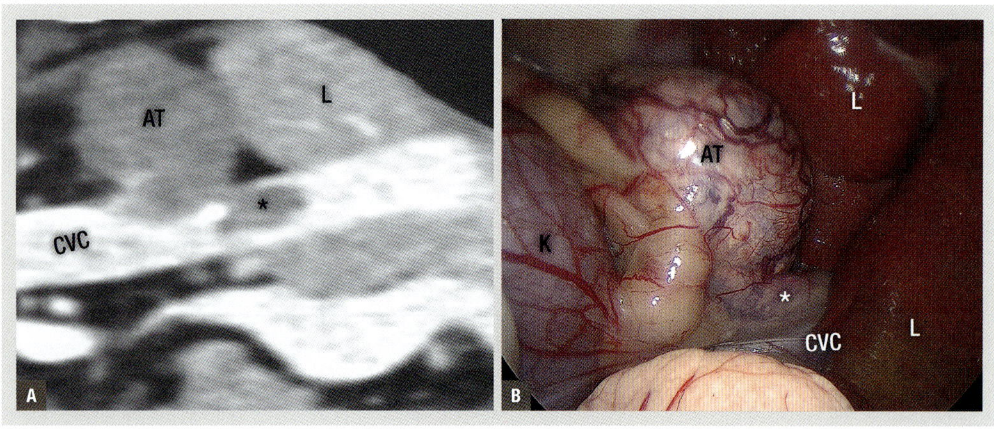

FIG. 34.29 (A) Contrast-enhanced CT and (B) in situ image of a right-sided adrenocortical tumor (AT) with vascular invasion of the phrenicoabdominal vein and small tumor thrombus (*) in the caudal vena cava (CVC). The right kidney (K) is retracted caudally. Approach through paracostal celiotomy. L, liver.

tumor protrusions or "tumor thrombi", primarily following adrenal venous drainage into the PAV and beyond, entering the CVC (left and right ATs) and/or left renal vein (left AT).

Disease staging preferably includes contrast-enhanced computed tomography (CECT) to evaluate 3D anatomy of the AT, involvement of surrounding tissues, vascular invasion, localize possible metastatic disease (abdominal lymph nodes, liver, kidneys, pancreas, omentum, small intestines, and lungs),[144-147] and comorbidities. Knowing the anatomic situation will guide the surgical procedure and reduce complications (Fig. 34.29).

Complications and perioperative measures

Perioperative complications are frequently reported (Table 34.8), and apart from surgically-induced hypocortisolism, disease-specific comorbidities may occur, including a hypercoagulable state and hypertension. Therefore, surgical treatment of cortisol-secreting AT requires a multidisciplinary team of experienced endocrinologists, surgeons, anesthetists, and intensivists to prevent, monitor, and treat potential complications before, during, and after adrenalectomy. Perioperative death without a diagnosed cause is reported in 4% of cases,[54,144,148,149] stressing the need for intensive monitoring. Abnormal clinical findings, such as dyspnea, hypoxemia, or hypotension, warrant diagnostic measures to diagnose or exclude hemorrhage, pulmonary thromboembolism (PTE), pneumonia, pancreatitis, hypocortisolism, renal failure, cardiac arrhythmia, etc. and start treatment accordingly. Despite presumed immunosuppression and delayed wound healing from chronic cortisol excess, there is no evidence of increased risk of wound complications in dogs after adrenalectomy.

The risk of intraoperative hemorrhage increases with tumor size and invasive growth. Blood product transfusions have been reported in 25-64% of patients with large or invasive tumors necessitating CVC venotomies.[150,151] Therefore, preoperative complete blood count, coagulation profile, and blood type determination is advised in these cases. Surgical trauma to the renal vein or severe compromise of renal vasculature or kidney by an AT were reasons for nephrectomy in 18-26% of invasive AT cases.[150,151]

Thromboembolic complications may occur due to a paraneoplastic hypercoagulable state. Reported incidence of postoperative PTE is 2-8% and associated mortality is high.[144,145,149,151,152] There is no evidence that medical pretreatment to normalize cortisol levels before surgery reduces coagulation abnormalities nor reduces the risk of perioperative complications, such as PTE.[153,154] Anticoagulation therapy has also not been proven effective to prevent PTE. Therefore, conservative preventative measures are advised: keep anesthesia duration short, apply analgesic protocols that promote patients to be ambulatory within 2-4 hours after surgery, and implement frequent physical exercise to avoid venous stasis.[153] Reduced tissue trauma and shorter recovery associated with laparoscopic adrenalectomy may further reduce the risk of thromboembolism and other potential complications such as pancreatitis (Table 34.8).

Surgical approach

The surgical approach is based on tumor-related anatomy on CECT. Adrenalectomy is performed by dissection close to the adrenal capsule, freeing the AT from attached peritoneal and retroperitoneal tissues, taking care to minimize trauma to nearby blood vessels and nerves. Electrosurgical instruments, including advanced vessel sealer/dividers are routinely used to improve hemostasis and dissection close to the AT capsule.

A minimally invasive laparoscopic approach is preferred over celiotomy because of reduced tissue trauma, improved access and visibility, and significantly faster recovery.[54,155] Criteria for laparoscopic adrenalectomy include a well-defined AT, without vascular invasion beyond the PAV (no CVC involvement), minimal interference with renal vein and renal hilus, and relatively small size. Reported mean tumor diameter in laparoscopic adrenalectomy is 2.5-3 cm.[54,152,155,156] Maximum tumor diameters usually do not exceed 5 cm.[54] The same criteria apply to bilateral ATs, which are preferably excised in a single session, single preparation, bilateral flank laparoscopic approach in sternal recumbency.[54]

Larger ATs without involvement of organs or blood vessels medial to the tumor or right-sided tumors with prehepatic CVC invasion are best approached via paracostal celiotomy, enabling the improved access to the adrenal gland and dissection of right-sided ATs from the dorsal CVC wall. Left-sided tumors with suspicion of CVC or renal vein invasion and bilateral adrenalectomies with at least one AT not being amenable for laparoscopic excision are best approached through a ventral midline celiotomy.

Laparoscopic adrenalectomy is performed through three 5 mm portals in the abdominal flank caudal to the last rib at the level of the kidney

TABLE 34.8 Reported perioperative complications of laparoscopic adrenalectomy, open adrenalectomy in general, and surgical treatment of large and/or vascular invasive tumors in specific.

Perioperative complications		Laparoscopic adrenalectomy[54,157,160]	Open adrenalectomy[54,150,154,159,160]	Large adrenal tumors and/or CVC venotomy[151-154,155,156]
Intraoperative	Hypertension	0-17%	0-8%	11-41%
	Hypotension	0-5%	0-29%	62-73%
	Hemorrhage	0-5%	0-15%	5-32%*
	Arrhythmia	0-2%	0-25%	16%
	AT capsule penetration	19-32%**	4-20%	N.R.
	Nephrectomy	0%	0-8%	8-26%
	Death	0-2%	0%	3-8%
Postoperative	Pancreatitis	0-2%	0-8%	4-11%
	Pulmonary thromboembolism	0-3%	0-8%	0-6%
	Dyspnea	0-2%	0-12%	0-14%
	Pneumonia	0-5%	0-8%	0-6%
	Cardiac arrest	0-2%	0-4%	4-9%
	Acute renal failure	0%	0-2%	2-14%
	Death of unknown cause	0%	0-4%	0-4%
	Death	0%	0-8%	0-19%
Venotomy/thrombectomy incidence		0%	0-10%	16-100%
Blood product transfusion		0%	0-11%	2-64%*
Perioperative mortality		0-5%	2-8%	21-26%

*Reported intraoperative hemorrhage was lower than reported use of blood product transfusion, which may be related to missing data because of the retrospective nature of the current case series. **Data on capsular penetration is usually recorded in reports of laparoscopic surgery while often lacking in reports of open surgery, making retrospective comparison difficult.[155] N.R., not reported; caudal vena cava (CVC); adrenal tumor (AT).

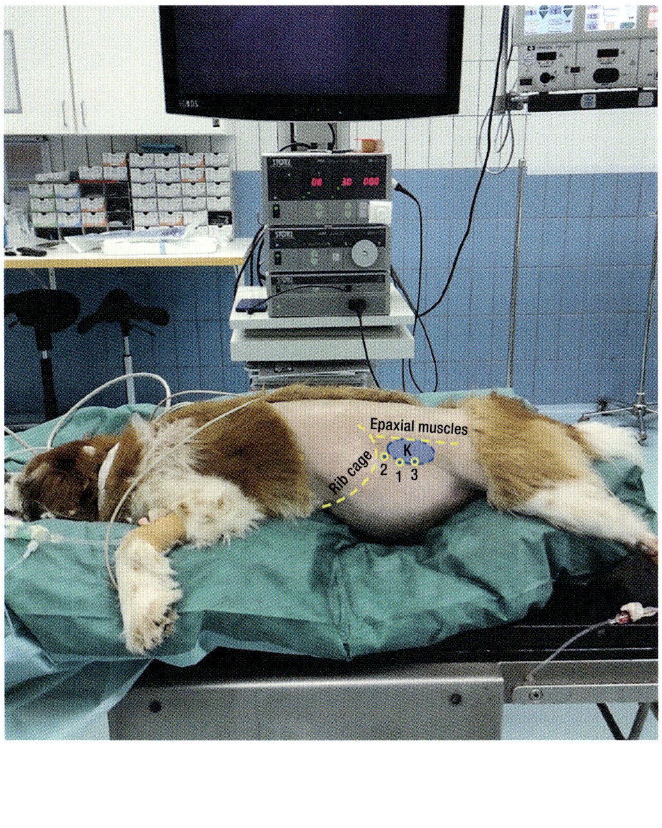

FIG. 34.30 Sternal position of patient prepped for left-sided flank laparoscopic adrenalectomy with the indication of the three instrument portal locations (numbers 1,2,3). Elevation of the sternum and pubic bone with vacuum cushions allows a "hanging belly" with abdominal organs moving ventrally. K, kidney.

with the patient in sternal recumbency (up to 30° contralateral oblique) (**Fig. 34.30**). This gives superior access to the adrenal gland, including dissection dorsal to the CVC for right-sided tumors.[54] Patients are supported by moldable vacuum cushions lifting the sternum and pubic bone, allowing abdominal organs to move dependently and creating space in the paralumbar fossa (**Fig. 34.27** and **Fig. 34.28**).[156] Small tumor thrombi in the PAV are excised *en bloc* with the AT. The excised AT is removed from the abdomen through an enlarged portal using a retrieval bag or glove-finger to prevent contamination with tumor cells.[54,156]

Open adrenalectomy is performed through a paracostal or midline celiotomy. In right-sided ATs or ATs with PAV invasion, the tumor is freed from surrounding attachments until the attachment to the CVC (or sometimes left renal vein) through PAV remains, which can be ligated or clipped, or sealed and transected near its entry into the CVC. Invasion of the kidney, renal hilus, or renal blood vessels may necessitate nephrectomy.[148,150]

Tumor thrombectomy

Intravenous tumor thrombi are usually not attached to the vessel walls and can be pulled out of the lumen through a venotomy to be removed *en bloc* with the AT. Three types of thrombectomies are distinguished for the removal out of the CVC:

- Small CVC thrombi can sometimes be milked back into the PAV, followed by ligation or sealing of the PAV at its junction with the CVC.
- Small-diameter thrombi may be pulled out through a PAV incision at some distance to its junction with CVC, either under partial or complete occlusion of the dependent CVC segment. The PAV stump is ligated.
- Large CVC thrombi are removed through a caval venotomy under complete occlusion using Rummel tourniquets on all associated veins. After excising the base of the PAV around the thrombus, the venotomy in the CVC wall is enlarged until the thrombus can be pulled out. For thrombi reaching the hepatic hilus or beyond, the thoracic CVC can be reached by increasing the celiotomy to a caudal sternotomy or diaphragmatic incision.

In the case of CVC wall involvement, partial cavectomy may sometimes be feasible in a dilated CVC. Complete excision of an obstructed CVC segment may be possible if CVC blood flow already follows an alternative route via azygos vein and/or vertebral venous sinuses.

Cortisol supplementation

Chronic inhibition of the pituitary ACTH feedback loop by cortisol causes atrophy of the normal adrenal gland cortex. Thus, adrenalectomy of a unilateral functional AT causes a state of hypocortisolism. Glucocorticoids have to be supplemented temporarily until the contralateral adrenal gland regains physiologic cortisol production. In the author's institution, ADHC patients receive hydrocortisone 1 mg/kg IV over 6h after induction of anesthesia for unilateral adrenalectomy. Postoperatively, glucocorticoid supplementation is continued with oral cortisone acetate 1 mg/kg q12h PO. In unilateral cases, cortisone acetate is tapered over 6-8 weeks and discontinued thereafter.[148] Alternatively, prednisone 0,5 mg/kg q24h PO can be administered in a tapered fashion over 6-8 weeks.[148] After bilateral adrenalectomy, glucocorticoid and mineralocorticoid supplementation is prescribed for life as described for primary hypoadrenocorticism (see chapter 33).

Outcome and prognosis

The reported median survival times (MST) of dogs with ADHC after adrenalectomy are 953 to 1641 days.[54,144,157] Current perioperative mortality rates range from 1.5-8%.[54,145,149,152,154,155] Higher perioperative mortality rates of 21-26% are linked to large tumors or extensive tumor invasion in the CVC.[146-148,150,151] However, patients with larger ATs or (prehepatic) CVC invasion are often good surgical candidates in the hands of experienced surgeons, and after surviving the perioperative period, the long-term prognosis is relatively good. Therefore, perioperative mortality is the most important risk factor for long-term survival, dictated by anatomic features such as tumor size, shape, and involvement of adjacent tissues.

The current favorable perioperative mortality rates and MST after adrenalectomy may follow improved disease staging, case selection, and perioperative management.[54,145,149,154,155] Reported one-, two-, and three-year disease-specific survival percentages are 83-95%, 76-89%, and 81-89% respectively.[54,149] Clinical recurrence rates range from 9-38%.[54,148,152,157] However, recurrence occurs relatively late after treatment, with clinical signs being detected after a mean of 533 days[54] in one report and median survival time for dogs with recurrent disease being 507 days in another report.[157] No significant differences were found for short- and long-term outcomes between laparoscopic and open adrenalectomy, except for a shorter hospital stay after laparoscopic adrenalectomy.[54,155] Laparoscopic adrenalectomy was successful in dogs of 5.9 kg up to 50 kg body weight but seems more challenging in small/miniature dogs since conversion to open adrenalectomy (7%) was necessary in two miniature dogs (5.1 and 5.9 kg) and one obese dog of 9.4 kg[54] (Video 34.9). In a multi-institutional case series of 255 dogs undergoing laparoscopic adrenalectomy for ATs, capsular penetration (19%) and major hemorrhage (5.5%) were the most prevalent intraoperative complications. Conversion rate was 9% and perioperative mortality was 5.1%. Complication rates were low (Table 34.8). Increased surgeon experience was related to a decreased risk of death prior to discharge. Capsular penetration was related to a 6.5 times higher rate of disease recurrence.[152]

Significant prognostic factors in dogs operated for ATs are listed in Table 34.9. Notably, tumor type and vascular invasion limited to the prehepatic CVC were not prognostic for survival.[54,147,150,151,158] Emergency surgery for AT rupture-induced hemoperitoneum was associated with an increased risk of (29-50%) mortality in two studies.[145,158] However, delayed surgery after stabilization of patients significantly reduced short-term mortality (17%).[158]

Video 34.9

Laparoscopic adrenalectomy of a right-sided adrenocortical tumor in a 6.5 kg Maltese dog with adrenal-dependent hypercortisolism.

TABLE 34.9 Significant prognostic factors for adrenalectomy of cortisol-secreting adrenocortical tumors.

Prognostic factors for adrenalectomy of adrenal tumors	
Tumor size	Increased tumor size is significantly related to increased perioperative mortality,[145,152] long-term disease recurrence,[54] and reduced median survival time (MST)[54,144,157]
Extent of caudal vena cava invasion*	Caval tumor thrombus beyond the hepatic hilus/diaphragm is related to a significantly increased risk of perioperative death[147,150]
Capsular penetration	Capsular penetration/rupture during surgery is related to an increased risk of long-term tumor recurrence[152]
Surgeon's experience	Increased experience in laparoscopic adrenalectomy is related to lower surgical times, conversion rates, and risk of perioperative death[152]

* Tumor type (cortical vs pheochromocytoma), bilateral tumors, and prehepatic caval invasion were not prognostic for perioperative mortality or MST[54,145,147-149,154]

Radiation therapy

Maurice Zandvliet and Jérôme Benoit

Radiotherapy as a treatment option for a patient with pituitary-dependent hypercortisolism (PDH), tends to effectively control tumor growth from the time of treatment onwards (slow volume regression over months), whereas hormone production typically continues following completion of the radiation treatment for at least a year. This delay in hormonal response is typical and should not be considered a lack of treatment response. Clinically, this implies that patients will require further medical treatment to control the patient's hypercortisolism while being monitored until an endocrine response is observed.[2,57]

Human patients whose pituitary gland was included in the radiation field will potentially develop late severe combined endocrine dysfunction (panhypopituitarism), with the most important risk factors being the total radiation dose the gland receives and the time interval since the completion of the radiation treatment. In humans, the production of growth hormone (GH) is usually the first to be affected, followed by that of the gonadotrophins (LH, FSH) and adrenocorticotropic hormone (ACTH), while thyroid-stimulating hormone (TSH) production appears least impaired.[159] This suggests that GH, FSH, and LH-producing cells are more sensitive to radiation damage than those producing ACTH and TSH. Production of antidiuretic hormone is not typically affected by radiotherapy.

The role of radiation therapy in the management of adrenal tumours is, to date, poorly described in veterinary medicine[160] and will not be addressed.

Types of radiation therapy

The goal of radiation therapy is generally to deliver the highest possible dose to the tumor to obtain a maximum cytotoxic effect with the lowest possible dose to the healthy surrounding tissues to reduce the adverse effects. To this end, there are two different treatment approaches. The first and most used approach is to apply conventionally fractionated radiotherapy; the second, a more advanced technique, is called stereotactic therapy.

In the case of conventionally fractionated radiotherapy, the total radiation dose is divided into multiple smaller (sublethal) doses or fractions, and for canine pituitary lesions, this implies typically 10 to 16 fractions. This approach allows healthy tissues to repair their DNA damage and replace healthy cells (repopulate), minimizing damage to healthy tissue while allowing at the same time for reoxygenation of the tumor and redistribution of the tumor cells in the cell cycle synchronizing them in the more radiosensitive phases of the cell cycle, thereby increasing the effect on the tumor.

In stereotactic radiotherapy, a high (radioablative) dose of radiation is given as a single fraction (stereotactic radiosurgery or SRS) or as 3-5 fractions (stereotactic radiotherapy or SRT) to a well-defined tumor volume with minimal margins and steep dose gradients to limit toxic radiation dose to the surrounding non-neoplastic tissues, thereby limiting adverse effects. While the benefits of fewer treatments and the necessity for fewer sedations are attractive, a higher fractional radiation dose requires more advanced technical equipment and does not allow for the repair of healthy irradiated tissues, which may increase the risk of late radiation toxicity. This consideration is important in pituitary irradiation due to the pituitary's proximity to nearby structures, so-called organs at risk e.g. the optic chiasm, that are particularly sensitive to larger dose fractions.

Treatment considerations

Radiotherapy can be used in dogs with PDH as both a primary treatment as well as in an adjuvant setting in dogs with incompletely resected pituitary tumors.[57] When considering radiotherapy as a possible treatment option, a minimum database should include an assessment of the dog's general health status (screening for comorbidities affecting the dog's life expectancy and fitness to undergo multiple anesthetic episodes), comprehensive endocrine testing, and advanced imaging of the pituitary gland (CT and/or MRI). Staging is not routinely indicated since pituitary adenomas do not metastasize. However, prior to initiating radiotherapy in an older patient, full body screening (CT or thoracic radiographs and abdominal ultrasound) should be considered to exclude other unrelated conditions the patient might have, which could potentially impact the prognosis or treatment decision.

Dogs are routinely started on prednisolone (1 mg/kg PO q24h) in preparation for their radiation treatment. This implies that dogs treated with trilostane could temporarily discontinue their medication, only to reinitiate it if needed (i.e., by showing clinical signs consistent with hypercortisolism) once prednisolone treatment has been completely stopped.

Radiotherapy treatment planning requires CT acquisition with the patient in the exact same position as for treatment (indexed flat couch, positioning aids, reference markers). Pituitary lesions usually show a very marked contrast intake on CT, yet T1-weighted post-contrast MRIs are considered most accurate for delineating tumor mass and will typically result in a larger gross tumor volume (GTV) than post-contrast CT images.[161] Some treatment planning software packages will allow for fusion imaging of MRI and CT studies; however, the actual plan (contouring and dose calculation) is made on the CT study.

Following the delineation of the GTV, additional margins are needed for compensation for imaging technique limitations (depending on level of equipment, and imaging modality [CT vs. MRI]), microscopic tumor extension, the so-called clinical target volume (CTV), and compensation for positioning uncertainty (positioning technique, on-board imaging patient quality assurance techniques) leading to an additional margin known as planning target volume (PTV). In pituitary tumors, margins will typically imply extensions of 1-2 mm for CTV and an additional 1-5 mm for PTV (Table 34.10, Fig. 34.31).

TABLE 34.10 Definitions of volumes used in radiotherapy.

Volume	Definition	Practical
Gross tumor volume (GTV)	Position and extent of the primary tumor	Tumor as visualized with advanced imaging (post-contrast T1W MRI or CT)
Clinical target volume (CTV)	GTV extended with a margin to include subclinical (microscopic and/or nonimageable) tumor spread	An expansion of the GTV, size depending on tumor type, taking into account possible biological barriers (e.g., skull)
Planned target volume (PTV)	CTV extended with a margin to allow for uncertainties in treatment planning or treatment delivery	An isometric expansion of the CTV, size depending on the type of position aids and verification mode used; may cross biological barriers and can extend beyond the patient

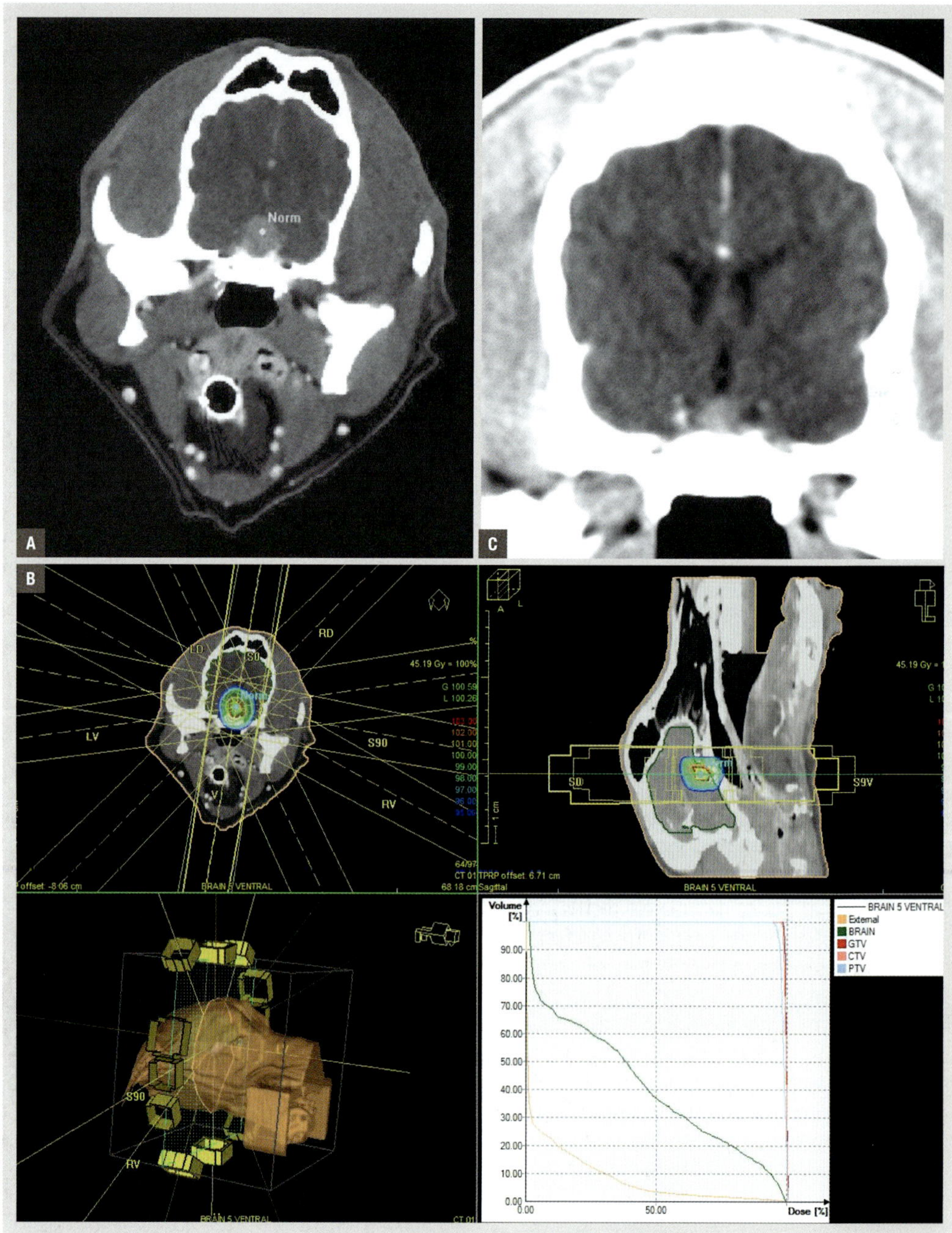

FIG. 34.31 Post-contrast CT images of an 8-year-old dog with pituitary-dependent hypercortisolism prior to (**A**) and 20 months following (**C**) curative-intent radiotherapy and its treatment plan (**B**) The treatment plan shows 4 panels representing the beam configuration and dose distribution in a transverse CT slice (upper left panel), reconstructed sagittal CT slice (upper right), a 3D reconstruction of the dog in treatment position with the beam setup (lower left) and the corresponding dose-volume histogram for the brain, GTV: gross tumor volume; CTV: clinical target volume; PTV: planned target volume.

Radiation-associated toxicity

While radiotherapy for intracranial targets is generally well-tolerated by dogs, various forms of radiation-induced neurotoxicity can occur. Radiation-induced brain injury may include:

- Acute changes that occur during or shortly after completing a course of radiotherapy that are attributed to transient disruption of the blood-brain barrier.
- Early delayed or subacute effects that occur anywhere from weeks up to about 5 months after radiotherapy and which are thought to be a result of transient and generally reversible demyelination.
- Late effects that occur many months to years after radiotherapy and are largely attributed to irreversible brain necrosis.[162]

Acute radiation toxicity

Acute radiation toxicity results from damage to rapidly proliferating tissues, such as skin and mucous membranes in the radiation field, and may occur 10-14 days after starting radiotherapy. Acute toxicities associated with pituitary irradiation are rare but may include radiation-induced dermatitis (otitis externa), mucositis (pharyngitis), and ocular toxicity (keratoconjunctivitis, keratoconjunctivitis sicca in some smaller breeds). These signs are more commonly seen with nonconformal radiotherapy and are rare with modern conformal or stereotactic radiation techniques. Damage to the pituitary gland and surrounding nervous system is also rare but appears more common with both nonconformal and/or hypofractionated treatments (palliative 3D nonconformal or stereotactic treatments). Acute neurological deterioration may be seen from a few weeks to a couple of months after radiotherapy is completed.

Acute radiation toxicity is typically mild and, in most cases, self-limiting but may require supportive therapy and/or (temporary) treatment with steroids. Most veterinary radiation oncologists routinely prescribe anti-inflammatory doses of oral glucocorticoids (e.g., prednisolone 0.5-1 mg/kg PO q24h) prophylactically when treating canine PDH patients, with the intention to taper steroids slowly between 2 to 8 weeks following completion of radiotherapy.

Late radiation toxicity

Late radiation toxicity is generally rare with standard protocols, relatively small target volumes, moderate dose to brain and sensitive structures, but may become more prevalent with hypofractionation, including stereotactic techniques, in the future. It is caused by irreversible, unrepairable damage to slowly dividing or nondividing healthy tissues such as neurons and blood vessels. Signs of late toxicity to the skin would include persistent alopecia, skin hyperpigmentation and/or leukotrichia but do not seriously affect the patient's quality of life. In PDH patients, the residual dose to the skin is minimal, and skin changes may only be seen within the ear canals in smaller breeds and/or dogs receiving radiotherapy with poorly conformal techniques (limited number of beams).

However, impaired vision due to optic nerve neuropathy, cataracts (if lenses are exposed), hearing loss, and progressive pituitary and brain dysfunction have a more significant impact on the patient's quality of life. Damage to the pituitary gland and surrounding nervous system structures is more common than extraneuronal structures and results from radiation-induced necrosis of nervous tissue, vascular damage (hemorrhage, infarction), damage to the blood-brain barrier, and progressive neuronal demyelination or necrosis. Typical signs would include depression (obtundation), reduced awareness (apathy), and potentially seizures. These signs may, to some extent, mimic those arising from tumor recurrence or vascular damage, and the underlying cause may only be differentiated by repeating advanced imaging. However, advanced MRI studies, including perfusion or diffusion-weighted series, are not always characteristic, and only a presumptive diagnosis may be given. Monitoring of clinical signs in combination with imaging findings may eventually help to differentiate between these conditions.[162]

Pituitary dysfunction will show as a progressive loss of pituitary hormone production and may ultimately result in clinically relevant hypothyroidism and/or hypocortisolism. In order to treat this appropriately, dogs need to be intermittently monitored following the completion of their radiation treatment.

Outcomes of pituitary radiotherapy

The veterinary literature on pituitary radiotherapy is limited and consists mostly of case series (**Table 34.11**) using either conventionally fractionated radiotherapy[57,163-168] or stereotactic radiotherapy.[161,169] The majority of these cases are dogs with a suspected pituitary macroadenoma (possibly carcinoma), and although many are diagnosed with PDH, most dogs presented with (concurrent) neurological signs. This selection bias is easily explained since in dogs PDH clinical signs may be solely attributable to their endocrine hyperfunction. As a result, most of these dogs receive only medical treatment to control the signs of hypercortisolism but may, in selected cases, be referred for hypophysectomy. Dogs with larger and/or inoperable functioning pituitary tumors or primarily neurological signs are more often referred for radiotherapy.

Conclusion

Despite the obvious limitations (various protocols, various machines, multiple institutions, retrospective studies), the analysis of the published treatment results appears to favor 3D conformal definitive-intent treatment protocols. Although regularly fractionated treatment protocols require multiple anesthesias, these protocols appear to yield the longest survivals with the lowest frequency of radiation-induced toxicity. Radiation will, in most cases, reduce or even completely control both signs of hypercortisolism as well as neurological signs. However, most dogs will ultimately be euthanized due to progressive neurological signs, and although in most cases, tumor progression is thought to account for this deterioration, late radiation toxicity cannot be ruled out as a contributing factor.

Follow-up for dogs with PDH treated with radiotherapy is partly based on the reduction of clinical signs, but can be more objectively assessed by means of serial measurement of endogenous ACTH levels and/or urinary corticoid-creatinine ratio's, once supplementary glucocorticoids have been discontinued. It is also recommended to monitor for radiation toxicity, both acute (ocular signs, otitis) as well as late toxicity (hypothyroidism, diabetes insipidus, and other brain damage).

For information on the radiobiological and technical considerations of radiotherapy, see Box 34.2.

TABLE 34.11 Reported case series on dogs with pituitary tumors treated with radiotherapy.*

Radiation source	n	Fractionation	D_{total} (Gy)	mOST (d)	Remarks	Reference
^{60}Co	6	11 × 4Gy (3 × /W)	44	N.R.	■ 6 detectable tumors ■ 6 PDH, 0 neuro ■ 1/6 long-term control PDH ■ 1 year post-treatment imaging showed 4 × CR, 2 × SD	168
MV (nonconformal)	24	12 × 4Gy (3 /W)	48	360	■ 24 macrotumors ■ 19 PDH, 24 neuro ■ 3 dogs did not complete therapy	169
Linac (2D-RT; 6 MV)	24	1 × 5Gy + 4 × 8.25 Gy 1 × /W (12 dogs) or 10 × 3.8 Gy 3 × /W (12 dogs)	38	235	■ 24 macrotumors (≥1 cm) ■ 13 PDH, 11 neuro	170
Linac (3D-CRT)	13	16 × 2.5-4 Gy (5 × /W)	35-52.5	688		171
^{60}Co (5x) & Linac (7×; 5 MV)	12	12 × 3Gy (2 or 3 × /W)	36	539	■ 12 macrotumors ■ 12 PDH, 4 neuro ■ 11 reductions in tumor size ■ Recurrence neuro signs in 4 dogs	172
Linac (3D-CRT; 4 MV)	19	16 × 3 Gy (5 × /W)	48	1,405 (mean)	■ Median P/B value 0.10, median height 1.3 cm ■ 2 dogs did not complete RT ■ 14 PDH, 11 neuro ■ 5/14 PDH signs resolved ■ 0 acute, 1 potential late toxicity	173
Linac (3DCRT; MV)	94	Median 43Gy (12-50)	± 44 (12-50)	514	■ 94 macrotumors ■ 47 PDH, 67 neuro ■ 12/37 trilostane discontinued after radiation ■ 20 acute, 5 late toxicity	57
Linac (SRS/SRT; 6 MV)	45	1 15 Gy (32 ×) 3 × 8 Gy (12)	15 24	311	■ 29 PDH, 33 neuro ■ 37/45 clinical improvement ■ 9/21 improved control PDH ■ 10 acute, 35 potential late toxicities	174
Linac (SRS; 6 MV)	13	1 × 16Gy	16	357	■ 3 PDH, 13 neuro ■ 9 potential late toxicities	166

* Note: not all dogs showed signs of pituitary-dependent hypercortisolism (PDH). The definition of a macrotumor varies between references and is not always supported by the pituitary/brain value (P/B); neurological signs (neuro).

Box 34.2 Radiobiological and technical considerations of radiotherapy.

Radiobiological considerations

Radiotherapy uses ionizing radiation to treat tumors by causing nonselective DNA damage in both the neoplastic and surrounding non-neoplastic cells. DNA damage arises mostly through indirect radiation effects, meaning that DNA damage is caused by free radicals generated by the interaction of ionizing radiation with water molecules, which in turn cause DNA damage. A smaller part of the DNA damaging effect results from a direct interaction of the ionizing radiation with the cell's DNA, as well as other cellular structures. The effect of ionizing radiation varies throughout the cell cycle, with proliferating cells, and in particular, those in the G2-phase and the mitosis, being most susceptible.

The resulting DNA damage leads to cellular responses, mostly the failure to complete multiple cell divisions due to the accumulation of chromosomal abnormalities (mitotic death) but also planned cell death (apoptosis). Ionizing radiation also affects the microenvironment through effects on the (micro)vasculature and the induction of fibrosis, which, together with the cellular effects on the non-neoplastic cells, are responsible for the late toxicity associated with radiation therapy.

The radiosensitivity of a tumor or normal tissue depends on several factors, including the tissue of origin (histological type), tumor volume/clonogenic tumor cells, proliferative activity, and its microenvironment, including its oxygenation status. Nervous tissue is generally considered to be relatively radiosensitive, specifically to higher fractional doses, due to its low proliferation. Benign pituitary tumors tend to be relatively small and have relatively low proliferative activity. The radio sensitivity of any tumor or normal tissue can be estimated by using the linear-quadratic (LQ) model. The basic LQ model describes the surviving fraction (SF) of clonogenic or stem cells as a function of the radiation dose D.

$$SF(D) = e^{(-\alpha \cdot D - \beta \cdot D^2)}$$

The main parameters of this model, α and β, represent the intrinsic radiosensitivity of the irradiated cells. The ratio of the two parameters, α/β, is a measure of the fractionation sensitivity of the cells: cells with a higher α/β are less sensitive to the sparing effect of fractionation. On the other hand, cells with a lower α/β (e.g., CNS) will be more sensitive to the dose fraction and experience more damage when exposed to higher dose fractions.

The LQ model has shown its clinical usefulness in predicting the treatment outcome, as well as the sparing effect of fractionated radiotherapy, and in comparing the equivalent total dose of different fractionation schedules.[170]

The radiosensitivity of benign neoplasms is not as well documented as the sensitivity of malignant tumors; however, it is admitted that they possibly have a lower α/β ratio which would make them less sensitive to dose fractionation.[170]

In the specific context of pituitary tumors, the optimal treatment dose prescription remains empirical. However, concerns arise from the dose tolerance to other organs at risk in direct proximity to the pituitary gland.[171] For pituitary tumors in humans, the radiation dose required to control tumor growth was found to be lower than the dose needed to control hormone production in the long-term.[172]

Technical considerations

Radiotherapeutic treatment of pituitary tumors can only be provided with megavoltage (MV) photon beam radiation produced by a linear accelerator (Linac), mostly with energy of 6 MV in the veterinary field. The depth of the tumor within the skull precludes the use of lower-intensity radiation produced by orthovoltage units.

Treating pituitary neoplasia requires precise treatment planning and delivery techniques and necessitates a combination of advanced pretreatment imaging (CT and/or MRI scan), a multileaf collimator (MLC), planning software, and a portal imaging modality, such as MV portal imaging or kV on-board imaging (2D or 3D with a cone-beam CT) for patient position verification. This setup allows for so-called 3D-conformal radiotherapy (3DCRT) but, depending on further specifications, will also allow for more advanced treatment options such as intensity-modulated radiotherapy (IMRT), volumetric modulated arc therapy (VMAT), and stereotactic radiotherapy (SRT).

To best conform to tumor volumes and limit therapy-related toxicity, the radiation dose absorbed in healthy tissue needs to be minimized, and to this end, the development of the multileaf collimator (MLC) has been a major step forward. In the past, nonconformal radiotherapy, as provided by cobalt machines and Linacs without an MLC, used conventional collimator jaws that only allowed for shaping rectangular treatment fields. Since treatment volumes are typically not rectangular, additional shaping would require the use of individualized beam blocks. An MLC consists of multiple (80-120) movable tungsten leaves, each blocking part of the radiation beam. Moving these narrow, closely abutting leaves individually allows for generating any desired field shape.

While 3D-conformal radiotherapy (3D-CRT) allows for more conformal treatment, the dose intensity is the same throughout the entire treatment field. By combining multiple smaller fields (beamlets) into larger treatment fields or arcs, dose intensity may vary within the treatment fields, and this technique is called IMRT or VMAT, respectively. It allows for a highly conformal dose shaping of the tumor target versus organs at risk. While 3D-CRT plans can be made by means of forward planning, more complex treatment plans will require reverse planning where the complex beam modulation is calculated by the treatment planning software based on the radiation oncologist dose prescription to the target and dose constraints to organs at risk (Fig. 34.32).

The above-described advances in diagnostic imaging, hardware, and software have allowed for more precise treatment planning, which in turn requires more precise quality assurance (QA) methods, from regular machine QA to pretreatment (or plan) QA and patient (position)- specific QA procedures.

Radiation biology and dose fractionation schemes

Radiation dose (D) to the patient is currently typically reported in Gray (Gy; 1 Gy = 1 J/kg = 100 cGy) and equals the number of fractions (n) by the fractional dose (d). Although, in general, a higher total dose will have a stronger effect on the tumor, a significant part of the biological effect is determined by the fractional dose and the fractionation schedule.

Conventionally fractionated protocols in veterinary medicine will typically consist of five or three once-daily treatments per week with a fractional dose of 2.5-3 Gy, for a total of 12-20 fractions (D up to 42-50 Gy) given over 3 to 4 weeks. A low fractional dose reduces the risk for late radiation toxicity to the CNS (nervous tissue has a low α/β and is therefore sensitive to large fractional doses) but will require multiple sessions to reach a sufficiently high dose for a therapeutic effect.

With a higher fractional dose (hypofractionation), the number of fractions is reduced, but the risk of delayed reaction to normal tissues significantly increases. There is also a compromise on the total dose given over a 3-to-4-week period and this approach is considered palliative for most cases. In order to reduce the acute side effects in this setting, longer intervals between fractions are needed, and treatment frequency is reduced to once or twice weekly. In the context of pituitary tumors, the median survival with 5 once-weekly radiation fractions (total dose 38 Gy) was found to be short, with a 15% risk of delayed complications for dogs surviving >6 months.[173]

Since a higher fractional dose increases the risk of late toxicity, to which normal brain and pituitary tissue are particularly sensitive, hypofractionated protocols are not recommended in a definitive setting. However, a moderately hypofractionated protocol of 10 daily fractions of 4 Gy (40 Gy) has been described as effective and appears generally well tolerated.[174] This fractionation scheme may not be considered a standard but an alternative to more fractionated protocols.

However, if the treatment planning and delivery techniques allow better sparing of the normal tissues, specifically with stereotactic techniques, an effective therapeutic dose may be reached with a lower total dose, and fractions may be given on consecutive days. In this particular setting margin doses of 14-16 Gy in a single fraction or 20-25 Gy in fractionated SRT (3-5 fractions).

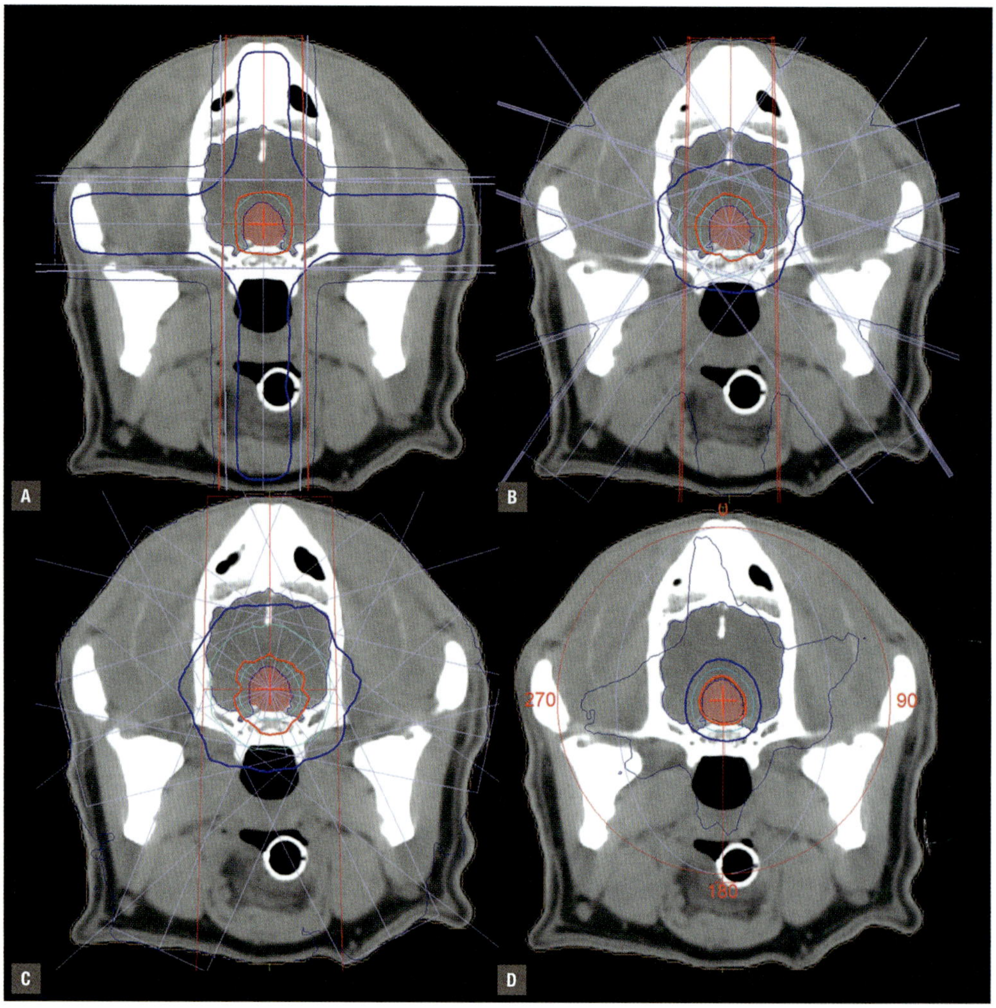

FIG. 34.32 Transverse CT images showing the pituitary tumor (gross tumor volume, GTV) (red area) and 100% (red line), 75% (green line), 50% (thick blue line), and 10% (thin blue line) isodose lines for a 3D nonconformal (**A**), a 3D conformal radiotherapy (**B**), intensity-modulated radiotherapy (**C**) and stereotactic radiotherapy (**D**) plan.

KEY POINTS

Pathogenesis and clinical manifestations

Carolina Arenas, Carlos Melián

- Pituitary-dependent hypercortisolism (PDH) is caused by an corticotroph tumor and is the most common form of AT.
- Less common is adrenal-dependent hypercortisolism (ADHC), caused by an autonomously secreting adrenocortical tumor.
- The most common clinical signs of HC are polyuria and polydipsia, polyphagia, abdominal distension, alopecia, panting, and muscle weakness.
- The most common clinicopathological abnormalities include stress leukogram, elevated alkaline phosphatase (ALP), alanine aminotransferase (ALT), hypercholesterolemia, hypertriglyceridemia, hyperglycemia, a low urine specific gravity, and proteinuria.

Endocrine testing

Sara Galac

- The suspicion of HC, based on patient history, clinical manifestations, and clinicopathological findings, necessitates confirmation by endocrine testing.
- The LDDST is the most recommended test for confirming the diagnosis of HC.
- Circulating concentrations of endogenous ACTH are useful for differentiating between PDH and ADHC.

Diagnostic imaging

Henk van den Broek and Stefanie Veraa

- Diagnostic imaging of preferentially both pituitary and adrenal glands should be included in the diagnostic evaluation of every dog with HC.
- Diagnostic imaging allows to differentiate between PDH and ADHC, helps in choosing the most optimal treatment, and estimates prognosis.
- A CT scan allows for the assessment of the pituitary gland, adrenal glands, and potential metastasis.

Medical treatment

Stefania Golinelli

- Trilostane is the medical treatment of choice for PDH, while both trilostane and mitotane can be considered for ADHC.
- Evaluation of clinical signs is the initial step in monitoring trilostane treatment.
- The ACTH stimulation test is the only monitoring test that can evaluate adrenal reserve, while prepill cortisol shows the best correlation with clinical signs in dogs treated with trilostane.
- Mitotane is indicated in inoperable and metastatic ADHC; the ablation protocol should preferably be used.

Surgical treatment: trans-sphenoidal hypophysectomy

Björn Meij and Sara Del Magno

- Trans-sphenoidal hypophysectomy is an effective treatment for PDH and addresses both the hormonal excess and the mass effect.
- Complete hypophysectomy results in panhypopituitarism and central diabetes insipidus. The latter usually regresses in weeks or months after surgery but remains permanent in 22% of dogs.
- Life-long hormone supplementation with cortisone acetate and levothyroxine is necessary and requires professional guidance.

Surgical treatment: adrenalectomy

Sebastiaan A. van Nimwegen

- Adrenalectomy is the treatment of choice for ADHC as it will cure the clinical signs of HC and prevent potential malignancy.
- Laparoscopic adrenalectomy is preferred over open surgery.
- In unilateral cortisol-secreting adrenocortical tumors, temporary supplementation with glucocorticoids is needed postoperatively.
- The most important prognostic factors are adrenal tumor size and extensive vascular invasion.

Radiation therapy

Maurice Zandvliet and Jérôme Benoit

- Radiotherapy, as a treatment option for a PDH, tends to effectively control tumor growth from the time of treatment onwards.
- ACTH production typically continues for at least a year, requiring additional medical treatment in dogs with PDH.
- Radiotherapy is well-tolerated by dogs; however, various forms of radiation-induced neurotoxicity can occur.

References

1. Pérez-Alenza MD, Melián C. Hyperadrenocorticism in dogs. In Ettinger SJ, Feldman EC, Côté E (editors). Textbook of Veterinary Internal Medicine 8th edition. St. Louis, Saunders Elsevier, 2017, pp. 1795-1811.
2. Behrend EN. Canine hyperadrenocorticism. In Feldman EC, Nelson RW, Reusch CE, Scott-Moncrieff R, Behrend EN (editors). Canine and Feline Endocrinology and Reproduction 4th edition. Philadelphia, WB Saunders, 2015, pp. 377-451.
3. Bennaim M, Shiel RE, Mooney CT. Diagnosis of spontaneous hyperadrenocorticism in dogs. Part 1: Pathophysiology, aetiology, clinical and clinicopathological features. *Vet J* 252:105342, 2019.
4. Sungin L, Aeri L, Suh-Hyun C, Seulji L, Oh-Kyeong K, Wan Hee K. Ectopic Cushing's syndrome associated with a pheochromocytoma in a dog: a case report. *BMC Vet Res* 16:35, 2020.
5. Soler Arias EA, Castillo VA, Louiset E, Lefebvre H. Cushing's syndrome caused by intra-adrenocortical adrenocorticotropic hormone in a dog. *J Vet Intern Med* 36(1):264-271, 2022.
6. Galac S, Kars VJ, Voorhout G, Mol JA, Kooistra HS. ACTH-independent hyperadrenocorticism due to food-dependent hypercortisolemia in a dog: a case report. *Vet J* 177(1):141-143, 2008.
7. Espiñeira IM, Vidal PN, Ghersevich MC, Soler Arias EA, Bosetti F, Cabrera Blatter MF, et al. Adrenal cortex stimulation with hCG in spayed female dogs with Cushing's syndrome: is the LH-dependent variant possible? *Open Vet J* 11(2):319-329, 2021.
8. Carotenuto G, Malerba E, Dolfini C, Brugnoli F, Giannuzzi P, Semprini G, et al. Cushing's syndrome –An epidemiological study based on a canine population of 21,281 dogs. *Open Vet J* 9(1):27-32, 2019.
9. O'Neill DG, Scudder C, Faire JM, Church DB, McGreevy PD, Thomson PC, et al. Epidemiology of hyperadrenocorticism among 210,824 dogs attending primary-care veterinary practices in the UK from 2009 to 2014. *J Small Anim Pract* 57(7):365-373, 2016.
10. Schofield I, Brodbelt DC, Niessen SJM, Church DB, Geddes RF, O'Neill DG. Frequency and risk factors for naturally occurring Cushing's syndrome in dogs attending UK primary care practices. *J Small Anim Pract* 63(4):265-274, 2022.
11. Hoffman JM, Lourenço BN, Promislow DEL, Creevy KE. Canine hyperadrenocorticism associations with signalment, selected comorbidities and mortality within North American veterinary teaching hospitals. *J Small Anim Pract* 59(11):681-690, 2018.
12. Machado L, de Oliveira MC, Barbieri CR, Riboldi CI, Leotti VB, González FHD, et al. Clinical and microbiological characterization of subclinical bacteriuria and sporadic bacterial cystitis in dogs with spontaneous hypercortisolism. *Comp Immunol Microbiol Infect Dis* 75:101624, 2021.
13. Wood FD, Pollard RE, Uerling MR, Feldman EC. Diagnostic imaging findings and endocrine test results in dogs with pituitary-dependent hyperadrenocorticism that did or did not have neurologic abnormalities: 157 cases (1989-2005). *J Am Vet Med Assoc* 231(7):1081-1085, 2007.
14. Berry CR, Hawkins EC, Hurley KJ, Monce K. Frequency of pulmonary mineralization and hypoxemia in 21 dogs with pituitary-dependent hyperadrenocorticism. *J Vet Intern Med* 14(2):151-156, 2000.
15. Doerr KA, Outerbridge CA, White SD, Kass PH, Shiraki R, Lam AT, et al. Calcinosis cutis in dogs: histopathological and clinical analysis of 46 cases. *Vet Dermatol* 24(3):355-61, e78-e9, 2013.
16. Mooney CT, Shiel RE, Sekiya M, Dunning M, Gunn E. A preliminary study of the effect of hyperadrenocorticism on calcium and phosphate concentrations, parathyroid hormone and markers of bone turnover in dogs. *Front Vet Sci* 7:311, 2020.
17. Benchekroun G, Desquilbet L, Herrtage ME, Jeffery ND, Rosenberg D, Granger N. Dogs with macroadenomas have lower body temperature and heart rate than dogs with microadenomas. *Vet J* 227:42-45, 2017.
18. Menchetti M, De Risio L, Galli G, Bruto Cherubini G, Corlazzoli D, Baroni M, et al. Neurological abnormalities in 97 dogs with detectable pituitary masses. *Vet Q* 39(1):57-64, 2019.
19. Woelfel CW, Mariani CL, Nolan MW, Keenihan EK, Topulos SP, Early PJ, et al. Presumed pituitary apoplexy in 26 dogs: clinical findings, treatments, and outcomes. *J Vet Intern Med* 37(3):1119-1128, 2023.
20. García San José P, Arenas Bermejo C, Clares Moral I, Cuesta Alvaro P, Pérez Alenza MD. Prevalence and risk factors associated with systemic hypertension in dogs with spontaneous hyperadrenocorticism. *J Vet Intern Med* 34(5):1768-1778, 2020.
21. García San José P, Arenas Bermejo C, Alonso-Miguel D, Clares Moral I, Cuesta-Alvaro P, Pérez Alenza MD. Changes in systolic blood pressure in dogs with pituitary-dependent hyperadrenocorticism during the first year of trilostane treatment. *J Vet Intern Med* 35(1):130-141, 2021.
22. Behrend EN, Kooistra HS, Nelson R, Reusch CE, Scott-Moncrieff JC. Diagnosis of spontaneous canine hyperadrenocorticism: 2012 ACVIM consensus statement (small animal). *J Vet Intern Med* 27(6):1292-1304, 2013.
23. Golinelli S, Fracassi F, Bianchi E, Pöppl Á, Miceli DD, Benedicenti L, et al. Clinical features of muscle stiffness in 37 dogs with concurrent naturally occurring hypercortisolism. *J Vet Intern Med* 37(2):578-585, 2023.
24. Swinney GR, Foster SF, Church DB, Malik R. Myotonia associated with hyperadrenocorticism in two dogs. *Aust Vet J* 76(11):722-724, 1998.
25. Jaffey JA, Pavlick M, Webster CR, Moore GE, McDaniel KA, Blois SL, et al. Effect of clinical signs, endocrinopathies, timing of surgery, hyperlipidemia, and hyperbilirubinemia on outcome in dogs with gallbladder mucocele. *Vet J* 251:105350, 2019.
26. Bennaim M, Shiel RE, Mooney CT. Diagnosis of spontaneous hyperadrenocorticism in dogs. Part 2: Adrenal function testing and differentiating tests. *Vet J* 252:105343, 2019.
27. Del Baldo F, Corsini A, Tardo AM, Tirolo A, Sapignoli A, Tumbarello M, Vasylyeva K, Fracassi F. Hypothalamic-pituitary-adrenal axis recovery after intermediate-acting glucocorticoid treatment in client-owned dogs. *J Vet Intern Med* 38(2):942-950, 2024.
28. Zeugswetter FK, Carranza Valencia A, Glavassevich K, Schwendenwein I. Patterns of the low-dose dexamethasone suppression test in canine hyperadrenocorticism revisited. *Vet Clin Pathol* 50:62-70, 2021.
29. Bennaim M, Shiel RE, Forde C, Mooney CT. Evaluation of individual low-dose dexamethasone suppression test patterns in naturally occurring hyperadrenocorticism in dogs. *J Vet Intern Med* 32:967-977, 2018.
30. Lim Lim L, Hulsebosch SE, Gilor C, Reagan KL, Kopecny L, Maggiore AD, Phillips KL, Kass PH, Vernau W, Nelson RW. Re-evaluation of the low-dose dexamethasone suppression test in dogs. *J Small Anim Pract* 64:12-20, 2023.
31. Bennaim M, Shiel RE, Forde C, Mooney CT. Evaluation of individual low-dose dexamethasone suppression test patterns in naturally occurring hyperadrenocorticism in dogs. *J Vet Intern Med* 32:967-977, 2018.
32. Galeandro L, Sieber-Ruckstuhl NS, Riond B, Hartnack S, Hofmann-Lehmann R, Reusch CE, Boretti FS. Urinary corticoid concentrations measured by 5 different immunoassays and gas chromatography-mass spectrometry in healthy dogs and dogs with hypercortisolism at home and in the hospital. *J Vet Intern Med* 28:1433-1441, 2014.
33. Schäfer I, Rehbein S, Holtdirk A, Kottmann T, Klein R, Müller E, Thoren-Tolling K. Diagnostic cut-off values for the urinary corticoid:creatinine ratio for the diagnosis of canine Cushing's syndrome using an automated chemiluminescent assay. *Vet Clin Pathol* 52:443-451, 2023.
34. Galac S, Kooistra HS, Teske E, Rijnberk A. Urinary corticoid/creatinine ratios in the differentiation between pituitary-dependent hyperadrenocorticism and hyperadrenocorticism due to adrenocortical tumour in the dog. *Vet Q* 19:17-20, 1997.
35. Behrend EN, Kemppainen RJ, Bruyette DS, Busch KA, Lee HP. Intramuscular administration of a low dose of ACTH for ACTH stimulation testing in dogs. *J Am Vet Med Assoc* 229(4):528-530, 2006.
36. Aldridge C, Behrend EN, Kemppainen RJ, Lee-Fowler TM, Martin LG, Ward CR, Bruyette D, Pannu J, Gaillard P, Lee HP. Comparison of 2 doses for ACTH stimulation testing in dogs suspected of or treated for hyperadrenocorticism. *J Vet Intern Med* 30:1637-1641, 2016.

37. Melián C, Pérez-López L, Saavedra P, et al. Ultrasound evaluation of adrenal gland size in clinically healthy dogs and in dogs with hyperadrenocorticism. *Vet Rec* e80, 2021. doi:10.1002/vetr.80
38. Benchekroun G, Fornel-Thibaud P, Rodriguez Piñeiro MI, et al. Ultrasonography criteria for differentiating ACTH dependency from ACTH independency in 47 dogs with hyperadrenocorticism and equivocal adrenal asymmetry. *J Vet Intern Med* 24(5):1077-1085, 2010. doi:10.1111/j.1939-1676.2010.0559.x
39. Bargellini P, Orlandi R, Dentini A, et al. Use of contrast-enhanced ultrasound in the differential diagnosis of adrenal tumors in dogs. *J Am Anim Hosp Assoc* 52(3):132-143, 2016. doi:10.5326/JAAHA-MS-6363
40. Bargellini P, Orlandi R, Paloni C, et al. Contrast-enhanced ultrasonographic characteristics of adrenal glands in dogs with pituitary-dependent hyperadrenocorticism. *Vet Radiol Ultrasound* 54(3):283-292, 2013. doi:10.1111/vru.12018
41. Burti S, Zotti A, Rubini G, et al. Contrast-enhanced ultrasound features of adrenal lesions in dogs. Vet Rec e2949, 2023. doi:10.1002/vetr.2949
42. Vlugt-Meijer RH, Meij BP, Voorhout G. Intraobserver and interobserver agreement, reproducibility, and accuracy of computed tomographic measurements of pituitary gland dimensions in healthy dogs. *Am J Vet Res* 67(10):1750-1755, 2006. doi:10.2460/ajvr.67.10.1750
43. Vlugt-Meijer RH, Meij BP, Ingh TSGAM, et al. Dynamic computed tomography of the pituitary gland in dogs with pituitary-dependent hyperadrenocorticism. *J Vet Intern Med* 17(6):773-780, 2003. doi:10.1111/j.1939-1676.2003.tb02514.x
44. Del Magno S, Grinwis GCM, Voorhout G, et al. Dynamic computed tomography of the pituitary gland using a single slice scanner in dogs with pituitary-dependent hypercortisolism. *Res Vet Sci* 107:42-49, 2016. doi:10.1016/j.rvsc.2016.04.00
45. Pollard RE, Reilly CM, Uerling MR, et al. Cross-sectional imaging characteristics of pituitary adenomas, invasive adenomas and adenocarcinomas in dogs: 33 cases (1988-2006). *J Vet Intern Med* 24(1):160-165, 2010. doi:10.1111/j.1939-1676.2009.0414.x
46. Galli G, Bertolini G, Dalla Serra G, et al. Suspected pituitary apoplexy: clinical presentation, diagnostic imaging findings and outcome in 19 dogs. *Vet Sci* 9(4):191, 2022. doi:10.3390/vetsci9040191
47. Bertolini G, Furlanello T, De Lorenzi D, et al. Computed tomographic quantification of canine adrenal gland volume and attenuation. *Vet Radiol Ultrasound* 47(5):444-448, 2006. doi:10.1111/j.1740-8261.2006.00164.x
48. Rodríguez Piñeiro MI, Fornel-Thibaud P, Benchekroun G, et al. Use of computed tomography adrenal gland measurement for differentiating ACTH dependence from ACTH independence in 64 dogs with hyperadenocorticism. *J Vet Intern Med* 25(5):1066-1074, 2011. doi:10.1111/j.1939-1676.2011.07773.x
49. Bokhorst KL, Kooistra HS, Boroffka SAEB, et al. Concurrent pituitary and adrenocortical lesions on computed tomography imaging in dogs with spontaneous hypercortisolism. *J Vet Intern Med* 33(1):72-78, 2019. doi:10.1111/jvim.15378
50. Taoda T, Hara Y, Masuda H, et al. Magnetic resonance imaging assessment of pituitary posterior lobe displacement in dogs with pituitary-dependent hyperadrenocorticism. *J Vet Med Sci* 73(6):725-731, 2011. doi:10.1292/jvms.10-0192
51. Auriemma E, Barthez PY, Vlugt-Meijer RH, et al. Computed tomography and low-field magnetic resonance imaging of the pituitary gland in dogs with pituitary-dependent hyperadrenocorticism: 11 cases (2001-2003). *J Am Vet Med Assoc* 235(4):409-414, 2009. doi:10.2460/javma.235.4.409
52. Sanders K, Kooistra HS, Galac S. Treating canine Cushing's syndrome: current options and future prospects. *Vet J* 241:42-51, 2018.
53. Hanson JM, van't Hoofd MM, Voorhout G, et al. Efficacy of transsphenoidal hypophysectomy in treatment of dogs with pituitary-dependent hyperadrenocorticism. *J Vet Intern Med* 19(5):687-694, 2005.
54. van Bokhorst KL, Galac S, Kooistra HS, de Grauw JC, Teske E, Grinwis GCM, et al. Laparoscopic vs. open adrenalectomy: perioperative data and survival analysis in 70 dogs with an adrenal tumor. *Front Vet Sci* 10, 2023.
55. Sieber-Ruckstuhl NS, Boretti FS, Wenger M, Maser-Gluth C, Reusch CE. Cortisol, aldosterone, cortisol precursor, androgen and endogenous ACTH concentrations in dogs with pituitary-dependant hyperadrenocorticism treated with trilostane. *Domest Anim Endocrinol* 31:63-75, 2006.
56. Galac S, Buijtels JJ, Mol JA, et al. Effects of trilostane on the pituitary-adrenocortical and renin-aldosterone axis in dogs with pituitary-dependent hypercortisolism. *Vet J* 183:75-80, 2010a.
57. Rapastella S, Morabito S, Sharman M, et al. Effect of pituitary-dependent hypercortisolism on the survival of dogs treated with radiotherapy for pituitary macroadenomas. *J Vet Intern Med* 37(4):1331-1340, 2023. doi:10.1111/jvim.16724.
58. Golinelli S, de Marco V, Leal RO, et al. Comparison of methods to monitor dogs with hypercortisolism treated with trilostane. *J Vet Intern Med* 35(6):2616-2627, 2021.
59. Potts GO, Creange JE, Hardong HR, et al. Trilostane, an orally active inhibitor of steroid biosynthesis. *Steroids* 32:257-267, 1978.
60. Witt AL, Neiger R. Adrenocorticotropic hormone levels in dogs with pituitary-dependent hyperadrenocorticism following trilostane therapy. *Vet Rec* 154:399-400, 2004.
61. Sieber-Ruckstuhl NS, Boretti FS, Wenger M, et al. Serum concentrations of cortisol and cortisone in healthy dogs and dogs with pituitary-dependent hyperadrenocorticism treated with trilostane. *Vet Rec* 163:477-481, 2008.
62. Griebsch C, Lehnert C, Williams GJ, et al. Effect of trilostane on hormone and serum electrolyte concentrations in dogs with pituitary-dependent hyperadrenocorticism. *J Vet Intern Med* 28:160-165, 2014.
63. Johnston L, Chohan A, Chapman E. Absorption of trilostane in the fasted and non-fasted healthy dog [abstract]. Proceedings of the 15th ECVIM Congress, 2005, p. 223.
64. Ruckstuhl NS, Nett CS, Reusch CE. Results of clinical examinations, laboratory tests, and ultrasonography in dogs with pituitary-dependent hyperadrenocorticism treated with trilostane. *Am J Vet Res* 2002;63:506–512.
65. Neiger R, Ramsey I, O'Connor J, et al. Trilostane treatment of 78 dogs with pituitary-dependent hyperadrenocorticism. *Vet Rec* 150:799-804, 2002.
66. Braddock JA, Church DB, Robertson ID, et al. Trilostane treatment in dogs with pituitary-dependent hyperadrenocorticism. *Aust Vet* J 81:600-607, 2003.
67. Benchekroun G, de Fornel-Thibaud P, Lafarge S, et al. Trilostane therapy for hyperadrenocorticism in three dogs with adrenocortical metastasis. *Vet Rec* 163:190, 2008.
68. Eastwood JM, Elwood CM, Hurley KJ. Trilostane treatment of a dog with functional adrenocortical neoplasia. *J Small Anim Pract* 44:126-131, 2003.
69. Helm JR, McLauchlan G, Boden LA, et al. A comparison of factors that influence survival in dogs with adrenal dependent hyperadrenocorticism treated with mitotane or trilostane *J Vet Int Med* 25:251-260, 2011.
70. Arenas C, Melián C, Pérez-Alenza MD. Long-term survival of dogs with adrenal-dependent hyperadrenocorticism: a comparison between mitotane and twice daily trilostane treatment *J Vet Intern Med* 28:473-480, 2014.
71. Arenas C, Melián C, Pérez-Alenza MD. Evaluation of 2 trilostane protocols for the treatment of canine pituitary-dependent hyperadrenocorticism: twice daily versus once daily. *J Vet Intern Med* 27:1478-1485, 2013.
72. Vaughan MA, Feldman EC, Hoar BR, et al. Evaluation of twice-daily, low-dose trilostane treatment administered orally in dogs with naturally occurring hyperadrenocorticism. *J Am Vet Med Assoc* 232:1321-1328, 2008.
73. Feldman EC, Kass PH. Trilostane dose versus body weight in the treatment of naturally occurring pituitary-dependent hyperadrenocorticism in dogs. *J Vet Intern Med* 26:1078-1080, 2012.
74. Nam S, Kim T, Song K, Feldman EC, Seo K. Evaluation of compounded trilostane packets for dogs with naturally occurring hyperadrenocorticism. *J Vet Intern Med* 35(4):1729-1732, 2021.
75. Arenas Bermejo C, Pérez Alenza D, García San José P, et al. Laboratory assessment of trilostane treatment in dogs with pituitary dependent hyperadrenocorticism. *J Vet Intern Med* 34:1413-1422, 2020.
76. Smets PM, Lefebvre HP, Meij BP, et al. Long-term follow-up of renal function in dogs after treatment for ACTH-dependent hyperadrenocorticism. *J Vet Intern Med* 26:565-574, 2012.

77. Tebb AJ, Arteaga A, Evans H, et al. Canine hyperadrenocorticism: effects of trilostane on parathyroid hormone, calcium and phosphate concentrations. *J Small Anim Pract* 46:537-542, 2005.
78. Wehner A, Glöckner S, Weiss B, et al. Association between ACTH stimulation test results and clinical signs in dogs with hyperadrenocorticism treated with trilostane. *Vet J* 276:105740, 2021.
79. Midence JN, Drobatz KJ, Hess RS. Cortisol concentrations in well-regulated dogs with hyperadrenocorticism treated with trilostane. *J Vet Intern Med* 29:1529-1533, 2015.
80. Macfarlane L, Parkin T, Ramsey I. Pre-trilostane and three-hour post trilostane cortisol to monitor trilostane therapy in dogs. *Vet Rec* 179:597-601, 2016.
81. Boretti FA, Holzthuem J, Reusch CE, et al. Lack of association between clinical signs and laboratory parameters in dogs with hyperadrenocorticism before and during trilostane treatment. *Schweiz Arch Tierheilkd* 158:631-638, 2016.
82. Galac S, Buijtels JJ, Kooistra HS. Urinary corticoid:creatinine ratios in dogs with pituitary-dependent hyperadrenocorticism during trilostane treatment. *J Vet Intern Med* 23:1214-1219, 2009.
83. Arteaga A, Dhand NK, McCann T, et al. Monitoring the response of canine hyperadrenocorticism to trilostane treatment by assessment of acute phase protein concentrations. *J Small Anim Pract* 51:204-207, 2010.
84. Cook AK, Bond KG. Evaluation of the use of baseline cortisol concentration as a monitoring tool for dogs receiving trilostane as a treatment for hyperadrenocorticism. *J Am Vet Med Assoc* 237:801-805, 2010.
85. Burkhardt WA, Boretti FS, Reusch CE, Sieber-Ruckstuhl NS. Evaluation of baseline cortisol, endogenous ACTH, and cortisol/ACTH ratio to monitor trilostane treatment in dogs with pituitary-dependent hyperadrenocorticism. *J Vet Intern Med* 27:919-923, 2013.
86. Woolcock AD, Bugbee AC, Creevy KE. Evaluation of baseline cortisol concentration to monitor efficacy of twice-daily administration of trilostane to dogs with pituitary-dependent hyperadrenocorticism: 22 cases (2008–2012). *J Am Vet Med Assoc* 248:814-821, 2016.
87. Boretti F, Musella C, Burkhardt W, et al. Comparison of two prepill cortisol concentrations in dogs with hypercortisolism treated with trilostane. *BMC Vet Res* 14:417, 2018.
88. McGrotty YL, Arteaga A, Knottenbelt CM, et al. Haptoglobin concentrations in dogs undergoing trilostane treatment for hyperadrenocorticism. *Vet Clin Pathol* 34:255-258, 2005.
89. Bonadio CM, Feldman EC, Cohen TA, Kass PH. Comparison of adrenocorticotropic hormone stimulation test results started 2 versus 4 hours after trilostane administration in dogs with naturally occurring hyperadrenocorticism. *J Vet Intern Med* 28:239-1243, 2014.
90. King JB, Morton JM. Incidence and risk factors for hypoadrenocorticism in dogs treated with trilostane. *Vet J* 230:24-29, 2017.
91. Appleman E, Schrage A, Lamb KE, et al. Evaluation of iatrogenic hypocortisolemia following trilostane therapy in 48 dogs with pituitary-dependent hyperadrenocorticism. *J Am Anim Hosp Assoc* 57:217-224, 2021.
92. Lamoureux A, Cadoré JL, Hugonnard M, et al. Iatrogenic symptomatic hypoadrenocorticism after treatment with trilostane for hyperadrenocorticism in dogs: eight cases (2008-2019). *J Small Anim Pract* 64:409-414, 2023.
93. Burkhardt WA, Guscetti F, Boretti FS, et al. Adrenocorticotropic hormone, but not trilostane, causes severe adrenal hemorrhage, vacuolization, and apoptosis in rats. *Domest Anim Endocrinol* 40:155-164, 2011.
94. García San José P, Arenas Bermejo C, Alonso-Miguel D, et al. Changes in systolic blood pressure in dogs with pituitary-dependent hyperadrenocorticism during the first year of trilostane treatment. *J Vet Intern Med* 35:130-141, 2021.
95. Barker EN, Campbell S, Tebb AJ, et al. A comparison of the survival times of dogs treated with mitotane or trilostane for pituitary-dependent hyperadrenocorticism. *J Vet Intern Med* 19:810-815, 2005.
96. Fracassi F, Corradini S, Floriano D, et al. Prognostic factors for survival in dogs with pituitary-dependent hypercortisolism treated with trilostane. *Vet Rec* 176:49, 2015.
97. Clemente M, De Andrés PJ, Arenas C, et al. Comparison of non-selective adrenocorticolysis with mitotane or trilostane for the treatment of dogs with pituitary-dependent hyperadrenocorticism. *Vet Rec* 161:805-809, 2007.
98. Teshima T, Hara Y, Takekoshi S, et al. Trilostane-induced inhibition of cortisol secretion results in reduced negative feedback at the hypothalamic-pituitary axis. *Domest Anim Endocrinol* 36:32-44, 2009.
99. Sbiera S, Leich E, Liebisch G, et al. Mitotane inhibits sterol-o-acyl transferase 1 triggering lipid-mediated endoplasmic reticulum stress and apoptosis in adrenocortical carcinoma cells. *Endocrinology* 156:3895-3908, 2015.
100. Kintzer PP, Peterson ME. Mitotane (o, p'DDD) treatment of 200 dogs with pituitary-dependent hyperadrenocorticism *J Vet Intern Med* 5:182-190, 1991.
101. Galac S, Reusch CE, Kooistra HS, Rijnberk A. Adrenals. In Rijnberk AD, Kooistra HS (editors). Clinical Endocrinology of Dogs and Cats. Schlütersche, 2010, pp. 93-154.
102. Feldman EC, Bruyette DS, Nelson RW, et al. Plasma cortisol response to ketoconazole administration in dogs with hyperadrenocorticism. *J Am Vet Med Assoc* 197:71-78, 1990.
103. de Bruin, C, Hanson JM, Meij BP, et al. Expression and functional analysis of dopamine receptor subtype 2 and somatostatin receptor subtypes in canine Cushing's disease. *Endocrinology* 149:4357-4366, 2008.
104. Castillo V, Gómez NV, Lalia JC, et al. Cushing's disease in dogs: cabergoline treatment. *Res Vet Sci* 85:26-34, 2008.
105. Golinelli S, Fracassi F, Pöppl AG, et al. Addition of cabergoline to trilostane treatment for dogs with pituitary-dependent hypercortisolism. Proceeding ECVIM Congress (abstract), 2023.
106. Castillo V, Theodoropoulou M, Stalla J, et al. Effect of SOM230 (Pasireotide) on corticotropic cells: action in dogs with Cushing's disease. Neuroendocrinology 94:124-136, 2011.
107. Lottati M, Bruyette DS Outcomes of the addition of pasireotide to traditional adrenal-directed treatment for dogs with pituitary-dependent hyperadrenocorticism secondary to macroadenoma: 9 cases (2013-2015). *J Am Vet Med Assoc* 252:1403-1408, 2018.
108. Bicknell AB. The tissue-specific processing of pro-opiomelanocortin. *J Neuroendocrinol* 20:692-699, 2008. doi:10.1111/j.1365-2826.2008.01709.x
109. Nguyen JB, Kusnetzow AK, Reinhart G, et al. In vitro pharmacological characterization of CRN04894: the first reported oral, selective nonpeptide melanocortin 2 receptor antagonist evaluated in phase 1 first-in-human clinical trials. *FASEB J* 36, 2022.
110. Trainer P, Ferrara-Cook C, Ayala A, et al. CRN04894: an oral, nonpeptide adrenocorticotropic hormone (ACTH) receptor antagonist decreases basal and stimulated cortisol secretion in healthy volunteers. *Endocrine Abstracts Bioscientifica* 86, 2022.
111. Sanders K, Mol JA, Kooistra HS, et al. Melanocortin 2 receptor antagonists in canine pituitary-dependent hypercortisolism: in vitro studies. *Vet Res Commun* 42:283-288, 2018.
112. Puglisi S, Cosentini D, Grisanti S, et al. Activity of abiraterone acetate in the management of Cushing syndrome associated to advanced adrenocortical carcinoma: results of the ABACUS trial. *Endocrine Abstracts Bioscientifica* 81, 2022.
113. Sanders K, Mol JA, Kooistra HS, et al. New insights in the functional zonation of the canine adrenal cortex. *J Vet Intern Med* 30:741 750, 2016.
114. Sanders K, de Wit WL, Mol JA, et al. Abiraterone acetate for Cushing syndrome: study in a canine primary adrenocortical cell culture model. *Endocrinology* 159: 3689-3698, 2018.
115. Galac S, Kool MMJ, van den Berg MF, et al. Expression of steroidogenic factor 1 in canine cortisol-secreting adrenocortical tumors and normal adrenals. *Domest Anim Endocrinol* 49:1-5, 2014.
116. Sanders K, Mol JA, Slob A, et al. Steroidogenic factor-1 inverse agonists as a treatment option for canine hypercortisolism: in vitro study. *Domest Anim Endocrinol* 63: 23-30, 2018.
117. Buhman KF, Accad M, Farese RV. Mammalian acyl-CoA: cholesterol acyltransferases. *Biochim Biophys Acta* 1529:142-154, 2000. doi:10.1016/S1388-1981(00)00144-X.

118. Dominick MA, McGuire EJ, Reindel JF, et al. Subacute toxicity of a novel inhibitor of acyl-CoA: cholesterol acyltransferase in Beagle dogs. *Fundam Appl Toxicol* 20:217-224, 1993. doi: 10.1006/faat.1993.1029.
119. Burns VE, Kerppola TK. ATR-101 inhibits cholesterol efflux and cortisol secretion by ATP-binding cassette transporters, causing cytotoxic cholesterol accumulation in adrenocortical carcinoma cells. *Br J Pharmacol* 174:3315-3332, 2017. doi: 10.1111/bph.13951.
120. LaPensee CR, Mann JE, Rainey WE, et al. ATR-101, a selective and potent inhibitor of Acyl-CoA acyltransferase 1, induces apoptosis in H295R adrenocortical cells and in the adrenal cortex of dogs. *Endocrinology* 157:1775-1788, 2016. doi:10.1210/en.2015-2052.
121. Langlois DK, Fritz MC, Schall WD, et al. ATR-101, a selective ACAT1 inhibitor, decreases ACTH-stimulated cortisol concentrations in dogs with naturally occurring Cushing's syndrome. *BMC Endocr Disord* 18:24, 2018. doi:10.1186/s12902-018-0251-5.
122. Sanders K, Kooistra HS, van den Heuvel M, et al. Transcriptome sequencing reveals two subtypes of cortisol-secreting adrenocortical tumours in dogs and identifies CYP26B1 as a potential new therapeutic target. *Vet Comp Oncol* 21:100-110, 2023.
123. Pivonello R, Ferrigno R, De Martino MC, et al. Medical treatment of Cushing's disease: an overview of the current and recent clinical trials. *Front Endocrinol* 11:648, 2020.
124. Duggan S. Osilodrostat: first approval. *Drugs* 80:495-500, 2020.
125. Weckbecker G, Briner U, Lewis I, et al. SOM230: a new somatostatin peptidomimetic with potent inhibitory effects on the growth hormone/insulin-like growth factor-I axis in rats, primates, and dogs. *Endocrinology* 143:4123-4130, 2002.
126. Colao A, Petersenn S, Newell-Price J, et al. A 12-month phase 3 study of pasireotide in Cushing's disease. *N Engl J Med* 366:914-924, 2012.
127. Robben JH, van den Brom WE, Mol JA, et al. Effect of octreotide on plasma concentrations of glucose, insulin, glucagon, growth hormone, and cortisol in healthy dogs and dogs with insulinoma. *Res Vet Sci* 80:25-32, 2006.
128. Biermasz NR. New medical therapies on the horizon: oral octreotide. *Pituitary* 20:149-153, 2017.
129. Castillo V, Giacomini D, Páez-Pereda M, et al. Retinoic acid as a novel medical therapy for Cushing's disease in dogs. *Endocrinology* 147:4438-4444, 2006.
130. Ciato D, Mumbach AG, Paez-Pereda M, et al. Currently used and investigational drugs for Cushing's disease. *Expert Opin Investig Drugs* 26:75-84, 2017.
131. Occhi G, Regazzo D, Albiger NM, et al. Activation of the dopamine receptor type-2 (DRD2) promoter by 9-cis retinoic acid in a cellular model of Cushing's disease mediates the inhibition of cell proliferation and ACTH secretion without a complete corticotroph-to-melanotroph transdifferentiation. *Endocrinology* 155:3538-3549, 2014.
132. Meij BP, Voorhout G, van den Ingh TSGAM, et al. Results of transsphenoidal hypophysectomy in 52 dogs with pituitary-dependent hyperadrenocorticism. *Vet Surg* 27(3):246-261, 1998.
133. Tanaka S, Suzuki S, Oishi M, Soeta S, Namiki R, Hara Y. Adrenocorticotropic hormone-producing pituitary adenoma with pituitary apoplexy treated by surgical decompression: a case report. *BMC Vet Res* 18:397, 2022.
134. Meij BP, Voorhout G, Van den Ingh TS, et al. Transsphenoidal hypophysectomy in beagle dogs: evaluation of a microsurgical technique. Vet Surg 26(4):295-309, 1997.
135. Escauriaza L, Fenn J, McCue J, et al. A 3-dimensional printed patient-specific surgical guide to facilitate transsphenoidal hypophysectomy in dogs. *Front Vet Sci* 9, 2022. doi:10.3389/fvets.2022.930856.
136. Roh J, Kim D, Jeong S, Lee H. Evaluation of the accuracy of three-dimensionally printed patient-specific guides for transsphenoidal hypophysectomy in small-breed dogs. *J Am Vet Med Assoc* 83(5):465-472, 2022.
137. Owen Tj, Chen AV, Frey S, et al. Transsphenoidal surgery: accuracy of an image-guided neuronavigation system to approach the pituitary fossa (sella turcica). *Vet Surg* 47(5):664-671, 2018.
138. Mamelak AN, Owen TJ, Bruyette D. Transsphenoidal surgery using a high definition video telescope for pituitary adenomas in dogs with pituitary-dependent hypercortisolism: methods and results. *Vet Surg* 43(4):369-379, 2014.
139. Van Stee L, Van Rijn SJ, Sara Galac, et al. Challenges of transsphenoidal pituitary surgery in severe brachycephalic dogs. *Front Vet Sci* 20:10, 2023. doi:10.3389/fvets.2023.1154617.
140. Sato A, Teshima T, Ishino H, et al. A magnetic resonance imaging-based classification system for indication of trans-sphenoidal hypophysectomy in canine pituitary-dependent hypercortisolism. *J Small Anim Pract* 57(5):240-247, 2016.
141. Hanson JM, Teske E, Voorhout G, et al. Prognostic factors for outcome after transsphenoidal hypophysectomy in dogs with pituitary-dependent hyperadrenocorticism. *J Neurosurg* 107(4):430-440, 2007.
142. Van Rijn SJ, Galac S, Tryfonidou MA, et al. The influence of pituitary size on outcome after transsphenoidal hypophysectomy in a large cohort of dogs with pituitary-dependent hypercortisolism. *J Vet Intern Med* 30(4):989- 995, 2016.
143. Van Rijn SJ, Hanson JM, Zierikzee D, et al. The prognostic value of perioperative profiles of ACTH and cortisol for recurrence after transsphenoidal hypophysectomy in dogs with corticotroph adenomas. *J Vet Intern Med* 29(3):869-876, 2015.
144. Massari F, Nicoli S, Romanelli G, Buracco P, Zini E. Adrenalectomy in dogs with adrenal gland tumors: 52 cases (2002-2008). *J Am Vet Med Assoc* 239(2):216-221, 2011.
145. Lang JM, Schertel E, Kennedy S, Wilson D, Barnhart M, Danielson B. Elective and emergency surgical management of adrenal gland tumors: 60 Cases (1999-2006). *J Am Anim Hosp Assoc* 47(6):428-435, 2011.
146. Schwartz P, Kovak JR, Koprowski A, Ludwig LL, Monette S, Bergman PJ. Evaluation of prognostic factors in the surgical treatment of adrenal gland tumors in dogs: 41 cases (1999-2005). *J Am Vet Med Assoc* 232(1):77-84, 2008.
147. Barrera JS, Bernard F, Ehrhart EJ, Withrow SJ, Monnet E. Evaluation of risk factors for outcome associated with adrenal gland tumors with or without invasion of the caudal vena cava and treated via adrenalectomy in dogs: 86 cases (1993-2009). *J Am Vet Med Assoc* 242(12):1715-1721, 2013.
148. Kyles AE, Feldman EC, De Cock HEV, Kass PH, Mathews KG, Hardie EM, et al. Surgical management of adrenal gland tumors with and without associated tumor thrombi in dogs: 40 cases (1994-2001). *J Am Vet Med Assoc* 223(5):654-662, 2003.
149. Cavalcanti JVJ, Skinner OT, Mayhew PD, Colee JC, Boston SE. Outcome in dogs undergoing adrenalectomy for small adrenal gland tumours without vascular invasion. *Vet Comp Oncol* 18(4):599-606, 2020.
150. Mayhew PD, Boston SE, Zwingenberger AL, Giuffrida MA, Runge JJ, Holt DE, et al. Perioperative morbidity and mortality in dogs with invasive adrenal neoplasms treated by adrenalectomy and cavotomy. *Vet Surg* 48(5):742-50, 2019.
151. Knight RC, Lamb CR, Brockman DJ, Lipscomb VJ. Variations in surgical technique for adrenalectomy with caudal vena cava venotomy in 19 dogs. *Vet Surg* 48(5):751-759, 2019.
152. Mayhew PD, Massari F, Araya FL, Nimwegen SA van, Goethem B Van, Singh A, et al. Laparoscopic adrenalectomy for resection of unilateral noninvasive adrenal masses in dogs is associated with excellent outcomes in experienced centers. *J Am Vet Med Assoc* 1(aop):1-8, 2023.
153. Séguin B, Brownlee L (editors). Endocrine System. Veterinary Surgical Oncology 2nd edition Wiley Blackwell, 2022, pp. 569-623.
154. Appelgrein C, Hosgood G, Drynan E, Nesbitt A. Short-term outcome of adrenalectomy in dogs with adrenal gland tumours that did not receive pre-operative medical management. *Aust Vet J* 98(9):449-454, 2020.
155. Mayhew PD, Culp WTN, Hunt GB, Steffey MA, Mayhew KN, Fuller M, et al. Comparison of perioperative morbidity and mortality rates in dogs with noninvasive adrenocortical masses undergoing laparoscopic versus open adrenalectomy. *J Am Vet Med Assoc* 245(9):1028-1035, 2014.
156. Naan EC, Kirpensteijn J, Dupré GP, Galac S, Radlinsky MG. Innovative approach to laparoscopic adrenalectomy for treatment of unilateral adrenal gland tumors in dogs. *Vet Surg* 42(6):710-715, 2013.

157. Sanders K, Cirkel K, Grinwis GCM, Teske E, van Nimwegen SA, Mol JA, et al. The Utrecht Score: A novel histopathological scoring system to assess the prognosis of dogs with cortisol-secreting adrenocortical tumours. *Vet Comp Oncol* 17(3):329-337, 2019.
158. Traverson M, Zheng J, Tremolada G, Chen CL, Cray M, et al. Adrenal tumors treated by adrenalectomy following spontaneous rupture carry an overall favorable prognosis: retrospective evaluation of outcomes in 59 dogs and 3 cats (2000-2021). *J Am Vet Med Assoc* 1(aop):1-9, 2023.
159. Toogood AA. Endocrine consequences of brain irradiation. *Growth Horm IGF Res* 14 (Suppl A):S118-124, 2004. doi:10.1016/j.ghir.2004.03.038.
160. Dolera M, Malfassi L, Pavesi S, et al. Volumetric-modulated arc stereotactic radiotherapy for canine adrenocortical tumours with vascular invasion. *J Small Anim Pract* 57(12):710-717, 2016. doi:10.1111/jsap.12592.
161. Gieger TL, Nolan MW. Treatment outcomes and target delineation utilizing CT and MRI in 13 dogs treated with a uniform stereotactic radiation therapy protocol (16 Gy single fraction) for pituitary masses: (2014-2017). *Vet Comp Oncol* 19(1):17-24, 2021. doi:10.1111/vco.12627.
162. Rossmeisl JH, Garcia PA, Daniel GB, et al. Invited review –neuroimaging response assessment criteria for brain tumors in veterinary patients. *Vet Radiol Ultrasound* 55(2):115-132, 2014.
163. Goossens MM, Feldman EC, Theon AP, et al Efficacy of cobalt 60 radiotherapy in dogs with pituitary-dependent hyperadrenocorticism. *J Am Vet Med Assoc* 212(3):374-376, 1998.
164. Théon AP, Feldman EC. Megavoltage irradiation of pituitary macrotumours in dogs with neurologic signs. *J Am Vet Med Assoc* 213(2):225-231, 1998.
165. Marcinowska A, Warland J, Brearley M, et al. Comparison of two coarse fractionated radiation protocols for the management of canine pituitary macrotumour: an observational study of 24 dogs. *Vet Radiol Ultrasound* 56(5):554-562, 2015. doi:10.1111/vru.12270.
166. Bley CR, Sumova A, Roos M, et al. Irradiation of brain tumours in dogs with neurologic disease. *J Vet Intern Med* 19(6):849-854, 2005. doi:10.1892/0891-6640(2005)19[849:iobtid]2.0.co;2.
167. de Fornel P, Delisle F, Devauchelle P, et al. Effects of radiotherapy on pituitary corticotroph macrotumours in dogs: a retrospective study of 12 cases. *Can Vet J* 48(5):481-486, 2007.
168. Kent MS, Bommarito D, Feldman E, et al. Survival, neurologic response, and prognostic factors in dogs with pituitary masses treated with radiation therapy and untreated dogs. *J Vet Intern Med* 21(5):1027-1033, 2007. doi:10.1892/0891-6640(2007)21[1027:snrapf]2.0.co;2.
169. Hansen KS, Zwingenberger AL, Théon AP, et al. Long-term survival with stereotactic radiotherapy for imaging-diagnosed pituitary tumours in dogs. *Vet Radiol Ultrasound* 60(2):219-232, 2019. doi:10.1111/vru.12708.
170. van Leeuwen CM, Oei AL, Crezee J, et al. The alfa and beta of tumours: a review of parameters of the linear-quadratic model, derived from clinical radiotherapy studies. *Radiat Oncol* 13(1):96, 2018. doi:10.1186/s13014-018-1040-z.
171. Speckter H, Santana J, Lara G, et al. Assessment of the alpha/beta ratios of pituitary adenomas and craniopharyngiomas for the quantification of single fraction equivalent dose benefits from hypofractionated radiosurgery. *Int J Rad Oncol* 108(3):e714, 2020.
172. Milker-Zabel S, Debus J, Thilmann C, et al. Fractionated stereotactically guided radiotherapy and radiosurgery in the treatment of functional and non-functional adenomas of the pituitary gland. *Int J Rad Oncol Biology Physics* 50:1279-1286, 2001.
173. Brearley MJ, Jeffery ND, Phillips SM, et al. Hypofractionated radiation therapy of brain masses in dogs: a retrospective analysis of survival of 83 cases (1991-1996). *J Vet Intern Med* 13(5):408-412, 1999. doi:10.1892/0891-6640(1999)013<0408:hrtobm>2.3.co;2.
174. Schwarz P, Meier V, Soukup A, et al. Comparative evaluation of a novel, moderately hypofractionated radiation protocol in 56 dogs with symptomatic intracranial neoplasia. *J Vet Intern Med* 32(6):2013-2020, 2018. doi:10.1111/jvim.15324.

CHAPTER 35

Adrenal tumors (all but cortisol-secreting and pheochromocytoma)

Viviani De Marco
DVM, PhD

Canine adrenal tumors (ATs) originate from either the adrenal cortex or medulla. They may be functional (i.e., synthesizing and secreting hormones) or nonfunctional (hormonally silent). Functional ATs that secrete aldosterone, sex steroids, or steroid precursors will be addressed in this chapter, together with nonfunctional or hormonally silent ATs. During diagnostic imaging, these are typically serendipitously detected as an adrenal incidentaloma because affected dogs do not exhibit clinical signs. Both functional and nonfunctional ATs can be benign or malignant, which should be considered when finding the most optimal treatment option.[1,2]

Hyperaldosteronism

Aldosterone-secreting ATs causing hyperaldosteronism are extremely rare in dogs, with only a few cases published to date.[3,4] Aldosteronomas primarily produce and secrete aldosterone, leading to increased sodium reabsorption and increased potassium excretion. Dogs present with weakness, polyuria and polydipsia, hypokalemia, and hypertension. Serum sodium concentrations are usually at the upper end or mildly above the reference range.

Inappropriately elevated serum aldosterone concentrations should ideally make a diagnosis of hyperaldosteronism in the presence of hypokalemia. Renin concentration within the reference range or lower is expected. The plasma aldosterone-to-renin ratio is the most reliable in diagnosing hyperaldosteronism. However, currently, canine renin assay is not available.[2]

Tumors secreting nonaldosterone mineralocorticoids, e.g., deoxycorticosterone or corticosterone may occur and cause a clinical picture of hyperaldosteronism, but with low aldosterone levels.[5,6] Mixed tumors secreting both mineralocorticoids and glucocorticoids can occur as well.[7]

When the diagnosis of hyperaldosteronism is confirmed, treatment typically involves oral potassium supplementation and the administration of mineralocorticoid receptor blockers, such as spironolactone. Hypertension should be managed with antihypertensive medications, such as calcium channel blocker amlodipine, and titrated to effect. Medical therapy should be given as required until surgery, with electrolytes and blood pressure monitored regularly, ideally every 7 or 14 days. Adrenalectomy is the most optimal treatment for aldosteronoma, as removing the adrenal mass not only alleviates clinical signs but also mitigates the risk of potential malignancy. After unilateral adrenalectomy, mineralocorticoid suppression of the residual adrenal gland can occur. If hyperkalemia and hyponatremia develop postoperatively, temporary fludrocortisone acetate therapy is needed, but it can usually be tapered and discontinued within a week.[2] When surgery is not possible due to comorbidities, metastasis, or invasive growth of the tumor, medical treatment addressing mineralocorticoid excess in combination with antihypertensive drugs is indicated. However, this is only a palliative treatment as it does not suppress the AT growth. Consequently, the prognosis may not be as favorable as it is with complete surgical removal of an aldosterone-producing tumor.[2]

Steroid precursors and sex hormone-secreting adrenal tumors

Adrenocortical tumors possess the capacity to synthesize and secrete excessive amounts of precursors of aldosterone and cortisol (progesterone, 17-alpha-hydroxyprogesterone [17OHP]) as well as sex steroids (dehydroepiandrostenedione [DHEAS], androstenedione, testosterone, and estradiol).[8-10]

Progestins can exert a glucocorticoid effect by binding to glucocorticoid receptors or displacing cortisol from its binding proteins, which leads to elevated levels of free cortisol in the bloodstream. This results in negative feedback on the pituitary-adrenal axis and suppressed endogenous plasma ACTH concentration.[8-10] In dogs with ATs secreting steroid precursors such as progesterone and 17OHP, clinical presentation may mimic hypercortisolism. However, endocrine testing reveals normal results on low-dose dexamethasone suppression test (LDDST) or urinary cortisol to creatinine ratio (UCCR). The ACTH stimulation test gives a subnormal cortisol response but increased levels of progesterone and 17OHP.[11-13]

Secretion of steroid precursors, instead of the end-product cortisol, is presumably the result of malignant

dedifferentiation of the adrenocortical cells or aberrant pathways. In humans, advanced diagnostic techniques such as urine steroid metabolomic profiling with mass spectrometry are utilized to detect the entire spectrum of adrenocortical steroidogenesis precursors.[14] Through this method, differentiation between malignant and benign adrenal masses can be made based on a steroidogenic profile, guiding the treatment approach. This technique, however, has not been applied to dogs yet.
The treatment of choice for steroid-precursors secreting ATs is adrenalectomy. Temporary supplementation with glucocorticoids after surgery may be necessary in cases with suppressed endogenous ACTH. Adrenocortical tumors associated exclusively with symptoms of hyperandrogenism (virilization syndrome) or hyperestrogenism (feminization syndrome) are extremely rare.[2]

Adrenal incidentaloma: hormonally silent adrenal tumors

A hormonally silent AT is typically discovered incidentally on diagnostic imaging in a patient that is not suspected of having adrenal disease.[11] An incidentally found adrenal mass can originate from the cortex or medulla and may present as either benign or malignant, as well as functional or nonfunctional. A retrospective study of case series identified an adrenal incidentaloma in 9.3% of cases undergoing abdominal CT[12] and in 4% of cases undergoing abdominal ultrasound.[13]
After the discovery of an adrenal incidentaloma, a more comprehensive medical history and physical examination should be performed or retaken with knowledge of the presence of the adrenal mass. This approach ensures that any potential symptoms and signs associated with the adrenal mass are evaluated and addressed. Routine blood and urine tests, along with blood pressure measurement, should be performed, and a complete endocrine workup to assess hypercortisolism and pheochromocytoma is needed in every case. Additional testing for other differentials is recommended based on the clinical presentation.[2,11] If endocrine tests yield negative results, a diagnosis of a hormonally silent AT is made. In humans, 20-30% of adrenal incidentalomas may exhibit mild autonomous cortisol secretion without specific clinical signs of hypercortisolism. These patients may experience metabolic disturbances, including dyslipidemia, insulin resistance, arterial hypertension, hyperglycemia, and visceral fat accumulation. This condition has recently been termed "mild autonomous cortisol syndrome" (MACS)[11] and has not yet been identified in dogs.
The management of a hormonally silent AT depends on its etiology. A benign AT can be left untreated, while a malignant type requires timely intervention (Fig. 35.1).

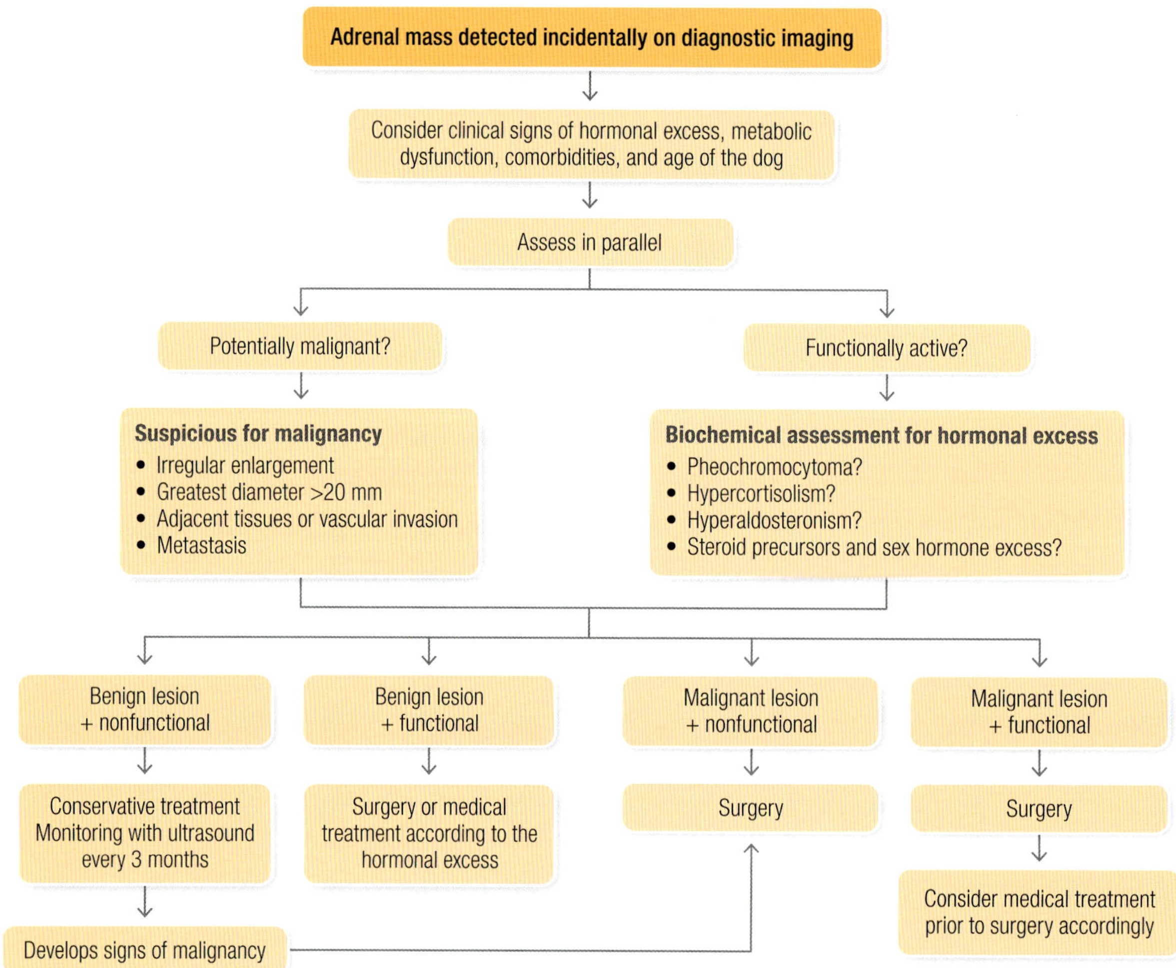

FIG. 35.1 Approach to an incidentally discovered adrenal mass.

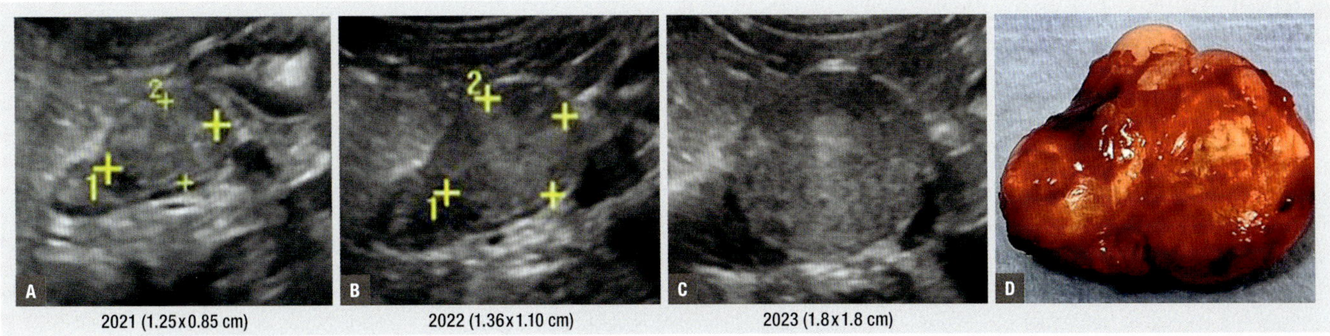

FIG. 35.2 Evolution of the left adrenocortical mass during a 3-year follow-up of a 12-year-old male Lhasa Apso. (**A-C**) Ultrasonographic images show a gradual increase in size. (**D**) The adrenal mass has been successfully removed, and histopathology revealed an adrenocortical carcinoma. Images courtesy of: (A,B,C) Dr. Mariangela Zanini and (D) Dr. Rodrigo Ubukata.

Fine-needle aspiration biopsy is not reliable in differentiating between malignant and benign adrenal mass, and the diagnostic imaging characteristics of the AT remain the most relevant aspects in treatment decision-making for hormonally silent AT.[2] A diameter exceeding 20 mm, irregular structure, invasive growth, and the presence of metastasis are indicative of malignancy. However, none of these characteristics, except metastasis, serves as a solitary predictor of malignancy. Even more, an adrenal mass with a diameter of less than 20 mm can still be malignant. Sometimes, even histopathology is inconclusive about malignancy.

A conservative approach is recommended for hormonally silent ATs that exhibit benign characteristics on diagnostic imaging. This typically involves regular rechecks of the AT size every 3 months (Fig. 35.2). If the disease remains stable, the interval between check-ins may be extended to 6 months. When the malignant nature of the AT is suspected, adrenalectomy is indicated.

As for now, there are no specific guidelines for peri- and postoperative management of hormonally silent ATs in dogs. Based on endocrine testing, patients with hormonally silent ATs may not require hormone supplementation postadrenalectomy. Hence, it is at the discretion of the veterinarian whether to administer preventive glucocorticoid supplementation during the perioperative period and to reduce the postoperative medication. The author's advice is to conduct an ACTH stimulation test after surgery to assess the need for glucocorticoid supplementation. If treatment with glucocorticoids is deemed necessary, a protocol for cortisol-secreting adrenocortical tumors can be applied (see chapter 34).

The prognosis of hormonally silent ATs remains largely unknown. However, insights have been gained from two retrospective studies. One such study evaluated 22 dogs with adrenal incidentalomas who underwent adrenalectomy. Among them, five dogs had biochemically undiagnosed pheochromocytoma. The remaining dogs had hormonally silent ATs, and histopathology disclosed adrenocortical carcinoma in ten dogs (one bilateral) and adrenocortical adenoma in seven dogs.[15] Another study describes the clinical features and survival of non-cortisol-secreting AT, presumably hormonally silent, as none of the dogs presented with clinical signs.[16] The median survival without surgery was found to be 17.8 months. Notably, dogs with large ATs and metastasis had a poorer prognosis, as expected.

Large case studies are needed to establish an evidence-based approach to hormonally silent ATs in both diagnosis and treatment. This can lead to the development of standardized diagnostic protocols, treatment guidelines, and prognostic indicators, ultimately improving the care and outcomes for dogs with these tumors.

KEY POINTS

- Canine adrenal tumors originate from the adrenal cortex or medulla and may be benign or malignant, functional or nonfunctional.
- Aldosterone-secreting adrenal tumors causing hyperaldosteronism are extremely rare in dogs.
- Adrenocortical tumors can also secrete excessive amounts of steroid precursors and sex hormones (alpha-hydroxyprogesterone, progesterone, estradiol, testosterone, androstenedione and dehydroepiandrosterone sulfate).
- Non-functional or hormonally silent AT are usually detected as an adrenal incidentaloma during diagnostic imaging in dogs when adrenal disease was not suspected.

References

1. Melian C. Investigation of adrenal masses. In Mooney CT, Peterson ME (editors). BSAVA Manual of Canine and Feline Endocrinology 4th edition. UK, British Small Animal Veterinary Association, 2012, pp. 272-277.
2. Behrend EN, Wasik B. Non-cortisol-secreting adrenocortical tumors. In Côté E, Ettinger SJ, Feldman EC (editors). Textbook of Veterinary Internal Medicine 9th edition. Philadelphia, Elsevier, 2024.
3. Rijnberk A, Kooistra HS, van Vonderen IK, Mol JA, Voorhout G, van Sluijs FJ, et al. Aldosteronoma in a dog with polyuria as the leading symptom. *Domest Anim Endocrinol* 20(3):227-240, 2001.
4. Johnson KD, Henry CJ, McCaw DL, Turnquist SE, Stoll MR, Kiupel M, et al. Primary hyperaldosteronism in a dog with concurrent lymphoma. *J Vet Med A Physiol Pathol Clin Med* 53(9):467-470, 2006.
5. Reine NJ, Hohenhaus AE, Peterson ME, Patnaik AK. Deoxycorticosterone-secreting adrenocortical carcinoma in a dog. *J Vet Intern Med* 13(4):386-390, 1999.
6. Behrend EN, Weigand CM, Whitley EM, Refsal KR, Young DW, Kemppainen RJ. Corticosterone- and aldosterone-secreting adrenocortical tumor in a dog. *J Am Vet Med Assoc* 226(10):1662-1666, 2005.
7. Machida T, Uchida E, Matsuda K, Hirayama K, Yoshii K, Takiguchi M, et al. Aldosterone-, corticosterone- and cortisol-secreting adrenocortical carcinoma in a dog: case report. *J Vet Med Sci* 70(3):317-320, 2008.
8. Syme HM, Scott-Moncrieff JC, Treadwell NG, Thompson MF, Snyder PW, White MR, et al. Hyperadrenocorticism associated with excessive sex hormone production by an adrenocortical tumor in two dogs. *J Am Vet Med Assoc* 219(12):1725-1728, 2001.
9. Norman EJ, Thompson H, Mooney CT. Dynamic adrenal function testing in eight dogs with hyperadrenocorticism associated with adrenocortical neoplasia. *Vet Rec* 144(20):551-554, 1999.
10. Ristic JM, Ramsey IK, Heath EM, Evans HJ, Herrtage ME. The use of 17-hydroxyprogesterone in the diagnosis of canine hyperadrenocorticism. *J Vet Intern Med* 16(4):433-439, 2002.
11. Fassnacht M, Tsagarakis S, Terzolo M, Tabarin A, Sahdev A, Newell-Price J, et al. European Society of Endocrinology clinical practice guidelines on the management of adrenal incidentalomas, in collaboration with the European Network for the Study of Adrenal Tumors. *Eur J Endocrinol* 189(1):G1-G42, 2023.
12. Baum JI, Boston SE, Case JB. Prevalence of adrenal gland masses as incidental findings during abdominal computed tomography in dogs: 270 cases (2013-2014). *J Am Vet Med Assoc* 249(10):1165-1169, 2016.
13. Cook AK, Spaulding KA, Edwards JF. Clinical findings in dogs with incidental adrenal gland lesions determined by ultrasonography: 151 cases (2007-2010). *J Am Vet Med Assoc* 244(10):1181-1185, 2014.
14. Arlt W, Biehl M, Taylor AE, Hahner S, Libé R, Hughes BA, et al. Urine steroid metabolomics as a biomarker tool for detecting malignancy in adrenal tumors. *J Clin Endocrinol Metab* 96(12):3775-3784, 2011.
15. Sant'Anna IM, Ubukata R, Kahvegian M, Galac S, De Marco V. Adrenal incidentaloma: clinical and histopathological characteristics. *J Vet Intern Med* 33(5):1841-2551, 2019.
16. Arenas C, Pérez-Alenza D, Melián C. Clinical features, outcome and prognostic factors in dogs diagnosed with non-cortisol-secreting adrenal tumours without adrenalectomy: 20 cases (1994-2009). *Vet Rec* 173(20):501, 2013.

CHAPTER 36

Pheochromocytoma

Marit F. van den Berg
DVM, DECVIM-CA
(Internal Medicine)

Etiology

Pheochromocytomas (PCCs) are neuroendocrine tumors that originate from the chromaffin cells of the adrenal medulla. According to the fifth series of the World Health Organization (WHO) classification of endocrine and neuroendocrine tumors, PCCs are part of the paraganglioma family of tumors that develop in sympathetic and parasympathetic paraganglia. A PCC is classified as an intra-adrenal sympathetic paraganglioma.[1] While the true prevalence of PCC in dogs remains unknown, it is estimated that PCCs account for approximately 0.01% to 0.1% of all canine tumors.[2] This estimation is likely underestimated as it is primarily based on autopsy findings rather than the more recently available biochemical diagnosis.

Genetics

In dogs with PCC, sequencing of succinate dehydrogenase subunits B and D (*SDHB* and *SDHD*) has revealed mutations in these genes that are likely pathogenic.[3,4] In people, mutations in one of the *SDH* genes are seen in approximately 20% of patients with PCCs and paragangliomas. Specifically, *SDHB* mutations have been identified as the strongest genetic risk factor for metastatic disease and contribute to radioresistance. Future studies are expected to offer further insights into the genetic background of PCCs in dogs.

Multiple endocrine neoplasia

In human medicine, multiple endocrine neoplasia (MEN) is characterized by the development of tumors within two or more endocrine glands and is classified into several types. MEN-2 is associated with mutations in the RET proto-oncogene and is characterized by medullary thyroid carcinoma, PCC, and primary hyperparathyroidism.[5] While concurrent endocrine neoplasms are relatively common in dogs, the combinations of these neoplasias differ from those observed in humans, and the genetic background is unknown. Therefore, the term "concurrent endocrine neoplasia" (CEN) has been introduced. The most common tumor combinations are those affecting the adrenal glands (PCCs, adrenocortical tumors) and the pituitary gland.[6,7] In addition, dogs with PCC can present with non-endocrine tumors, such as osteosarcoma and lymphoma.[7-9] This highlights the importance of a thorough evaluation for concurrent (endocrine) neoplasia in patients with a PCC.

Clinical features

PCCs occur mostly in middle-aged to older dogs (with a mean age that varies between 10.5 and 12 years) without a clear breed or sex predilection.[7-10] Clinical signs are related to excessive catecholamine secretion and, less commonly, to the space-occupying or invasive nature of the tumor.[2]

Hormone secretion from PCCs is highly variable, resulting in a wide variability in the severity and range of clinical symptoms. The symptoms may be constant or may occur occasionally due to the episodic secretion of catecholamines. Clinical manifestations are often nonspecific (e.g., lethargy, weight loss, hyporexia, weakness), but can also be related to the cardiorespiratory system (e.g., panting, tachycardia, arrhythmias, collapse) or the neuromuscular system (e.g., seizures, muscle tremors).[2,7,8] Seizures may arise from various factors, including hypertensive encephalopathy, catecholamine-induced vasospasms, or the presence of brain metastasis. Miscellaneous clinical signs include polyuria/polydipsia, abdominal pain, vomiting, and diarrhea.[2,7-11] Polyuria/polydipsia can be attributed to catecholamine-induced effects, resulting in a secondary decrease in the release and activity of antidiuretic hormone, or they may stem from primary polydipsia associated with abdominal mass effect or abdominal pain.[2] Nausea and vomiting can result from catecholamine-induced effects involving the activation of α-adrenergic receptors in the chemoreceptor trigger zone, while diarrhea can be catecholamine- or hypertension-induced.

Hypertension, one of the key features in humans with PCCs, is present in approximately 50% of affected dogs at the time of investigation.[7-9]

Dogs with "clinically silent" PCCs are reported to exhibit no symptoms associated with catecholamine excess. Nevertheless, in many cases, patients might show subtle

TABLE 36.1 Most common clinical signs and physical examination findings derived from four larger case series of dogs with PCC.[8-11]

Clinical signs and physical examination findings	Percentage of dogs
Lethargy/weakness/depression	32%
Vomiting	28%
Polyuria/polydipsia	25%
Abdominal pain	22%
Panting/tachypnea/dyspnea	22%
Anorexia/hyporexia	21%
Collapse/weakness	21%
Palpable abdominal mass	17%
Weight loss	15%
Cardiac arrhythmias	14%
Pale mucous membranes	10%
Abdominal distension (ascites/hemoperitoneum)	10%
Diarrhea	7%
Seizures	5%

Asymptomatic dogs were excluded. The provided percentages should be regarded as approximate numbers due to differences in history-taking and physical examination protocols, which were not standardized across the studies. In addition, it is worth noting that concurrent disease was present in some dogs and could have contributed to the observed clinical signs.

or nonspecific signs that clinicians could easily overlook, particularly in the case of comorbidities.
PCCs often invade surrounding structures, especially the caudal vena cava. This can result in occlusion of the caudal vena cava, which may cause ascites and hind limb edema.[2,8] Spontaneous tumor rupture with intra-abdominal or retroperitoneal hemorrhage has been described in a small number of dogs with PCC.[9] Table 36.1 shows the most common clinical signs in dogs with PCC.

Clinicopathological findings

There are no consistent abnormalities in routine clinicopathological tests that are specific for canine PCC. In some dogs, the routine bloodwork can be completely normal.[2,10] Most reported hematological findings include anemia and leukocytosis or stress leucogram. Both thrombocytopenia and thrombocytosis are reported, with the latter being associated with chronically bleeding tumors.[2,7,8]
Among serum biochemical abnormalities, an increase in liver enzymes is the most common, occurring in about 70% of afflicted dogs in one study.[7] Hypertension-induced hepatopathy could be an explanation, although concurrent disease is likely contributing (as 20% of these dogs were diagnosed with concurrent hypercortisolism).[7] Additional reported biochemical abnormalities include azotemia, hypercholesterolemia, hypoalbuminemia, hyperphosphatemia, hyperglycemia, hypokalemia, and hyponatremia.[7,8] Hypercholesterolemia may occur due to catecholamine-induced lipolysis and conversion of excess mobilized fatty acids to cholesterol in the liver or may be associated with concurrent disease.[2,8]

Proteinuria, hematuria, and low urine specific gravity are the most consistent abnormalities on urinalysis and may be caused by hypertension-induced glomerular damage and polyuria/polydipsia.[2,8]

Diagnostic imaging

Abdominal ultrasonography

Abdominal ultrasonography is the primary method for evaluating PCC in dogs due to its widespread availability and noninvasive nature, eliminating the need for anesthesia. It is not uncommon for PCC to be diagnosed when an incidental adrenal mass is detected during abdominal ultrasonography for an unrelated problem.
Pheochromocytomas may present as rounded masses with irregular or well-defined margins or as solitary or multiple adrenal nodules.[12,13] The majority of PCCs in dogs are unilateral, while approximately 10% are bilateral. Tumor size is highly variable, ranging from 2 mm to 16 cm in diameter.[2,9,12] The echogenicity of canine PCC exhibits significant variability; hypoechoic, isoechoic, or hyperechoic patterns may be seen, and echogenicity may be heterogeneous or homogenous.[7,12,13] Mixed patterns with anechoic areas may represent foci of necrosis and hemorrhage.[12,13] During ultrasonography, it is important to assess for local invasion into surrounding structures and the presence of metastasis. Vascular invasion into the phrenicoabdominal vein and the caudal vena cava is described in up to 82% of dogs with PCC (Figs. 36.1 and 36.2).[9,14-16] It is probable that the lumen of the phrenicoabdominal vein overlying the affected adrenal gland is infiltrated and that a so-called tumor thrombus subsequently extends into the caudal vena cava without involvement of the caval wall.[16] There might be an association between tumor size and thrombosis, although this needs further investigation in a larger number of dogs.
Because canine PCCs do not exhibit a characteristic sonographic appearance, other adrenal masses, specifically cortisol-secreting adrenocortical tumors, remain an important differential diagnosis. Definitive differentiation between adrenal masses is not possible by ultrasonographic criteria alone.

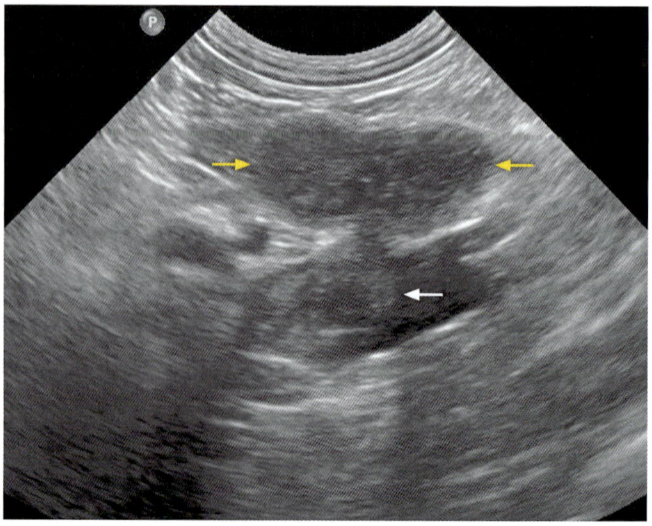

FIG. 36.1 Long-axis ultrasonographic image of a PCC of the left adrenal gland (yellow arrows) with vascular invasion (white arrow) of the caudal vena cava.

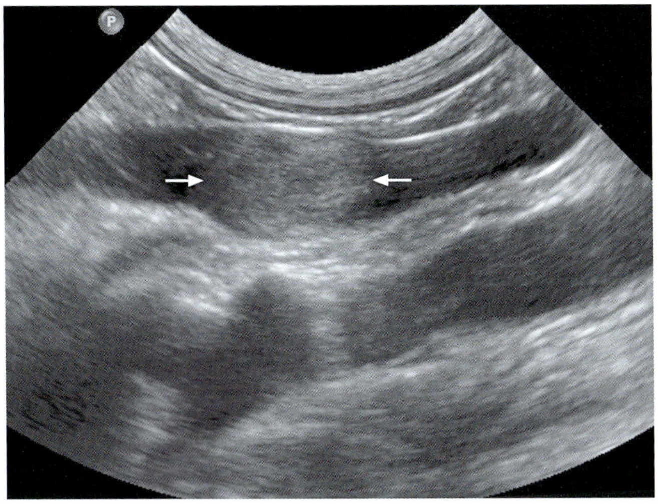

FIG. 36.2 Ultrasonographic image of vascular invasion of the caudal vena cava of the same patient as in Fig. 36.1. The tumor thrombus (arrows) almost completely occludes the caudal vena cava lumen.

Contrast-enhanced ultrasound (CEUS) has gained in popularity in veterinary medicine, and recent studies suggest that this technique can be utilized for distinguishing between adrenocortical tumors and PCCs.[17,18] Characteristic CEUS findings of PCC include a shorter mean transit time and a rapid wash-in and wash-out.[17,18]

Computed tomography

Computed tomography (CT) is highly recommended for surgical planning as it enables accurate assessment of the size, shape, and architecture of the tumor, is superior to ultrasound to detect vascular invasion, and is more sensitive for the detection of pulmonary metastasis compared to thoracic radiographs.[2,16,19] On CT, PCCs present as soft tissue masses in the mid-dorsal abdomen and can demonstrate irregular margins and heterogeneous contrast enhancement (Figs. 36.3 and 36.4).[19]

Efforts have been made to distinguish between adrenocortical tumors and PCCs based on CT criteria. Although not helpful in guiding diagnosis on an individual basis, PCCs have higher precontrast attenuation values, are rarely mineralized, are more often associated with vascular invasion, and demonstrate longer tumor thrombi compared to adrenocortical carcinomas.[19,20]

Nuclear imaging

Functional imaging with ^{123}I-metaiodobenzylguanidine (MIBG) has been used once to successfully image a PCC in a dog.[21] In addition, PET imaging using ^{18}F-PFBG has been described in two dogs with PCC.[22] An increasing amount of literature consistently shows that (68Ga)-DOTATATE PET/CT outperforms other functional imaging techniques in the detection of PCCs.[23] While studies in dogs are currently lacking, this technique holds great diagnostic potential.

Diagnosis

Overview

The diagnosis of PCC is based on clinical suspicion, diagnostic imaging, and biochemical testing. The final confirmation is made by histopathology. Biochemical testing involves the measurement of catecholamines (norepinephrine and epinephrine) or catecholamine metabolites, of which normetanephrine and metanephrine (together referred to as "metanephrines") are the major metabolites.

Biochemical testing

Catecholamine synthesis and metabolism

Catecholamines are synthesized from tyrosine, which is converted to L-dihydroxyphenylalanine (L-DOPA) by the enzyme tyrosine hydroxylase. This conversion is the rate-limiting step in catecholamine synthesis.[24] The formed L-DOPA is converted to dopamine by L-aromatic amino-acid decarboxylase, which is translocated into storage vesicles. Here, dopamine-β-hydroxylase is responsible for the intravesicular conversion

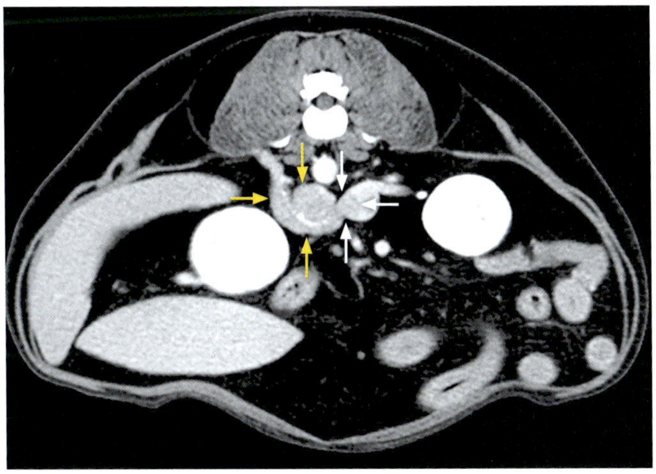

FIG. 36.3 Transverse post-contrast CT image in soft tissue window at the level of the mid-abdomen. The left adrenal gland is markedly enlarged and demonstrates heterogeneous contrast enhancement (yellow arrows). A well-defined filling defect in the caudal vena cava is observed due to the presence of a tumor thrombus (white arrows).

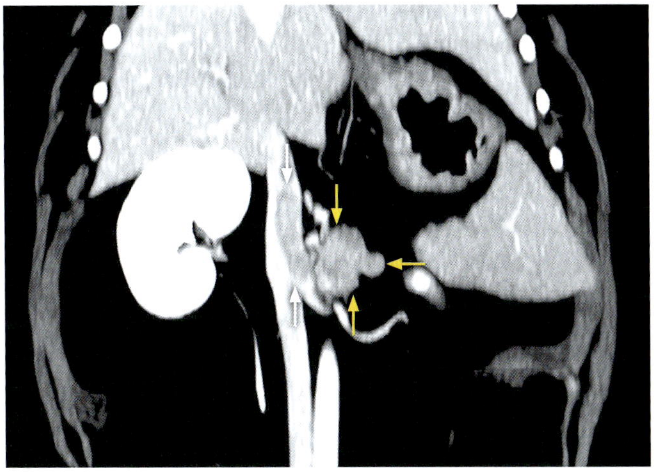

FIG. 36.4 Dorsal reconstruction of the post-contrast CT study of the PCC shown in Fig. 36.3. The yellow arrows point to the tumor, and the white arrows show the vascular invasion into the caudal vena cava.

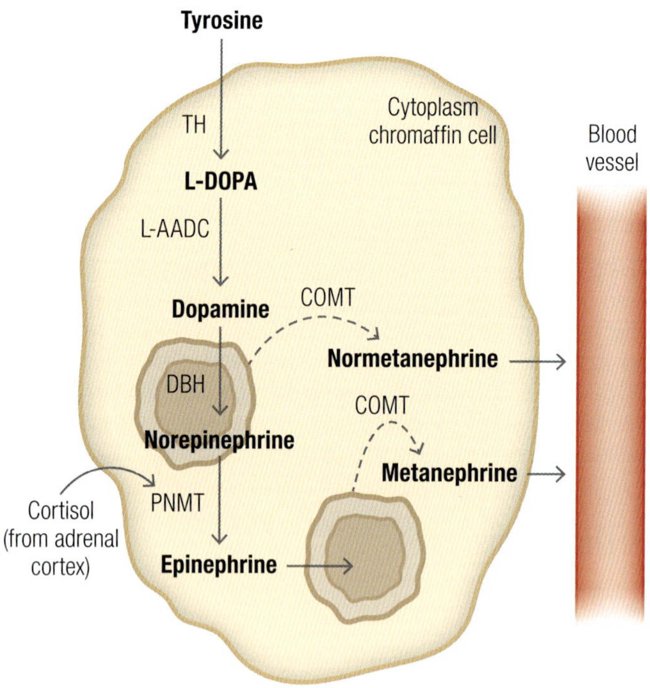

FIG. 36.5 Schematic illustration of the biosynthesis and metabolism of catecholamines within adrenal medullary chromaffin cells. COMT, catechol-O-methyltransferase; DBH, dopamine-β-hydroxylase; L-AADC, L-aromatic amino-acid decarboxylase; PNMT, phenylethanolamine-N-methyltransferase; TH, tyrosine hydroxylase.

of dopamine to norepinephrine. In adrenal medullary chromaffin cells, norepinephrine is released from the vesicles into the cytoplasm, where the enzyme phenylethanolamine-N-methyltransferase (PNMT) further converts it into epinephrine. Epinephrine is then transported into another storage vesicle (Fig. 36.5). Upon sympathetic stimulation, catecholamines are secreted into the circulation from their storage vesicles by exocytosis. The expression of PNMT is dependent on glucocorticoids, and it is primarily found in the adrenal medulla. Therefore, the vast majority of circulating epinephrine is derived from the adrenal medulla.[24]
Within adrenal medullary chromaffin cells, there is a continuous leakage of norepinephrine and epinephrine from their storage vesicles into the cytoplasm, where they are metabolized to normetanephrine and metanephrine by the enzyme catechol-O-methyltransferase (COMT), and subsequently released into the circulation (Fig. 36.5).[24] This contrasts with the release of catecholamines, which is usually highly variable and episodic. Due to the absence of the enzyme COMT in sympathetic nerves, the O-methylated metabolites demonstrate higher specificity for chromaffin cells and PCCs compared to their parent catecholamines or any other catecholamine metabolites.

Biochemical diagnosis of PCC

Biochemical testing is essential for the diagnosis of PCC. In dogs, it has only been conducted for the past 10-15 years and includes evaluation of plasma and urinary catecholamines and metanephrines, as well as urinary vanillylmandelic acid (VMA).[25-28] Measurement of metanephrines in plasma or urine is superior to catecholamines,[25] and measurement of normetanephrine has better diagnostic performance than measurement of metanephrine, both in plasma and urine.[25,26,28] For this reason, to date, the measurement of plasma or urinary normetanephrine is considered the best diagnostic method to investigate canine PCC. In view of diagnostic accuracy, there is currently no consensus on whether to use plasma or urine for metanephrine measurements.[25]
The primary techniques for measuring catecholamine metabolites are high-pressure liquid chromatography with electrochemical detection and liquid chromatography-tandem mass spectrometry (LC-MS/MS). Currently, LC-MS/MS is the preferred method due to its cost-effectiveness and high throughput, precise and accurate measurement of metanephrines.[24]
Traditionally, it was recommended to stabilize urinary metanephrines by acidification of urine, but it has been shown that acidification is not required for adequate measurement of urinary metanephrines.[26] Determination of urinary VMA has the advantage of wide availability, although the reported sensitivity and specificity are lower compared to plasma metanephrines, and urinary acidification is necessary.[27,28]
Reference intervals for plasma, urinary, and salivary-free metanephrines and 3-methoxytyramine (3MT) in healthy dogs have been recently established.[28] Measuring 3MT, the metabolite of dopamine, can aid in detecting primarily dopamine-secreting PCCs and has been reported to be associated with metastatic potential and genetics of PCC in people.[29] Although the diagnostic performance of salivary metanephrines and 3MT has not been evaluated in dogs, the availability of dog-specific reference intervals facilitates further research in this area.
Some medications, notably α-blockers, β-blockers (e.g., atenolol), calcium channel blockers (e.g., amlodipine), metoclopramide, and sympathomimetics (e.g., ephedrine, phenylpropanolamine), may influence catecholamine and metabolite measurements, potentially leading to false-positive test results.[24] However, their impact on catecholamines and metanephrines in dogs has not been studied. Phenoxybenzamine, a nonselective α-blocker used in preoperative medical management of PCCs, is a well-known cause of false-positive results for plasma normetanephrine. Consequently, biochemical testing for PCC should be performed prior to the start of this drug.

Fine-needle aspiration (FNA) of the adrenal glands

Two studies have evaluated the safety of percutaneous ultrasound-guided FNAs of adrenal lesions.[30,31] In a study involving 10 dogs with PCC, ventricular tachycardia developed in one dog, but this dog was also diagnosed with pericardial effusion.[30] In another study involving 50 dogs

Video 36.1

CT of invasive pheochromocytoma. Video of transverse post-contrast CT images of a large, invasive pheochromocytoma. The right adrenal gland is severely enlarged and demonstrates heterogeneous contrast enhancement with irregular and ill-defined margins, especially at the level of the sublumbar musculature and major vessels.

Video 36.2

CT of pheochromocytoma with caudal vena cava invasion. Video of transverse post-contrast CT images of a pheochromocytoma of the right adrenal gland. A large filling defect in the caudal vena cava is observed due to the presence of a tumor thrombus.

with adrenal lesions, complications were reported in four dogs (three hemorrhages and one death due to acute respiratory distress syndrome, possibly related to a concurrent laryngeal paralysis).[31] The diagnostic accuracy of FNAs for differentiation between PCCs and adrenocortical tumors ranges from 87-100%.[31,32] In human medicine, biopsy by FNA or core needle biopsy of PCCs is contraindicated because it can result in serious complications (such as hematoma, severe pain, or severe hypertension) and increased operative difficulty.[33] While FNAs can be valuable for the diagnosis of PCC, the decision to perform FNAs should be made on a case-by-case basis, taking into account the potential benefits and risks.

Histopathology

The definitive diagnosis of PCC is based on histopathology and immunohistochemistry (IHC). Histologically, PCCs are characterized by neoplastic cells arranged in a nest pattern separated by fibrovascular septa. Differentiation between adrenocortical and adrenomedullary origin may be challenging, and IHC using several neuroendocrine markers, including synaptophysin and chromogranin A, is used to support the diagnosis of PCC (Fig. 36.6).[2,11]

The WHO no longer classifies PCCs as either benign or malignant, as any lesion can exhibit metastatic potential, and there are no definitive features that can predict metastatic behavior.[1] A histopathological scoring system used in humans to predict metastatic behavior, the Pheochromocytoma of the Adrenal gland Scaled Score (PASS), and several IHC markers were evaluated in dogs with PCC in relation to surgical outcome and were found to be unable to differentiate between dogs that survived to discharge and dogs that died following adrenalectomy.[34] However, no studies have evaluated the association between these scoring systems and long-term survival in dogs so far.

Therapy

Adrenalectomy

Adrenalectomy is the treatment of choice for dogs with PCC but may be prevented by extensive local invasion, concurrent disorders, or distant metastasis. Undergoing adrenalectomy may still be an option for patients with vascular invasion since several studies reported that tumor invasion into the vena cava does not affect perioperative mortality.[14,16,35] However, extensive vascular invasion, particularly tumor thrombi extending cranial to the liver, may be associated with higher perioperative mortality.[15]

Resection of PCCs can be performed laparoscopically or by an open laparotomy. The choice of an open versus a laparoscopic approach depends on tumor size, the presence of vascular invasion, and the surgeon's experience.[36] Regardless of vascular invasion, long-term survival is common in dogs surviving the perioperative period.[9,15,35] Reported survival rates at 1, 2, and 3 years are 83%, 60%, and 60%, respectively.[15] In a study assessing long-term outcomes of 53 dogs that underwent adrenalectomy for pheochromocytoma, a median survival time of 1,150 days was reached.[9] A favorable outcome relies on a skilled surgeon, an experienced anesthesia team, and diligent postoperative care.[11]

Preoperative medical management

Intraoperative tumor manipulation can cause cardiovascular instability due to episodic hypersecretion of catecholamines, which can result in life-threatening complications such as cardiac arrhythmias and hypertensive crisis.[2] Preoperative medical management aims to prevent these complications by blocking the α-adrenergic response to circulating epinephrine and norepinephrine. Phenoxybenzamine, an irreversible antagonist of α-adrenergic receptors that binds to both α-1 and α-2 adrenergic receptors, is most often used.

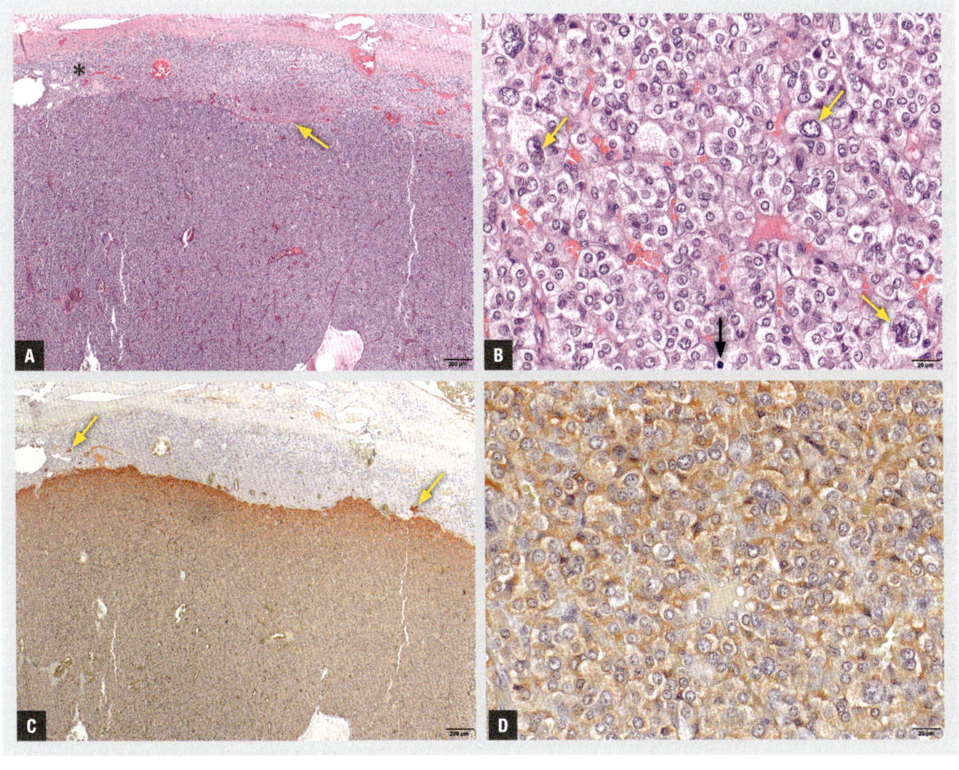

FIG. 36.6 Histology of a PCC of a dog. The neoplasm is separated from the compressed adrenal cortex (asterisk) by a thin fibrous capsule (arrow). (A) Hematoxylin and eosin stain, 4× objective). The neoplastic cells are arranged in sheets and lobules with several cells that contain a large pleomorphic nucleus (arrows) and a mitotic figure (black arrow). (B) Hematoxylin and eosin stain, 40× objective). Tumor cells show marked to moderate immunoreactivity with a few small positive cell clusters within the preexisting adrenal cortex (arrows). (C) Chromogranin A immunohistochemistry, 4× objective). The immunoreactivity is finely granular and cytoplasmic. (D) Chromogranin A immunohistochemistry, 40× objective). (Courtesy of Dr. Guy Grinwis, Department of Biomolecular Health Sciences, Faculty of Veterinary Medicine, Utrecht University, Utrecht, The Netherlands).

In a study involving 48 dogs undergoing adrenalectomy for PCC, perioperative mortality was significantly lower in dogs receiving pretreatment with phenoxybenzamine compared to untreated dogs (13 versus 48%, respectively), although there were no differences in perioperative blood pressure characteristics between the two groups.[14] In contrast, pretreatment with an α-blocker was not correlated with survival in another study involving 53 dogs with PCC.[9] A separate study involving 13 dogs undergoing adrenalectomy for PCC revealed a low mortality rate and minimal perioperative complications despite the absence of prior α-blocker therapy.[10] Randomized controlled clinical trials are warranted to evaluate whether preoperative α-blockade is necessary. Currently, preoperative α-blockade is still recommended at the author's institution (see the protocol below on "medical treatment"). Clinicians should be aware that intraoperative cardiovascular instability can occur despite optimal blockade, emphasizing the importance of an experienced surgical and anesthesia team.

Medical treatment

In cases where surgery is not deemed feasible or is hindered by financial or other constraints of the owner, medical treatment with phenoxybenzamine is indicated to control the clinical signs of catecholamine excess and hypertension. The starting dose of pheonoxybenzamine is 0.25 mg/kg PO q12h. In the case of hypertension, the dose is gradually increased every 2-3 days until blood pressure is effectively controlled. A maximal dose of phenoxybenzamine is approximately 1 mg/kg PO q12h.[2] Before each dose escalation, blood pressure should be monitored. If hypotension is detected, the dose should be reduced back to the last dose the patient was receiving. No studies have investigated the impact of phenoxybenzamine treatment alone on survival.

The use of the tyrosine kinase inhibitor (TKI) toceranib phosphate has been described in a retrospective series of 5 dogs with metastatic, recurrent, or inoperable PCC, showing partial response in one dog and stable disease in four dogs for a period of 11 to 61 weeks.[37] While the information on TKIs is limited in dogs with PCC, several TKIs are currently under evaluation in phase II clinical trials in humans with PCCs. The most significant benefits may be observed in patients with mutations in the *SDH* family or RET proto-oncogene.[38]

At present, no other tumor-targeted drugs are available for dogs with PCC. Dopamine receptor D2 (*DRD2*) antagonists are being evaluated in phase II clinical trials in human patients with metastatic PCC and paraganglioma. In dogs, RNA sequencing revealed overexpression of DRD2, making it a promising therapeutic target.[39]

Treatment with ^{131}I-MIBG has been reported in one dog and resulted in clinically stable disease for 4 months.[21]

Radiation therapy

A recent study evaluated the use of stereotactic body radiation therapy for the treatment of PCC in 8 dogs, which resulted in a favorable outcome with complete resolution of clinical signs in all dogs and, based on tumor size, complete remission in 2/8 dogs and partial remission in 2/8 dogs.[40]

Prognosis

Several factors, such as tumor size, the endocrine activity of the tumor, the extent of vascular invasion, and the presence of metastasis, influence the prognosis of PCC. Dogs that undergo adrenalectomy and survive the perioperative period can live for several years.

KEY POINTS

- Pheochromocytoma is a catecholamine-secreting adrenal tumor.
- The diagnosis is based on clinical suspicion, biochemical testing, diagnostic imaging, and histopathological confirmation.
- Biochemical testing primarily relies on measurements of plasma or urinary metanephrines, which are produced continuously within tumor cells, independent of tumoral catecholamine secretion.
- Measurement of normetanephrine is superior to metanephrine, both in plasma and urine.
- The treatment of choice is adrenalectomy, but a favorable outcome relies on an experienced surgical and anesthesia team and intensive postoperative care.
- Vascular invasion into the phrenicoabdominal vein and the caudal vena cava is frequently observed but does not necessarily preclude surgery.
- Randomized controlled clinical trials are warranted to evaluate whether preoperative medical management with α-blockers (e.g., phenoxybenzamine) is necessary.
- Current medical treatment options include tyrosine kinase inhibitors, but there is an urgent need to identify additional novel therapeutics.

References

1. Mete O, Asa SL, Gill AJ, et al. Overview of the 2022 WHO Classification of paragangliomas and pheochromocytomas. *Endocrine Pathol* 33:90-114, 2022. doi:10.1007/s12022-022-09704-6.
2. Reusch CE. 2015. Pheochromocytoma and multiple endocrine neoplasia. In Feldman E, Nelson R, Reusch C, Scott-Moncrieff J, Behrend E (editors). Canine and Feline Endocrinology 4th edition. St. Louis, Elsevier, 2015, pp. 521-554.
3. Holt DE, Henthorn P, Howell VM, et al. Succinate dehydrogenase subunit D and succinate dehydrogenase subunit B mutation analysis in canine phaeochromocytoma and paraganglioma. *J Comp Pathol* 151(1):25-34, 2014. doi:10.1016/j.jcpa.2014.03.007.
4. Korpershoek E, Dieduksman DAER, Grinwis GCM, et al. Molecular alterations in dog pheochromocytomas and paragangliomas. *Cancers (Basel)* 11(5), 2019. doi:10.3390/cancers11050607.
5. Moline J, Eng C. Multiple endocrine neoplasia type 2: an overview. *Genet Med* 13:755-764, 2011. doi:10.1097/GIM.0b013e318216cc6d.
6. Beatrice L, Boretti FS, Sieber-Ruckstuhl NS, et al. Concurrent endocrine neoplasias in dogs and cats: a retrospective study (2004-2014). *Vet Rec* 182(11):323, 2018. doi:10.1136/vr.104199.
7. Barthez PY, Marks SL, Woo J, et al. Pheochromocytoma in dogs: 61 cases (1984-1995). *J Vet Intern Med* 11(5):272-278, 1997. doi:10.1111/j.1939-1676.1997.tb00464.x
8. Gilson SD, Withrow SJ, Wheeler SL, et al. Pheochromocytoma in 50 dogs. *J Vet Intern Med* 8(3):228-232, 1994. doi:10.1111/j.1939-1676.1994.tb03222.x.
9. Enright D, Dickerson VM, Grimes JA, et al. Short- and long-term survival after adrenalectomy in 53 dogs with pheochromocytomas with or without alpha-blocker therapy. *Vet Surg* 51(3):438-446, 2022. doi:10.1111/vsu.13771.
10. Appelgrein C, Hosgood G, Drynan E, et al. Short-term outcome of adrenalectomy in dogs with adrenal gland tumours that did not receive pre-operative medical management. *Aust Vet J* 98(9):449-454, 2020. doi:10.1111/avj.12991.
11. Galac S, Korpershoek E. Pheochromocytomas and paragangliomas in humans and dogs. *Vet Comp Oncol* 15:1158-1170, 2017. doi:10.1111/vco.12291.
12. Besso JG, Penninck DG, Gliatto JM. Retrospective ultrasonographic evaluation of adrenal lesions in 26 dogs. *Vet Radiol Ultrasound* 38(6):448-455, 1997. doi:10.1111/j.1740-8261.1997.tb00870.x.
13. Pagani E, Tursi M, Lorenzi C, et al. Ultrasonographic features of adrenal gland lesions in dogs can aid in diagnosis. *BMC Vet Res* 12(1):267, 2016. doi:10.1186/s12917-016-0895-1.
14. Herrera MA, Mehl ML, Kass PH, et al. Predictive factors and the effect of phenoxybenzamine on outcome in dogs undergoing adrenalectomy for pheochromocytoma. *J Vet Intern Med* 22(6):1333-1339, 2008. doi:10.1111/j.1939-1676.2008.0182.x.
15. Barrera JS, Bernard F, Ehrhart EJ, et al. Evaluation of risk factors for outcome associated with adrenal gland tumors with or without invasion of the caudal vena cava and treated via adrenalectomy in dogs. *J Am Vet Med Assoc* 1715-1721, 2013. doi:10.2460/javma.242.12.1715.
16. Kyles AE, Feldman EC, De Cock HE, et al. Surgical management of adrenal gland tumors with and without associated tumor thrombi in dogs–40 cases (1994-2001). *J Am Vet Med Assoc* 654-662, 2003. doi:10.2460/javma.2003.223.654.
17. Nagumo T, Ishigaki K, Yoshida O, et al. Utility of contrast-enhanced ultrasound in differential diagnosis of adrenal tumors in dogs. *J Vet Med Sci* 82(11):1594-1601, 2020. doi:10.1292/jvms.20-0427.
18. Burti S, Zotti A, Rubini G, et al. Contrast-enhanced ultrasound features of adrenal lesions in dogs. *Vet Rec* 193(3):e2949, 2023. doi:10.1002/vetr.2949.
19. Gregori T, Mantis P, Benigni L, et al. Comparison of computed tomographic and pathologic findings in 17 dogs with primary adrenal neoplasia. *Vet Radiol Ultrasound* 56(2):153-159, 2015. doi:10.1111/vru.12209.
20. Pey P, Specchi S, Rossi F, et al. Prediction of vascular invasion using a 7-point scale computed tomography grading system in adrenal tumors in dogs. *J Vet Intern Med* 36(2):713-725, 2022. doi:10.1111/jvim.16371.
21. Bommarito DA, Lattimer JC, Selting KA, et al. Treatment of a malignant pheochromocytoma in a dog using 131I metaiodobenzylguanidine. *J Am Anim Hosp Assoc* 47(6):e188-194, 2011. doi:10.5326/JAAHA-MS-5605.
22. Berry CR, DeGrado TR, Nutter F, et al. Imaging of pheochromocytoma in 2 dogs using p-[18F]fluorobenzylguanidine. *Vet Radiol Ultrasound* 43(2):183-186, 2002. doi:10.1111/j.1740-8261.2002.tb01667.x.
23. Patel D, Phay JE, Yen TWF, et al. Update on pheochromocytoma and paraganglioma from the SSO endocrine/head and neck disease-site work group. Part 1 of 2: Advances in pathogenesis and diagnosis of pheochromocytoma and paraganglioma. *Ann Surg Oncol* 27(5):1329-1337, 2020. doi:10.1245/s10434-020-08220-3.
24. Eisenhofer G, Pamporaki C, Lenders JWM. Biochemical assessment of pheochromocytoma and paraganglioma. *Endocrine Rev* 44(5):862-909, 2023. doi:10.1210/endrev/bnad011.
25. Salesov E, Boretti FS, Sieber-Ruckstuhl NS, et al. Urinary and plasma catecholamines and metanephrines in dogs with pheochromocytoma, hypercortisolism, nonadrenal disease and in healthy dogs. *J Vet Intern Med* 29(2):597-602, 2015. doi:10.1111/jvim.12569.
26. Sasaki N, Ikenaka Y, Inoue Y, et al. Urinary free metanephrines measurement in dogs with adrenal gland diseases using a new simple liquid chromatography tandem mass spectrometry method. *J Vet Med Sci* 83(4):648-655, 2021. doi:10.1292/jvms.20-0508.
27. Soler Arias EA, Trigo RH, Miceli DD, et al. Urinary vanillylmandelic acid:creatinine ratio in dogs with pheochromocytoma. *Domest Anim Endocrinol* 74:106559, 2021. doi:10.1016/j.domaniend.2020.106559.
28. van den Berg MF, Kooistra HS, Grinwis GCM, et al. Reference intervals for plasma, urinary, and salivary concentrations of free metanephrines in dogs: Relevance to the diagnosis of pheochromocytoma. *J Vet Intern Med* 37(1):173-183, 2023. doi:10.1111/jvim.16624.
29. Eisenhofer G, Lenders JWM, Siegert G, et al. Plasma methoxytyramine: A novel biomarker of metastatic pheochromocytoma and paraganglioma in relation to established risk factors of tumour size, location and SDHB mutation status. *European J Cancer* 48(11):1739-1749, 2012. doi:10.1016/j.ejca.2011.07.016.
30. Sumner JA, Lacorcia L, Rose AM, et al. Clinical safety of percutaneous ultrasound-guided fine-needle aspiration of adrenal gland lesions in 19 dogs. *J Small Anim Pract* 59(6):357-363, 2018. doi:10.1111/jsap.12829.
31. Pey P, Diana A, Rossi F, et al. Safety of percutaneous ultrasound-guided fine-needle aspiration of adrenal lesions in dogs: perception of the procedure by radiologists and presentation of 50 cases. *J Vet Intern Med* 34(2):626-635, 2020. doi:10.1111/jvim.15743.
32. Bertazzolo W, Didier M, Gelain ME, et al. Accuracy of cytology in distinguishing adrenocortical tumors from pheochromocytoma in companion animals. *Vet Clin Pathol* 43(3):453-459, 2014. doi:10.1111/jvim.15743.
33. Vanderveen KA, Thompson SM, Callstrom MR, et al. Biopsy of pheochromocytomas and paragangliomas: Potential for disaster. *Surgery* 146(6):1158-1166, 2009. doi:10.1016/j.surg.2009.09.013.
34. Zini E, Nolli S, Ferri F, et al. Pheochromocytoma in dogs undergoing adrenalectomy. *Vet Pathol* 56(3):358-368, 2019. doi:10.1177/0300985818819174.
35. Lang JM, Schertel E, Kennedy S, et al. Elective and emergency surgical management of adrenal gland tumors: 60 cases (1999-2006). *J Am Anim Hosp Assoc* 47(6):428-435, 2011. doi:10.5326/JAAHA-MS-5669.
36. van Bokhorst KL, Galac S, Kooistra HS, et al. Laparoscopic vs. open adrenalectomy: perioperative data and survival analysis in 70 dogs with an adrenal tumor. *Front Vet Sci* 10:1156801, 2023. doi:10.3389/fvets.2023.1156801.
37. Musser ML, Taikowski KL, Johannes CM, et al. Retrospective evaluation of toceranib phosphate (Palladia®) use in the treatment of inoperable, metastatic, or recurrent canine pheochromocytomas: 5

dogs (2014-2017). *BMC Vet Res* 14(1):272, 2018. doi:10.1186/s12917-018-1597-7.

38. Nölting S, Ullrich M, Pietzsch J, et al. Current management of pheochromocytoma/paraganglioma: A guide for the practicing clinician in the era of precision medicine. *Cancers (Basel)* 11(10):1505, 2019. doi:10.3390/cancers11101505.
39. van den Berg MF, Kooistra HS, Grinwis GCM, et al. Whole transcriptome analysis of canine pheochromocytoma and paraganglioma. *Front Vet Sci* 10:1155804, 2023. doi:10.3389/fvets.2023.1155804.
40. Linder T, Wakamatsu C, Jacovino J, et al. Stereotactic body radiation therapy as an alternative to adrenalectomy for the treatment of pheochromocytomas in 8 dogs. *Vet Comp Oncol* 21(1):45-53, 2023. doi:10.1111/vco.12859.

CHAPTER 37

Anatomy and physiology of the canine endocrine pancreas

Thomas A. Lutz
Prof. Dr. med. vet., PhD

Anatomy of the canine pancreas[1]

The pancreas develops from the endoderm of the foregut, and the endocrine and exocrine pancreas develop at the same time and from the same precursor cells.[1] In dogs, the pancreas is eventually divided into the right lobe, body, and left lobe. The right (duodenal) lobe extends along the duodenum, the left lobe extends from the body to the hilum of the spleen[1,2] (Fig. 37.1). Most endocrine cells will cluster in the islets of Langerhans[3] and in total only comprise approximately 1.5-2% of the pancreas. The pancreas receives its blood supply from the celiac and cranial mesenteric arteries, and venous blood drains into the hepatic portal vein. The pancreas receives sympathetic and parasympathetic innervation and is also supplied by sensory nerves. Sympathetic postganglionic neurons reside in the celiac and cranial mesenteric, and paravertebral ganglia. Parasympathetic innervation is received from neurons in the dorsal motor nucleus of the vagus. In addition to the classic adrenergic and cholinergic transmitters of the sympathetic and parasympathetic nervous systems, immunohistochemical studies have identified a large number of neuropeptides in intrapancreatic ganglia, e.g., cholecystokinin (CCK), neuropeptide Y (NPY), calcitonin gene-related peptide (CGRP) and substance P (SP). The exact role of these peptides in the physiological control of pancreatic hormone release and general homeostasis is unknown. Sensory neurons project to the dorsal root ganglia, mainly in the lower thoracic and upper lumbar regions.

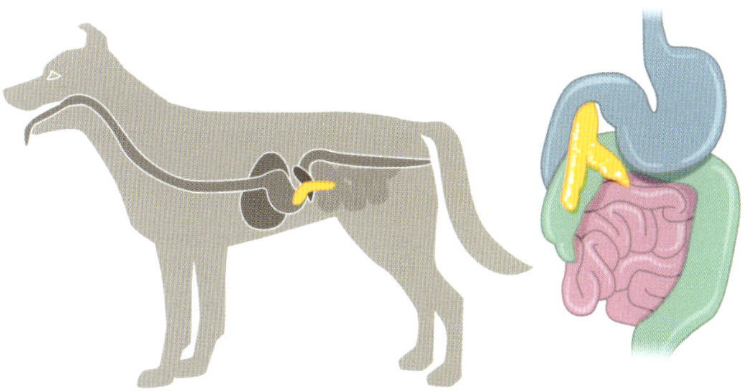

FIG. 37.1 The pancreas is located along the stomach and the proximal part of the small intestine.

Endocrine cell types

The endocrine tissue consists of the islets of Langerhans, but scattered endocrine cells can also be found across the exocrine tissue.[2] Islets are composed of several cell populations, most importantly the alpha- or A-cells that express the preproglucagon gene and that release glucagon and glucagon-like peptide-1 (GLP-1),[4-7] and the beta- or β-cells that express proinsulin and proamylin genes and that corelease insulin and amylin. Scattered islet cells express somatostatin (delta- or D-cells) and pancreatic polypeptide (PP- or F-cells) (Fig. 37.2). The non-beta-cells play an important role in the communication processes within the islets and, therefore, contribute to the well-controlled release of the respective hormones.[8] The localization of the different cell types within the islets differs across different species. In dogs, islets in the body and left lobe contain beta-cells that are distributed in all parts of the islets, with alpha-cells and fewer delta-cells being located in the periphery or scattered through the islets' center. Islets in the right lobe contain mainly beta-cells with few scattered delta-cells.[1] Overall, the volume of beta-cells in the right lobe seems to be lower than in the body and left lobe.[2]

Function of islet hormones

Insulin increases glucose uptake primarily in skeletal muscle and adipose tissue by the insulin-dependent glucose transporter GLUT4, which is translocated into the plasma membrane under the influence of insulin. Glucose uptake in other tissues (e.g., the liver [via GLUT2] or the central nervous system [via GLUT1 or GLUT3]) is insulin-independent. Insulin increases glycogen stores in the liver and skeletal muscle, promotes adipogenesis, and enhances protein storage in various tissues. Activation of lipoprotein lipase allows the uptake of fatty acids from the circulation, followed by the synthesis of triglycerides. Insulin also reduces lipolysis by inhibiting

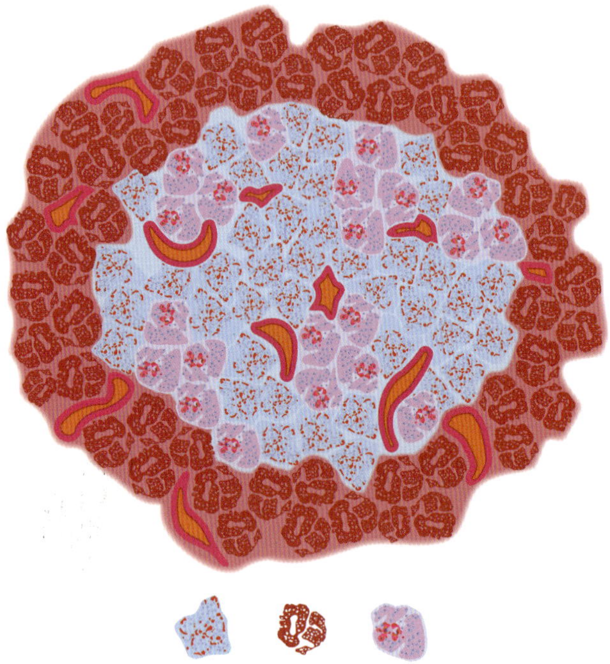

FIG. 37.2 The endocrine cells of the pancreas form the Langerhans islets. The three major cell types are A cells, which produce glucagon and GLP-1; β cells, which produce insulin and amylin; and D cells, which produce somatostatin.

hormone-sensitive lipase and, hence, the release of acetyl-CoA from adipose tissue. Because acetyl-CoA acts as an allosteric regulator of pyruvate carboxylase in the liver, the latter effect seems to be at least in part responsible for the reduction of hepatic gluconeogenesis by insulin.[9]

Part of the effect of insulin to reduce hepatic gluconeogenesis may also be mediated by insulin action in the brain and efferent signaling, possibly via the parasympathetic nervous system.[10,11] while the effects of insulin to increase hepatic glycogenesis seems to be direct via insulin receptors in hepatocytes.[9]

The second beta-cell hormone, amylin (also called islet amyloid polypeptide [IAPP]), complements insulin's action in nutrient metabolism by inhibiting gastric emptying and reducing pancreatic glucagon secretion.[12-15] Glucagon is considered the classical functional antagonist to insulin action. Glucagon action includes stimulating glycogenolysis, hepatic gluconeogenesis, lipolysis in adipose tissue, and amino acid release from skeletal muscle.[16]

GLP-1 is derived from the same preproglucagon gene as glucagon. GLP-1 is expressed in intestinal L-cells and the caudal hindbrain but also in pancreatic alpha-cells.[17] GLP-1's best studied metabolic actions are an incretin effect, i.e., it enhances glucose-stimulated insulin release, and an effect to enhance proliferation and reduce apoptosis of pancreatic beta-cells, but the physiological relevance of these effects in dogs has not yet been consistently confirmed.[18-20] GLP-1 also has beneficial effects on lipid and lipoprotein metabolism,[21,22] and GLP-1 reduces pancreatic glucagon release.

Somatostatin is synthesized in delta-cells, which make up about 5% of the total number of islet cells in dogs. Somatostatin's effect is mainly inhibitory, i.e., it inhibits insulin and glucagon secretion and, as such, probably contributes to the fine-tuning of glycemic control.[16] Because somatostatin analogs have been used in the treatment of neuroendocrine tumors, the relative affinity to somatostatin receptor subtypes and subsequent differential effects on pancreatic alpha- versus beta-cells may explain why some of these compounds lead to hyperglycemia.[23]

Secretory control of islet hormones

Direct control of hormone secretion

Insulin and glucagon release is, in part, directly mediated by the prevailing glucose concentration, but these effects are modulated by other factors, e.g., by incretin hormones, paracrine effects by other pancreatic hormones, or the autonomic nervous system. The release of insulin from beta-cells and glucagon from alpha-cells is a very well-coordinated phenomenon, i.e., the processes seem to be linked reciprocally even with small changes in the level of glycemia.[24] Similar to many peptide hormones, insulin secretion occurs in a pulsatile manner, and this release pattern seems to be important for full metabolic efficiency. The "pacemaker" for pulsatile release seems to reside within beta-cells, and its activity is, e.g., modulated by external stimuli like nutrient concentration or the autonomic nervous system.[25-27] Pulsatile insulin release seems to be disturbed in people with diabetes, but whether the same is true in diabetic dogs is currently unknown.

Glucagon release is triggered when glucose levels fall below a certain threshold, e.g., approximately 68 mg/dL (3.8 mmol/L) in dogs.[28] Interestingly, glucose entry into alpha-cells is insulin-dependent; hence, glucose sensing in alpha-cells is often disturbed in insulin-deficient states, which explains the prevailing hyperglucagonemia in most cases of diabetes mellitus. On the other hand, glucagon secretion is very sensitively inhibited by insulin, even in a state of (induced) slight hypoglycemia,[28] most likely at least in part by a direct effect of insulin in the islets.[29]

The mutual control of pancreatic hormone secretion is critical for fine-tuning metabolic control. Insulin, amylin, and GLP-1 all reduce alpha-cell secretion, but glucagon seems to stimulate insulin and amylin release. It is important to note that none of these effects have been specifically studied for their (patho)physiological relevance in dogs.

Central nervous system control of hormone secretion

Coordinated metabolic control of islets requires more than direct effects of nutrients on pancreatic endocrine cells; a major part of the control system is exerted by the autonomic nervous system.[30-32] Insulin and amylin release are triggered by the parasympathetic nervous system, and an increased sympathetic tone increases glucagon but inhibits insulin release.[33] When this coordinated reaction to metabolic challenges becomes dysfunctional, impaired central glucose sensing and, hence, disrupted feedback to the endocrine pancreas may be the reason for impaired glucose homeostasis in diabetes mellitus or defective counter-regulatory responses to hypoglycemia.

The central nervous system (CNS) is also responsible for part of the meal-induced coordinated releases of insulin, amylin, glucagon, and GLP-1. This meal-dependent stimulation may seem paradoxical, but glucagon, similar to amylin and GLP-1, is a classical satiation hormone.[7,34] So far, none of these hormones have been tested systematically for their eating inhibitory effect in dogs.

KEY POINTS

- The canine pancreas is divided into the right lobe, the body, and the left lobe.
- The endocrine pancreas is organized in the islets of Langerhans, where the alpha- or A-cells (which release glucagon and glucagon-like peptide-1) and the beta- or β-cells (which express proinsulin and proamylin genes and which corelease insulin and amylin) are present.
- Insulin increases glycogen stores in the liver and skeletal muscle, promotes adipogenesis, enhances protein storage in various tissues, and also reduces lipolysis by inhibiting hormone-sensitive lipase.
- Glucagon stimulates glycogenolysis, hepatic gluconeogenesis, lipolysis in adipose tissue, and amino acid release from skeletal muscle.
- Amylin induces satiation, inhibits glucagon release, and slows gastric emptying.

References

1. Tsuchitani M, Sato J, Kokoshima H. A comparison of the anatomical structure of the pancreas in experimental animals. *J Toxicol Pathol* 29(3):147-154, 2016.
2. Govendir M, Canfield PJ, Church DB. Morphometric study of the beta-cell volume of the canine pancreas with consideration of the axis of tissue transection. *Anat Histol Embryol* 28(5-6):351-354, 1999.
3. Dyce KM, Wensing CJG. The pancreas. Textbook of Veterinary Anatomy 4th edition. St. Louis, Saunders, 2010. pp. 139, 448.
4. Holst JJ, Holland W, Gromada J, Lee Y, Unger RH, Yan H, et al. Insulin and glucagon: partners for life. *Endocrinology* 158(4):696-701, 2017.
5. Unger RH, Dobbs RE, Orci L. Insulin, glucagon, and somatostatin secretion in the regulation of metabolism. *Annual Rev Physiol* 40:307-343, 1978.
6. Chambers AP, Sorrell JE, Haller A, Roelofs K, Hutch CR, Kim KS, et al. The role of pancreatic preproglucagon in glucose homeostasis in mice. *Cell Metab* 25(4):927-934.e3, 2017.
7. Woods SC, Lutz TA, Geary N, Langhans W. Pancreatic signals controlling food intake; insulin, glucagon and amylin. *Philos Trans R Soc Lond B Biol Sci* 361(1471):1219-1235, 2006.
8. Brereton MF, Vergari E, Zhang Q, Clark A. Alpha-, delta- and PP-cells: are they the architectural cornerstones of islet structure and co-ordination? *J Histochem Cytochem* 63(8):575-591, 2015.
9. Petersen MC, Vatner DF, Shulman GI. Regulation of hepatic glucose metabolism in health and disease. *Nat Rev Endocrinol* 13(10):572-587, 2017.
10. Schwartz MW, Seeley RJ, Tschop MH, Woods SC, Morton GJ, Myers MG, D'Alessio D. Cooperation between brain and islet in glucose homeostasis and diabetes. *Nature* 503(7474):59-66, 2013.
11. Bruning JC, Gautam D, Burks DJ, Gillette J, Schubert M, Orban PC, et al. Role of brain insulin receptor in control of body weight and reproduction. *Science* 289(5487):2122-2125, 2000.
12. Fineman M, Weyer C, Maggs DG, Strobel S, Kolterman OG. The human amylin analog, pramlintide, reduces postprandial hyperglucagonemia in patients with type 2 diabetes mellitus. *Horm Metab Res* 34(9):504-508, 2002.
13. Lutz TA. Control of energy homeostasis by amylin. *Cell Mol Life Sci* 69(12):1947-1965, 2012.
14. Weyer C, Maggs DG, Young AA, Kolterman OG. Amylin replacement with pramlintide as an adjunct to insulin therapy in type 1 and type 2 diabetes mellitus: a physiological approach toward improved metabolic control. *Curr Pharm Des* 7(14):1353-1373, 2001.
15. Young A. Inhibition of glucagon secretion. *Adv Pharmacol* 52:151-171, 2005.
16. Goff JP. The endocrine system. In Reece WO, Erickson HH, Goff JP, Uemura EE (editors). Dukes' Physiology of Domestic Animals 13th edition. Ames, Wiley & Sons, pp. 640-643, 2015.
17. Model JFA, Rocha DS, Fagundes ADC, Vinagre AS. Physiological and pharmacological actions of glucagon like peptide-1 (GLP-1) in domestic animals. *Vet Anim Sci* 16:100245, 2022.
18. Baggio LL, Drucker DJ. Biology of incretins: GLP-1 and GIP. *Gastroenterology* 132(6):2131-2157, 2007.
19. Drucker DJ. Glucagon-like peptides: regulators of cell proliferation, differentiation, and apoptosis. *Mol Endocrinol* 17(2):161-171, 2003.
20. Johnson KM, Farmer T, Schurr K, Patrick Donahue E, Farmer B, Neal D, Cherrington AD. Endogenously released GLP-1 is not sufficient to alter postprandial glucose regulation in the dog. *Endocrine* 39(3):229-234, 2011.
21. Farr S, Baker C, Naples M, Taher J, Iqbal J, Hussain M, Adeli K. Central nervous system regulation of intestinal lipoprotein metabolism by glucagon-like peptide-1 via a brain-gut axis. *Arterioscler Thromb Vasc Biol* 35(5):1092-100, 2015.
22. Lutz TA, Osto E. Glucagon-like peptide-1, glucagon-like peptide-2, and lipid metabolism. *Curr Opin Lipidol* 27(3):257-263, 2016.
23. Tarasco E, Seebeck P, Pfundstein S, Daly AF, Eugster PJ, Harris AG, et al. Effect of AP102, a subtype 2 and 5 specific somatostatin analog, on glucose metabolism in rats. *Endocrine* 58(1):124-133, 2017.
24. Flattem N, Igawa K, Shiota M, Emshwiller MG, Neal DW, Cherrington AD. Alpha- and beta-cell responses to small changes in plasma glucose in the conscious dog. *Diabetes* 50(2):367-375, 2001.
25. Juhl CB, Porksen N, Sturis J, Hansen AP, Veldhuis JD, Pincus S, et al. High-frequency oscillations in circulating amylin concentrations in healthy humans. *Am J Physiol Endocrinol Metab* 278(3):E484-490, 2000.
26. Matveyenko AV, Veldhuis JD, Butler PC. Measurement of pulsatile insulin secretion in the rat: direct sampling from the hepatic portal vein. *Am J Physiol Endocrinol Metab* 295(3):E569-574, 2008.
27. Polonsky KS, Given BD, Van CE. Twenty-four-hour profiles and pulsatile patterns of insulin secretion in normal and obese subjects. *J Clin Invest* 81(2):442-448, 1988.
28. Igawa K, Mugavero M, Shiota M, Neal DW, Cherrington AD. Insulin sensitively controls the glucagon response to mild hypoglycemia in the dog. *Diabetes* 51(10):3033-3042, 2002.
29. Gustavson SM, Nishizawa M, Farmer B, Neal D, Brissova M, Powers AC, Cherrington AD. A fall in portal vein insulin does not cause the alpha-cell response to mild, non-insulin-induced hypoglycemia in conscious dogs. *Metabolism* 52(11):1418-1425, 2003.
30. Furuzawa Y, Ohmori Y, Watanabe T. Immunohistochemical studies of neural elements in pancreatic islets of the cat. *J Vet Med Sci* 58(7):641-646, 1996.
31. Furuzawa Y, Ohmori Y, Watanabe T. Anatomical localization of sympathetic postganglionic and sensory neurons innervating the pancreas of the cat. *J Vet Med Sci* 58(3):243-248, 1996.
32. Chen XH, Itoh M, Sun W, Miki T, Takeuchi Y. Localization of sympathetic and parasympathetic neurons innervating pancreas and spleen in the cat. *J Auton Nerv Syst* 59(1-2):12-16, 1996.
33. Thorens B. Brain glucose sensing and neural regulation of insulin and glucagon secretion. *Diabetes Obes Metab* 13 Suppl 1:82-88, 2011.
34. Drucker DJ. Mechanisms of action and therapeutic application of glucagon-like peptide-1. *Cell Metab* 27(4):740-756, 2018.

CHAPTER 38

Diabetes mellitus

Lucy Davison
MA, VetMB, PhD, DSAM, DECVIM-CA (Internal Medicine), MRVCS

Federico Fracassi
DVM, PhD, DECVIM (SAIM)

Chen Gilor
DVM, PhD, DACVIM

Linda Fleeman
BVSc, PhD, MANZCVS

Charlotte Bjørnvad
DVM, PhD, DECVCN

Francesca Del Baldo
DVM, MRCVS, PhD, DECVIM-CA (Internal Medicine)

Diego Miceli
DVM, PhD

Álan G. Pöppl
DVM, MSc, DSc

Eleonora Malerba
DVM, PhD

Pathogenesis, clinical manifestations, and diagnosis

Lucy Davison

Diabetes mellitus (DM) is a condition of chronic hyperglycemia arising due to a relative or absolute deficiency of insulin. It is one of the most common canine endocrinopathies, affecting approximately 1 in 300 dogs.[1-3] In recent years, it has become clear that canine DM is a heterogeneous condition with many different pathophysiological routes to hyperglycemia.[4,5] In most dogs, insulin deficiency is caused by dysfunction or death of insulin-producing beta-cells in the pancreas. In some dogs, this may be preceded or accompanied by peripheral insulin resistance and/or exocrine pancreatic inflammation. Regardless of the route by which glucose homeostasis is disrupted, the resultant classical clinical signs of polyuria, polydipsia, polyphagia, and weight loss are the same. However, as practitioners develop a greater understanding of the spectrum of conditions covered by a diagnosis of diabetes mellitus, more precise and tailored treatment options are likely to become available. Delayed diagnosis and treatment will result in the progression of clinical signs to inappetence, nausea, collapse, coma, and death as the result of ketosis and, eventually, ketoacidosis.[6]

Pathogenesis

Several studies have attempted to examine the pathogenesis of canine diabetes in detail. The most recent attempt to define diagnostic criteria and a classification scheme for canine diabetes was undertaken by the European Society of Veterinary Endocrinology in cooperation with the Society of Comparative Endocrinology,[7] adapted from a human diabetes classification scheme.[7] A summary view of the classification scheme proposed by Project ALIVE is shown below (Table 38.1), but notably, this does not indicate the relative proportion of canine diabetes cases falling into each category, and in addition, current published evidence for diabetes caused by some of the mechanisms listed is scarce or absent.

In the healthy dog, the pancreatic beta-cells, contained within the pancreatic islets of Langerhans, produce insulin in direct response to an elevation in blood glucose. Insulin release is triggered when glucose enters the beta-cell, ATP is produced, and as a result, the ATP-sensitive potassium channel in the beta-cell membrane closes, leading to depolarization. This triggers the release of calcium from intracellular stores, which in turn triggers insulin release. Insulin acts in the peripheral tissues to enable glucose uptake into cells, but where there is insulin deficiency or resistance, glucose remains in the bloodstream, leading to hyperglycemia, whilst cells are starved of an important energy source.

Genetic susceptibility is suspected in dogs due to the consistently increased prevalence of diabetes mellitus in particular breeds, including the Samoyed, Tibetan Terrier, and West Highland White Terrier. Notably, some breeds are recognized to be at a much lower risk of diabetes, including the Boxer, German Shepherd dog, and Golden Retriever.[8] Juvenile onset diabetes at less than 6 months of age has also been reported in some breeds, including the Labrador Retriever and Keeshond,[9-11] but typically, diabetes onset in dogs is at age 7 years or older. Genetic studies suggest that the inheritance of canine diabetes is complex and likely to differ among breeds. The results of genetic studies to date implicate immune and inflammatory mechanisms, as well as increased susceptibility to stress-induced beta-cell death in disease pathogenesis.[12,13] However, similar to human diabetes, there are also likely to be environmental triggers in canine diabetes, and changes in such triggers may be a contributing factor in the rising incidence of diabetes in veterinary practice.

Histological examination of the canine diabetic pancreas is complicated by the fact that many studies have used postmortem tissue from long-standing diabetic cases, representing an end-stage of the disease.[14-16] Detail about the mechanisms involved in beta-cell death can only be observed in pancreas tissue from dogs euthanased around the time of diagnosis.

TABLE 38.1 Summary of proposed causes of canine diabetes mellitus disease complex – adapted from the classification proposed by the ALIVE project.[7]

Insulin-deficient diabetes mellitus (IDDM) (β-cell-related disorders)	Insulin-resistant diabetes mellitus (IRDM) (target organ disorders)
■ Reduced insulin secretion due to β-cell destruction ■ ß-cell loss associated with exocrine pancreatic disease* ■ Immune-mediated ■ Toxicity (e.g., diazoxide) ■ Infection ■ Idiopathic* ■ Reduced insulin secretion due to β-cell death (apoptosis) ■ Glucotoxicity* ■ Lipotoxicity* ■ Idiopathic* ■ Reduced insulin secretion due to β-cell aplasia/abiotrophy/hypoplasia ■ Production of defective insulin	■ Endocrine influence ■ Growth hormone (endogenous/exogenous) ■ Steroids (glucocorticoids/progestogens/other)* ■ Catecholamines ■ Thyroid hormone ■ Obesity ■ Drugs ■ Thiazide diuretics ■ Beta-adrenergic agonists ■ Inflammatory mediators ■ Disorders of receptor and intracellular signaling

*Conditions considered to be the most common are highlighted with an asterisk.

Typically the pancreas of the canine diabetic patient demonstrates extreme beta-cell deficiency, although a heterogeneous picture has been reported, with lymphocytic and/or neutrophilic inflammation around beta-cells being described, as well as fibrosis and exocrine pancreatic inflammation in some patients.

The islets containing the beta-cells are scattered throughout the exocrine tissue, which contains stores of digestive enzymes and makes up the majority of the pancreatic mass. The relationship between canine diabetes mellitus and acute or chronic exocrine pancreatitis is complex and likely to reflect both cause and consequence.[17] There are also diagnostic challenges associated with canine pancreatitis, particularly in the chronic form, which can be difficult to recognize clinically.[18] However, reduced beta-cell function has been demonstrated in dogs with confirmed chronic pancreatitis using insulin measurement following glucagon stimulation testing.[19] Therefore, exocrine pancreatic inflammation undoubtedly plays a role in beta-cell dysfunction and death in some canine diabetic cases, and these dogs are also at risk of developing exocrine pancreatic deficiency as a consequence of chronic inflammation and exocrine cell damage.

The hypothesis that canine diabetes results from autoimmune pancreatic beta-cell destruction, similar to type 1 diabetes in humans, has also been explored.[20] However, evidence for autoimmunity to beta-cell antigens such as GAD65, proinsulin, and IA-2 has only been documented in a small proportion of canine diabetic cases.[21,22] In addition, the lymphocytic infiltration of islets known as insulitis, which is present in most cases of human type 1 (autoimmune) diabetes, is not commonly observed in dogs. Taken together, these findings make an autoimmune pathogenesis unlikely in most canine diabetic patients.

More commonly, diabetes mellitus can develop in canine patients in the presence of hormones that antagonize insulin. Such hormones include progesterone, corticosteroids, and growth hormone. High levels of antagonistic hormones can result in hyperglycemia and diabetes, whether administered exogenously or present endogenously in a normal physiological state such as pregnancy or diestrus. A recent canine epidemiological study demonstrated that exposure to glucocorticoids is associated with a substantial increase in developing diabetes within the following 6 weeks, with diabetes associated with steroid use being more common in some breeds than others, such as the West Highland White Terrier and the Tibetan Terrier.[23] Potential endogenous hormonal triggers for canine diabetes include diestrus-related elevations in progesterone and growth hormone,[24] or elevations in corticosteroids due to pituitary or adrenal hypercortisolism.[25] Cases of diestrus and gestational diabetes are more common in countries where neutering of female dogs is performed less frequently.[26]

Epidemiological and physiological studies have demonstrated that obesity can also lead to insulin resistance in dogs,[27] and may play a role in diabetes risk, but the relationship is not as clear or consistent as the relationship between obesity and type 2 diabetes in humans.

Regardless of the underlying cause, prolonged insulin resistance or inflammation and hyperglycemia will usually result in canine beta-cell death. This means that even when a cause of insulin resistance or pancreatic inflammation is identified and managed in a newly diagnosed canine diabetic patient, it is unlikely that insulin-dependent diabetes will be reversible even when normoglycemia is restored. This is in marked contrast to cats and may reflect relatively increased beta-cell fragility in dogs. Figure 38.1 summarises several potential routes by which canine pancreatic beta cells may be dysfunctional or put under stress, which may contribute to beta-cell death and eventually result in a diagnosis of permanent insulin-dependent diabetes mellitus.

Clinical manifestations

Owners usually note excessive thirst and urination as the first signs of diabetes mellitus. Polyuria, with compensatory polydipsia, occurs secondary to the osmotic diuresis caused by glycosuria. Glycosuria results when blood glucose exceeds the renal threshold for reabsorption (220-270 mg/dL [12-15 mmol/L]).

In many cases, reduced energy availability to cells can also lead to weight loss, muscle loss, and lethargy. Lack of insulin can also have a negative central effect on satiety, resulting in polyphagia. If diabetes is complicated by or secondary to another condition, such as pancreatitis or hypercortisolism, clinical signs of those conditions may also complicate the clinical manifestation.

If left untreated, one form of metabolic compensation for lack of glucose transport into cells is the production of ketone bodies as an alternative energy source. Untreated or unstable treated diabetic dogs are therefore also at risk of ketosis, which results in a characteristic smell of acetone

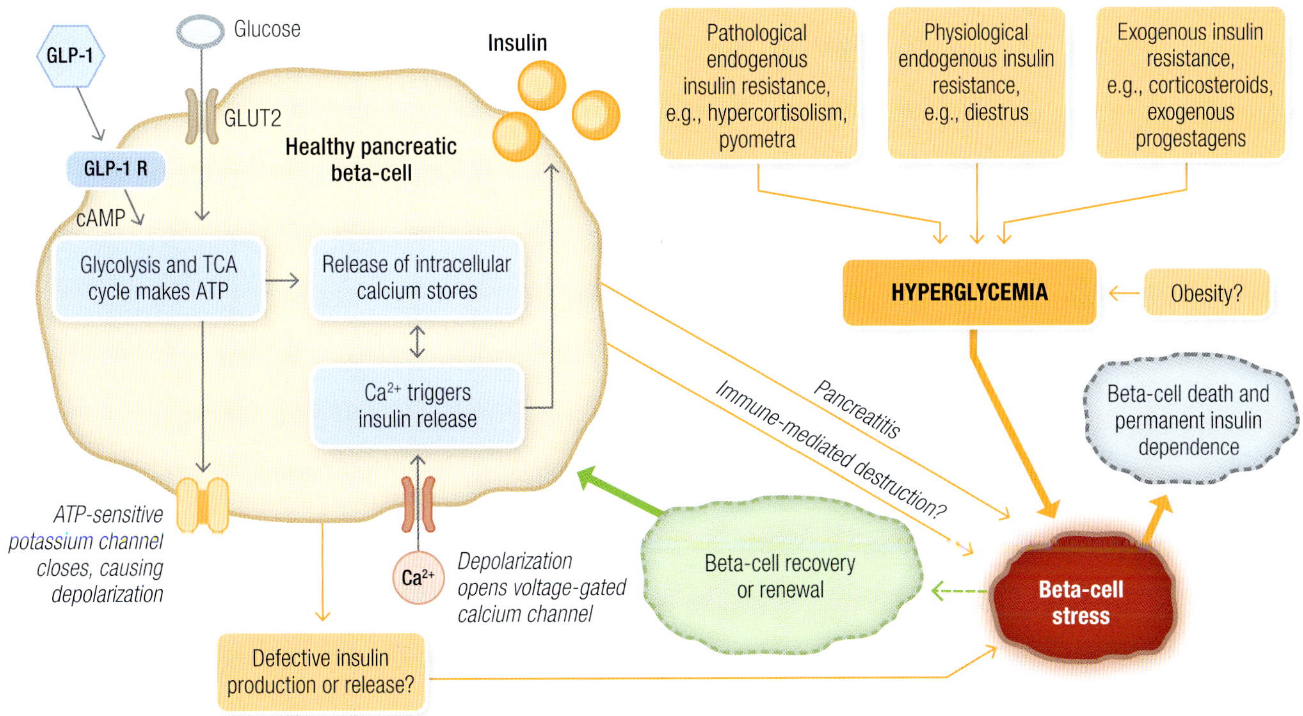

FIG. 38.1 Potential routes by which beta cell function may be disrupted or beta cells subjected to stress, eventually leading to canine diabetes mellitus. Adapted from O'Kell and Davison, VCNA, 2023.

on the breath. Ketosis can progress to ketoacidosis, which can cause vomiting, an elevated respiratory rate, severe dehydration, and collapse.[6] In epidemiological studies, variables associated with an increased hazard of death after diagnosis of diabetes included dogs that were ≥10 years of age at diagnosis, un-neutered, previously on glucocorticoids, or having had a blood glucose level >700 mg/dL (40 mmol/L) at diagnosis.[2] Un-neutered females are at particular risk of diabetes because of the progesterone-dominated phase of diestrus and the subsequent release of growth hormone from the mammary glands.[24] Here, the presentation may also be complicated by pyometra. Chronic hyperglycemia can also lead to the development of cataracts, which occasionally can develop very early in the course of the disease and, therefore, be present at the time of diagnosis.

Diagnosis

The agreed Project ALIVE definition of diabetes in dogs is a random (fasted or unfasted) blood glucose concentration (BGc) ≥200 mg/dL (≥11.1 mmol/L) with classic clinical signs of hyperglycemia (with no other plausible cause) or hyperglycemic crisis.[7] Where the diagnosis is uncertain, repeated blood glucose measurements to prove the persistence of blood glucose >126 mg/dL (7 mmol/L) over 24 hours and documentation of elevated glycated proteins in the blood can be used to confirm the diagnosis. Documentation of persistent glycosuria can also be supportive of a diagnosis but is not sufficient on its own to make the diagnosis of diabetes.

When measuring blood glucose in a veterinary patient, it is recommended to use a glucometer calibrated for veterinary species and a fresh sample. Stored samples, unless collected in a fluoride oxalate tube, will demonstrate a reduction in glucose concentration with time, as glucose is consumed by the erythrocytes.

The most commonly utilized glycated blood protein for confirmation of diagnosis is fructosamine, with an elevated serum fructosamine concentration demonstrating hyperglycemia for the previous 1-2 weeks.[28] However, care must be taken to use the same laboratory consistently for serial fructosamine measurements since reference ranges can vary considerably across different laboratories and assays. Glycosylated hemoglobin demonstrates average blood glucose over a longer period (approximately 2 months), but the assay is less widely available than fructosamine and may give a misleading result in a newly diagnosed patient that might only have been hyperglycemic for 2-3 weeks.[29]

When making a diagnosis of diabetes mellitus in a dog, several other tests should also be considered to establish the presence of underlying disease that may complicate future management so that a detailed and personalized treatment plan can be made. A characterization checklist (Table 38.2) has been proposed by the Project ALIVE group, although it must be noted that some methods of characterization, such as insulin C-peptide measurement and autoantibody measurement, are not currently commercially available.

Recommended diagnostic investigations for newly diagnosed canine diabetic patients include urinalysis and cytology, with culture if an inflammatory sediment, hematuria, or clinical suspicion of a urinary tract infection is present, since glycosuric patients are more susceptible to urinary tract infections. Similarly, evaluation of renal function and biochemical evidence of pancreatitis should also be considered, as the presence of chronic kidney disease or pancreatitis will make treatment more challenging. As well as management of pancreatitis with appropriate fluid,

TABLE 38.2 ALIVE diabetes characterization checklist for dogs.[7]

	Yes	No	Unknown
Female intact			
Pregnant			
Diestrus			
Onset of signs <12 months of age			
History of exogenous diabetogenic drug therapy			
Overweight/obese			
Underweight			
Current pancreatitis			
Historic pancreatitis			
Cushing's syndrome			
Exocrine pancreatic insufficiency			
Ketoacidosis			
Ketonuria			
Ketonemia			
Additional (unlisted above) comorbidity			
Additional research steps			
Insulin (or C-peptide) present at diagnosis			
Pancreatic autoantibody-positive			

analgesic, and antiemetic therapy, documentation of elevated pancreatic inflammatory markers in a diabetic patient should also prompt future measurement of trypsin-like immunoreactivity should signs of weight loss, ravenous appetite, and poor glycemic control persist. This is because diabetic patients with pancreatitis are also at risk of developing exocrine pancreatic insufficiency.

Most diabetic patients, particularly at the time of diagnosis, will demonstrate elevations in liver enzymes and cholesterol, but additional measurement of other blood lipids, such as triglycerides, should also be performed in high-risk breeds such as the Miniature Schnauzer and dogs where lipemia is very prominent.[30] Should there be suspicion of any other underlying conditions, including infection or neoplasia, hematology and diagnostic imaging (chest radiograph and abdominal ultrasound) should also be considered in the newly diagnosed patient.

If the dog is inappetant or lethargic, measurement of ketones should be performed, and ideally blood gases to assess pH. Ketone measurement in urine can be poorly sensitive, detecting only one form of ketone present in diabetic ketoacidosis (acetoacetate) but not beta-hydroxybutyrate. Therefore, where available, measurement of beta-hydroxybutyrate in blood is recommended.[6]

Management of any contributory conditions should be performed as promptly as possible, including neutering entire females as soon as they are considered stable for surgery.

Once insulin treatment has been instigated and intact female diabetic patients neutered, further consideration should also be given to the diagnosis and management of underlying conditions or risk factors such as hypercortisolism. However, diagnostic tests for other underlying endocrine conditions can yield false positive results if performed too close to the diagnosis of diabetes; therefore, at least 3 weeks of insulin therapy is recommended prior to endocrine tests such as ACTH stimulation test/low dose dexamethasone suppression test or measurement of serum T_4 and TSH.

A summary algorithm to assist with the diagnosis of canine diabetes mellitus is shown in Fig. 38.2.

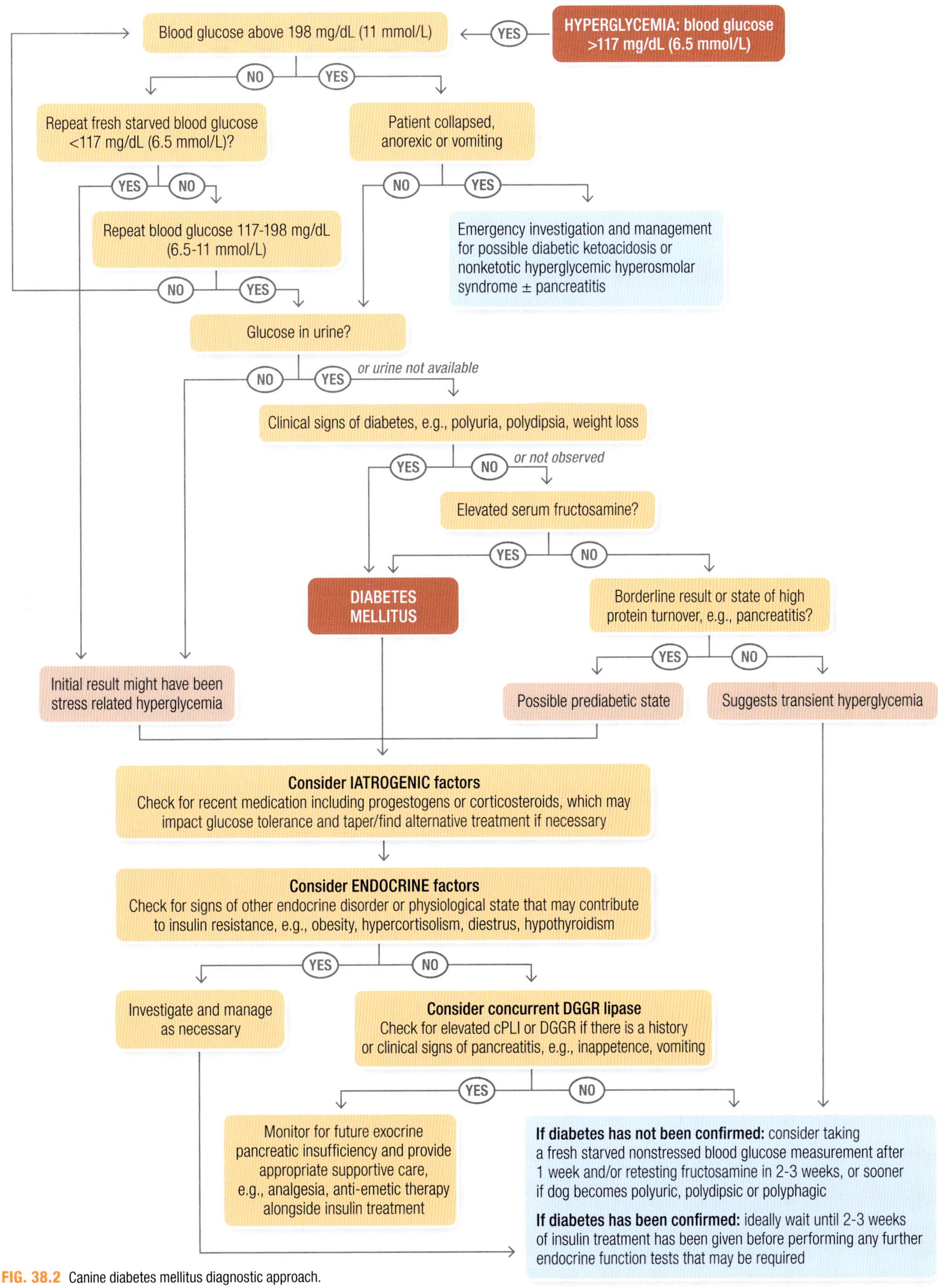

FIG. 38.2 Canine diabetes mellitus diagnostic approach.

General treatment considerations

Federico Fracassi

The importance of the owner and therapeutic goals

Successful treatment of DM in a dog requires excellent owner compliance and owner/veterinary team interaction. The "owner" may be one person or several, while the veterinary team involved in the long-term care of these dogs should include veterinarians, technicians, and non-technical personnel. The owner should be thoroughly educated regarding DM, how it is managed differently in dogs when compared with people, and the goals of therapy. The diagnosis of diabetes mellitus can have a significant negative impact on the dog's owner. The veterinarian must be able to communicate with the owner in the most appropriate way and should try to modify the therapeutic strategy as much as possible to achieve success as defined by the dog's owner. Open dialogue provides the best chance for owner compliance and will help avoid cessation of therapy or euthanasia. A survey involving 1192 veterinarians reported that a median of one in 10 pets with DM are euthanized at diagnosis; a further median of one in 10 within one year because of lack of success or compliance.[57] One study described the social and psychological impact of diabetes mellitus on the quality of life of both dogs and owners.[56] Aspects reported as most negatively impacting the owners' quality of life included: general worry about the disease, difficulties in leaving the dog with friends or family, worry about the dog's vision, boarding difficulties, worry about hypoglycemia, changed social and working life, costs related to the disease, worry about future care, and owners wanting more control of diabetes mellitus. Knowing these aspects can help veterinarians address their key issues and concerns to adapt a treatment and monitoring protocol specific to each owner. For example, one can introduce intensive glucose monitoring (i.e., the use of continuous glucose monitoring devices) for owners who want to have more control. On the other hand, the clinician should simplify treatment for owners worried about their social or working lives. Review expenses carefully for owners concerned about costs. Avoid tight glucose regulation if owners are worried about hypoglycemia. Establishing and agreeing on the definition of "successful management" is extremely important. For most veterinarians, their primary goal in the long-term management of DM should be to have the owner pleased with their dog's status. This is usually achieved if PU can be eliminated or significantly reduced, body weight is stable and acceptable, PP is tolerable, and the dog normally interacts with others at home. A more detailed definition of therapeutic objectives is presented in the "Insulin therapy and other treatment options" sub-chapter.

Initiating insulin therapy

Once diagnosed, treatment for DM should begin. Dogs in good condition and with an excellent appetite can be managed as "uncomplicated diabetics" even in the presence of ketonuria. The goals of therapy are to reduce or resolve clinical signs, prevent short-term complications (e.g., hypoglycemia, DKA), achieve the previously discussed areas of clinical improvement, and have a good quality of life. In DM dogs, this can be accomplished with exogenous insulin therapy, an appropriate diet, exercise, prevention or control of concurrent inflammatory, infectious, neoplastic or hormonal disorders, and avoidance of insulin-antagonistic drugs. Aiming for normal or near-normal blood glucose concentrations is not recommended, as it increases the risk of hypoglycemia, a common, serious, and potentially life-threatening complication. Hypoglycemia is usually the result of overzealous insulin therapy. Most diabetic dogs are described as well if their blood glucose is maintained between 80 to 250 mg/dL (4.4-13.9 mmol(L). However, the glycemic target can vary from dog to dog and depends on various factors (see "Insulin therapy and other treatment options" sub-chapter).

Owner education

Owners should be familiar with the clinical signs of DM. They should be aware of changes in water intake, urine output, appetite, and body weight. Poor appetite, vomiting, diarrhea, or unusual lethargy is always worrisome and worth veterinary consultation. It should be emphasized that consistency in the timing of injections, meals, type and amount of food, and exercise will make control of DM easier. Owners must learn the signs of hypoglycemia and DKA. Treatment should follow a precise and understandable protocol (see "Monitoring a diabetic patient" sub-chapter). While owners are the key to good DM control, decisions regarding insulin, dose and frequency of administration must always be made by the owner/veterinary team. Insulin should be stored in a refrigerator. Some insulin products must be mixed and this procedure should be done correctly. Some insulins should be shaken, some insulins do not require mixing, and some insulin products should be gently rolled. Owners must use appropriate syringes (40 U/mL for veterinary insulin products and 100 U/mL for most human insulin products), learn to eliminate air bubbles and administer the insulin SC over the lateral wall of the chest. The use of nonmatching syringes based on conversion tables for U40 and U100/mL, or the owner's own calculation, should be avoided as it can be confusing. Often, U40 insulin syringes have scales in both mL and Units; the owner must be instructed to use the unit scale. The injection technique should be demonstrated until the owner is familiar with it. If an insulin pen device is used for insulin administration, owners must be specifically trained with this tool (see "Insulin therapy and other treatment options" sub-chapter). Written instructions are useful. Owners of DM dogs should be encouraged to keep detailed records of their dogs' blood glucose, urine glucose, urine ketones, and any change in other parameters.

Dietary recommendations

Food given to DM dogs must be palatable to ensure regular consumption. Diets must be nutritionally complete and have day-to-day consistency with regard to composition, ingredients, and calories. These factors improve the chance for consistent insulin requirements and consistent response. Ideally, near-optimal body condition is achieved and maintained. A dog with DM may be overweight or underweight. In either, near-ideal weight is a reasonable goal. Insulin is an anabolic hormone, and insulin-treated diabetics gain weight easily. Since insulin is anabolic, having an obese dog with DM lose weight is far more difficult. Weight loss diets should be considered for obese DM dogs as they are typically rich in insoluble fiber, low in fat, and have decreased caloric density. Such diets should not be fed to underweight DM dogs.

Exercise

Consistent exercise can make the management of canine DM easier and should be encouraged. Physical activity decreases glucose concentrations by increasing the absorption of insulin from its injection site, increasing blood flow and insulin delivery to exercising muscles, stimulating translocation (i.e., upregulation) of glucose transporters (primarily GLUT-4) in muscle cells, and increasing glucose disposal despite basal insulin concentrations.[159,160] Strenuous and sporadic exercise can induce hypoglycemia and should be avoided. On the day a DM dog is expected to be involved in intense or unusual exercise (i.e., hunting), it is important to reduce that morning dose of insulin. The percent reduction necessary to prevent hypoglycemia is not predictable; thus, an initial reduction of 50% is reasonable. Further adjustments should be based on experience with issues like symptomatic hypoglycemia or PU during or after exercise. Owners of DM dogs should always have a glucose source readily available in case signs of hypoglycemia are observed while doing physical activity.

Insulin therapy and other treatment options

Chen Gilor, Linda Fleeman

Insulin therapy is required for the survival of most diabetic dogs, but it is associated with many inherent challenges that must be overcome for treatment to be safe, effective, and sustainable. These challenges arise from factors related to the complex nature of glycemic control, pharmacological limitations of available insulin formulations, and from life-long burden on nonprofessional caregivers. These issues have been significantly diminished in human medicine with the movement away from traditional insulin suspensions that require the use of syringes and needles multiple times a day and towards the use of recombinant insulin analogs, novel application methods such as injection pens and insulin pumps, and continuous glucose monitoring systems.

Goals of therapy for the individual patient

Clinical decisions regarding treatment strategies should align with goals for the individual diabetic dog and its owner. The factors that influence those decisions are outlined in Fig. 38.3. Current criteria developed by international consensus for treatment goals for diabetic animals are provided in Table 38.3. The clinical decisions on treatment and monitoring methods must also take into account potential long-term attrition in client and pet compliance. What seems like an ideal treatment and monitoring scheme in the short term might backfire in the long run if owners have maximized their financial capabilities, especially when concurrent diseases develop. In that respect, minimalist treatment and monitoring approaches might be better in the long run.

Avoidance of hypoglycemia

Avoidance of insulin-induced hypoglycemia is an important treatment goal, although the worry about potential hypoglycemia can often have a greater negative impact on the owner's quality of life than any occurrences of clinical hypoglycemia. Fortunately, episodes of hypoglycemia are rarely fatal in dogs and usually do not result in brain damage.[33] Because of continuous glucose monitoring, hypoglycemic events with insulin treatment are now known to be more common than previously realized, and most are subclinical. Dogs usually recover to normal after clinical hypoglycemia, although transient or permanent brain damage can result from severe episodes, and there is low risk of death due to misadventure or brain damage. Of note, there are currently no guidelines in veterinary medicine regarding acceptable levels of hypoglycemia (both in terms of absolute concentrations or duration) and how they translate to low interstitial glucose.

In people, hyperglycemia, hypoglycemia, and increased glycemic variability, together and separately, are risk factors for clinical hypoglycemia.[34] It is unknown whether or not that is also the case in dogs. In healthy animals, hypoglycemia initially causes an autonomic nervous system response, which may manifest as tremors, anxiety, panting, or hunger. If

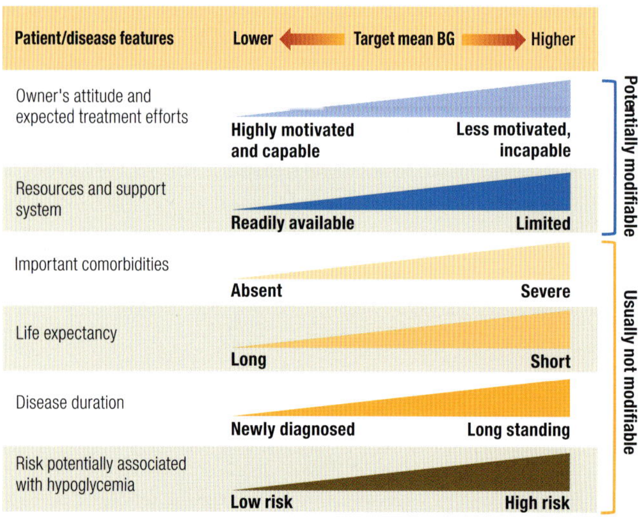

FIG. 38.3 Factors that influence clinical decisions regarding glycemic targets when treating diabetic dogs and cats.[31]

TABLE 38.3 ALIVE* criteria for treatment goals for diabetes mellitus in dogs and cats.

The ALIVE* consensus recommends the following goals to be considered:

- Good quality of life for pets and owners.
- Resolution of the classic clinical signs of diabetes mellitus.
- Avoidance of hypoglycemia and DKA.
- Normalization of body condition score.

The physiological mechanisms through which these aims are achieved include:

- Decreasing hepatic glucose output.
- Improving insulin sensitivity.
- Ensuring appropriate insulin availability.
- Reducing postprandial hyperglycemia.
- Attending underlying causes or comorbidities.

The success of the therapy can be assessed through:

- Systematic and standardized assessment of classic clinical signs of diabetes mellitus ideally incorporating a scoring system.
- Assessment of glycemic parameters in blood, interstitium, and/or urine.
- There is no prospective high-level evidence that setting a specific glycemic goal is correlated with a specific treatment outcome, including remission.
- Glycemic parameters within the reference interval of nondiabetic animals commonly indicates diabetic remission or insulin overdosing and, therefore, implies possibility of episodes of hypoglycemia in a treated diabetic patient.

The ALIVE consensus emphasizes the need for appreciation that:

- Serial glucose assessment shows substantial day-to-day variation.
- Fructosamine evaluation suffers from reliability problems and the use of the same validated assay in the same patient is recommended if this parameter is chosen to be used.
- Negative urine glucose can indicate periods of hypoglycemia in a treated diabetic patient.
- Comorbidities are common and should especially be considered when there are clinical signs which are not classic clinical signs of diabetes mellitus.
- Specific blood glucose targets are not a goal.

* Project ALIVE (Agreeing Language In Veterinary Endocrinology) was founded by the European Society of Veterinary Endocrinology in 2016 and endorsed by the Society for Comparative Endocrinology in 2017, and focuses on creating agreement over the definition of common terminology in veterinary endocrinology.

hypoglycemia persists, neuroglycopenic signs develop. Individuals experiencing hypoglycemia, even if episodes do not cause clinical signs, might lose their "protective" autonomic response (hypoglycemic unawareness), and neuroglycopenic signs may then develop quickly without warning. Multiple well-established mechanisms that explain this phenomenon have been described in people and rodents, with some recent, though still scarce, evidence in dogs.[35,36]

Avoidance of diabetic ketoacidosis and other complications

For most diabetic dogs, the insulin dose required to avoid diabetic ketoacidosis (DKA) is substantially lower than the insulin dose required to control clinical signs (e.g., 25% of the "optimal" dose). Therefore, the goal of fine-tuning of insulin therapy is not to avoid DKA but to control clinical signs.

It is currently unknown if the risk of diabetic cataract formation in dogs is proportional to the level of hyperglycemia, related to a certain threshold of hyperglycemia, glycemic variability, or other factors. Therefore, although it is likely that cataract formation is associated with hyperglycemia, it cannot be assumed that the risk of cataract formation is reduced by lower glycemic targets and the corresponding increased risk of hypoglycemia.

In summary, glycemic targets are not absolute but rather are tailored to the patient, taking into account the disease, comorbidities, monitoring method, compliance, etc.

Choosing the best insulin

Insulin formulations vary in their average time-action profile, day-to-day variability, cost, method of administration, and more. There are currently two "veterinary" insulin formulations labeled for use in dogs, but more than a dozen other "human" formulations are available on the market. Some of these "human" formulations are routinely used in dogs. A smart choice between insulin formulations would depend on interdependent factors that differ between patients and between different times for the same patient:

- Disease pathophysiology (including concurrent diseases).
- Insulin-related factors (including insulin pharmacology, cost, regional prescribing regulations).
- Pet and owner compliance.
- Diet (composition and frequency).
- Monitoring strategy.
- Goals of therapy for the specific patient (taking into account hypoglycemic risk) (Fig. 38.4).

Therefore, no insulin formulation should be considered "best" by default. Rather, it is more appropriate to seek the "best fit" insulin choice tailored to the specific clinical situation. Often, opposing needs will result in compromise.

Caveat to insulin pharmacology

In this chapter, pharmacodynamic parameters, such as duration of action and time to peak action, will be presented when data from glucose clamps are available. These pharmacodynamic data will be supplemented with pharmacokinetic data when available. Otherwise, when only data from serial blood glucose curves are available, the effect of insulin will be described in more vague terms describing its perceived appropriateness

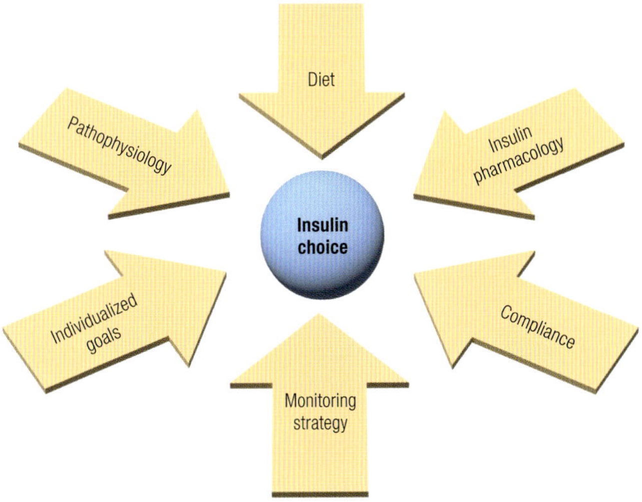

FIG. 38.4 Factors influencing insulin choice: the choice between insulin formulations depends on interdependent factors that will differ between patients and between different times for the same patient.[31]

for clinical use, such as recommended frequency of administration. The common terminology that assigns duration of action ("short-", "intermediate-", and "long-acting") will be used for convenience, considering the above caveat. In addition, it is important to note that this terminology is problematic because, for most insulin formulations, the duration of action can be extended to some degree by increasing the insulin dose (Fig. 38.5).[33] The unique pharmacodynamic characteristics of all of the commercial formulations described in this chapter are only relevant to SC injections. When administered intravenously, dilution in the blood leads to immediate dissociation of insulin hexamers, resulting in the same ultrarapid action as intravenously administered regular insulin.

The ultimate goal of insulin therapy: mimic physiologic insulin delivery

Endogenous insulin secretion can be divided into two phases: the "basal" phase, in which insulin is secreted continuously at a relatively constant rate throughout the day, and the "bolus" phase, in which insulin is secreted in response to nutrients digested and absorbed from the gut. Basal insulin secretion changes over time in response to changes in insulin sensitivity; it increases when insulin resistance develops (e.g., with obesity or other diseases) and decreases when insulin sensitivity increases (e.g., with exercise). "Bolus" insulin secretion is largely determined by factors such as the carbohydrate, fat, and protein contents of the meal, gastrointestinal transit time, and the effects of incretin hormones. In people, the "bolus" phase usually lasts only 2-4 hours with five-fold increases from baseline in insulin peak concentrations. In healthy dogs, the "bolus" phase also varies significantly in shape and magnitude with diet. Although insulin also increases within minutes after feeding and often peaks within 30 minutes at five to seven times the baseline concentration, it can remain increased for 6-9 hours in dogs, depending on the diet (Table 38.4).[36-38] Most people with type 1 diabetes are treated with a combination of a "basal" insulin (typically long-acting with a flat time-action profile and administered once

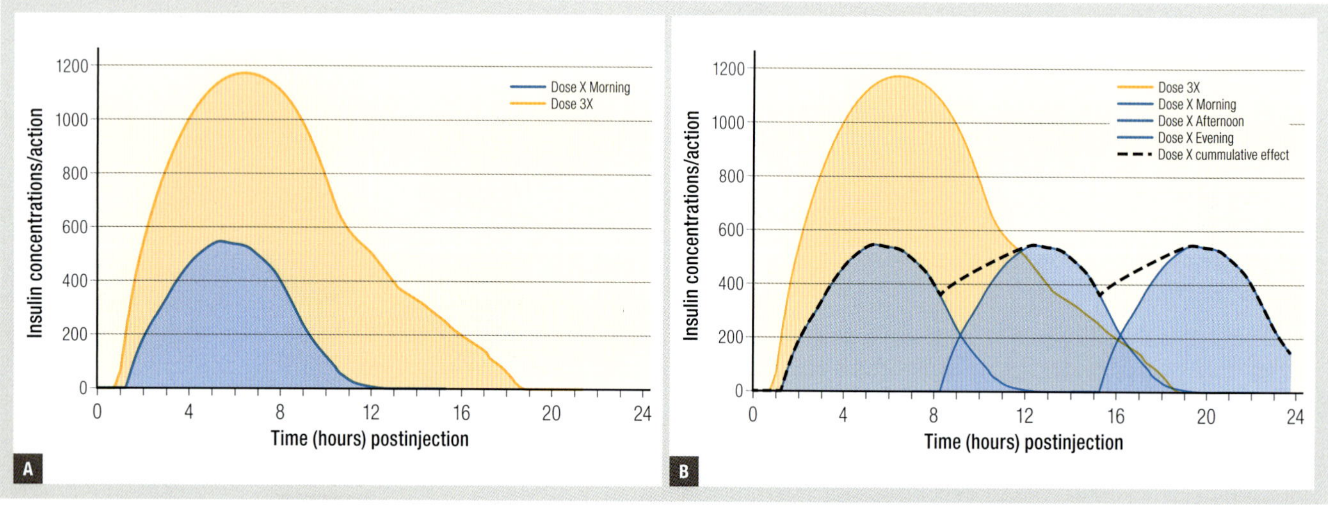

FIG. 38.5 Effects of changing the dose and frequency of administration of an "intermediate-acting" insulin: (A) A three-fold dose increase of a typical "intermediate-acting" insulin formulation nearly doubles the duration of action but also doubles peak action and increases the risk of hypoglycemia. (B) Decreasing the dose and tripling the frequency of administration decreases the risk of hypoglycemia and achieves lesser intraday variation.

daily) and a "bolus" insulin (typically rapid and short-acting and administered at the time of the meals, with the number of injections depending on the number of meals) (Fig. 38.6). The dose of "basal" insulin is dependent on the interaction between residual beta-cell function and background insulin resistance. The dose of "bolus" insulin is based on the premeal interstitial or blood glucose concentration, the carbohydrate content of the meal, and anticipated physical activity. The delivery of a "basal-bolus" pattern can be achieved with subcutaneous insulin injections or by using an insulin pump that is programmed to deliver insulin at variable rates. Insulin pumps are widely used in human medicine, but their cost and other practical considerations limit their use in pets.

TABLE 38.4 Comparison of "bolus" insulin secretion in humans, dogs, and cats.

	Duration of "bolus" insulin secretion	Magnitude of increase of "bolus" insulin secretion
Human	2-4 hours	5-fold
Dog	6-9 hours	5-7-fold
Cat	6->12 hours	0-3-fold

Note that this is a rough guide only as there is large individual variability depending on meal composition, quantity consumed, and frequency of feeding.[39]

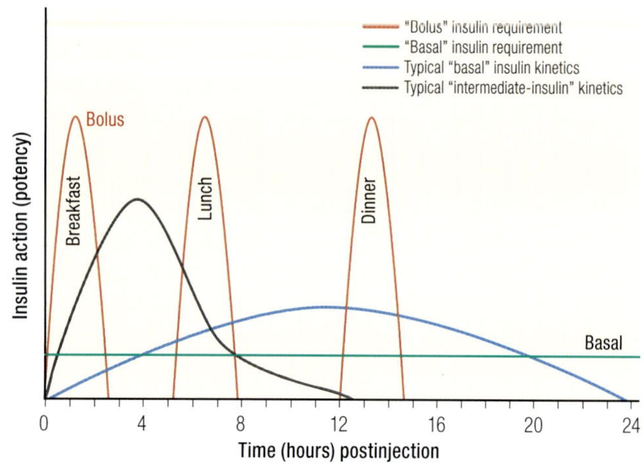

FIG. 38.6 Combination of "basal-bolus" insulin therapy.[31]

A basal-bolus perspective for insulin treatment in dogs

Ideally, insulin therapy in most diabetic dogs should mimic a "basal-bolus" pattern (Fig. 38.6),[39] although this will not always be a practical option because of cost and the need for multiple injections daily. The alternative is one of two compromises:

- Choose either a "basal" or a "bolus" insulin.
- Choose an "intermediate-acting" formulation that has a duration long enough to be administered only once or twice daily but also has a curved time-action profile with a peak that is somewhat congruent with peak insulin requirement postprandially.

If choosing a strategy that employs the administration of a "bolus" insulin alone, the time action profile of the exogenous "bolus" insulin should mimic the physiologic "bolus" secretion required by the individual. Considering the differences in physiologic "bolus" insulin secretion in dogs and people (Table 38.4), the "intermediate-acting" insulin formulations might provide a better approximation of "bolus" insulin secretion in many dogs than the rapid-acting formulations that are typically used for this purpose in diabetic people.

Using basal insulin as monotherapy –Why?

The main advantage of using a basal insulin is the uncoupling of injections from feeding, which creates flexibility and reduces owners' anxiety. Owners are free to choose the time of injection that is most convenient to them and will administer the insulin whether or not the dog has been fed or is vomiting. Most diabetic dogs can be well-managed by using a basal insulin alone. Postprandial hyperglycemia is then expected, but most often it is mild and not associated with clinical signs and so does not require specific treatment. Sometimes a diet change may be used to moderate the postprandial glucose excursions.

Using basal insulin as monotherapy –How?

Another advantage of basal insulin therapy is that rapid dose titration using continuous glucose monitoring (CGM) guidance is possible if using a formulation with low day-to-day variability (e.g., glargine U300, degludec). Dose titration of a basal insulin relies on fasting blood glucose concentrations: the target nadir is euglycemia and so the dose can be increased as long as fasting blood glucose is in the hyperglycemic range. If using a formulation with low day-to-day variability, the dose may be increased every 1-3 days as long as a stable pattern is observed on the CGM. Table 38.5 provides guidelines for dose titration of glargine U300 insulin.[40]

"Intermediate-acting" formulations versus "basal" formulations

Side-by-side clinical trials comparing the efficacy and safety of "intermediate-acting" formulations to "basal" or "bolus" insulin formulations are rare. In one small study in dogs, there was no difference in mean daily blood glucose concentrations or in the frequency of hypoglycemic events when an "intermediate-acting insulin" (porcine lente) was compared to "basal" insulin formulations insulin degludec and insulin glargine U300.[41] In another study, the mean blood glucose concentrations were higher when four diabetic dogs were treated with "intermediate-acting" NPH insulin twice daily compared with 'basal' insulin degludec twice daily, even though NPH was used at a higher dose, and postprandial hyperglycemia and lower preprandial glycemia were observed with insulin degludec.[42]

TABLE 38.5 Guidelines for insulin glargine U300 (IGla300) dose adjustments based on continuous interstitial glucose monitoring during induction of therapy.[40]

IG nadir and/or mean	Graphic illustration of interstitial glucose pattern	Recommended dose adjustments for: Dogs >8 kg	Recommended dose adjustments for: Dogs <8 kg
Nadir 150-350 mg/dL (8.3-19 mmol/L)		↑10-30% once daily	↑1U once daily
Nadir 80-150 mg/dL (4.4-8.3 mmol/L), or nadir <80 mg/dL (<4.4 mmol/L) and mean IG >120 mg/dL (>6.6 mmol/L)	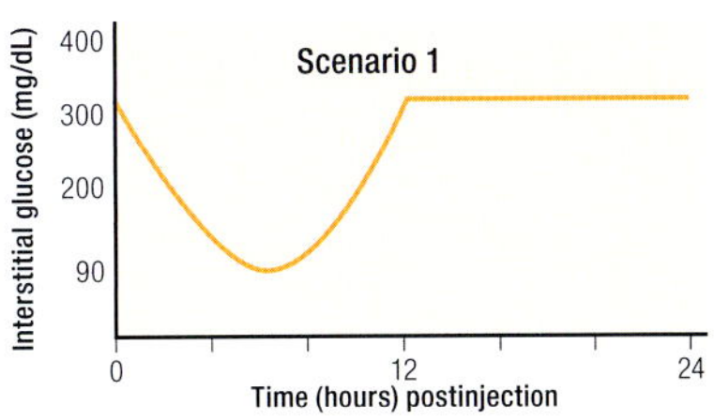 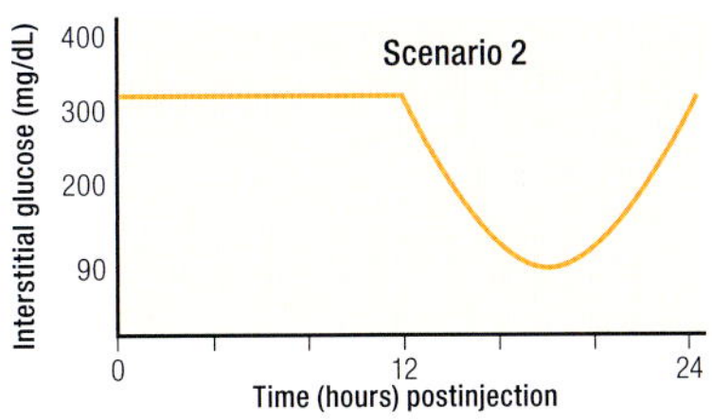	Switch to twice daily dosing (with a 30% dose reduction per injection) and re-evaluate the following 3-5 days. Adjust Toujeo dose to achieve nadir between 90-300 mg/dL (5-17 mmol/L)	
	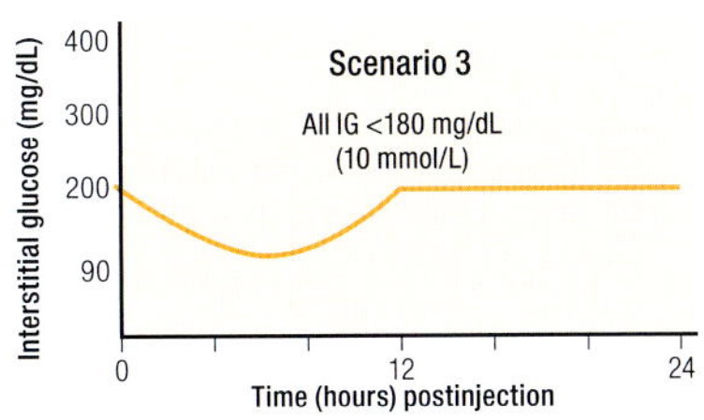	No change	
	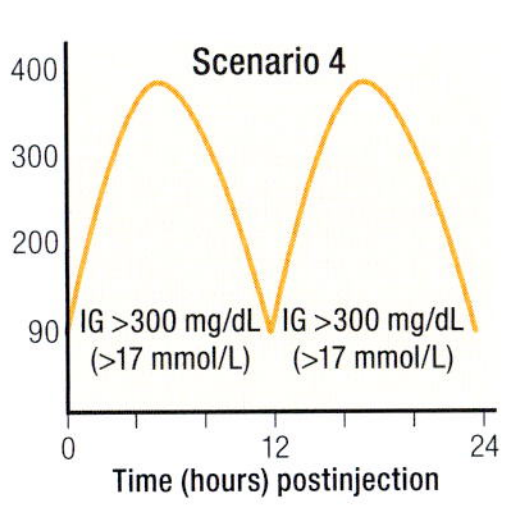 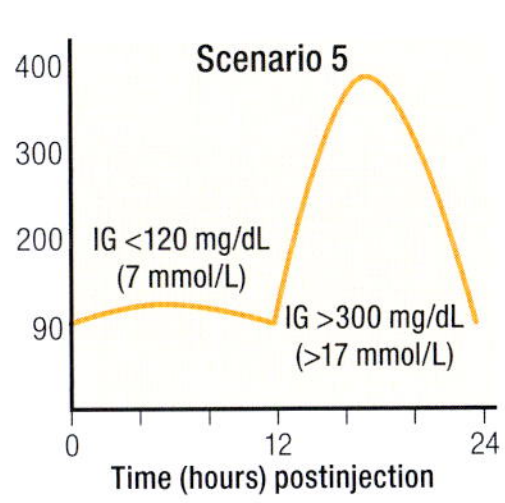 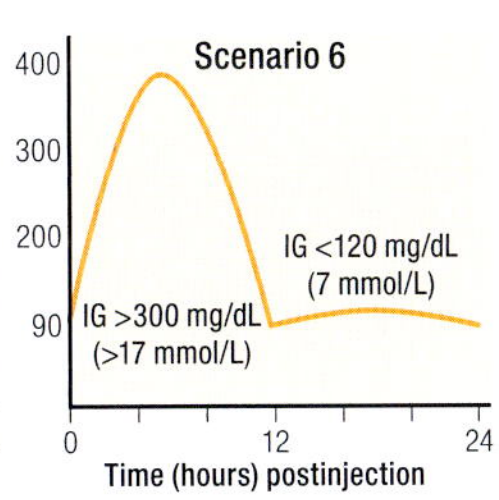	Maintain IGla300 once daily and add meal-time bolus injections ■ Scenario 4: at hours 0 and 12 ■ Scenario 5: at hour 12 ■ Scenario 6: at hour 0 OR changing the timing and/or quantities fed at meals	
Nadir <80 mg/dL (<4.4 mmol/L) and mean IG <120 mg/dL (<6.6 mmol/L)		↓10-30% once daily	↓1U once daily

Combination "basal-bolus" treatment in dogs

There are two clinical scenarios in which a "basal-bolus" insulin combination may be indicated in dogs:

- "Intermediate-acting" insulin has achieved good control of postprandial hyperglycemia, but there is underlying insulin resistance causing a short duration of action of injected insulin, resulting in marked hyperglycemia 6-12 hours after injections.
- "Basal" insulin has achieved good glycemic control for most of the day, but substantial postprandial hyperglycemia is present 1-6 hours after meals.

In the first scenario, "basal" insulin can be added to the existing insulin treatment. When making this change, it is recommended that the total insulin dose that the dog is currently receiving every 12 hours is not changed. This requires that the dose of the "intermediate-acting" insulin is reduced (by about 50%) and the remainder of the 12-hourly dose delivered by the "basal" insulin. It is obviously crucial that there is very clear communication with owners regarding the dose of each of the insulin formulations. In the second scenario, it is recommended that the same dose of the "basal" insulin is continued and an "intermediate-acting" insulin is added at 0.25 U/kg at meal times (Table 38.5).

Insulin pharmacology in dogs

Pharmacodynamics, pharmacokinetics, and guidelines for frequency of administration of specific insulin formulations are presented in Table 38.6. Characteristics of "basal" and "intermediate-acting" insulin formulations are summarized in Box 38.1 and Box 38.2, respectively.

TABLE 38.6 Pharmacodynamics (PD), pharmacokinetics (PK), and guidelines for frequency of administration of specific insulin formulations.

Formulation	Concentration Syringe/pen	Starting dose	Frequency	PD (for X U/kg): T_{DA} (hours) T_{PEAK} (hours)	Comments
hr NPH Suspension	U100 Syringe/pen	0.25-0.5 U/kg	q8-12h	■ 0.5 U/kg:[15] ■ N = 3 ■ DA ≈12 ■ T_{Peak} ≈6	PK data on 0.6 U/kg in DM:[16] Insulin returned to baseline in 8 ± 2h, peak at 1.5h (N =10)
Porcine lente Suspension	U40 Syringe/pen	0.25-0.5 U/kg	q12h or higher		PK data on 1.0-2.8 U/kg in DM:[48] Insulin first peak at 4-6h, second peak (half of the first peak) at 11h (8-14h) returned to baseline in 16h (14-24), in 8/10 dogs (N = 10) PK data on 0.64-1.12 U/kg:[48] (N = 8) Peak at 3 and 9 hour, return to baseline by 16h
hr PZI Suspension	U40 Syringe	0.5 U/kg	q12-24h		PK data on 0.8 U/kg:[19] Insulin peak at 7 (1-22)h, returned to baseline in 22 (12->24)h, (N = 10). Time-action profile markedly variable between dogs
hr insulin detemir Solution	U100/U200 Syringe/Pen	0.1 U/kg	q12h or higher	■ 0.1 U/kg:[44] ■ N = 8 ■ DA ≈11 ± 2 ■ T_{Peak} ≈5 ■ 0.5 U/kg:[50] ■ N = 3 ■ DA ≈17 ■ T_{Peak} ≈9	
hr insulin glargine Solution	U100 Syringe/pen	0.5 U/kg	q12h or higher	■ 0.5 U/kg:[46] ■ N = 3 ■ DA ≈21 ■ T_{Peak} ≈7	
hr insulin glargine Solution	U300 Pen	0.5 U/kg	q12-24h	■ 0.4 U/kg:[44] ■ N = 8 ■ DA ≈15 ± 5 ■ T_{Peak} ≈10	PD estimated from clamp and lowering of endogenous insulin
hr insulin degludec Solution	U100/U200 Pen	0.5 U/kg	q12h or higher	■ 0.5 U/kg:[42] ■ N = 5 ■ DA >20 ■ T_{Peak} ≈10	Clamp discontinued at 20h

Arrows represent potentially longer or shorter interval. Abbreviations: hr = human recombinant; DA = duration of action; T_{Peak} = Time to peak.[39]

Box 38.1 Characteristics of "basal" formulations: insulin degludec and insulin glargine U300

- Low within-day variability of action, that is, its action should be roughly the same every hour of the day. Currently, two formulations meet this standard in dogs: insulin glargine U300, and insulin degludec.[42,43]
- Low day-to-day variability[11] (an important feature in prevention of hypoglycemic events).
- Solutions that do not need to be resuspended (no rolling or shaking).
- In the authors' opinion, basal insulin formulations should not be used in dogs unless the dose can be titrated with the help of continuous glucose monitoring.[40]
- In client-owned dogs, both insulin glargine U300 and insulin degludec have been used successfully and extensively. With a starting dose of 0.5 U/kg q24h, dose escalation over 1-2 weeks results in good or excellent glycemic control in the majority of cases with about half requiring twice-daily injection and half being well maintained on once daily injections. The final dose in which good control is achieved ranged from 0.2-5.2 U/kg/day (median 1.9) for glargine U300 and 0.7-2.2 U/kg/day (median 1.7) for insulin degludec.[44] Of 95 dogs treated with the dose titration protocol outlined in Table 38.5, less than 5% needed the addition of a bolus insulin to achieve good glycemic control.[40]
- Critically, the use of these two formulations usually does not require that the dog consumes food at the time of insulin injections.
- Of the two formulations, while degludec seems to last longer (more consistently reaching a 24h mark), it also seems less "flat", often resulting in a substantial difference in action between the first and second halves of the day.
- Insulin glargine U300 is biochemically identical to insulin glargine U100 but it is three times more concentrated. Because the same number of units are delivered as a smaller droplet with smaller surface area, its absorption is slower, its duration is longer, its time-action profile is flatter, and it is associated with decreased day-to-day variability when compared to insulin glargine U100. Because of its high concentrations, it is available only in a pen.
- In diabetic people, insulin glargine U300 is superior to insulin glargine U100 in maintaining glycemic control while also reducing the risk of hypoglycemia. Emerging evidence from a handful of small studies that are supported by clinical experience suggests similar advantages of insulin glargine U300 compared to insulin glargine U100 in dogs although its duration of action is not sufficient for once daily administration in all canine patients.[40,43,44]

Box 38.2 Characteristics of "intermediate-acting" insulin formulations

- This group includes insulin suspensions (neutral protamine Hagedorn [NPH], NPH/regular mixes, lente, and protamine zinc insulin [PZI]) as well as insulin solutions like glargine U100 and detemir.
- Usually recommended for q12h administration.[43,45-50]
- It is recommended to feed a meal at the time of insulin injections to avoid hypoglycemia. When fasting is planned, a dose that is 50% or less of maintenance is typically administered.
- Incongruity between required and delivered insulin often results in wide and frequent intraday fluctuations in blood glucose concentrations. It is usually recommended to aim for blood glucose concentrations around 250-350 mg/dL (14-19 mmol/L) preinjection with a nadir (on average at 6 hours postinjection but highly variable) of about 80-100 mg/dL (4.5-5.5 mmol/L).[48,49,51,52]
- With a renal threshold for glucose at about 180-200 mg/dL (10-11 mmol/L),[53] this treatment strategy usually results in dogs spending about half the time above the renal threshold and having residual clinical signs of increased water intake and urination. Glycated protein concentrations above the reference interval are to be expected.
- In the absence of polyuria and polydipsia, or if glycated proteins are normal and/or the blood glucose nadir is <80 mg/dL (<4.5 mmol/L), it is assumed that the animal might be overcontrolled and experiencing hypoglycemia, at least intermittently.
- Porcine lente, PZI, and insulin detemir tend to have a duration of action that is longer than observed with NPH.[46,48,49]
- Decreasing the dose and increasing the frequency to three times daily, coupled with three meals per day, will decrease the likelihood of hypoglycemia and can lead to better glycemic control (Figure 38.5B).
- Once-daily injection of a higher dose of porcine lente, PZI or detemir (but not NPH) might result in acceptable level of clinical control.[51,54] but with an increased risk of hypoglycemia.
- Insulin detemir in dogs, on a unit-by-unit basis is more potent compared to other formulations and should be started at a much lower dose (0.05-0.10 U/kg). At a dose range in which it is safe and effective (0.05-0.35 U/kg), it should be administered at least q12h.[43,55] Therefore, the use of this insulin is not recommended for dogs <10 kg, unless substantial insulin resistance is present. It is not recommended to dilute insulin detemir (or any other insulin) because dilution decreases the lipophilic interactions between insulin detemir molecules and might dramatically change the pharmacodynamic profile in undesired ways.
- Insulin suspensions (lente, NPH, PZI) have several disadvantages compared with insulin solutions:
  - Insulin has to be resuspended evenly before each dose. The recommendation is to resuspend the insulin by gently rolling then inverting the vial or, in the case of lente, to vigorously shake the vial until completely mixed. However, the process of resuspension is often inconsistent and leads to inaccuracy in dosing.
  - The deprecipitation in the injection site is highly variable and unpredictable, which leads to considerable variation in insulin absorption.
  - These formulations have time-action profiles that are usually not congruent with physiological insulin secretion patterns. The onsets of action may be too slow and durations of action too long to mimic the "bolus" phase, whereas insulin action profiles are often too peaked and durations may not be long enough to mimic "basal" secretion. Better congruency might be achieved with formulations that mix "short-" and "intermediate-acting" suspensions such as the premixed combinations of 30% regular and 70% NPH insulin, or porcine lente insulin, which is a mix of 35% amorphous semilente insulin and 65% crystalline ultralente insulin. However, absorption of the "short-acting" component might still sometimes be too slow in these formulations. In addition, there is inability with the commercial insulin mixes to separately fine-tune the "short-" and "intermediate-acting" components; a limitation that may be overcome by administering the "short-" and "intermediate-acting" insulin by separate injections.

Guidelines for starting insulin therapy and adjusting the dose

Insulin is a unique drug because its therapeutic range and its toxic range completely overlap. For any given insulin in a given population, the range of doses associated with good glycemic control overlaps with the range of doses reported to cause hypoglycemia. For most insulin formulations, this range is about 0.25-1.0 U/kg twice daily. For insulin detemir in dogs, this range is about 0.05-0.3 U/kg twice daily. Starting a patient on a dose at the low end of the therapeutic/toxic range will result in a low risk of hypoglycemia but a high risk of less-than-optimal glycemic control. Using a higher starting dose minimizes the interval to achieving good glycemic control but might increase the risk of hypoglycemia. Therefore, the choice of a starting dose should be based on individual patient and owner factors, such as the owner's tolerance of polyuria or the cost of more intensive monitoring in the first few weeks of treatment. Using predictable formulations with low day-to-day variability (glargine U300, degludec) and the dose titration protocol outlined in **Table 38.5** allows for very rapid dose escalation and achieving reasonable clinical control in just a few days.[40] This protocol allows for a low starting dose while minimizing the period of uncontrolled diabetes. When using less predictable formulations, and especially when not using continuous glucose monitoring, more time is required to appreciate the full spectrum of responses to any given dose, and therefore, dose escalation should be done more slowly. With less predictable formulations, the dose of insulin is increased by 20-25% at 1-2 week intervals. The dog's response to each dose change should be assessed using a clinical scoring system such as the ALIVE diabetic clinical score (**Table 38.7**) with the goal of determining the lowest insulin dose that achieves good clinical control.

A troubleshooting checklist for when there seems to be an insufficient response to insulin is provided in **Box 38.3**. The most common causes of insulin resistance in dogs are diestrus in intact bitches and Cushing's syndrome (**Box 38.4**). Information about the recognition and management of hypoglycemia is included in **Box 38.5**. When hypoglycemia is observed, it is recommended to decrease the dose by 25-50% and then reassess. Assuming no change in factors that might increase insulin requirement (weight gain, increased carbohydrates in diet, concurrent disease), the dose of insulin should never be increased back to the dose previously associated with hypoglycemia.

TABLE 38.7 ALIVE diabetic clinical score.

Factor	Score
Unintended weight loss 0 = None, or gained since last examined 1 = Mild (<5% loss) 2 = Moderate (5-10% loss) 3 = Severe (>10% loss)	
Polyuria and polydipsia 0 = Normal 1 = Mild (some increase noted by owner) 2 = Moderate (increased filling of water bowl) 3 = Severe (constantly at bowl)	
Appetite 0 = Normal or decreased appetite (if decreased appetite exclude DKA or concurrent disease) 1 = Mild polyphagia (finishes eagerly) 2 = Moderate polyphagia (finishes eagerly and begs for more) 3 = Severe polyphagia (obsessed with food)	
Attitude/activity 0 = Normal 1 = Mild decrease (a bit less running and jumping) 2 = Moderate decrease (a lot less running and jumping) 3 = Severe decrease (lying about all the time) (*consider DKA in the ill patient with diabetes mellitus)	
Total score	

Total score range: 0-12
Treatment aim: lowest score possible without unacceptably high risk of hypoglycemia

Box 38.3 Cheklist for perceived insufficient response to insulin

Improper insulin administration and poor compliance

- Handling of insulin and syringe, poor administration technique (watch owners administer the injection using their own syringe!); incorrect dosing (e.g., use of U100 syringes with U40 insulin formulations).
- Handling of insulin dosing pen (watch owners administer the injection!); check that the pen will prime (the "air shot"), for air bubbles in the insulin, cracks or chips in the glass insulin cartridge, and/or poor administration technique.
- Check type, dose, and expiration date
  - Insulin suspensions should be resuspended before drawing a dose either by roling the vial (PZI, NPH) or shaking it. Insulin solutions (glargine, detemir, degludec, etc.) do not require rolling or shaking before drawing a dose.
- Use of diluted insulin (this is not recommended because it will alter the pharmacologic characteristics of the formulation)
- Check storage of insulin (insulin should be stored <30°C and protected from heat and light; it should never be frozen; note that continuous refrigeration at 4°C is not essential).

Insulin resistance and/or increased glycemic variability (the most common conditions are italicized)

- Circulating insulin antagonists
  - Increased counterregulatory hormones (epinephrine, norepinephrine, glucagon, cortisol, growth hormone):
    - Organ failure (e.g., renal failure, heart failure).
    - Endocrine tumors (e.g., *hypercortisolism*, hyperthyroidism, glucagonoma).
    - Diestrus ± hypersomatotropism, pregnancy.
    - Iatrogenic (progestins, *glucocorticoids*).
  - Increased cytokines (TNF-α, IL-6): *inflammatory diseases, obesity.*
  - Neutralizing insulin antibodies (rare in contrast to the presence of non-neutralizing antibodies that do not interfere with glycemic regulation).
- Target tissue defects
  - Insulin-receptor defects (*obesity*, genetic mutations).
  - Postreceptor defects (*obesity*, genetic mutations).

Short-acting insulin (might be associated with episodes of hypoglycemia)

Compliance, adherence, convenience, and cost

Human patients consider insulin injections to be a serious burden and have a negative impact on quality of life. In contrast, surveys of owners of diabetic dogs identified few concerns relating to the administration of insulin injections.[56] The greatest concerns were associated with the owners' quality of life, rather than the pet's, with worry about who would care for their pet when they were unavailable near the top of the list. Therefore, it may be surmised that it might be helpful for veterinarians to be flexible and offer insulin treatment options that are client-focused, particularly with respect to the timing of injections. In many cases, it might be more important to incorporate measures to reduce the impact of the pet's treatment on the owner's lifestyle than to focus on specific treatment goals for the pet. It is also unknown how the act of injection itself affects pets' compliance and the owners' short- and long-term decisions to treat. While not exclusively associated with this problem, it is reasonable to assume that the high euthanasia rate (40%) upon diagnosis of diabetes is associated with owner concerns regarding compliance.[57,58]

Studies in people show that adherence declines with increasing dosing frequency. Other reasons for poor adherence include the pain of injection, forgetfulness and having other priorities, regimen complexity (more than one medication or the need to draw up insulin doses), and cost of medication. Treatment strategies that minimize these barriers would likely result in greater treatment success, improved quality of life for pets and owners, and increased patient survival. In this context, it is also important to consider not just the treatment choice *per se* but also how it affects monitoring intensity and cost. For example, using a human recombinant "basal" insulin has the potential to achieve reasonably good glycemic control with q24 h dosing; using a convenient and stress-free insulin pen might result in minimal day-to-day variability, allowing less monitoring and simplifying recommendations regarding episodes of inappetence, while lessening the concern regarding hypoglycemia.

Cost and availability are also factors in treatment adherence. For example, in most countries, veterinary-labeled formulations are relatively more expensive than formulations labeled for people. The opposite is true in the USA. In the UK and parts of Europe, the regulation requires that veterinary-labeled products are used first in the prescribing cascade. It is noted that insulin products labeled for human use are not backed up by official pharmacovigilance programs for veterinary species.

Syringe versus pen administration

Multiple studies have found various advantages to using insulin-dosing pens over the traditional combination of multidose vial and syringe-needle, including increased patient adherence, a significant reduction in hypoglycemic events, and overall healthcare cost savings. Most people preferred the pen over vial-syringe[59] and considered it easier to use. It is important for clinicians to familiarize themselves with the correct use of insulin dosing pens and to provide clear instructions for diabetic dog owners (**Box 38.6**). Insulin pens are especially easier to use by those with visual impairments or dexterity problems and overall they lead to better patient satisfaction and improved quality of life. Also, injection pens are consistently shown to have better dosing accuracy and precision compared to insulin syringes.[60] This effect is most pronounced at lower dosages, up to 5 U. The relative

Box 38.4 The special case of diabetes associated with other endocrinopathies in dogs

- Insulin resistance caused by hypercortisolism or hyperprogesteronism often leads to glucose dysregulation and sometimes is associated with clinical diabetes.
- Medical treatment of these conditions rarely leads to diabetic remission.
- Early spay combined with insulin treatment increases the chances of diabetic remission to about 10% in bitches suffering from diestrus-related diabetes.

Box 38.5 Recognition and management of insulin-induced hypoglycemia

- Hypoglycemia can manifest as increased appetite, lethargy, altered mentation, ataxia, bed wetting, and, if advanced, seizures or loss of consciousness.
- It is better to prevent hypoglycemia than to treat it. Hypoglycemia is often subclinical. When clinical episodes occur, signs are usually very mild initially, but repeated episodes increase the risk of future, more severe signs. Therefore, even if hypoglycemia is not clinical, insulin dose reduction and other management modifications (such as a change in the feeding regimen) should be considered.
- If the clinical signs are mild and the patient is conscious and can be safely fed, feed glucose-rich food. Once fully recovered, feed a small meal of the dog's usual food.
- In an outpatient that is unconscious or unable to be safely fed, glucose or other sugars can be applied to the gums in the form of honey or glucose solution.
- In hospital, treat severe hypogylcemia with IV dextrose (50% at 1 mL/kg), followed by infusion of 5% dextrose as required to raise blood glucose. If the patient is suffering from severe hypoglycemia and is seizuring or unconscious, glucagon powder can be administered intra-nasal or per rectum or glucagon solution (1 mg) can be administered IV/IM.

Box 38.6 Steps for proper use and storage of insulin with a pen device[62]

- Place a new needle for every injection.
- Prime the pen prior to every injection once the needle is attached.
- Hold the pen in place for the recommended (manufacturer's) time during administration *(note: this does not appear to be essential for doses <20 U)*.
- Store the pen with no needle attached.
- Store the pen at the recommended (manufacturer's) temperature.
- Dispose of the pen vial or pen after the recommended (manufacturer's) days of use.

Video 38.1

How to use an insulin dosing pen.

imprecision of vial-syringe method can be critical in contributing to increased day-to-day variability which subsequently makes monitoring more complicated and more expensive. When using a traditional insulin syringe, for a target dose of 1 U, 50% of actual drawn doses were >20% different than the target dose. This frequency and magnitude of inaccuracy can have substantial consequences on the management of diabetic patients. Importantly, most syringe-measured doses exceed the intended dose.[61]

To avoid dosing errors, it is recommended to always administer 40 U/mL insulin with either U-40 syringes or the manufacturer's insulin dosing pen. There is currently one insulin dosing pen for use in veterinary patients containing 40 U/mL lente insulin. Initial pilot studies on this device have shown that the device is easy to use in dogs, is well tolerated under real-life conditions, is more accurate compared to the traditional syringe-vial system and is preferred over syringe use by many owners.[59]

In the past, high cost was an important barrier to using insulin pens. However, depending on country and region, cost is usually no longer a barrier. For example, insulin degludec pens are the second least expensive formulation (on a unit-by-unit basis) in the USA, second only to certain NPH vials. Moreover, for pens that are still on the expensive side, with some minor deviations from the manufacturers' blanket recommendations (**Box 38.6** and **Video 38.1**), cost can be substantially reduced without sacrificing safety and efficacy.

Managing inappetence and gastrointestinal signs

In health, about half of the daily insulin requirement is "basal" and the other half is "bolus", leading to the recommendation to lower the dose of "intermediate-acting" insulin by 50% in a patient that skips a meal or in a patient that is vomiting. There are two potential problems with this strategy. First, the 50% "basal-bolus" ratio is a general estimate, and might lead to significant over- or underdosing in any particular patient. Second, it is common for diabetic pets to be "picky eaters" or to have concurrent gastrointestinal disease, pancreatitis, or other disease that affects their appetite. The need to adjust the dose of insulin in these instances can have a significant impact on glycemic control and on the owners' stress level. This problem is generally avoided entirely when using "basal" insulin monotherapy. Some of this might also be alleviated by using a "basal-bolus" insulin combination in which the dose and frequency of the "basal" insulin are unaltered during episodes of decreased appetite and the "bolus" insulin is simply skipped.

Dietary management of diabetes

Linda Fleeman, Charlotte Bjørnvad

Nutritional management is an integrated part of the treatment of diabetes mellitus in dogs. When coordinated with the insulin treatment strategy, it can aid in improving both glycemic control and quality of life for the dog.

Recommendations regarding diet choice

Recently, there has been an increasing focus on possible benefits from limiting starch-containing ingredients because starch is readily digested and absorbed as glucose. However, limiting the starch-containing ingredients will necessitate that energy is derived from either protein or fat, which may not be warranted in dogs with concomitant chronic kidney disease, hyperlipidemia, or pancreatitis. Therefore, tailor-made diet recommendations should be made for diabetic dogs, taking into account the dog's age, appetite, food preferences, body composition, activity level, insulin treatment strategy, and concomitant conditions.

Nutritional considerations and recommendations regarding diet choice for uncomplicated and complicated diabetic dogs are provided in Table 38.8 and Table 38.9.

Management of postprandial hyperglycemia in diabetic dogs

Endogenous insulin secretion in healthy individuals can be divided into two phases: the "basal" phase, in which insulin is secreted continuously at a relatively constant rate, and the "bolus" phase, in which insulin is secreted in response to nutrients absorbed from the gut. In dogs, the "bolus" phase usually increases within minutes after feeding, often peaks within 30 minutes at five to seven times the baseline concentration, and can remain increased for 6-9 hours depending on the diet.[36-38] Factors other than diet composition can also influence "bolus" insulin requirement. These include high total food intake (for example, due to compensatory polyphagia in response to weight loss) and insulin resistance (for example, due to Cushing's syndrome). Excessive postprandial hyperglycemia and substantial within-day and day-to-day glycemic variability are some of the most pronounced effects of dysglycemia in Cushing's syndrome.[25]

Postprandial hyperglycemia occurs when there is insufficient insulin action to match "bolus" insulin requirement. This is commonly an issue in diabetic dogs treated with exogenous insulin. This mismatch will be ameliorated in dogs with residual beta cell function because endogenous secretion can fill at least some of the gap during the postprandial phase. In addition, relatively mild postprandial hyperglycemia (<350 mg/dL; <19 mmol/L) is typically not associated with unacceptable clinical signs in dogs. Therefore, although postprandial mismatch between insulin action and requirement is common in diabetic dogs, it does not always present a management problem. For example, supplemental "bolus" insulin treatment was required in only a minority (5%) of a heterogeneous population of diabetic dogs treated with "basal" insulin monotherapy.[40]

Changes in diet composition and/or feeding method can be stressful for both dog and owner. Given the high risk of euthanasia for diabetic dogs if their owner feels unable to cope with the requirements of treatment,[57] and that six of the top ten concerns reported by owners of diabetic dogs relate to the impact of the daily management schedule on their quality of life,[56] caregiver burden may be considerably reduced if diet change is not routinely recommended at the start of diabetes treatment. Instead, clinicians and owners are encouraged to first focus on insulin treatment and the dietary requirements of any concurrent health conditions. Once the owner is accustomed to insulin administration and reasonably good control of the clinical signs of diabetes is achieved, the clinical impact of postprandial hyperglycemia, if present, may then be assessed and managed.

Insulin treatment options and their effects on postprandial hyperglycemia in diabetic dogs are outlined in Video 38.2.

Case examples of different strategies to manage postprandial hyperglycemia in insulin-treated diabetic dogs are presented here:

Case 1

10-year-old neutered male Labrador Retriever mix

Physical features: body weight 51.7 kg; body condition score 7/9; muscle score 2/3.

Current insulin treatment: 37 units of insulin glargine U300 SC q24h at 6.00 pm.

Current diet per 24 h: 200 g of a commercial therapeutic dry dog food formulated for weight loss + 200 g cooked chicken breast or fish + as much zucchini and cucumber as the dog wants to eat.

Current feeding routine: daily portion fed as five meals throughout the day at 5.00 am, 10.00 am, 3.00 pm, 6.00 pm, and 9.00 pm.

Current ALIVE diabetic clinical score:[63] 0/12.

Concurrent health conditions: overweight; osteoarthritis.

Other medications: carprofen PO q24h and acetaminophen (paracetamol) PO q12h for management of osteoarthritis.

Assessment of postprandial hyperglycemia: postprandial hyperglycemia is not excessive, does not exceed 350 mg/dL (19 mmol/L), and is not associated with any noticeable clinical signs (Fig. 38.7).

Strategy to manage postprandial hyperglycemia: no change to the diet or feeding routine is required, except to continue the weight loss program to achieve and then maintain a lean body condition score of 4-5/9.

Case 2

11-year-old neutered male Maltese mixed with Poodle.

Physical features: body weight 6.3 kg; body condition score 4.5/9; muscle score 2/3.

Current insulin treatment: 7 units of insulin glargine U300 SC twice daily at 7.00 am and 5.00 pm.

Current diet per 24 h: 200 g of a commercial therapeutic wet dog food formulated for gastrointestinal support + 80 g of a commercial dry dog food formulated for adult maintenance.

TABLE 38.8 Nutritional considerations for the uncomplicated diabetic dog

Factors		Nutritional considerations
Insulin choice	Intermediate-acting insulin	Feed the majority of the daily ration in relation to insulin injections that are usually administered twice a day. Sometimes the duration of effect of the insulin is too short, consider to split feeding into three equal meals or two major meals and several smaller meals depending on the individual insulin action profile. Consider dosing insulin three times daily and split meals accordingly.
	Basal insulin	Feed twice daily or split the feedings into smaller meals according to the owner's preference and the individual insulin action profile.
	Feeding regimen	Consistency in daily routines is desirable, and includes consistent feeding times, diet composition and amount in relation to insulin injections. Avoid hasty transitions and ensure diet palatability to avoid inappetence and food aversion.
Body composition	Underweight (BCS 3/9)	Underweight condition may be due to uncontrolled diabetes or concurrent disease. In case of concurrent diseases that require nutritional management, this should be prioritized, and insulin dose and regimen adjusted according to this feeding. High-fiber/low energy diets are NOT recommended for underweight diabetic dogs while diets for adult maintenance are often advisable.[36]
	Normal weight (BCS 4-5/9)	Diet composition can be adjusted to improve insulin – diet interaction and glucose control. Adjustments depend on the individual insulin action profile, the patient's appetite, and the owner's preference, but may include changing feeding intervals and amounts, increasing protein and/or fiber and decreasing starch content. Monitor weight change and address if necessary.
	Overweight (BCS 6-7/9)	Overweight condition causes insulin resistance, counteracting insulin action and impairing glycemic control.[37] Avoid further weight gain and, when insulin treatment has started and the owner is ready, a weight loss program should be initiated using a purpose made weight loss diet.
Macronutrients	Water	Fresh drinking water must be available at all times. Whether diabetic dogs benefit from wet food compared to dry is uncertain, but wet foods generally contain less carbohydrate/starch, provide additional water, and may improve satiety. Feeding only with wet/canned foods is often expensive and may not be economically feasible, but combining dry and wet feeding in the daily routine may work for some dogs.
	Protein	Protein provides essential amino acids and can be used for hepatic gluconeogenesis. High protein diets substitute carbohydrates as a glucose and energy source and may improve satiation. Currently, there is limited evidence on whether high protein diets improve glycemic control in dogs, but they may benefit some diabetic dogs.
	Fat	Fat is an effective energy source, provides essential fatty acids and improves palatability. Fat can be used to adjust energy concentration according to the dog's body composition and appetite. Prioritizing vegetable and fish oil sources when limiting dietary fat content ensures provision of essential fatty acids.
	Carbohydrate	Carbohydrates as starch provide an easily digestible glucose source that significantly impacts postprandial blood glucose concentrations.[38] Carbohydrate-containing ingredients are categorized based on how quickly their intake affects blood glucose levels – the glycemic index. Carbohydrate sources such as rice and corn generally have a high glycemic index. Complex carbohydrates are found in ingredients such as peas, beans, lentils, whole grains, and vegetables, where the sugar molecules are integrated in long complex chains. This slows the intestinal digestion and absorption of glucose resulting in a lower glycemic index. Recently, there has been an increasing focus on possible benefits from limiting starch-containing ingredients for diabetic dogs. However, limiting the starch-containing ingredients will necessitate that energy is derived from either protein or fat, which may not be warranted in dogs with concomitant chronic kidney disease, hyperlipidemia, or pancreatitis.
	Fiber	Fiber is a diverse nutrient group spanning from highly fermentable fiber sources like pectin, guar gum, and beet pulp to indigestible variants like bran, psyllium, and cellulose. However, in general, fiber decreases energy concentration and delays nutrient digestion and absorption, often resulting in slower and more prolonged glucose absorption and decreased blood glucose fluctuations.[25] Additionally, fermentable fibers serve as prebiotics, supporting the gastrointestinal microbiome while nonfermentable fiber improves fecal consistency. High fiber diets may, however, decrease palatability, result in inadequate nutrient uptake and unacceptable increase in fecal bulk, and may not be an appropriate choice for all diabetic dogs.
Treats and supplements	Treats and chews	Treats and chews are an integrated part of dog-owner interaction and should continue to be used in diabetic dogs. Many treats, however, contain large amounts of sugar and fats and owners should be advised on preferably using vegetable or protein treats and on using them consistently in the daily feeding regimen.
	Supplements	There is limited evidence on the use of supplements for diabetic dogs. Prebiotics, probiotics, and fish oil supplements may be used in limited and consistent amounts, based on individual response. Chromium has been hypothesized to improve glycemic control but has shown little benefit in dogs. Be aware of additives in supplements, such as sugars.

TABLE 38.9 Nutritional considerations for the complicated diabetic dog.

Complication		Nutritional recommendations
Body composition	Emaciated (BCS 1-2/9)	Consider that a concurrent disease causing weight loss or severe insulin resistance might be present. Increased energy intake will be needed to achieve weight gain, followed by reduction of calorie intake after a normal body weight is achieved. The insulin dose might need to be decreased when calorie intake is reduced after normal weight is achieved.
	Obese (BCS 8-9/9)	Obesity causes insulin resistance, counteracting insulin action and impairing glycemic control.[10] After diabetes-associated weight loss is arrested by insulin treatment, and when the owner is ready, initiate a weight loss program using a purpose made weight loss diet. Insulin dose typically will need to be decreased as insulin resistance is reduced with weight loss.
Concurrent disease	Pancreatitis	Prioritize a low fat diet, preferably using complex carbohydrate sources.
	Exocrine pancreatic insufficiency	Include pancreatic enzymes supplement; use a highly digestible diet containing low/medium fat, and consider prioritizing complex carbohydrates.
	Chronic enteropathy	Gastrointestinal diet or hypoallergenic diet, and consider prioritizing complex carbohydrates and fiber composition/content.
	Hyperlipidemia	Low-fat diet with moderate/high-fiber content and prioritize vegetable/fish oil fat sources.
	Cushing's syndrome	Consider moderate/high protein, complex carbohydrate sources, and moderate to low-fat content.
	Chronic kidney disease	Prioritize recommendations based on IRIS staging, medium/low protein content, medium fat, and complex carbohydrate sources that will also provide protein without increasing phosphorus.

Video 38.2

Insulin treatment options and their effects on postprandial hyperglycemia in diabetic dogs.

Current feeding routine: daily portion fed as two equal sized meals (100 g wet food + 40 g dry food) at 7.00 am and 5.00 pm.

Current ALIVE diabetic clinical score:[63] 2/12 (tends to be lethargic and thirsty after the morning meal).

Concurrent health conditions: episodic gastrointestinal signs attributable to pancreatitis, which sometimes require hospitalization; hypertriglyceridemia; and pituitary-dependent hypercortisolism, for which treatment has not yet commenced; keratoconjunctivitis sicca and lens-induced uveitis.

Other medications: fenofibrate PO q24h; a commercial probiotic and prebiotic formulation PO q24h; topical dexamethasone and cyclosporine eye treatments; plus maropitant, ondansetron, and metoclopramide PO as required to manage gastrointestinal signs.

Assessment of postprandial hyperglycemia: there is a consistent pattern of excessive postprandial hyperglycemia >500 mg/dL (>27.8 mmol/L) after the morning meal. This should be treated because it is associated with noticeable clinical signs. It is not appropriate to manage this by increasing the dose of the "basal" insulin glargine U300 because the interstitial glucose nadir is often in the euglycemic range (Figs. 38.8A and 38.8B).

Strategy to manage postprandial hyperglycemia: potential strategies were: 1) add an injection of supplemental "bolus" insulin at the time of the morning meal (usually an "intermediate-acting" insulin [e.g., NPH] at a starting dose of 0.25 U/kg), 2) feed a smaller meal in the morning and a larger meal in the evening, or 3) change the morning meal to one with lower total carbohydrate content. The dog's owners elected for the second option because this was most convenient for them. They did not want to give an additional insulin injection, and were concerned that changing the composition of the diet might trigger gastrointestinal signs.

Follow-up

New feeding routine: daily portion fed as a smaller meal (70 g wet food + 30 g dry food) at 7.00 am and a larger meal (130 g wet food + 50 g dry food) at 5.00 pm.

New insulin treatment: 8 units of insulin glargine U300 SC twice daily at 7.00 am and 5.00 pm. The insulin dose was increased after the change in the feeding routine to achieve an interstitial glucose nadir in the euglycemic range.

Current ALIVE diabetic clinical score:[63] 0/12.

Assessment of postprandial hyperglycemia: there is still a pattern of excessive postprandial hyperglycemia that exceeds 350 mg/dL (19 mmol/L) following at least one meal on most days. However, postprandial peaks that exceed 500 mg/dL (27.8 mmol/L) occur much less frequently and have a shorter duration than previously (Figs. 38.8C and 38.8D). Importantly, the dog was clinically improved following the change of the feeding routine and the signs previously associated with postprandial hyperglycemia were no longer noticeable.

Strategy to manage postprandial hyperglycemia: no further changes to the insulin and dietary routine were indicated. It was decided to commence treatment of pituitary-dependent hypercortisolism.

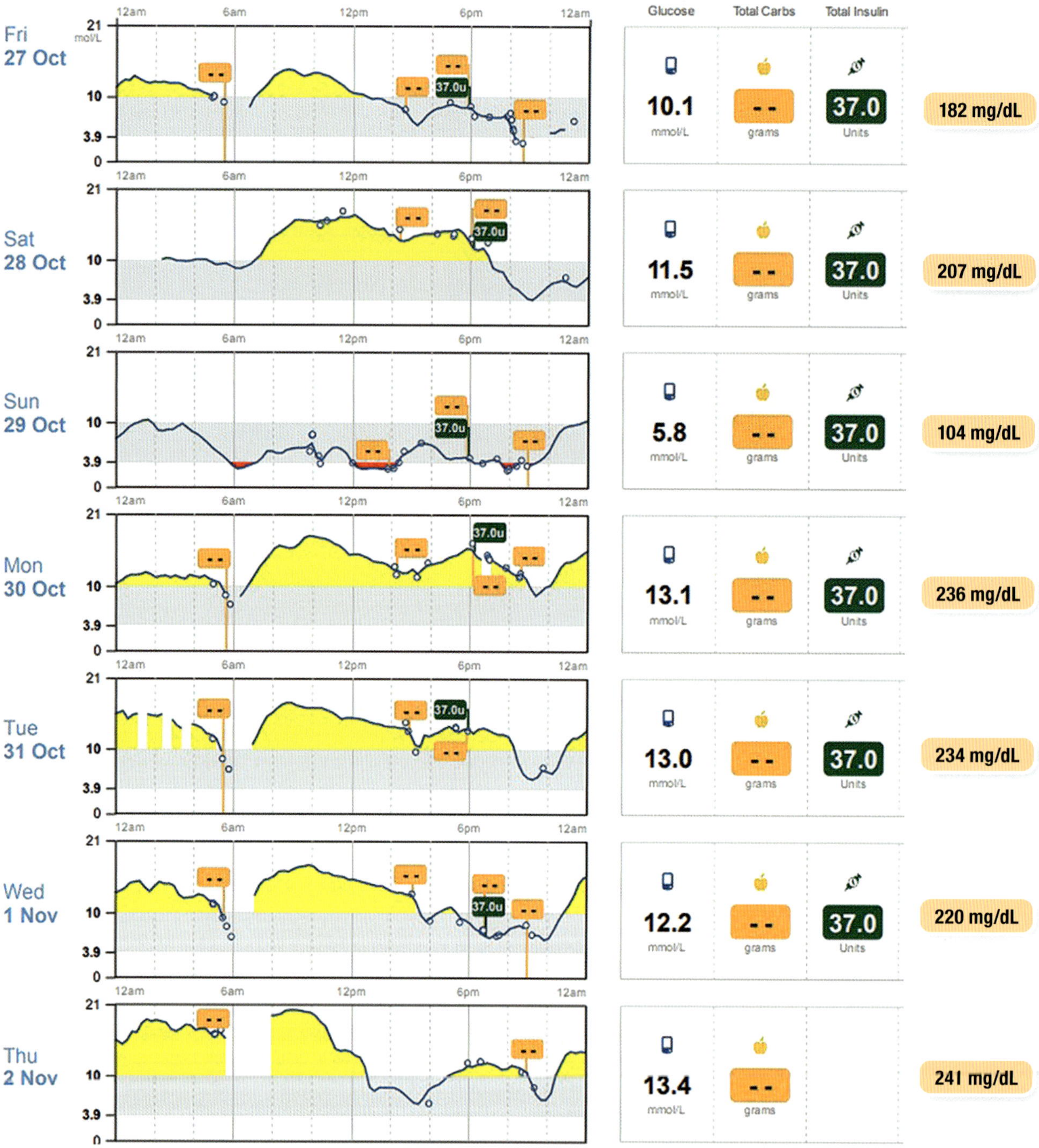

FIG. 38.7 Continuous glucose graph from case 1. Average daily interstitial glucose results are provided in the right panel. Assessment of postprandial hyperglycemia: postprandial hyperglycemia is not excessive and does not exceed 350 mg/dL (19 mmol/L).

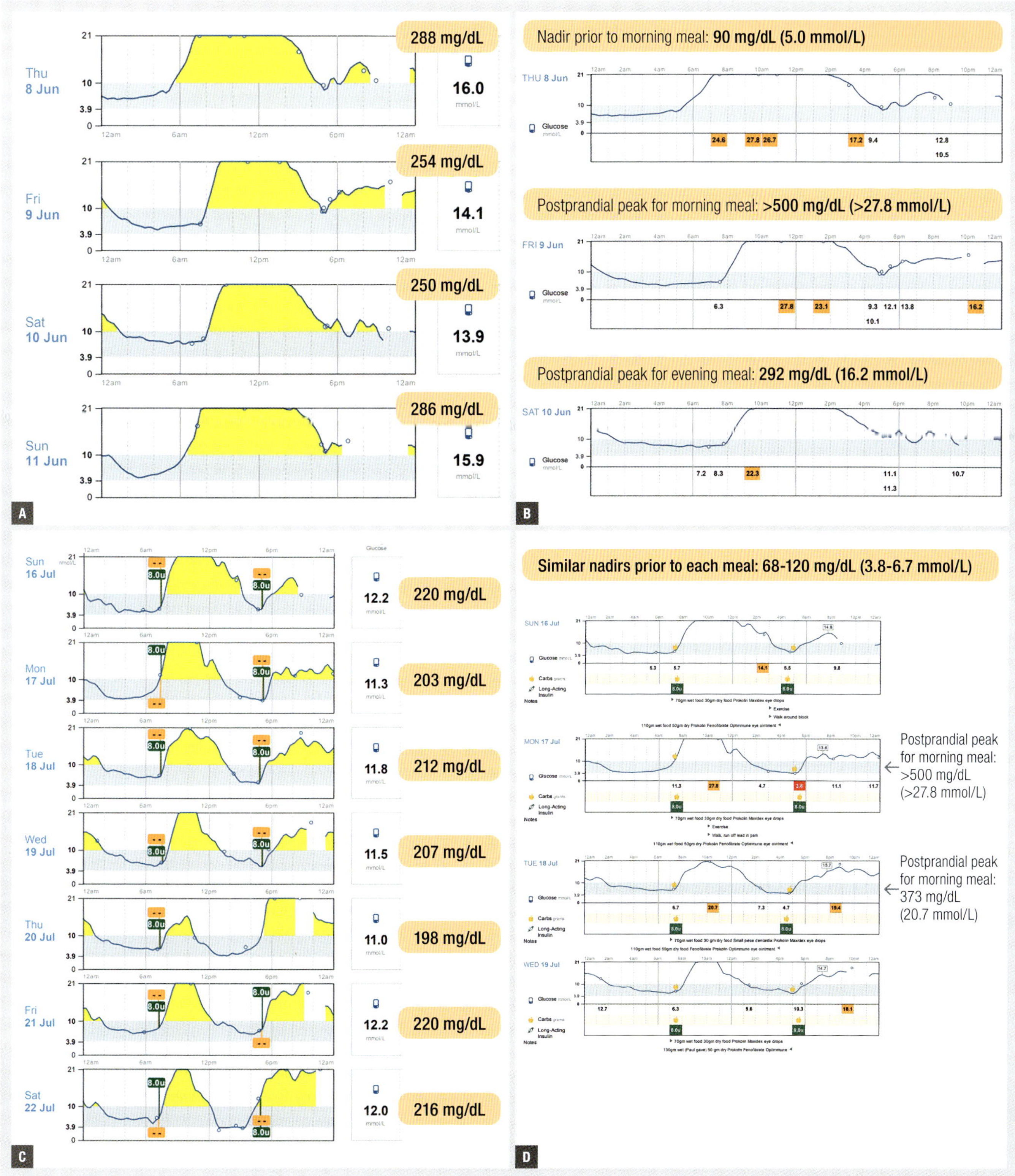

FIG. 38.8 Continuous glucose graphs from case 2. (**A**) Average daily interstitial glucose results are provided in the right panel. (**B**) A more detailed view of the same results from (**A**) showing the nadir and postprandial interstitial glucose peaks. Assessment of postprandial hyperglycemia: there is a consistent pattern of excessive postprandial hyperglycemia >500 mg/dL (>27.8 mmol/L) after the morning meal. (**C**) Average daily interstitial glucose results are provided in the right panel. (**D**) A more detailed view of the same results from (**C**) showing the nadir and postprandial interstitial glucose peaks. Assessment of postprandial hyperglycemia: there is still a pattern of excessive postprandial hyperglycemia that exceeds 350 mg/dL (19 mmol/L) following at least one meal on most days. However, postprandial peaks that exceed 500 mg/dL (27.8 mmol/L) occur much less frequently and have a shorter duration than previously.

Monitoring a diabetic patient

Francesca Del Baldo

Successful management of DM is indicated by minimal or no clinical signs, restoration of a normal body condition score, avoidance of complications such as diabetic ketoacidosis and hypoglycemia, and owner perception of a good quality of life for the animal.[7] Regular monitoring to ensure an appropriate insulin dose is vital to successfully achieving these aims. Monitoring options include clinical signs, continuous glucose monitoring systems (CGMSs) or blood glucose curves (BGCs), urinary glucose and glycated proteins (fructosamine and glycated hemoglobin). None of the monitoring options are perfect, and results from the different options may conflict. Decisions about monitoring options should consider the owner's financial situation, level of motivation, and overall expectations regarding their pet. Some owners are willing and able to monitor their pets regularly and are highly compliant with clinical recommendations. Others may approach their responsibilities as pet owners with a different philosophy and may be reluctant to follow suggested protocols if substantial cost or time is required. In these circumstances, the veterinarian must carefully advocate for the patient's needs while acknowledging the owner's position.

Clinical signs

The most important initial parameters to assess control of glycemia in a diabetic dog are the clinical signs observed by the owner, findings on physical examination, and stability of body weight. A diabetic dog in which polyuria, polydipsia, and polyphagia have resolved, the body weight is within the ideal range and physical examination reveals a good clinical condition is usually considered well controlled.[68] In contrast, the persistence of clinical signs and undesired weight loss is suggestive of inadequate glycemic control or the presence of another current condition. Although the evaluation of the clinical signs is an easy and fast way to determine the effectiveness of insulin treatment, they are subjective, and their reliability depends mainly on the owner's observational skills. Therefore, further monitoring options, such as the application of a CGMS or generation of a BGC, should be considered before adjusting the insulin therapy.

The Agreeing Language in Veterinary Endocrinology (ALIVE) diabetic clinical score can be used for the routine clinical assessment of diabetic veterinary dogs (Table 38.7).[7] This score helps objectively assess glycemic control and enables comparison with previous rechecks. The author advises completing the clinical score during the first evaluation and then at the following rechecks (see Table 38.10 for an overview of the monitoring protocol).

Blood glucose monitoring

Single blood glucose measurements

Measurement of a single blood glucose (BG) value is usually insufficient to assess glycemic control. The only exception is represented by the finding of a low BG value (<70 mg/dL, <3.9 mmol/L), which is most often due to an insulin overdosage but may also occur due to insufficient food intake (e.g., due to reduced appetite or vomiting/regurgitation episodes). In such instances, a detailed medical history is necessary to elucidate the underlying reason for the hypoglycemic event. To prevent further hypoglycemic episodes, it is advisable to decrease the insulin dosage by 25-50% and subsequently reevaluate the glucose concentration through a BGC or a CGMS.

Of note, measurement of a single BG value at the time of the presumed glucose nadir is not recommended because the timing of nadirs is unpredictable and can vary between dogs and within the same dog on different days (Fig. 38.9).

Blood glucose curves

Up to a few years ago, the BGCs were the most objective monitoring tool for making rational adjustments in insulin therapy. They allow the identification of subclinical hypoglycemia; thus, the insulin dose can be decreased before clinical signs develop. Moreover, when clinical signs suggest poor control of the disease, the BGCs may help to characterize the underlying problem (e.g., insulin doses are too low or insulin action is too short), thus allowing insulin changes. However, this monitoring method has several limitations, the most important of which is the inability to detect inter- and intraday glycemic variability (please refer to the Interday and intraday glycemic variability section). For this reason, the author recommends using this monitoring method only in situations where the use of a CGMS is not possible.

There are several situations when a BGC should be performed:

- At 5-7 days after the start of insulin therapy.
- At 7-14 days after an insulin dose change.
- At 5-7 days after the first dose of a new kind of insulin.
- At least every 3 months even in well-controlled diabetics.
- Any time clinical signs recur in a controlled patient.
- When hypoglycemia is suspected.[68]

BGCs are typically performed by measuring BG concentration on a capillary blood sample using a portable blood glucose meter (PBGM) validated for use in dogs. For technical aspects of capillary blood sampling and glucose measurement using a PBGM, the reader is referred to chapter 21.

Generation of blood glucose curves in the hospital

On the day of the planned BGC, a routine insulin treatment and feeding schedule must be maintained as much as possible. Dogs can be brought to the hospital early in the morning before administering insulin and food. Alternatively, owners can give insulin and food at home and bring the dog to the hospital as soon as possible. This last approach is particularly advisable for dogs with selective eating habits because the lack of appetite can significantly impact the results of the BGC. Also, this approach can be recommended when technical difficulties are suspected. In this case, the owner can be asked to carry out the entire administration procedure under the supervision of a veterinarian or a technician.

The first blood sample for BG measurement is obtained when the dog enters the hospital and subsequent blood samples are typically obtained every 2 hours throughout the day until the time of the next insulin dose.

TABLE 38.10 Overview of monitoring protocol used at the author's institution.

Initial presentation	
■ Diagnosis of diabetes mellitus (clinical signs, hyperglycemia, glucosuria, increased fructosamine or glycated hemoglobin) (ALIVE criteria). ■ Routine laboratory evaluation (CBC, biochemistry, urinalysis). ■ Abdominal ultrasonography and/or chest radiography (if indicated). ■ Cessation of diabetogenic drugs (if possible). ■ Start with intermediate insulin (NPH or lente insulin 0.25 U/kg SC q12h) or long-acting insulin (glargine 300U/ml 0.5 U/kg q24h). ■ Treatment of concurrent problems (if present/identified). ■ Dietary management ▪ High-fiber, low-calorie diet (except in cases in which other diseases have priority).	▪ Underweight dogs should be fed a high-quality maintenance diet or a diabetic diet that has both soluble and insoluble fiber and is not designed for weight loss. ▪ If overweight, aim for 1-2% weight loss per week. ■ Owner instruction regarding insulin preparation and administration (requires at least 1h). ■ Providing written instructions for the owner. ■ Information about the different monitoring options (ideally CGMS, second option BGCs) ■ Application of FreeStyle Libre sensor (if possible). ■ With intact bitches, make an appointment for spaying (as soon as possible).

Monitoring with CGMS (recommended method)	Monitoring with blood glucose curves
Remote re-evaluation 2 to 3 days after diagnosis ■ Evaluation of the interstitial glucose values using the Daily Log of the LibreView system. ■ Owners are asked to fill out an online form (e.g., Google form) to collect clinical information about their dog (alternatively, information about the clinical signs can be collected by phone or e-mail). ■ Adjustment of insulin dose if required (10% to 25%).	**Re-evaluation 1 week after diagnosis** ■ Option 1: administration of food and insulin at home, dog should be brought to hospital thereafter as soon as possible. ■ Option 2: food and insulin can be administered at the hospital. ■ History, physical examination and body weight. ■ Generation of the BGC. ■ Fructosamine. ■ Adjustment of insulin dose if required (10% to 25%).
Remote re-evaluation 7-10 days after diagnosis ■ Repeat all the procedures performed at the first re-evaluation.	**Re-evaluation 2-3 weeks after diagnosis** ■ Repeat all the procedures performed at the first re-evaluation. ■ Adjustment of insulin dose if required. ■ Introduction of the home monitoring (HM) and instruction on all relevant technical aspects (at least 30 minutes) (if the dog is being monitored with BGCs).
Remote re-evaluation 10-14 days after diagnosis ■ Repeat all the procedures performed at the first re-evaluation.	**Re-evaluation 3-4 weeks after diagnosis** ■ All procedures as during the first re-evaluation. ■ If the owner performs HM, possible technical issue should be assessed. If HM is done reliably, the generation of a BGC in the hospital is not necessary. ■ If glycemic control is not adequate or marked glycemic variability is present, consider the existence of concurrent diseases or technical errors in insulin administration (see Table 38.11). ■ Adjustment of insulin dose if required.
Re-evaluation in hospital 2 weeks after diagnosis (or before if a new sensor has to be applied) ■ History, physical examination and body weight. ■ Fructosamine measurement. ■ Application of a new FreeStyle Libre sensor.	**Re-evaluation of dogs without home monitoring** ■ Every 1-2 weeks until adequate glycemic control is reached; then approximately every 3 months. ■ At each re-evaluation repeat all the procedures done during the first re-evaluation and adjust the insulin dose as described above.

Re-evaluation in dogs monitored with FreeStyle Libre
■ Follow the previous scheme until the stabilization is achieved (no clinical signs, normal body weight, glucose values between 80 and 250 mg/dL); thereafter, apply a new sensor approximately every 3 months or whenever the dog is showing clinical signs suggestive of inadequate glycemic control.
	Re-evaluation of dogs with home monitoring
	■ Frequency of HM:
	  ▪ One BGC per week up to the stabilization of the dog (no clinical signs, normal body weight, glucose values between 80 and 250 mg/dL).
	  ▪ Thereafter, one BGC every 3 to 4 weeks.
	  ▪ 5-7 days after any change of insulin dose.
	■ Results should be sent to the hospital together with information on well-being, clinical signs, and body weight (owner can be asked to fill out a Google Form* or to keep a daily log recording this information).
	■ The veterinarian must perform adjustment of insulin dose on the basis of these data.
	■ Re-evaluation in the hospital approximately 2 and 3 months after diagnosis, thereafter once to twice per year. Re-evaluations should include history, physical examination, body weight, review of owner's log, fructosamine/glycated hemoglobin.

Goals of therapy ■ Resolution of the clinical signs (PU/PD, polyphagia, and normal body weight). ■ Glucose values between 80 and 250 mg/dL. ■ Fructosamine/glycated hemoglobin: slightly above the reference interval.	

HM, home monitoring; BGC, blood glucose curve; CGMS, continuous glucose monitoring system. *Link to the Google form used at the Veterinary Teaching Hospital of the University of Bologna: https://docs.google.com/forms/d/e/1FAIpQLSebLiZno6x0XYQqP2YvtY5S3MiFNLk3E6v4KsNlcco05G68SA/viewform?usp=sf_link

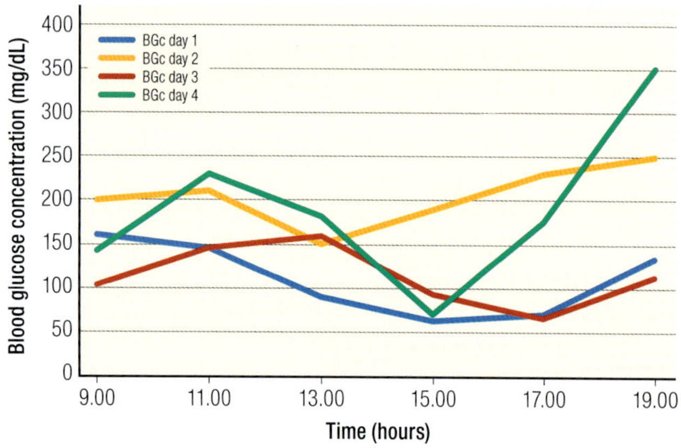

FIG. 38.9 Blood glucose curves generated on 4 consecutive days in a diabetic dog receiving lente insulin 0.6 U/kg at 8 a.m. On days 1 and 4, the nadir was 7 h after insulin injection; on day 2 the nadir was 5 h after insulin injection; on day 3 the nadir was 9 h after insulin injection.

In cases where the nadir has not been reached by then, insulin administration should be delayed and glucose measurements should continue to determine the duration of insulin action. If the BG moves down rapidly or approaches 100 mg/dL (5.5 mmol/L), the next sample should be collected within 60 minutes. In-hospital BGCs have some substantial limitations, including anorexia or hyporexia due to anxiety, disruption of normal exercise routines, and the effect of stress, aggression, or excitement on BG values. Moreover, diabetic pet owners can also be impacted by the inconvenience and expense of these visits and may postpone a recheck to avoid these issues.[57]

Generation of blood glucose curves at home

An alternative to hospital-generated BGCs is to have the client generate the BGCs at home. Most diabetic dog owners are nowadays able to collect capillary blood samples from their dogs and measure the BG concentration using a PBGM.[69,70] For most of them, the procedure is easy and quick to perform and is well tolerated by their dog.[69] The protocol for generating a BGC at home assumes that owners measure the BG concentration before the morning insulin injection and then every 2 hours until the evening insulin injection is given. One of the advantages of HM is that the owner can be asked to continue BG measurements if the glucose nadir is not reached during this time (e.g., 14-or 16-hour BGC instead of a 12-hour BGC).

Teaching the techniques (capillary blood sampling and use of PBGMs) requires at least 30 minutes and should be done by expert veterinarians or technicians who have done the procedure many times and know the details. Otherwise, the owner may not become confident enough to start HM or become frustrated after unsuccessful attempts at home and give up. Several websites on the internet explain capillary blood sampling in detail and provide information on clients' experiences with the technique and with different PBGMs. Owners should be encouraged to contact the hospital when problems or questions arise.

Problems with HM include overzealous clients who start monitoring BG concentration too frequently; interpretation of BGC results and adjusting insulin by the client without veterinarian input, a practice that results in insulin overdosing and poor control of DM; technical difficulties in obtaining capillary blood sampling (e.g., restraint of the dog, production of an adequate drop of blood, and correct use of the test strips and PBGM).[70]

Interpretation of blood glucose curves and adjustment of insulin dose

The evaluation of BGCs allows clinicians to determine glucose nadir, insulin efficacy, and duration of insulin effect. The goal of insulin therapy is to achieve BG concentrations that are below the renal threshold while avoiding hypoglycemia.[68] Thus, the BG concentration should stay between 80 and 250 mg/dL (4.4 and 13.9 mmol/L) most of the time, and the glucose nadir between 80 and 150 mg/dL (4.4 and 8.3 mmol/L). Lower nadirs might be due to insulin overdose, excessive overlap of the insulin action (common if long-acting insulin analogs are used), lack of food intake, or extreme exercise. In this case, the insulin dose should be decreased by 25 to 50% as hypoglycemia must always be avoided (regardless of other BG concentrations during the day). In contrast, a glucose nadir >150 mg/dL (8.3 mmol/L) can be caused by technical problems with insulin injections, insufficient insulin dose, insulin resistance, stress, and poor control of diabetes mellitus due to concurrent diseases (glycemic variability). In this case, the insulin dose may not necessarily be increased, but it is crucial to first rule out technical errors, especially if the dog is receiving a high dosage (e.g., >1.5 U/kg) (Table 38.11).

Insulin efficacy means the effectiveness of insulin in lowering the BG concentration. It can be determined by evaluating the difference between the highest and lowest glucose concentrations of a BGC. A small difference is acceptable if all BG concentrations are within the target range; however, it is not adequate if this is not the case. The shape of BGCs differs considerably according to the type of insulin used (e.g., lente insulin or NPH often give a bell-shaped BGC; in contrast, long-acting insulin analogs such as glargine or detemir, in theory, should keep BG concentration at a fairly constant level). Moreover, the shape of the BGC may change between dogs and even within the same dog.

Duration of action is defined as the time from the insulin injection through the nadir until the BG concentration exceeds approximately 180-250 mg/dL (10-13.9 mmol/L). It should be evaluated when the nadir is in the ideal range and should be approximately 12 hours for insulin products used twice daily and 24 hours for insulin used once daily. If the dog receives insulin twice a day and the duration of action is longer than 14 hours, the risk of insulin overdose rises. As BGC can vary from day to day[71,72] (see later), it is essential to interpret the results of the BGCs always together with clinical signs and it is advisable not to change the type of insulin after seeing an undesired BGC just once. Rather, if those changes occur repetitively, a change to longer or shorter-acting insulin should be considered.

As a general rule, if a dose change appears appropriate, it should not exceed 10 to 25% (except if hypoglycemia is identified; see above). During the initial phase of insulin therapy, mainly if an insulin solution is used (e.g., PZI, lente, NPH), and the dog is monitored with BGCs, dose adjustments are made approximately every 5-7 days (if needed). The number of dose adjustments needed to obtain reasonable glycemic control differs substantially between dogs.

Dose requirements to achieve reasonable glycemic control in an uncomplicated diabetic dog differ according to the type of insulin used (Table 38.12). When the insulin requirements exceed 1-1.5 U/kg, concurrent diseases or technical problems with insulin administration should be considered (Table 38.11).

Interday and intraday glycemic variability

In diabetic dogs, serial BGCs show significant day-to-day variability. In one study, significant differences in BG measurements were noted on 2 consecutive days when insulin dose and meals were kept constant. An

TABLE 38.11 Suggested protocol for re-evaluating insulin-resistant diabetic dogs (receiving >1.5 U/kg per dose but still showing clinical signs and unintended weight loss) and dogs with glycemic variability.*

1	**Rule out client and insulin-handling issues first** ■ Observe client's administration and handling of insulin, including type of syringes used. ■ Assess insulin product and replace if out of date or if the appearance of the insulin changes (i.e., becomes flocculent, discolored, or, in the case of glargine or detemir, cloudy).
2	**Review diet and weight loss plan**
3	**Rule out concurrent medications that could cause insulin resistance, such as glucocorticoids, cyclosporine, and progestins (of note, specifically ask owners about steroid-containing eye and ear drops and progestins that might be transferred from an owner via medicated cream used as hormone replacement therapy in women)** ■ If the concurrent medication can be discontinued, the patient should be reassessed 2 weeks later. ■ If the comedication cannot be discontinued within 2 weeks, the insulin dose may need to be increased.
4	**Rule out concurrent disease/conditions.** ■ Repeat a physical exam (specifically, evaluate the teeth and gums for dental disease; ovariohysterectomies must be performed in intact, diabetic female dogs). ■ Perform baseline laboratory testing (CBC, serum biochemistry, and urinalysis with culture, blood pressure, UPC). ■ Consider second-level diagnostics, such as abdominal and thoracic radiographs, abdominal ultrasound, species-specific pancreatic lipase immunoreactivity (specPLI), trypsin-like immunoreactivity (TLI), B_{12}/folate. ■ Consider specific diagnostics for hypercortisolism. ■ If the cause of insulin resistance is identified, the clinician should focus on resolving and treating that cause, then return to regulating the diabetes mellitus.
5	**If the patient has never been regulated and has only been administered one type of insulin thus far, consider switching insulin type (this may be attempted prior to considering second-level diagnostics, based on clinician preference).**

*The recommendation was published in the 2018 AAHA diabetes management guidelines for dogs and cats[57] and was slightly amended by the author.

TABLE 38.12 Dose requirements (U/kg) expressed as mean ± standard deviation or median (range) to achieve a good glycemic control in uncomplicated diabetic dogs.

NPH (U/kg/q12h)	Lente (U/kg/q12h)	Detemir (U/kg/q12h)	PZI (U/kg/q12h)	PZI (U/kg/q24h)	Glargine 100 U/mL (U/kg/q12h)	Glargine 300 U/mL (U/kg/q24h)
0.49±0.14[75]	0.61±0.14[75]	0.12 (0.05-0.34)[76]	0.75 (0.28-1.40)[77] 1.0 (0.4-1.5)[78]	1.09 (0.43–2.18)[77]	0.6 (0.11-1.07)[90] 0.5 (0.32-0.67)[91]	1.93 (0.2-5)*

NPH: neutral protamine Hagedorn; PZI: U-40 human recombinant protamine zinc insulin. * Internal data obtained on 100 cases

opposite or different but not opposite theoretical recommendation for adjustment of the dog's insulin dose on day 2, compared with day 1, was made on 27% and 17% of occasions, respectively.[85] In this study, day-to-day variability of serial BGCs was seen in a hospital environment with the same disadvantages as discussed before, although special attention was paid to keeping the amount of food constant each day.[72] A recent study looked at this aspect in a home environment using the FreeStyle Libre® flash glucose monitoring system.[71] When analyzing subsequent days, home-home, FreeStyle Libre® recorded interstitial glucose curves, an almost absent concordance was identified. Therefore, it seems that the reproducibility of the glucose curves produced at home is not better than that produced in a hospital environment, and this highlights the importance of performing and analyzing serial BGCs before making specific treatment decisions. Between-day glycemic variability is also reported in 93% of human diabetic patients,[77] and possible causes are reported in Table 38.13.

In addition to the interday glycemic variability (GV), an intraday day GV exists. This is defined as intraday glycemic excursions, including episodes of hypoglycemia and hyperglycemia.[78]

TABLE 38.13 Causes of glycemic variability.

Factors that can be improved
- Poor owner compliance with insulin
- Poor owner compliance with dietary recommendations
- Application of interfering drugs (e.g., steroids)
- Other diseases (e.g., infection, pancreatitis, endocrinopathies, renal disease)
- Different levels of activity or stress

Intrinsic factors that cannot be identified
- Variable amount of residual β-cell function
- Variable sensitivity to insulin
- Variable insulin absorption and degradation
- Defective counterregulation
- Impaired gastric emptying

Adapted from Reusch CE, Salesov E. Monitoring diabetes in cats. In Feldman EC, Fracassi F, Peterson M (editors). Feline Endocrinology 1st edition. Milan, Edra, 2019, pp. 522-539.

Somogyi

Nowadays, it is believed that the Somogyi phenomenon is not a special entity, but part of the GV complex. Indeed, contrary to a historic veterinary dogma, in recent years, overwhelming evidence accumulated contradicting the existence of the "Somogyi effect". The Somogyi effect is defined as a rebound hyperglycemia following a hypoglycemic episode or a rapid decrease of BG concentration that evokes the release of diabetogenic hormones, especially epinephrine and glucagon, and direct hypoglycemia-induced stimulation of hepatic glycogenolysis. However, up to date, there is no evidence in dogs or other species that DM counterregulatory hormones are released excessively in response to hypoglycemia. Instead, the opposite is true: hypoglycemia counterregulatory responses are impaired in DM.[33]

Glycemic variability: prognostic significance and management

In people, GV is an indicator of glycemic control.[78] A high GV is considered to be a risk factor for hypoglycemia, microvascular complications, neuropathy, nephropathy, retinopathy, stroke, and all-cause mortality.[78] In dogs, GV has not been studied yet. However, because the mechanisms leading to impaired counterregulatory responses in dogs are largely the same as in people,[91] it would be reasonable to hypothesize that, as in people, increased GV in dogs would also lead to increased frequency of hypoglycemia in the long run.

In dogs with high intraday or interday GV, as a first step, it is recommended to check for compliance with insulin and dietary therapy as well as technical issues related to insulin (e.g., syringe size, outdated insulin). After that, the dog should be evaluated for the presence of concurrent disorders/conditions (Table 38.11). If no reason is identified, the insulin dose should be set to a level that avoids hypoglycemia as much as possible, even if it means experiencing phases of hyperglycemia. Another option is switching to an insulin formulation associated with a lower GV (e.g., degludec or glargine 300U/ml).[41]

Continuous glucose monitoring systems

In recent years, glucose monitoring has been revolutionized by the development of CGMSs, wearable non-/minimally-invasive devices that measure glucose concentration almost continuously for several consecutive days/weeks, mitigating the need for repeated venipuncture and significantly increasing information regarding glucose fluctuations and trends. The technical and practical aspects of the different types of CGMSs are discussed in chapter 21.

In human diabetics, the use of CGMSs is advantageous, improving glycemic control, reducing hypoglycemic episodes and GV, and improving patient quality of life.[79] In veterinary medicine, up to date, some studies have investigated the clinical utility of these devices for monitoring DM in dogs, and the results are promising.[71,80] The use of a flash glucose monitoring system (FGMS) allowed more accurate identification of the glucose nadirs (79% vs. 41%) and hypoglycemic episodes (60% vs. 9%) as compared to the use of a PBGM.[71] Furthermore, it allowed detailed identification of the glycemic excursions occurring throughout the day, such as postprandial hyperglycemia and circadian fluctuations in glucose concentrations.[80] Moreover, they allow the assessment of GV on consecutive days, enabling the clinician to make a more informed decision regarding the insulin dose, taking into account day-to-day variations in glycemic control.[71]

These systems are nowadays used with increasing frequency to monitor canine diabetic patients and seem to offer a solution to the problem of interpreting a classical 12-hour-BGC and avoiding serial venipuncture. Fig. 38.10 shows a comparison between hypothetical BGC and CGMS-derived data. It is evident that BGCs, due to the low sampling frequency, fail to give a complete BG concentration profile and, therefore, cannot reveal all critical episodes occurring throughout the day. Moreover, BGCs are unable to detect glucose variability observed over several days.[5,6]

Up to date, the Abbott FreeStyle Libre® flash glucose monitoring system is the most commonly used CGMS. In the author's institution, the use of FreeStyle Libre® has nowadays replaced the use of BGCs for monitoring almost all diabetic patients. The sensor is easily placed, even in less cooperative patients, and is generally as affordable as a BGC, with significantly more useable information. The FreeStyle Libre® sensors can be purchased from a veterinary distributor, from a human pharmacy, or the official website. Owners should be aware that sensors do not always stay functional and attached for 14 days, but the information gained from even a few days of use is usually more helpful than a single BGC. It is advisable to apply the FreeStyle Libre® continuously from the time DM is diagnosed until stabilization is reached (the patient no longer shows clinical signs, body weight is stable and in the ideal range, and glucose values are between 80-250 mg/dL (4.4-13.9 mmol/L)

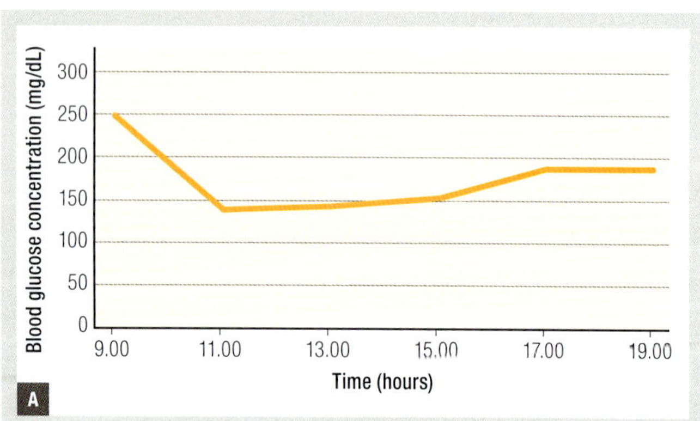

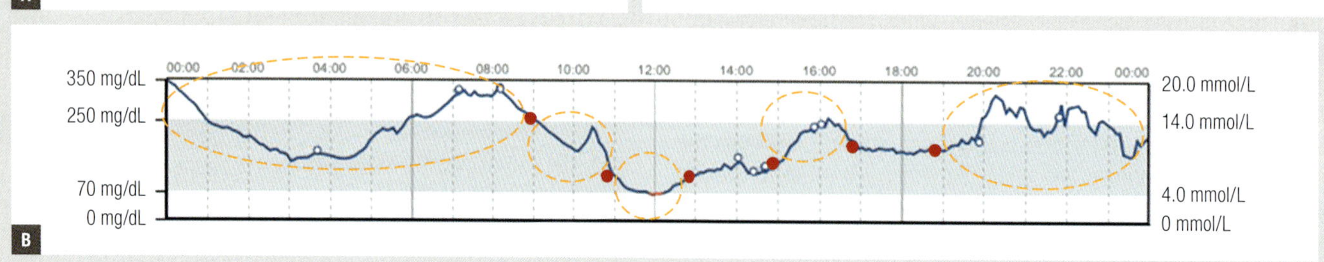

FIG. 38.10 Representative glucose monitoring data obtainable with intermittent measurements of blood glucose using a portable blood glucose meter (PBGM) (**A**) and red circles in (**B**) and using a continuous glucose monitoring system (CGMS)—blue line in (**B**). (**B**) Dotted circles denote glucose excursions which, using only intermittent PBGM measurements, are not detectable. BGC, blood glucose curve.

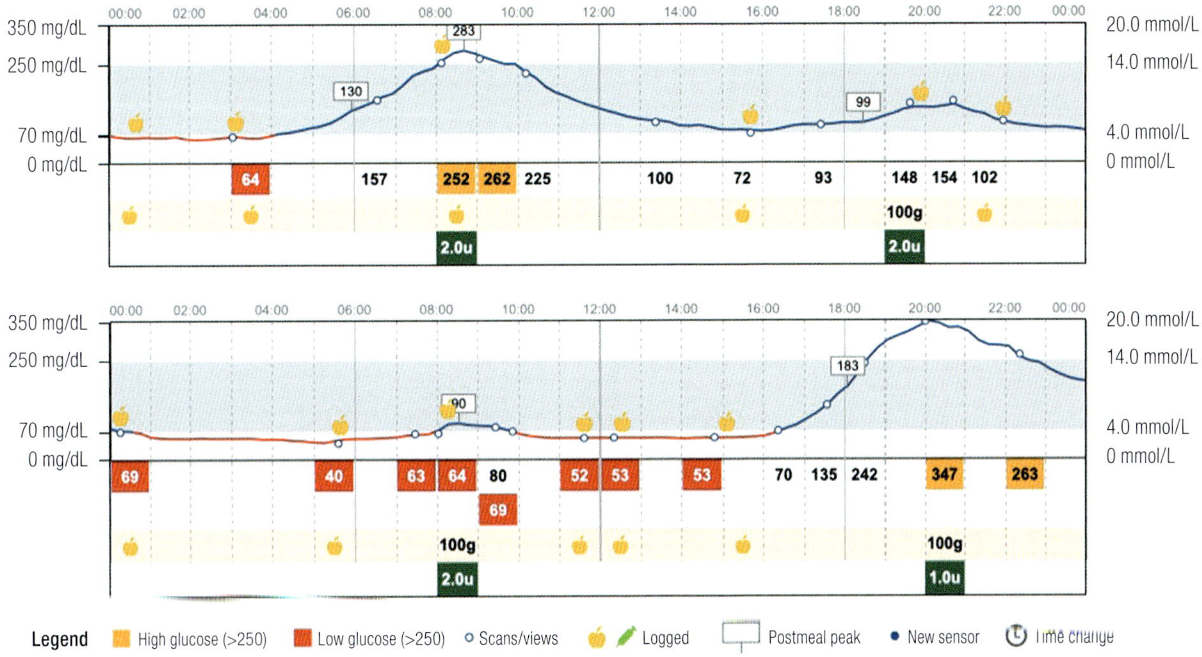

FIG. 38.11 Daily log report displayed when the data from the Freestyle Libre reader is downloaded to a computer or data automatically uploaded to the LibreView system when the sensor is scanned using the FreeStyle LibreLink app. Interstitial glucose (IG) fluctuations during 24-hour periods are depicted. The IG values detected by the scans are reported as numbers and are identified by the empty circles. The red box highlights the IG values <70 mg/dL (<3.9 mmol/L) while the yellow box highlights IG values >350 mg/dL (19.4 mmol/L). Using the reader or the mobile app, there is the possibility of adding notes to track food (yellow apple), insulin administration (green box), exercise and other events (not shown in this figure).

(Table 38.10). Once the dog has been stabilized, the device can be applied continuously or once every 2-3 months or whenever the dog shows any symptoms attributable to hyperglycemia or hypoglycemia. One of the main advantages of using such a device is that by allowing the patient to be monitored continuously, the insulin dose can be safely modified in a shorter time (every 1-3 days), mainly if an insulin analog is used (see Insulin therapy and other treatment options section). Therefore, the stabilization of the patient might be achieved more quickly, although, to date, no studies have supported this claim.

The author recommends the routine use of the LibreView System (see chapter 21, video 21.1 and the following website https://pro.libreview.io/articles/qsg for more specifications) to access patient glucose information from anywhere with an internet connection. Data from a compatible mobile app can automatically upload to LibreView if there is an internet connection. Alternatively, if the owner uses the reader to obtain glucose data, this can be uploaded on the LibreView system using the corresponding cable. Once the data is associated with a patient, it can be viewed anytime from the patient's profile by going to "glucose history" and clicking "glucose reports". Among the available glucose reports the "daily log", displaying IG fluctuations during 24-hour periods, is the most useful for making therapeutic decisions (Fig. 38.11).

Some case examples highlighting the clinical utility of FGMSs are reported in Fig. 38.12 and Fig. 38.13.

One drawback that authors have encountered when using the FGMS is that some owners become stressed with glycemic control (Fig. 38.14). A recent study has investigated the impact of FGMS on pet owners' quality of life and the satisfaction related to its usability using an online survey.[81] This study reports that the use of CGM increased anxiety in 12% of owners. In contrast, 88% of the owners reported a greater sense of control (88%) of the disease. The majority of diabetic pet owners considered the FGMS easier to use, and both less stressful, and painful for the animal, allowing them to obtain more glucose data with less effort as compared to BGCs. Overall, 92% of owners reported that the glycemic control of their pet was better when using an FGMS. The most challenging aspects of using the FGMS were ensuring proper sensor fixation during the wearing period, preventing premature detachment, and purchasing the sensor. Moreover, approximately a third of the owners reported that the device cost was difficult to afford in the long term.[81]

Urine glucose measurement

Glucose is freely filtered by the glomerulus and reabsorbed in the proximal tubules by the sodium-glucose-co-transporter 2 (SGLT2) up to the renal threshold, which is approximately 200 mg/dL (11.1 mmol/L) in dogs. The higher the BG, the more glucose is present in the urine, which would theoretically render urine testing a valuable monitoring tool. However, monitoring urine glucose can be misleading for several reasons:

- The test is semiquantitative.
- It does not reflect the BG concentration at any given time, since the bladder stores urine.
- A negative test does not differentiate between hypo-, normo- or mild hyperglycemia.
- A positive test does not differentiate between moderate and poor diabetic control and it does not exclude periods of hypoglycemia.
- Hydration status and urine concentration may affect the result. Therefore, relying solely on urine glucose monitoring to adjust the insulin dose is not recommended.

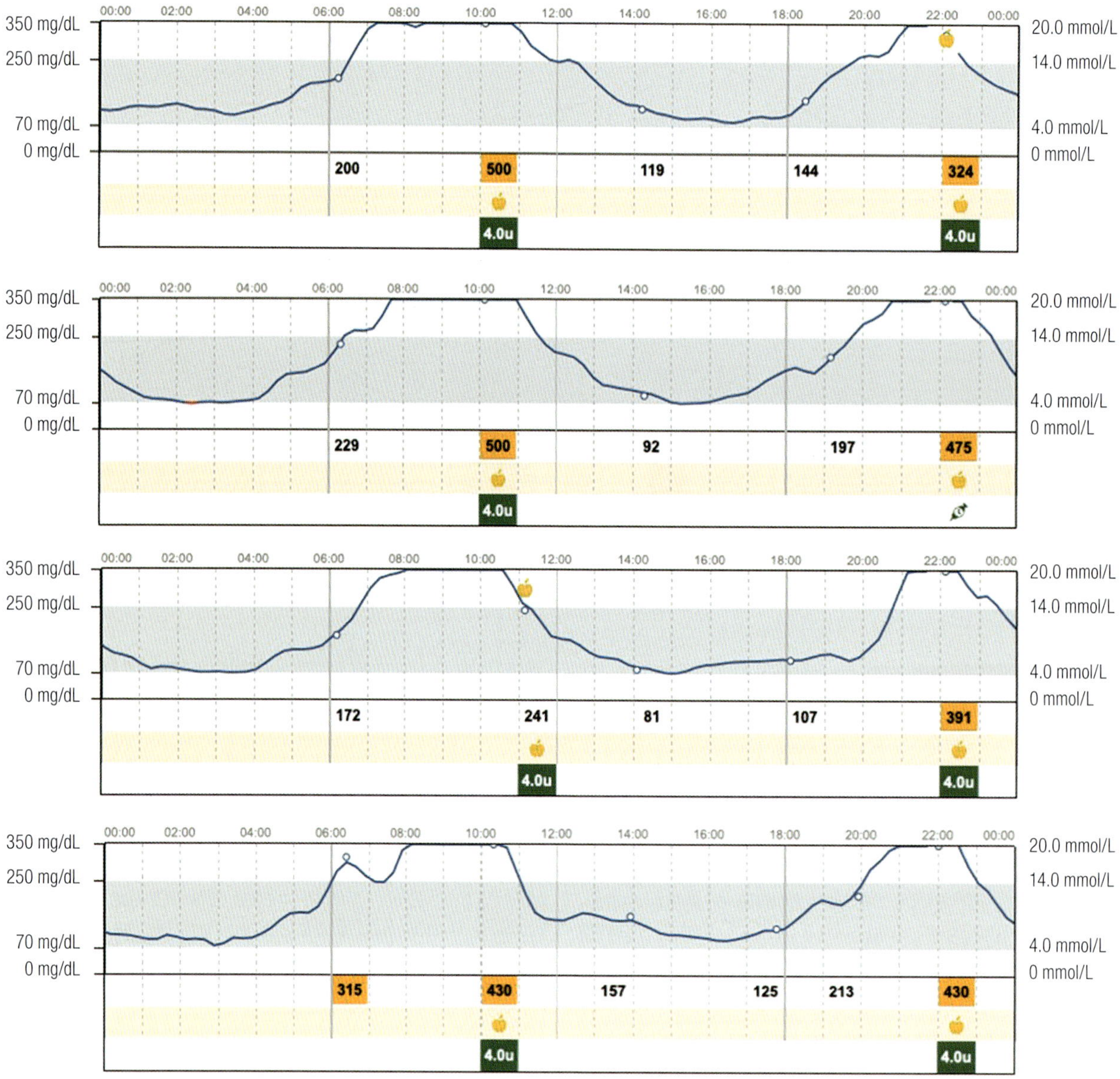

FIG. 38.12 Examples of one dog with no interday glucose variability (GV). The dog received porcine lente insulin (0.5 U/kg) and was fed a commercial diabetic diet twice daily.

Glycated proteins

Fructosamine

Fructosamine is formed by nonenzymatic, irreversible binding of glucose to amino groups of plasma proteins, mainly albumin. Its concentration depends on the BG concentration and the half-life of plasma proteins. As such, fructosamine reflects the mean BG concentration over the previous 1 to 2 weeks and is not affected by acute changes in BG concentration as occurs with stress or excitement. Fructosamine is usually measured on serum by an automated colorimetric assay using nitroblue tetrazolium chloride. The reference interval is approximately between 200 to 360 µmol/L but can differ slightly from laboratories. Therefore, it is advisable to use always the same laboratory. A linear relationship exists between serum total proteins, albumin, and fructosamine concentration. Hypoproteinemia and hypoalbuminemia can lead to a decrease in serum fructosamine concentration.[82] Furthermore, a decrease in serum fructosamine concentrations has been observed in cases of hyperlipidemia, azotemia, and hemolysis.[82] With some assays, hypertriglyceridemia/hyperlipidemia can also cause higher-than-expected high serum fructosamine concentration (personal communication). Conversely, an elevation in serum fructosamine concentration beyond the reference range has been demonstrated in dogs with hyperglobulinemia and dogs with naturally acquired hypothyroidism.[83,84] In most newly diagnosed diabetic dogs, fructosamine concentration ranged from 320 to 850 µmol/L, but some may reach values >1.500 µmol/L. The interpretation of fructosamine in diabetic-treated dogs should consider that most well-controlled diabetic dogs are slightly hyperglycemic for some hours throughout the day and, therefore, fructosamine will usually not be in the reference interval. Values in the reference interval (especially

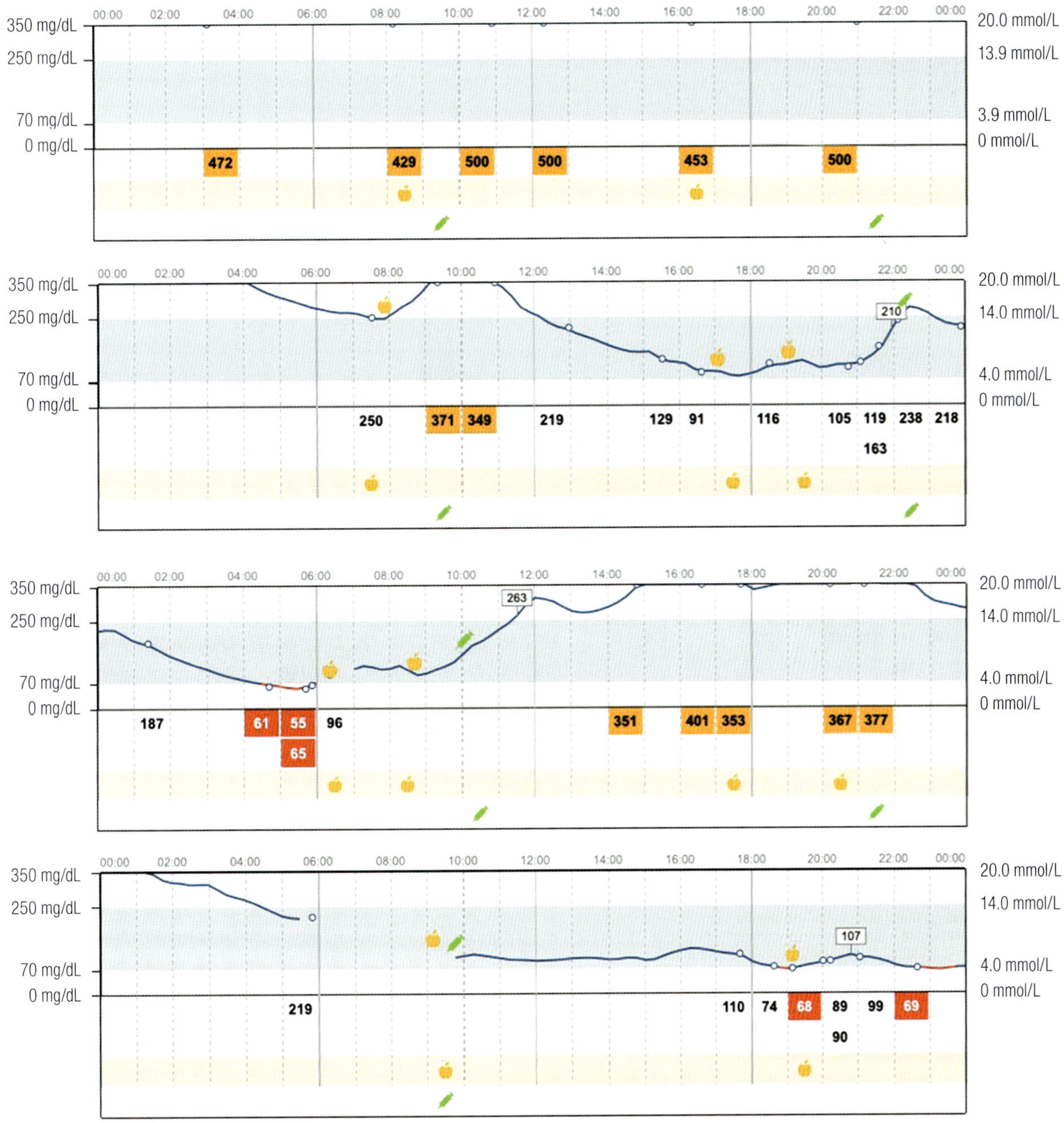

FIG. 38.13 Examples of one dog with marked interday GV. The dog received porcine lente insulin (0.8 U/kg) and was fed a commercial diabetic diet twice daily. A marked difference between interstitial glucose (IG) on 4 consecutive days is evident. On day 1, the IG was above 350 mg/dL for all the day. On day 2, the IG was within the ideal range for the major part of the day-time; vice versa, the IG was above 350 mg/dL (19.4 mmol/L) for most of the night-time. On day 3, an opposite IG trend is evident and low IG values were recorded between 4 a.m. and 6 a.m. Finally, on day 4, the IG was below the ideal range for the major part of the day-time. This highlights the importance of not considering the IG profile for only one day when making therapeutic decisions. Instead, it is recommended to consider the IG traces of several consecutive days before deciding to change the insulin dose.

in the lower half) suggest prolonged hypoglycemia. In this case, BGC or application of a CGMS should be considered.

Some authors have suggested the use of fructosamine to clarify discrepancies between the medical history, physical examination findings, and results of the BGC, and they propose specific cutoffs for differentiation of various degrees of diabetic control.[99] However, these unreferenced recommendations (e.g., 350-400 μmol/L = excellent control, 400-450 μmol/L = good control, 450-500 μmol/L = fair control, >500 μmol/L = poor control)[99] are imprecise and lack evidence of usefulness.[25-27] All studies so far found a substantial overlap of fructosamine concentrations between dogs with good, moderate, and poor or between good and poor control.[86,88] Based on these results, the cutoff values have an unproven clinical usefulness and fructosamine measurement cannot replace repeated glucose measurements and should not be used alone to guide insulin dose adjustments. Rather, it is advisable to monitor individual canine patients based on their previous values: increasing fructosamine in an individual dog usually indicates an increase in overall BG concentration and vice versa.

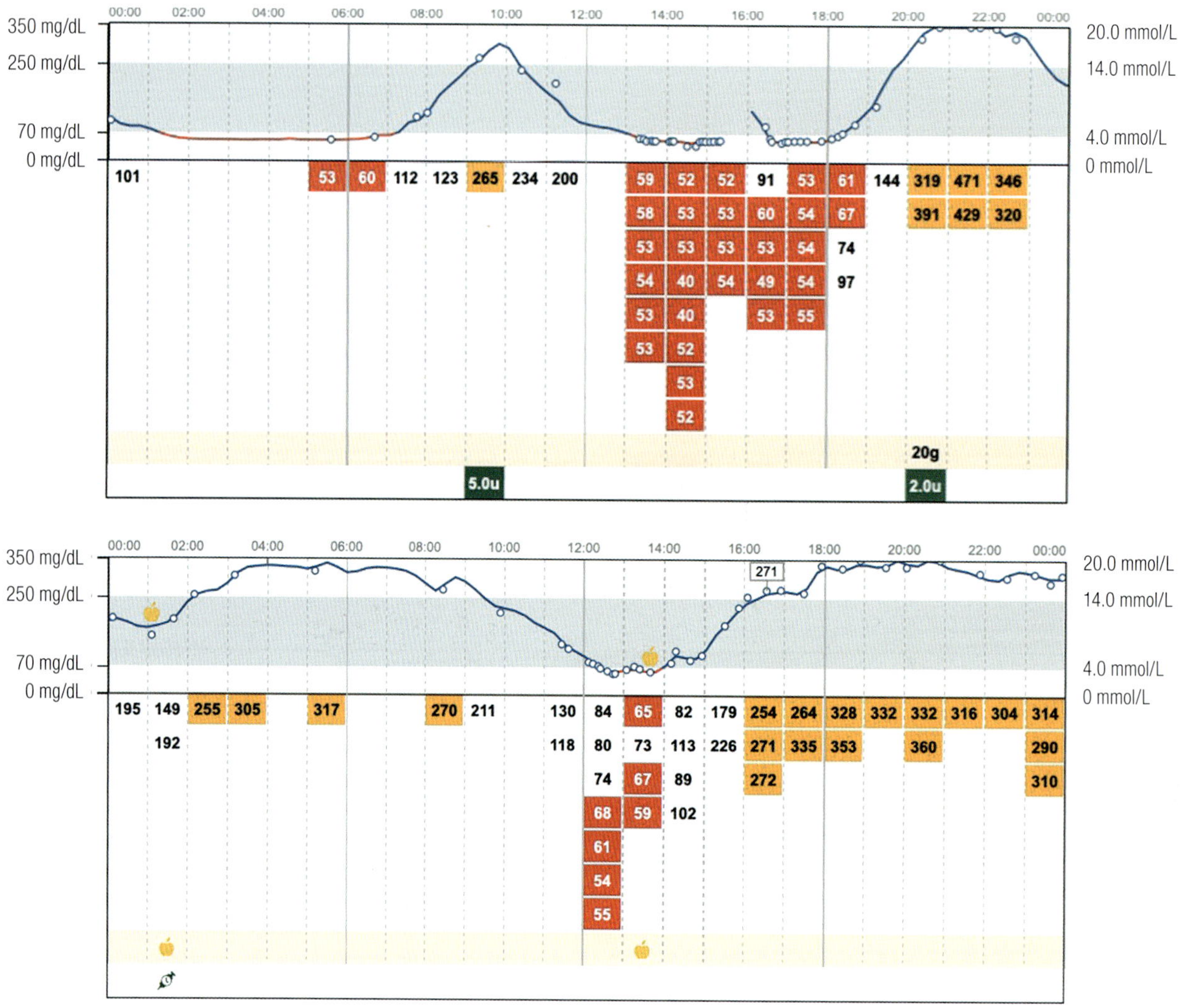

FIG. 38.14 Daily log report of a diabetic dog on porcine lente insulin. The number of individual scans (reported as numbers and identified by empty circles) that this diabetic pet owner performed daily, even during the night hours, should be noted.

Glycated hemoglobin

Glycated hemoglobin (GlyHb) is a glycated protein resulting from the irreversible, nonenzymatic binding of glucose to hemoglobin in erythrocytes. The extent of hemoglobin glycosylation depends on the erythrocytes' lifespan, erythrocytes' permeability to glucose, and the average BG concentration during the circulating lifespan of erythrocytes.[89] Consequently, in dogs, GlyHb reflects the average BG concentration over the preceding 2-3 months.[89] GlyHb is measured in whole blood collected in ethylenediaminetetraacetic acid (EDTA). Several methods have been implemented to determine GlyHb in dogs.[90-98] However, to date, no consensus gold standard has been defined. Thus, the routine use of GlyHb assays in clinical practice has not been adequately established. The reference interval differs considerably according to the method used, and it is therefore essential to refer to a laboratory that uses a GlyHb assay validated for use in the dog and established an internal reference interval. Any condition that affects the erythrocytes' lifespan can influence GlyHb concentration. In particular, GlyHb decreases in pathological conditions that shorten erythrocyte lifespan or are associated with increased erythrocyte turnover (e.g., blood loss anemia, hemolytic anemia).[99] In contrast, falsely increased GlyHb values might occur under conditions that prolong erythrocyte lifespan or are associated with decreased erythrocyte turnover (e.g., iron deficiency anemia).[99] Moreover, falsely elevated GlyHb values attributable to interference with the assay have been described in patients with extreme hypertriglyceridemia and hyperbilirubinemia.[99,100] GlyHb has been established as a highly specific and reliable biomarker for long-term control of both type 1 and type 2 diabetes mellitus.[101] Moreover, GlyHb is also used prognostically with increasing values corresponding to an increased risk of diabetic complications.[101]

In dogs, the clinical utility of GlyHb in classifying glycemic control has been investigated in a few studies.[86,88,92] GlyHb differs significantly between categories of clinical control, but there is substantial overlap among groups. As for SF, recent studies revealed that GlyHb is not accurate in classifying glycemic control,[86,88] and the use of the specific cutoffs provided by some authors[85] and commercial laboratories is not recommended. Rather, it is best to evaluate the trend in the individual patient. Up to date, no advantages have been demonstrated in using GlyHb instead of SF for monitoring dogs with DM.[86,88]

The unstable diabetic

Diego Miceli

The unstable diabetic is one of the most complex issues in the management of canine DM. Though a consensus regarding the terminology is yet to be reached, diabetic instability could be defined as a state of "uncontrollable" DM during insulin therapy, characterized by persistent difficulties in glycemic control or treatment goals achievement. This state is potentially reversible; however, in some cases, it may be permanent, and is associated with multiple patient, owner and management factors. Diabetic instability can also be defined in terms of a marked increase in GV. This emerging metric considers fluctuations in glucose levels or other glucose homeostasis-related parameters over a given period of time and has been associated with adverse outcomes in humans.[102]

The concept of "unstable diabetic" is often confused or overused due to the expectations of the clinicians/owners, which can be highly variable and, in some cases, overly ambitious. It is recommended to pursue agreed treatment goals for canine diabetology: minimal or no clinical signs of DM, good quality of life of the dog and the owner, body condition score normalization, and avoidance of diabetic ketoacidosis (DKA) and hypoglycemia.[7] Likewise, reasonable goals for each specific clinical situation should always be considered (e.g., glycemic targets tailored for each dog and owner's possibilities).

The causes of instability in dogs are numerous and can be categorized into two groups: management-related and insulin resistance (IR)-related. These causes may entail consistent day-to-day glycemic fluctuations or dramatic increases in insulin requirements. Besides, it is essential to highlight that the presence of comorbidities and failure to achieve adequate diabetic control are triggers for euthanasia of dogs with DM; therefore, it is of central importance to identify the cause of instability and, to the extent possible, approach them in a way that achieves treatment goals and avoids these unfortunate outcomes.[57]

Management factors

The umbrella term "management factors" includes instability causes both related to owner education and case management (Table 38.14). At first glance, management factors could create a scenario of apparent IR, while these are not causes of "true" IR. Failure to achieve glycemic control in dogs is usually associated with management, mainly owner-related. This could be prevented if clinicians provide owners with the appropriate theoretical/practical resources.

Owner education

Insulin storage and handling

Insulin preparations may denature and lose effectiveness if they are incorrectly stored (heated or frozen), expired, diluted, incompletely mixed, or vigorously shaken. It is recommended to store insulin in the fridge at 2-8°C (not in the freezer). If insulin is to be used within 4 to 6 weeks (depending on the type of insulin) and at room temperature (2-25°C), it can be stored outside the fridge. It is also recommended to protect insulin from sunlight and vibrations. Insulin dilutions are practical for small dogs, yet may exert unpredictable effects. Some insulin preparations require resuspension prior to administration, but this should be done carefully, avoiding vigorous shaking (except for porcine lente insulin).

Insulin administration

Several problems concerning insulin administration commonly arise in the early phase of insulin therapy: owners are often inexperienced, concerned, or scared, and may make various mistakes that lead to the incorrect administration of the indicated insulin dose, which results in under- or overdosing.

Problems with insulin administration may be related to the use of syringes that are inadequate for the concentration of insulin (40-100 IU/mL). It is recommended to employ a type of syringe that matches the insulin preparation used. Errors may also occur when switching from pen to syringe, using a new type of syringe, or changing the person administering the injection. Likewise, problems may be related to a poor injection technique: applications outside the subcutaneous tissue (e.g., hair or intradermal), inability to properly restrain the dog, or repetition of the injection site. Errors while drawing up insulin may also arise when owners have visual/motor difficulties, when drawing up air instead of insulin from the vial, or when discarding insulin prior to injection.

Many of these problems can be solved by administering the injections with pens. Several studies, most of them performed in humans, have shown the advantages of using insulin-dosing pens instead of vial-syringe, including better dosing accuracy/precision, hypoglycemic events reduction, increased adherence, and overall health care cost-saving.[103]

TABLE 38.14 Management factors that may potentially result in instability in diabetic dogs

Owner education	Case management
Insulin storage and handling ■ Expired solutions ■ Incorrect storage (heated or frozen) ■ Diluted preparations ■ Improper resuspension (incomplete or vigorous mixing)	**Insulin regimen** ■ Unsuitable type of insulin for the case ■ Inappropriate insulin dose (under-/overdosing) ■ Short/prolonged duration of insulin effect ■ Poor/variable insulin absorption
Insulin administration ■ Poor injection technique ■ Incorrect use of syringes ■ Inappropriate syringe type ■ Variable doses of insulin drawn up ■ Repetition of injection site	**Diet and exercise** ■ Inappropriate diet (composition and/or caloric content) ■ Switching diet types ■ Over-/underfeeding ■ Inconsistent exercise regimen
Owner compliance ■ Poor adherence to treatment/monitoring ■ Lack of treatment/monitoring persistence ■ Failure to adhere to a consistent regimen (insulin, diet and exercise)	**Monitoring** ■ Poor monitoring ■ Improper interpretation of monitoring

Owner compliance

Poor owner compliance represents a common obstacle to the achievement of glycemic control, not only due to lack of adherence to treatment and monitoring, but also failure to maintain it over time. Compliance issues can vary widely and include failure to adhere to a consistent regimen (variable timing of injections, feeding, or exercise), noncompliance with indications (e.g., ovariohysterectomy), poor monitoring and/or follow-up, among others. The most frequent compliance issues include adherence to feeding protocols and injection difficulties.[57,103]

The owners' quality of life is negatively affected following their dogs' diagnosis of DM. Approximately 10% of diabetic dogs are euthanized at diagnosis and 10% within a year due to lack of success or compliance.[57] Considering these factors, it would be ideal to reach an acceptable balance between treatment goals and the owner's possibilities. It is recommended to be flexible, assess each scenario individually, and propose owner-focused treatment and monitoring approaches. Likewise, owners should know that adherence to insulin therapy, even in a minimalist owner-focused approach, is critical for the survival of their dogs, and that adherence to a consistent daily regimen is recommended to achieve therapeutic success.[104]

Case management

Insulin regimen

Insulin type

The response to insulin therapy can often be unpredictable, and one type of insulin is not necessarily suitable for all cases. It should also be emphasized that no insulin formulation is "the best" by definition. Therefore, the choice of the type of insulin will depend mainly on each specific clinical situation (cause of DM, comorbidities, insulin pharmacology, cost, prescribing regulations, dog/owner compliance, diet, monitoring strategy, and treatment goals).[103,104]

Insulin suspensions (NPH, lente, and PZI) and insulin solutions (glargine, detemir, and degludec) exhibit several differences. In cases that need increased therapy predictability, insulin solutions are preferred over insulin suspensions because they are associated with less day-to-day variability.[103] Insulin detemir is not recommended for dogs <10 kg, unless they have IR.[104] If basal insulin (constant action throughout the day and low day-to-day variability) is required, insulin glargine U300 and insulin degludec are currently the preferred options.[104] Likewise, in basal-bolus protocols, the use of bolus with intermediate-acting insulin formulations is recommended.[104] It is also necessary to be aware of the fact that glycemic targets are different according to the type of insulin used.[103,104]

Insulin dose

Insulin dosing is a key factor in the management of DM in general, but especially in unstable DM. A fundamental principle of insulin therapy is that the dose should be safe to avoid complications and effective in controlling the diabetic condition (and sustainable).[103]

On the one hand, insulin underdosing may occur due to fear of hypoglycemia, inadequate monitoring, or the wrong assumption that "maximum doses" are excessive for a certain body weight.

On the other hand, there is the possibility of insulin overdosing. One of the effects traditionally described is the development of insulin-induced hyperglycemia (Somogyi overswing). Exceedingly high doses of insulin could generate an abrupt drop in glycemia, in which case the dog would theoretically react with a "rebound effect" with markedly increased glycemia (Fig. 38.15). This phenomenon occurs due to the effect of counterregulatory hormones (glucagon, cortisol, and adrenaline). However, in recent years, the veracity of this phenomenon has been questioned, as there is no consistent evidence for the "Somogyi effect" in dogs.[33] Another possibility is the development of insulin-induced hypoglycemia. Diabetic dogs show diminished sympathetic innervation to pancreatic islets, which may alter the counterregulatory response to hypoglycemia.[33] This event could promote glycemic instability, since the regulatory response to hypoglycemia is impaired. Episodes of subclinical insulin-induced hypoglycemia lower the threshold for sympathoadrenal defenses and increase the risk of future iatrogenic hypoglycemia. According to this paradigm, hypoglycemia begets hypoglycemia, not hyperglycemia (Fig. 38.15).[33]

Continuous glucose monitoring systems (CGMSs) are recommended to identify problems with insulin dosing, as blood glucose curves (BGC) can yield variable results and underestimate episodes of hypoglycemia.[102]

Insulin administration frequency

The use of intermediate-acting insulins in once-daily protocols may be problematic due to the shortened duration of insulin action. In these cases, dogs usually present clinical signs of DM in the latter part of the interinjection period. These fluctuation issues can be detected by using a CGMS or, if not available, performing a BGC. This short action could be compensated for by increasing insulin dose or switching to twice-daily or three times daily treatments. If the dose of intermediate-acting insulin suspensions (PZI and lente, but not NPH) is increased, an acceptable clinical control could be achieved, but with a concomitant increase in the risk of hypoglycemia.[104] Other options include switching to basal insulins or basal-bolus treatment.

For its part, the use of intermediate-acting insulins in twice-daily protocols may result in a prolonged duration of insulin effect (>12 hours). Decreasing the insulin dose or switching to a longer-acting insulin (e.g., basal insulin) given once daily could be a suitable option.

Insulin activity

Poor or variable insulin absorption and autoinsulin antibodies (AIAs) may entail inadequate insulin activity. Injections in scar tissue or areas with excessive adipose tissue (poorly perfused), or repeating the application site

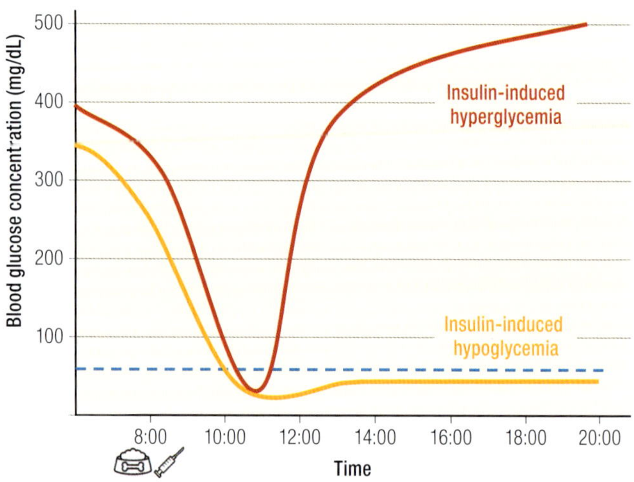

FIG. 38.15 Overdosing of insulin. Red line: insulin-induced hyperglycemia caused by the rebound effect (Somogyi overswing). Yellow line: insulin-induced hypoglycemia caused by the impairment of the counterregulatory response to hypoglycemia.

(with potential local inflammation) could lead to poor insulin absorption. Rotating the injection site daily is recommended, preferring lean areas if possible. Likewise, insulin absorption can be highly variable depending on the type of insulin used. In the case of insulin suspensions, the deprecipitation in the injection site could be unpredictable, leading to marked variations in insulin absorption.[103]

AIAs were described as a potential cause of IR in dogs. AIAs are present mainly in dogs treated with heterologous insulin (e.g., bovine insulin), but also in dogs treated with homologous insulin (porcine insulin) and, to a lesser extent, in dogs with newly diagnosed DM.[103] However, the clinical implications of these AIAs are currently unknown and there is no evidence of their interference with glycemic control. In fact, dogs are routinely treated with human-recombinant insulin with successful results.[103]

Dietary management and exercise

Poor adherence to a consistent diet and exercise regimen may promote instability. Problems can arise if owners use diets that are inappropriate for diabetic dogs (inadequate composition and caloric content), switch diet types, change feeding schedules, offer treats, over or underfeed their dogs, among others. It is generally recommended that the feeding time coincides with the time of insulin injection (except for basal insulin). It is important to mention that there is considerable day-to-day and interdog variability of dietary carbohydrate absorption, which may lead to incongruities between required and delivered insulin (particularly with intermediate-acting insulin) and result in fluctuations in glycemia.

Another hurdle in the dietary management of diabetic dogs is inappetence ("finicky eaters"), which entails difficulties in glycemic control and injection decisions. The concurrence of pancreatitis, gastrointestinal disease, or other conditions can affect appetite. In these cases, the basal-bolus protocol could be indicated: basal insulin administration is maintained, and the bolus insulin is skipped if the dog has decreased appetite.[103]

On the other hand, regimens with changing or lack of physical activity can cause instability in diabetic dogs, especially if the owners are not consistent with the daily regimen and are not strict with monitoring and the time of day for physical activity. It is common for owners not to exercise their dogs during the week and take them for long walks on weekends or holidays.

Monitoring

Adequate monitoring is helpful not only in achieving treatment goals but also in identifying whether the dog presents instability. Ideally, complete monitoring should include an integrated assessment of the owners' daily perception, regular glucose measurements, physical examination, and routine workup, including blood glycated proteins and lipid profile. Diabetic instability could be associated with poor monitoring, especially if owners are not good observers, do not perform glucose measurements and/or do not attend prescribed follow-ups.

In addition, proper interpretation of monitoring is decisive in identifying and controlling the unstable diabetic. Regular glucose monitoring is essential to successfully achieving treatment goals.[102] Each monitoring method has its advantages and disadvantages. Using single glycemia measurements is not an appropriate method in these cases, because a single time point does not represent the trend throughout the day. BGCs are useful to monitor blood glucose concentrations throughout the day but have several limitations (e.g., considerable variability). CGMSs are nowadays a widespread and accurate tool for diabetic dogs, with plenty of advantages over BGC.[102] GV is best appreciated using CGMSs.[102]

Causes of insulin resistance

Several comorbidities, physiological states with hormonal antagonism, and diabetogenic drugs could promote diverse IR states, thus resulting in diabetic instability (Table 38.15).[105] IR is characterized by varying degrees of interference of insulin action on target cells. This term is not defined by the exogenous insulin dose required or the glycemic response following insulin injection. However, when a high insulin dose is required to achieve glycemic control, IR should be considered, among other causes.[7] Treatment strategies should target the cause of IR and appropriately adjust insulin therapy.

Comorbidities

Endocrine conditions

Hypercortisolism

Glucocorticoids antagonize several physiological effects of insulin, potentially contributing to IR and DM development. Dogs with hypercortisolism may present mild to moderate hyperglycemia, decreased insulin sensitivity, hyperinsulinism, and dyslipidemia, all of which are characteristics of "prediabetes". Dogs with hypercortisolism that present fasting glycemia >100 mg/dL (>5.6 mmol/L), dyslipidemia, urinary cortisol creatinine ratio $>100 \times 10^{-6}$, pituitary-dependent hypercortisolism and noncastrated females are at high risk of developing DM.[106] It was reported that 5-22% of dogs with hypercortisolism had concurrent DM, whereas 23% of diabetic dogs had concurrent hypercortisolism.[106] Hypercortisolism is one of the most common causes of IR and is associated with the most severe cases of IR in diabetic dogs.[25,107]

Hypercortisolism diagnosis in unstable diabetic dogs is challenging. Firstly, early stage or mild cases of hypercortisolism do not always exhibit a typical clinical manifestation, and many clinical signs (PU/PD and polyphagia) and clinicopathological abnormalities are common to

TABLE 38.15 Causes of insulin resistance that may potentially result in instability in diabetic dogs

Comorbidities	Physiological states	Diabetogenic drugs
Endocrine conditions	Diestrus	Corticosteroids
Hypercortisolism	Pregnancy	Progestagens
Hypothyroidism		
Obesity		
Hypersomatotropism		
Dyslipidemia		
Glucagonoma		
Hypoadrenocorticism*		
Pheochromocytoma		
Nonendocrine conditions		
Inflammatory condition		
Infections		
Stress hyperglycemia		
Chronic kidney disease		
Hepatobiliary disease		
Cardiac disease		
Neoplasia		
Traumatic condition		

*Hypoadrenocorticism is not considered a cause of insulin resistance, yet it is a cause of diabetic instability.

both conditions. It is important to note that dogs with hypercortisolism show some abnormalities that are not seen in DM: abdominal distention, alopecia, thin skin, panting, calcinosis cutis, reproductive abnormalities, etc. (Fig. 38.16). Secondly, the hormonal test may have controversial results in dogs with hypercortisolism and concurrent DM. Though the ACTH-stimulation test and the low-dose dexamethasone suppression test can give false positive results in chronically stressed animals, these dynamic tests are recommended to confirm the diagnosis of hypercortisolism. A negative result is highly suggestive of the absence of hypercortisolism. A positive result should be interpreted cautiously. It is necessary to support the diagnosis of hypercortisolism with abdominal and/or intracranial diagnostic imaging. It is also relevant to consider that newly diagnosed diabetic dogs are often not stable. Therefore, it is recommended that the patient be stabilized and that the risk of DKA be avoided before performing hormonal tests.

The main therapeutic recommendation for this condition is to control the concurrent hypercortisolism. Mitotane treatment resulted in precipitous declines in insulin requirements in 8/11 cases.[108] Hypoglycemia was avoided by lowering the dosage of mitotane and supplementing with glucocorticoids. Trilostane treatment was evaluated in retrospective studies, and it was shown that fructosamine concentrations and insulin requirements do not consistently decrease, and may even increase, during trilostane treatment.[109,110] Hypophysectomy could resolve hypercortisolism and concurrent DM, leading to diabetic remission.

Insulin therapy may be difficult in diabetic dogs with hypercortisolism due to excessive postprandial hyperglycemia, short perceived duration of insulin action, and substantial GV.[25] In general, there is no need to reduce insulin dose after starting trilostane treatment; IR and GV seem to persist for a long time after successful control of hypercortisolism.[25] It is recommended to perform intensive glucose monitoring with CGMS to detect sudden changes in insulin requirements.

When dogs with hypercortisolism develop significant IR, the use of potent insulin formulations (e.g., insulin detemir) should be considered. Strategies to manage excess GV can also be tried, such as basal insulins or basal-bolus treatments.[25]

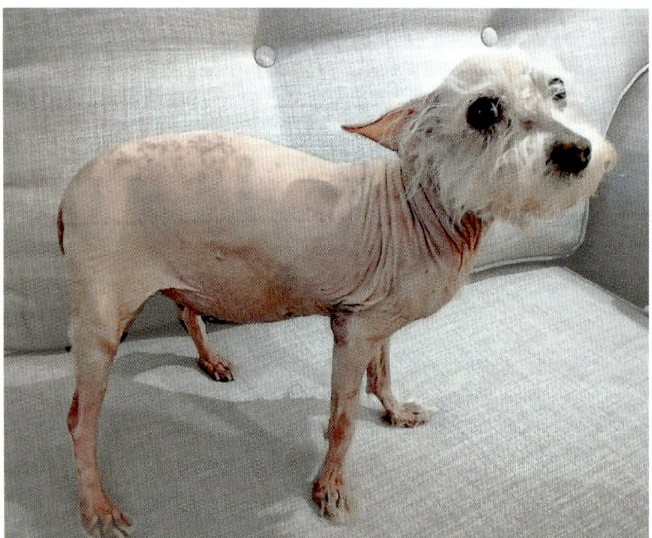

FIG. 38.16 A 9-year-old Poodle with DM and concurrent hypercortisolism. Note the alopecia, abdominal distension and thin skin, which are clinical signs not associated with DM.

Hypothyroidism

Canine hypothyroidism is commonly associated with marked IR. Hypothyroid dogs show reduced insulin sensitivity, but overall glucose tolerance is maintained by increased insulin secretion.[111] The cause of IR is presumed to be multifactorial. In hypothyroid dogs, IR is associated with obesity and increased serum leptin, growth hormone (GH) and IGF-1 concentrations.[111-113]

It has been reported that 1.5-10% of hypothyroid dogs have concurrent DM,[114,115] whereas 4% of diabetic dogs have concurrent hypothyroidism.[3] Concurrence of immune-mediated endocrine diseases, such as hypothyroidism, in diabetic dogs has been documented.[116] It is possible that these dogs' condition could be explained by a common immune-mediated etiology, similar to polyglandular autoimmune syndromes described in humans.

The diagnosis of hypothyroidism can be challenging in dogs with unstable diabetes, as some clinical signs (weakness, lethargy) and clinicopathological abnormalities are common to both conditions. It is important to note that hypothyroid dogs show some abnormalities that are not seen in DM: alopecia, "rat tail", tragic facial expression, etc. (Video 38.3). Ideally, the hormonal test should be performed once glycemic control has been achieved. Likewise, always consider the possibility of a nonthyroidal illness in a dog with unstable diabetes. It is also relevant to note that serum fructosamine should be interpreted cautiously in the hypothyroid dog, as it may be high due to a reduction in protein turnover.

Levothyroxine treatment reduces insulin requirements in diabetic dogs with hypothyroidism, since restoration of euthyroidism is associated with improvements in insulin sensitivity. Therefore, it is recommended that glucose concentrations be carefully monitored to adjust insulin dose accordingly.

Other endocrine conditions

Other potential endocrine causes of diabetic instability include obesity, dyslipidemia, hypersomatotropism, glucagonoma, hypoadrenocorticism, pheochromocytoma, honeymoon phase, juvenile-DM, insulinoma-DM cases, among others. Many of these causes are rare, and there is scarce information regarding them.

Obesity impairs insulin sensitivity in dogs, with the degree of IR positively correlated with adiposity severity.[25] Though some authors recognize obesity as DM-risk factor,[117] it does not necessarily result in overt DM because obese dogs compensate this state with hyperinsulinemia.[105] However, obesity may have a role in the etiology of pancreatitis. Also, it can have an additive effect on insulin requirements in diabetic dogs.[105]

Nonendocrine conditions

Many concurrent conditions can promote IR in diabetic dogs, probably by stimulating the secretion of diabetogenic or stress-related hormones. One study demonstrated an association between serum ketone concentrations and serum glucagon, cortisol, and norepinephrine concentrations

Video 38.3

A 6-year-old Labrador Retriever with DM and concurrent hypothyroidism. Note the dermatological abnormalities, which are clinical signs not associated with DM. Serum fructosamine concentration before and after levothyroxine supplementation was 670 and 313 µmol/L, respectively. Insulin requirements were consistently reduced after levothyroxine treatment.

in dogs with DM.[118] Theoretically, any focus of consistent inflammation or infection could potentially impair insulin sensitivity in dogs with DM.

Inflammation: exocrine pancreas disease

Pancreatitis and DM are two distinct and relatively common conditions in dogs that can occur concurrently. The prevalence of this concurrence is high, which might be related to shared risk factors or a causative relationship between both conditions. Although the relationship might be bidirectional, the most common direction of progression may be that DM occurs secondary to pancreatitis.[17]

Diabetic dogs with concurrent pancreatitis often show variable insulin requirements, and their stabilization can be challenging. Pancreatitis, whether acute or chronic, increases IR and is potentially associated with intermittent episodes of disease and risk of DKA, which complicates their dietary and insulin management.

The diagnosis of pancreatitis should consider a combination of history, physical examination, clinical signs, measurement of canine pancreatic lipase immunoreactivity and abdominal ultrasound. The appropriate identification and treatment of pancreatitis can make a relevant contribution to diabetic management; therefore, clinicians should be aware of this comorbidity. In hospitalized dogs, regular insulin (0.2 IU/kg) could be used every 2-4 hours, adjusting the requirements depending on glycemia and food eaten. In dogs that do not require hospitalization and present inappetence, the combination basal-bolus treatment may be indicated.[103]

Exocrine pancreatic insufficiency is another cause of instability in diabetic dogs, which can develop secondary to chronic pancreatitis.

Infections

Dogs with DM are at increased risk for urinary tract infections, probably due to glycosuria (substrate for bacterial growth) and decreased neutrophil adherence to antigens.[105] Other infections, such as dermatitis, otitis, pneumonia, dental disease and pyometra, have also been associated with IR in dogs.[105,119]

Other nonendocrine conditions

Other potential nonendocrine causes of diabetic instability include chronic kidney disease, stress hyperglycemia, hepatobiliary disease, inflammatory bowel disease, cardiac disease, neoplasia, traumatic conditions, among other diseases.[25,105]

Physiological states with hormonal antagonism: diestrus and pregnancy

The estrous cycle in female dogs includes a progesterone luteal phase of approximately 2 months. In dogs, progesterone stimulates GH hypersecretion from the mammary gland, substantially contributing to circulating GH concentration.[24] In some cases, this luteal phase may induce hypersomatotropism with physical changes compatible with acromegaly. The combined diabetogenic effect of progesterone and GH promotes DM during diestrus in susceptible bitches. Progesterone-induced hypersomatotropism is probably the most common cause of DM in populations in which female dogs are not routinely neutered.[25,58] This IR state can be worsened by pyometra or DKA.[58]

The mechanism whereby GH induces IR in dogs is not completely understood. Carnivores appear to be highly susceptible to the diabetogenic effects of GH.[24] In humans, excess GH promotes IR primarily through the stimulation of lipolysis and gluconeogenesis, and the inhibition of insulin signaling mediators.[120]

Luteal phase in dogs mimics pregnancy both in length and hormone pattern; however, pregnant dogs are more insulin resistant.[25,107] Despite the marked IR during pregnancy, DM is uncommon in bitches. In the few cases reported, difficulties in glycemic control, development of DKA, and death in puppies were described.[121]

The best treatment to control this type of DM is ovariohysterectomy. The chances of diabetic remission are presumably increased if surgery is performed as soon as possible after the diagnosis of DM. It has been described that approximately 9% of bitches achieve diabetic remission after ovariohysterectomy.[119] However, not all bitches undergo the surgical procedure during diestrus. Therefore, it is recommended to stabilize these dogs, increasing progressively the insulin dose according to the dog's requirements, and avoiding DKA. The use of potent insulins for dogs (e.g., detemir) should be evaluated in those cases. It is important to highlight that once the diestrus or pregnancy is over, insulin requirements may decrease substantially. Special attention should be paid to the monitoring and adjustment of insulin doses to avoid hypoglycemia. In some cases, diabetic remission could occur spontaneously at the end of diestrus.

In those cases in which ovariohysterectomy is not an option, a progesterone receptor antagonist (aglepristone) could be applicable.[122] Further studies of aglepristone in diabetic dogs are warranted.

Diabetogenic drugs

The two most renowned diabetogenic drugs in dogs are corticosteroids and progestogens; the mechanisms of action and metabolic consequences are the same as those mentioned above for naturally-occurring hypercortisolism and diestrus, respectively. Cyclosporin A, diazoxide, thiazide diuretics and β-adrenergic agonists could promote IR or the development of DM.[7,105]

Investigation of diabetic instability

Identifying and managing diabetic instability in dogs can be difficult and expensive, and requires time and good communication between the veterinary team and owners. The first step, and one of the most important ones, is to perform an exhaustive anamnesis. It should be determined whether the dog is unstable or not. Problems related to management factors can be assessed initially: clinicians should evaluate insulin handling and storage practices, injection technique, and all aspects of the treatment regimen (insulin, diet, and exercise), monitoring, and compliance (Fig. 38.17). It is essential to conduct a detailed questionnaire and to be aware of recent changes in management, since any modification in the treatment regimen can have an impact on glycemic control. These causes of instability should be ruled out before proceeding with more complex investigations. At this point, clinicians can also evaluate any potential causes of IR, such as comorbidities, diabetogenic drugs, or diestrus/pregnancy.

The investigation of diabetic instability should also include a complete physical examination and routine workup (hematology, serum biochemistry, fructosamine, lipid profile, urinalysis, and urine culture). It is recommended to perform an integrated assessment of all the information collected and a detailed analysis of each case, thus creating a problem list and reaching accurate differential diagnoses. In order to investigate possible comorbidities, more specific diagnostic tests may be requested according to the clinical suspicion. Once identified the possible cause of diabetic instability, the clinician can start making management adjustments and specific therapeutic decisions.

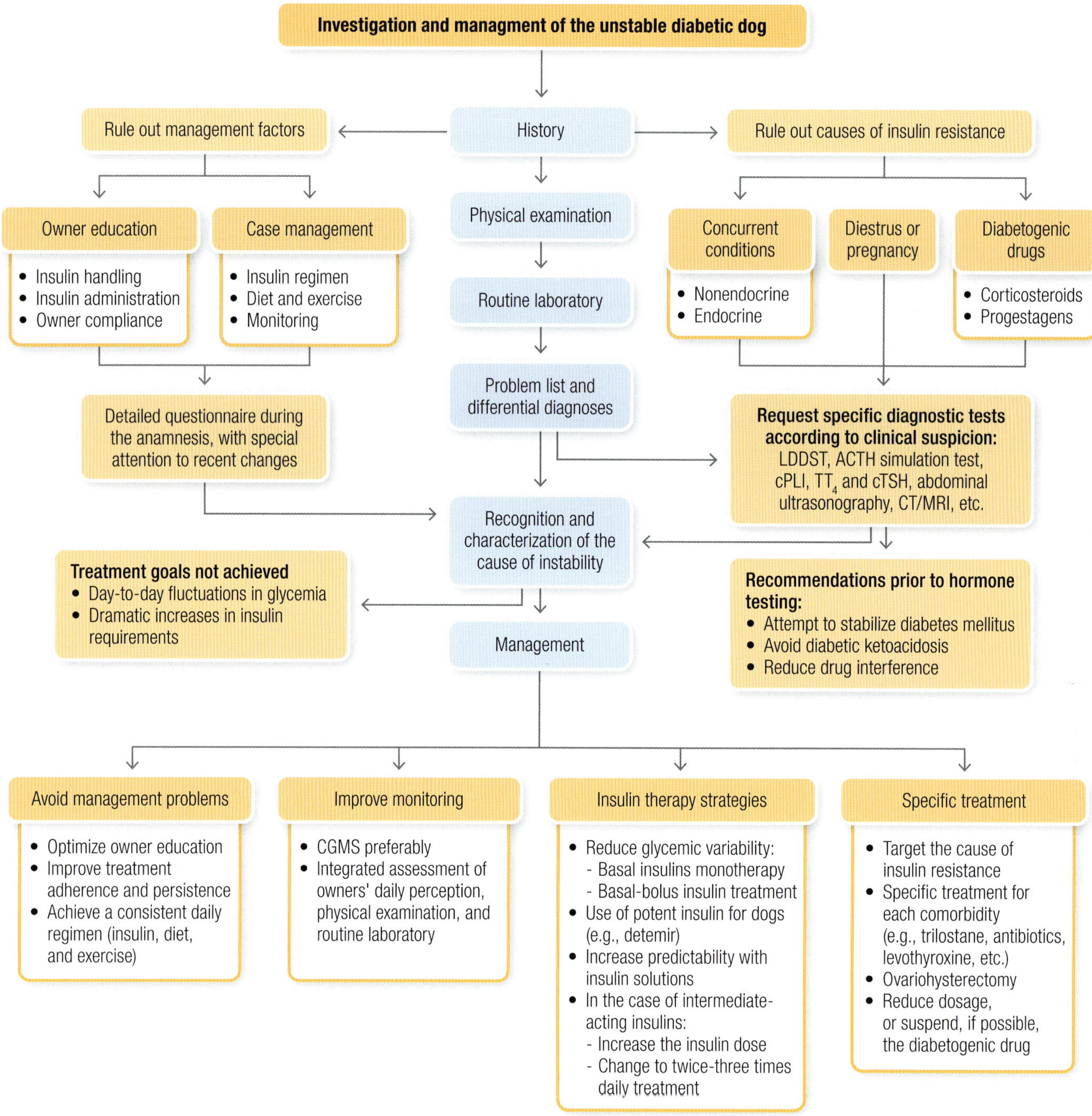

FIG. 38.17 An approach to the investigation and management of diabetic instability in dogs.

Long-term complications and prognosis

Álan G. Pöppl

Chronic hyperglycemia is associated with the overproduction of superoxide by the mitochondrial electron transport chain and glyceraldehyde-3-phosphate dehydrogenase inhibition. This key glycolytic enzyme inhibited leads to the accumulation of glycolytic intermediates that in turn can activate different mechanisms associated with long-term complications in humans, and potentially also in dogs: 1) increased alternative glucose metabolism pathways flux (polyol, hexosamine, and pentose phosphate), 2) increased intracellular formation of advanced glycation end products, and 3) activation of protein kinase C.[123,124]
Most classic chronic diabetic complications recognized in humans (i.e., myocardiopathy, microangiopathy) are poorly documented in dogs, probably because they took decades to develop. Diabetic dogs are often diagnosed in middle age, and even a dog diagnosed at a young will rarely live enough to experience the devasting clinical manifestation of the chronic complications described for humans.[123] Still, many long-term complications are well documented in diabetic dogs, especially ophthalmic issues.[125]

Ophthalmic long-term complications

Ocular long-term complications are diverse and warrant detailed ophthalmic monitoring of diabetic dogs. The most common ocular findings in a retrospective study with 75 dogs[125] were cataracts (97.3%), vitreous degeneration (45.9%), anterior uveitis (31.3%), aqueous deficiency dry eye (22%), diffuse corneal edema (20.7%), nonproliferative retinopathy (13.3%), and lipid keratopathy (6%).

Cataracts

Subtle bilateral cataract formation may be one of the clinical signs (blindness) observed by an owner before looking for a veterinary consult for a diabetic dog. However, cataracts are considered the most common long-term complication, being reported in 80% of diabetic dogs within 16 months of diagnosis.[126] The process of formation of cataracts is irreversible after it has started and can occur very quickly from normal vision to blindness in a frame of days, months, or years according to the ability to avoid chronically severe hyperglycemia and glycemic fluctuation, and individual metabolic characteristics of the dog's lens.[127]
Lens metabolism is supported by glucose and other metabolites, which freely penetrate through facilitated transport from aqueous humor. Glucose concentration within the lens is near 10% of the aqueous humor and is converted into lactate by hexokinase anaerobically. Lactate can easily leave the lens. When this system is saturated by higher glucose concentrations within the lens, aldose reductase activity increases converting glucose to sorbitol. Sorbitol can be further converted into fructose by sorbitol dehydrogenase. These metabolites are not freely permeable in the lens and act as potent hydrophilic agents causing water influx to the lens fiber with resultant intumescent cataracts, fiber rupture, and typical "Y" suture lines in the lens (Fig. 38.18).[127]
Topic use of the aldose reductase inhibitor q8h for a year has shown success in delaying cataract formation in diabetic dogs,[128] as well as oral alpha lipoic acid at 2 mg/kg PO q24h supplementation.[129] Strict glycemic control and minimal glucose variability are potential goals to delay cataract formation. Vision is restored in 75-80% of the dogs submitted to phacoemulsification surgery. However, factors such as poor glycemic control, retinal atrophy and degeneration, and the presence of lens-induced uveitis impact surgical success.[130]

Lens-induced uveitis

The intumescent features of diabetic cataracts can cause lens rupture and induce uveitis because the immune system does not recognize the lens proteins as proper.[127] Uveitis treatment consists of inflammatory reaction reduction and additional intraocular damage prevention using anti-inflammatory topics drugs, including glucocorticoids. However, these products can be systemically absorbed leading to insulin antagonism, especially in toy and miniature dogs. The use of nonsteroidal anti-inflammatories ophthalmic products, or cyclosporine can also be considered.[123,127]

Corneal ulceration and diabetic retinopathy

Chronic hyperglycemia has been associated with reduced corneal sensitivity and a negative impact on tear quality and quantity due to diffuse peripheric neuropathy, predisposing diabetic patients to corneal ulcers. Moreover, this scenario also impacts the ability of corneal healing and may be associated with recurrent or nonhealing corneal ulcers in diabetic dogs.[127,131] Multifactorial metabolic alterations due to the hyperglycemic insulin-deficiency state and the microvascular changes documented in diabetes are probably the cause of diabetic retinopathy. It is characterized by retinal hemorrhages and microaneurysms; however, early development of cataracts limits fundoscopic evaluation in many diabetic dogs.[127,131]

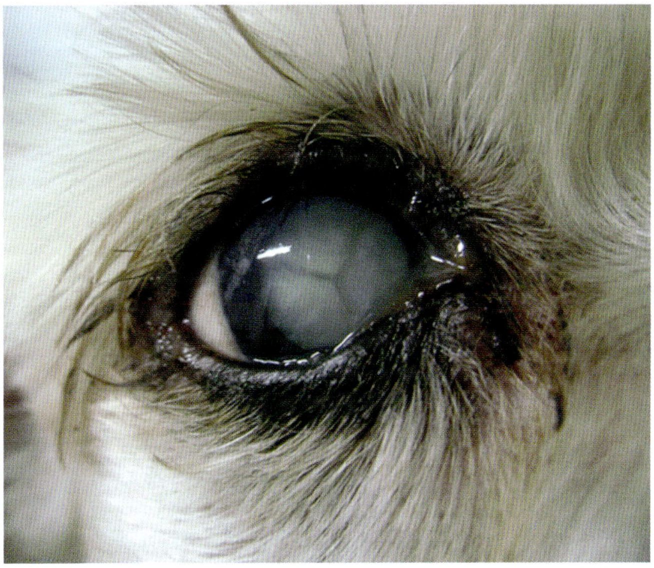

FIG. 38.18 Diabetic cataract aspect with the typical "Y-shape" suture lines.

Neurological long-term complications

In humans, diabetes is identified as a major risk factor for cognitive dysfunction due to multiple mechanisms related to the diabetic state that impact neuronal function and mental capacity (i.e., hypoxia due to cerebrovascular abnormalities, altered neuronal glucose uptake and metabolism, hypoglycemic episodes secondary to therapy).[132] Older dogs are prone to developing canine cognitive dysfunction (CCD). Long-term diabetic dogs may be at increased risk for CCD syndrome through the same mechanisms, or at least be susceptible to more severe cognitive dysfunction as observed anecdotally in some older diabetic dogs. As observed in humans, CCD negatively impacts diabetic treatment and can lead to reduced quality of life for both owner and patient.[133]

Diabetic neuropathy

As mentioned above, most diabetic dogs' ophthalmic complications result from peripheric neuropathy, including cranial nerves.[127] Despite uncommon, dogs can also develop distal polyneuropathy characterized by segmental demyelination and axonal degeneration. Pelvic limb lower motor neuron signs such as paresis, reduced muscle tone, muscular atrophy, reduced or delayed reflexes/postural testing responses, as well as gait abnormalities may be documentable in chronic diabetic dogs. Meticulous metabolic control of the diabetic state can reverse these signals.[123]

Autonomic impairment

In humans, diabetic autonomic neuropathy is associated with long-term cardiovascular complications (impairment of autonomic control of the cardiovascular system), as well as central control of breathing and sympathetic bronchial innervation can be impacted by the autonomic impairment. The same is observed in the gastrointestinal tract due to the remodeling of the enteric nervous system by diabetes, with associated dysmotility.[134] Despite being poorly characterized in veterinary medicine, autonomic impairment was documented as the main cause of impaired glucagon response in diabetic dogs exposed to hypoglycemia.[35]

Systemic hypertension and diabetic cardiomyopathy

Diabetes is assumed to be a common cause of systemic arterial hypertension in humans and affects 24 to 67% of diabetic dogs.[135] Vasculopathy and increased vascular peripheric resistance are some of the mechanisms potentially involved[136] as well as lipid metabolism disturbances leading to reduced vascular complacence and generalized glomerular hyperfiltration secondary to increased sodium absorption mediated by the sodium-glucose transporters (SGLTs) in the proximal convoluted tubules.[123,124] Despite the fact some diabetic dogs may exhibit hypertension due to subclinical kidney disease, is important to notice that exogenous insulin may also induce sodium retention.[137] Hyphema and retinal hemorrhage or detachment are potential additional ophthalmic complications due to systemic hypertension.[127]

Diabetes duration is associated with hypertension, increased proteinuria, and increased urinary albumin-to-creatine ratio.[138] Serum fructosamine concentration was positively correlated with systolic blood pressure in a study,[139] despite diabetes duration was not correlated with the cardiovascular parameters evaluated regarding cardiac function and structure. Also, troponin-I did not show increased values in diabetic dogs suggesting diabetic cardiomyopathy is uncommon in dogs.[138,139] Diabetic dogs ideally should have blood pressure routinely monitored at each clinical re-evaluation and treated if persistently hypertensive (i.e., >160 mmHg) according to guidelines recommendations (see chapter 9),[135] especially in the presence of proteinuria or other target organ damage evidence.

Diabetic nephropathy

Diabetic kidney disease is a well-known long-term diabetes complication in people and has been poorly characterized in dogs. The topic was extensively reviewed recently by Gal and Burchel, 2023.[124] Despite many components of human diabetic nephropathy being documented in diabetic dogs, diabetes is not recognized as a risk factor for chronic kidney disease development or progression in dogs. However, regular evaluation of kidney function using urine analysis and serum biochemistry in diabetic dogs is warranted.

Persistent hyperglycemia is a key factor for diabetic kidney abnormalities. Increased glucose and sodium reabsorption in the proximal convoluted tubule by SGLTs causes a reduction in sodium content in the distal tubules, inducing renin secretion by the macula densa cells of the juxtaglomerular apparatus. The net result is afferent arteriole dilatation and efferent arteriole vasoconstriction leading to glomerular hypertension, hyperfiltration, and renal hypoxia. Hyperglycemic-induced tubular hypertrophy substantially increases tubular oxygen consumption due to the increased activity of the Na-K ATPase in the basolateral membranes. In this way, an imbalance between oxygen delivery and oxygen consumption occurs.[124]

Chronic histological abnormalities found in diabetic kidneys may include glomerular hypertrophy with nodular (Kimmestiel-Wilson) and diffuse deposition of mesangial hyaline matrix, thickening of endothelial basement membranes with variable degree of capillary lumen narrowing, podocyte foot fusion and decreased podocyte density, and arteriolar hyalinosis. Mesangial expansion eventually is associated with abnormal glomerular-tubular junction (adhesion, proximal convoluted tubule obstruction, and tubular detachment leading to atubular glomerulus). The tubular lesions involve focal and diffuse proximal tubular atrophy and interstitial fibrosis.[124] In the long-term, these abnormalities can decline the glomerular filtration rate and evolve into a chronic (diabetic) kidney disease with azotemia and eventual oliguric/anuric end-stage outcome.[123]

Human diabetic nephropathy is associated with severe proteinuria and microalbuminuria due to glomerular dysfunction and may be present even in prediabetic patients. Despite some diabetic dogs also showing microalbuminuria the clinical significance and prognostic value of this finding is not clear. Since diabetic kidney disease in humans takes years to develop; the coexistence of CKD and DM in older dogs probably are independent events.[123]

There is no specific treatment for diabetic kidney disease beyond adequate glycemic control associated with standardized medical treatment of CKD. Hypertension and proteinuria monitoring and treatment are warranted in diabetic dogs according to published guidelines (i.e., angiotensin-converting enzyme inhibitors as initial potential treatment).[123]

Gastrointestinal complications

Besides the potential dysmotility secondary to gastrointestinal impairment discussed above, diabetes is associated with intestinal dysbiosis and a dysfunctional intestinal barrier.[140] The altered intestinal microbiome and mycobiome in diabetic dogs can influence insulin responsiveness, while intestinal barrier disruption can also be associated with increased bacterial translocation and systemic inflammation. Stimulation of the peroxisome proliferator-activated receptor-alpha (PPARα) signaling with fenofibrate 10 mg/kg, PO, q24h for three weeks was effective in repairing the intestinal barrier and reducing local and systemic inflammatory markers, while had a positive effect on fasting glucose and triglycerides. Pancreatitis is a well-known predisposing factor for diabetes mellitus in dogs; however, pathologic and metabolic consequences of diabetes can drive pancreatitis development in diabetic patients.[5]

Lipodystrophy

Lipodystrophy is the most common dermatologic complication of insulin therapy in humans, being classified as lipohypertrophy (LH –far more common) and lipoatrophy,[141] and probably underidentified in diabetic dogs. LH is characterized by local abnormal accumulation of fat tissue in the subcutaneous insulin injection site and appears as a thickened, swollen skin area with increased consistency on palpation (Video 38.4). The mechanism behind this condition probably involves local anabolic insulin effect on adipocytes. Improper or absence of site rotation for insulin administration predisposes to this condition in humans, and the same can be assumed for dogs. Insulin application into regions of LH can affect insulin pharmacokinetics (PK) increasing the likelihood of glucose variability, hypo-, and hyperglycemia when a site is changed. Lipoatrophy is clinically evidenced by depression at the site of repeated insulin injections and has a supposed immune-mediated basis.[141] Proper rotation of insulin injection sites is recommended to avoid these conditions.

Prognosis

Canine diabetes mellitus prognosis is extremely dependent on owner compromise in treating the condition, as well as the veterinarian's ability to propose individualized therapeutic measures to increase owner adhesion minimizing the impact of treatment on the owner's quality of life. In this way, good client-veterinary communication is highly desired. Diabetic dogs can have longer survival time accordingly with the ease of glycemic regulation, presence of comorbidities and reversibility of the ones documented, and avoidance and early identification of long-term complications.[123] However, survival curves for diabetic dogs can be dramatically affected by age at diagnosis, as well as other factors such as cultural issues within a particular region or country, the strength of the animal-client bond, and the owner's socioeconomic conditions. The first 6 months of treatment are critical for long-term survival due to increased deaths associated with initial presentation in diabetic ketoacidosis or inability to achieve adequate diabetic control due to factors related to the owner (poor compliance), the patient (comorbidities or poor cooperation), or the veterinarian (unfamiliarity with diabetes management).

Median survival time estimated in different studies varies from 2 to 3 years after diagnosis,[142,143] despite most diabetic dogs can live for many years according to the factors above mentioned. Periodic and timely re-evaluations are essential to achieve this goal. Diabetes *per se* does not reduce life span if the disease is well controlled and comorbidities are adequately identified and managed. Notwithstanding, factors such as the coexistence of hypercortisolism,[106] higher hematocrit, or hyperphosphatemia at diagnosis[143] were associated with reduced survival time among diabetic dogs. On the other hand, diabetic remission eventually can be achieved in particular cases (i.e., progesterone-related cases) after adequate treatment.[142] All these aspects emphasize the importance of the growing concept of an individualized approach and precision medicine in veterinary medicine.[5]

Video 38.4

Lipohypertrophy in a diabetic dog. The patient has a two-year history of well-controlled diabetes mellitus receiving 0,5U/kg of NPH insulin q12h, always applied above the scapulas. Unstable poorly-controlled diabetes was reported by the owners in the preceeding weeks and motivated a clinical review. In the physical exam, a focal abnormal accumulation of fat tissue in the subcutaneous insulin injection site was documented. Rotation of insulin injection sites over the dorsum avoiding the lipohypertrophy area was recommended and insulin dose was kept. Diabetes clinical control was quickly restored.

Diabetic ketosis, diabetic ketoacidosis and the hyperosmolar hyperglycemic state

Eleonora Malerba

Diabetic ketosis (DK), diabetic ketoacidosis (DKA) and the hyperosmolar hyperglycemic state (HHS) are challenging complications of uncontrolled diabetes mellitus (DM). Diabetic ketosis represents the early stage of DKA; a reversal of metabolic mechanisms which determine it can be obtained more easily when promptly managed. Otherwise, DKA and HHS are serious life-threatening emergencies, the management of which is very demanding and not without pitfalls. Mortality is rarely linked to the complications of hyperglycemia, but more often depends on the complications of the concomitant disease (if present), which precipitate metabolic decompensation, or on improper patient management and monitoring. Effective standardized treatment protocols, as well as prompt identification and treatment of the precipitating cause, are important factors affecting outcome.

Etiology

The etiopathogenetic mechanisms underlying these conditions are:

- Reduced insulin activity due to its absolute or relative deficiency.
- Increased production of stress counterregulatory hormones (glucagon, catecholamines, cortisol, and growth hormone).[144]

The reduced insulin activity causes the reduced availability of glucose for the cells and, consequently, a lack of energy which the body attempts to deal with by resorting to an alternative energy source: ketone bodies (KBs).

Subjects prone to developing this condition are patients with unknown DM not receiving insulin, patients with known DM receiving insulin treatment but at an inadequate dosage in relation to their needs or due to errors made by the owner in the way of administering the insulin and, finally, patients with known DM receiving an adequate insulin regimen but in which the equilibrium achieved is decompensated by the occurrence of a concomitant disease which interferes with the action of insulin by means of the phenomenon known as insulin resistance. The counterregulatory hormones that are produced in supraphysiological quantities in a wide range of pathological or even simply stressful conditions are responsible. Although these hormones exert protective action on the body by helping it to react to difficult conditions, in the specific case of a diabetic patient their action, antagonistic to that of insulin, contributes to the establishment of hyperglycemia and ketonemia during DKA (Fig. 38.19). Their hyperglycemic activity is justified by the stimulation of hepatic glycogenolysis and by the activation of protein catabolism in the muscle tissue, thus making a substrate for hepatic gluconeogenesis available. Furthermore, the excess of counterregulatory hormones, together with the lack of insulin, determines the activation of an enzyme, hormone-sensitive lipase, which stimulates the lipolysis of the adipose tissue, thus making free fatty acids (FFAs), used for hepatic ketogenesis, available. Ketone bodies represent an alternative form of energy to glucose when there is no glucose (prolonged fasting) or when, although available, it cannot be used (lack of insulin activity). The KB acetoacetate (AcAc) is the precursor from which acetone and beta-hydroxybutyrate (BHB) are derived. Under conditions of reduced insulin activity, BHB is the KB that plays the most important role since it is that is synthesized in the greatest quantity and that in which the blood concentration most faithfully reflects the entity of the ketonemia. The increased synthesis of KBs represents the first step of diabetic decompensation: diabetic ketosis.

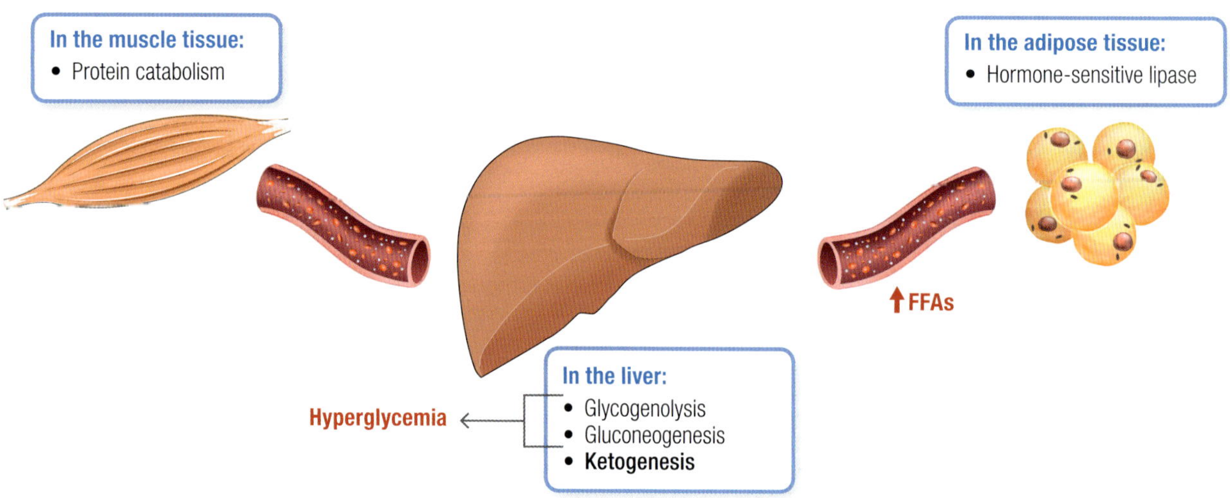

FIG. 38.19 Pathogenesis of hyperglycemia and ketonemia in diabetic ketoacidosis. Insulin deficiency and excess glucose counterregulatory hormones (i.e., glucagon, catecholamines, cortisol and growth hormone) cause hyperglycemia and ketosis. Hyperglycemia results from stimulation of hepatic glycogenolysis and protein catabolism in muscle tissue which provides the substrate for gluconeogenesis. Ketogenesis is the result of the activity of hormone-sensitive lipase which results in lipolysis of adipose tissue producing FFAs used for hepatic ketogenesis.

How the state of ketosis determines acidosis is very simple if one considers that a hydrogen ion is released for each KB synthesized in the liver. When the rate of production of hydrogen ions exceeds the buffer capacity of the organism, acidemia is established. Thus, DKA is a condition defined by the triad of hyperglycemia (or prior diagnosis of DM), ketonemia, and metabolic acidosis. In addition to acidosis, another consequence of hyperglycemia and ketonemia is cellular and interstitial dehydration proportional to the plasmatic concentration of glucose and KBs since these molecules have a powerful osmotic action. Furthermore, at the renal level, these molecules are completely ultrafiltered and, when their concentration inside the renal tubules exceeds the threshold reabsorption capacity, they remain in the ultrafiltrate by exerting a powerful osmotic diuresis. Finally, the anionic charge present on the KBs is responsible for the excretion of positively charged ions (Na^+, K^+, Ca^{2+}, Mg^{2+}) in order to maintain electroneutrality. The clinical features that characterize a patient with DKA are dehydration, hypovolemia, and electrolyte depletion, signs that additionally worsen when the dog develops symptoms secondary to acidemia (anorexia, vomiting, low water intake).

The situation is different in the case of HHS which is defined as a syndrome characterized by severe hyperglycemia, hyperosmolarity and dehydration in the absence of significant ketosis. The absence of ketosis is explained by these patients having a small amount of insulin sufficient to inhibit lipolysis (no availability of FFAs for ketogenesis) but not enough to prevent hyperglycemia (Fig. 38.20).[145] Hyperglycemia, together with hypernatremia, severely increases plasma osmolality generating an osmotic gradient which draws water from the cells into the bloodstream. At the cerebral level, the dehydration of cerebral cells causes progressive changes in mental status. Initially, the hyperglycemia is contained due to osmotic diuresis and glycosuria; however, as hypovolemia sets in, glomerular filtration is impaired, limiting renal glucose excretion and contributing to worsening hyperglycemia which is generally more severe than in DKA.

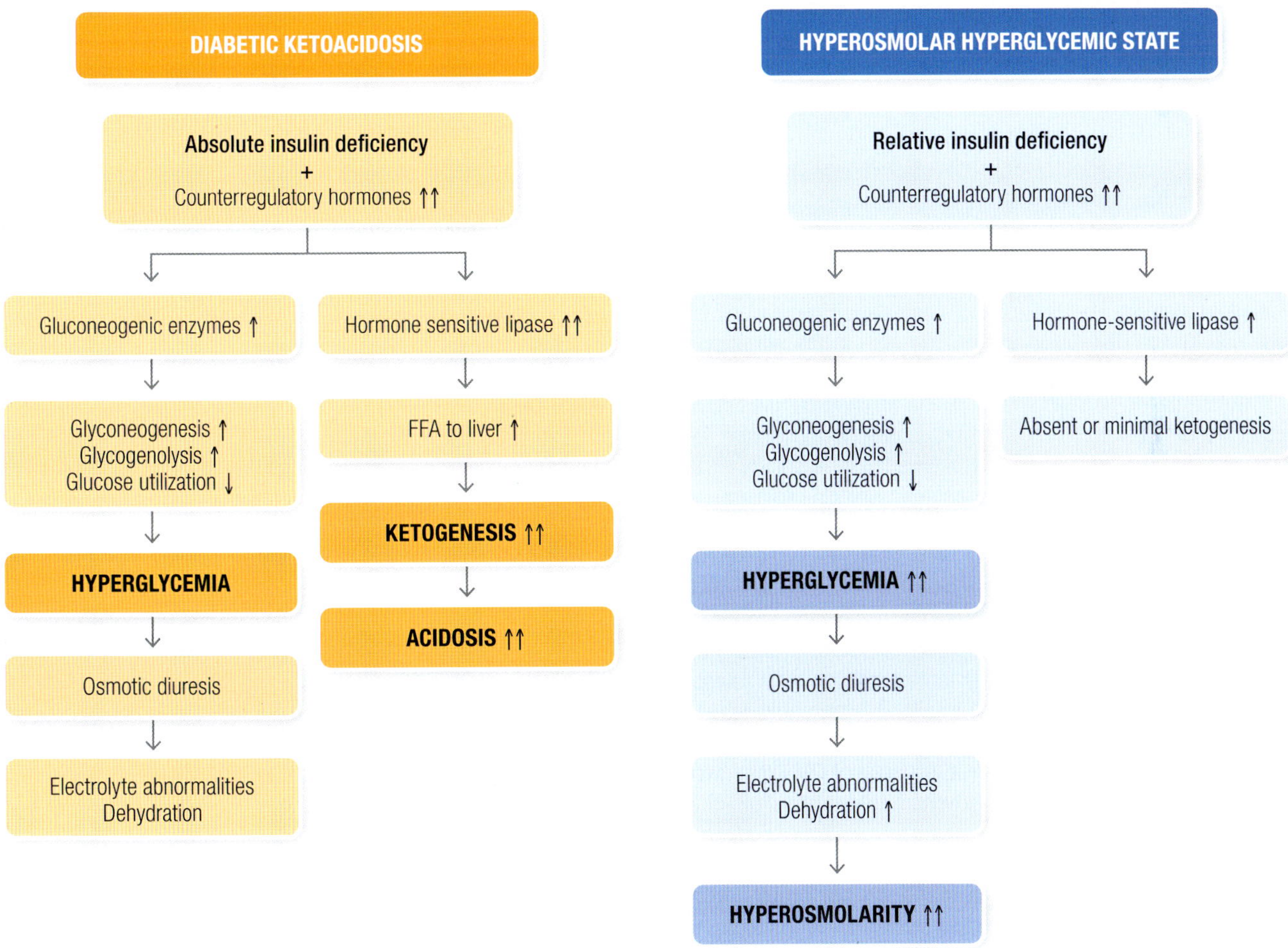

FIG. 38.20 Pathogenesis of diabetic ketoacidosis and hyperosmolar hyperglycemic state. In HHS, the presence of a small amount of insulin can inhibit the activity of hormone-sensitive lipase in adipocytes, thus decreasing the availability of FFAs for ketogenesis and preventing metabolic acidosis and systemic clinical manifestations, while hyperglycemia and hyperosmolarity progressively worsen as a result of increased gluconeogenesis, accelerated glycogenolysis, and inadequate utilization of blood glucose by peripheral tissues. On the contrary, in DKA, the absolute insulin deficiency does not allow the inhibition of the hormone-sensitive lipase and FFAs are mobilized by the adipocytes, reach the liver and are used for ketogenesis. The synthesis of KBs is associated with the release of hydrogen ions in the bloodstream resulting in metabolic acidosis and associated systemic clinical signs. (Adapted from French EK, Donihi AC, Korytkowski MT. Diabetic ketoacidosis and hyperosmolar hyperglycemic syndrome: review of acute decompensated diabetes in adult patients. *BMJ* 365:1114, 2019).

Clinical features

The signalment of dogs developing DK, DKA or HHS is the same as for patients with DM. These are middle-aged and elderly dogs without breed predisposition.
In the period of time (usually a few days) preceding the decompensation, clinical symptoms are the same as those of uncontrolled DM, namely polyuria/polydipsia, polyphagia, and weight loss. In DKA, following the onset of ketonemia, systemic signs appear, such as lethargy, anorexia, nausea, and vomiting, the severity of which depends on the extent of acidemia, hyperosmolality, and dehydration, and on the presence and severity of any concomitant disease. In addition to the symptoms already described, behavioral changes, abnormal mentation (dull, depressed mentation, coma) and respiratory abnormalities are more evident in patients with HHS due to the greater severity of dehydration/hypovolemia and the consequences of plasma hyperosmolality. Other clinical signs that may be reported by the owner or observed during physical examination may reflect the presence of a concomitant disease the recognition and resolution/management of which is critical to the patient's survival. In pets, the most common concomitant disorders include acute pancreatitis, bacterial pneumonia, hepatic lipidosis, cholangiohepatitis, urinary tract infection, acute kidney injury, and chronic kidney disease.

Diagnosis

The diagnosis of diabetic decompensation is quite simple once diagnostic suspicion has been raised. In this case, anamnesis represents an important support. The presence of compatible clinical signs in a patient with known DM should immediately lead to the suspicion of decompensation of the diabetic condition. In patients with unknown DM, it is essential to proceed with a careful anamnestic investigation aimed at revealing the presence of polyuria/polydipsia, polyphagia, and weight loss in the previous days/weeks, followed by a clinical worsening, mainly characterized by inappetence or anorexia, vomiting, lethargy, and abnormal mentation. Physical examination reveals nonspecific clinical signs. Patients are generally severely dehydrated, hypovolemic, and sometimes demonstrate slow deep breathing (i.e., Kussmaul respiration) with a strong odor of acetone on the breath. A thorough history and physical examination, to be interpreted in the context of laboratory and other diagnostic tests, are essential to identify concomitant disorders which need to be managed to reduce insulin resistance and increase the chances of therapeutic success.
The diagnostic criteria for DKA include a diagnosis of DM (hyperglycemia), ketonemia, and metabolic acidosis (venous/arterial blood pH <7.35 and decreased bicarbonate).
The diagnostic criteria for HHS have not been defined uniformly; they usually include severe hyperglycemia (blood glucose >600 mg/dL; 34 mmol/L), serum osmolality >325-330 mOsm/kg, dehydration, and the absence of significant ketosis.
Until a few decades ago, the tool used to estimate the status of ketosis was a urine reagent strip that provided a semiquantitative estimation of AcAc and acetone concentrations in the urine or plasma. The limitation of this tool is that it does not detect BHB, the predominant KB produced during DKA.[146] For this reason, direct measurement of blood BHB using a quantitative enzymatic assay or portable blood ketometer is now preferred.
Blood gas analysis, a complete blood count, a serum biochemistry panel and urinalysis are required to understand the patient's general status and to detect complications which need to be monitored or treated, but primarily to identify concomitant disorders. Other tests (e.g., urine culture, abdominal ultrasound, thoracic radiographs, serum pancreatic-specific lipase) may be indicated for this purpose.

Therapy and prognosis for diabetic ketoacidosis

The therapy for DKA has three objectives:

- To replace fluid and electrolyte deficits using appropriate fluid therapy, adequately supplemented with electrolytes.
- To allow the cells to use glucose to resolve the energy deficit and interrupt ketogenesis by means of the administration of insulin and, as needed, glucose supplementation.
- To resolve insulin resistance by identifying and managing/treating the concomitant disorders to avoid interference with treatment efficacy (**Fig. 38.21**).

Fluid therapy

The aim of IV fluid therapy is to hydrate the patient and restore blood volume, normalizing blood pressure and the heart rate, and ensuring adequate tissue perfusion. It also reduces the extent of hyperglycemia due to a simple dilution effect, partially corrects acidosis, and finally represents a tool to correct existing electrolyte imbalances and prevent additional imbalances secondary to insulin therapy.

Type of fluid

The fluid to be administered should be an isotonic crystalloid solution. Hypertonic or colloidal solutions are to be avoided as they restore volume but worsen the patient's dehydration state; hypotonic solutions are also to be avoided as they lower plasma osmolality too rapidly, increasing the risk of developing cerebral edema. Of the isotonic crystalloid solutions, those balanced with a buffer (e.g., Ringer's solution, Plasma-Lyte 148, Normosol-R) are preferred over a 0.9% saline solution since, in humans, it is associated with hyperchloremic metabolic acidosis that can prolong recovery from acidosis. Sodium bicarbonate therapy can be counterproductive when considering the risks associated with a too rapid correction of acidemia (exacerbation of hypokalemia, reduced dissociation of oxygen from hemoglobin, worsening of central nervous system function).

Rate of infusion

Fluid rates should be based on the assessment of the hydration, the degree of shock, and the presence of concomitant diseases that may limit the infusion rate. If the patient is in shock at the time of admission, boluses of fluids are to be administered at 5-10 mL/kg in 20 minutes until the heart rate and blood pressure are satisfactory. If shock is not present, the fluid deficit must be calculated, based on the estimation of the dehydration (with % dehydration expressed as decimal, e.g., 10% = 0.1):

$$\text{Fluid deficit (mL)} = \%\ \text{dehydration} \times \text{body weight (kg)} \times 1000\ \text{mL/kg}$$

1. DIAGNOSIS →

Once DKA is suspected based on history and physical examination, perform the following evaluations to confirm the diagnosis:

- Blood glucose
- BHB using a portable ketometer or urinary/plasma AcAc using urine reagent strip
- Venous/arterial blood gas analysis

Other:

- CBC, serum biochemistry panel, urinalysis
- Other diagnostic tests should be done based on clinical suspicion to identify concomitant diseases that may require additional therapy

→ Diagnostic criteria for diabetic ketoacidosis:

- Diagnosis of DM
- Demonstration of ketonemia/ketonuria
- Demonstration of metabolic acidosis (pH <7.35 and decreased bicarbonate)

2. FLUID THERAPY →

Begin as soon as possible using balanced crystalloid with a buffer (e.g., Ringer's solution, Plasma-Lyte 148, Normosol-R); proceed with caution in case of renal or cardiac disease, or chronic hyperosmolarity

- Insert an intravenous catheter (a central venous catheter is ideal as it allows for blood sampling)
- Calculate the fluid deficit
- Administer 60-80% of fluid deficit in first 12 hours and the remaining 20-40% in the next 12 hours, while also supplying maintenance fluid requirements and estimated ongoing fluid losses
- **Supplement potassium** (Table 38.16)

→ To avoid complications resulting from excessive or insufficient fluid therapy, it is advisable to frequently check:

- Mental status
- Heart rate and pulse characteristics
- Mucous membrane moisture
- Capillary refill time
- Vesicular murmure
- Blood pressure
- Urine output
- Body weight

3. INSULIN PROTOCOLS (beginning 2-4 hours after fluid therapy) →

MONITORING SCHEME DURING INSULIN PROTOCOL:

- Blood glucose concentration q1h during the first 24 hours and then q2h until DKA resolution (a continuous glucose monitoring system is ideal)
- BHB or urinary/plasma AcAc q4h until DKA resolution
- Venous/arterial blood gas analysis q8h during the first 24 hours and then q12h until DKA resolution

INTRAVENOUS ROUTE

- Insert a second venous catheter
- Prepare insulin infusion: 2.2 U/kg of regular, lispro or aspart insulin is added to 48 mL of 0.9% saline
- Insulin solution must be left in the line for 30 minutes and then run through the IV line
- Reprepare insulin solution and start infusion at a rate depending on blood glucose concentration

Blood glucose concentration (mg/dL) (mmol/L)	Fluids	Rate of administration of insulin solution (mL/h)
>250 (>13.9)	Crystalloid	2
150-250 (8.3-13.9)	2.5% dextrose†	1.5
100-150 (5.6-8.3)	5% dextrose‡	1
<100 (<5.5)	5% dextrose‡	Stop insulin infusion

† 2.5% dextrose composed of 25 mL dextrose 50% added to 475 mL of balanced crystalloid with a buffer or 0.9% saline
‡ 5% dextrose composed of 50 mL dextrose 50% added to 450 mL of balanced crystalloid with a buffer or 0.9% saline.

INTRAMUSCULAR/SUBCUTANEOUS ROUTE:

Option 1
REGULAR INSULIN:

- Initial bolus: 0.1-0.2 U/kg IM
- Maintenance: 0.1 U/kg IM q1-2h

When blood glucose <250 mg/dL (13.9 mmol/L):

- 0.1-0.3 U/kg IM q4-6h or SC q6-8h
- Add 5% dextrose to maintain blood glucose concentration between 150 and 300 mg/dL (8.3-16.7 mmol/L) until DKA resolution

Option 2
LISPRO INSULIN:

- Initial bolus: 0.25 U/kg IM q1h
- Maintenance: 0.25 U/kg IM q3h

When blood glucose <250 mg/dL (13.9 mmol/L):

- 0.125 U/kg IM or SC q3h
- Add 2.5-7.5% dextrose to keep blood glucose concentration between 150 and 300 mg/dL (8.3-16.7 mmol/L) until DKA resolution

↓

DKA is considered resolved, and it is possible to switch to maintenance insulin therapy with intermediate/long-acting insulin, when ketosis and acidemia are resolved, hydration status is adequate, electrolyte balance has been re-established, and appetite returns without vomiting

FIG. 38.21 Principles of care for dogs with diabetic ketoacidosis.

Approximately 60-80% of this deficit should be restored within the first 12 hours and the remaining 20-40% in the next 12 hours while also supplying maintenance fluid needs and matching ongoing losses due to polyuria, vomiting, and diarrhea. When the fluid deficit has been restored, the fluid rate should be adjusted to meet the patient's hemodynamic needs. Fluid rates 1.5 to 2 times maintenance (i.e., 60 to 100 mL/kg/24h) are usually used initially (**Fig. 38.21**).

Electrolytes

Although not always reflected in serum concentration, a patient with DKA should be assumed always potassium depleted, except in individuals with oliguric acute kidney injury. For this reason, fluid therapy must include potassium supplementation according to its serum concentration (**Table 38.16**), except when renal function impairment is suspected and urinary output is inadequate. During boluses administration, the dose of 0.5 mEq/kg/h of potassium should not be exceeded. Since changes in blood potassium concentration are unpredictable, during the first 24-48 hours of treatment, frequent assessments (q2-4h) and adjustments in treatment should be made accordingly.

TABLE 38.16 Guidelines for potassium, phosphate, and magnesium supplementations in dogs with diabetic ketoacidosis.

Electrolyte	Guidelines for electrolyte supplementation
Serum K^+ (mEq/L)	**Potassium supplementation mEq/L of fluids**
>5.0	wait
4.0-5.0	20 to 30
3.5-4.0	30 to 40
3.0-3.5	40 to 50
2.5-3.0	50 to 60
2.0-2.5	60 to 80
<2.0	80
	K^+ supplementation should not exceed 0.5 mEq/kg/h Frequency of monitoring: every 4 to 8 hours
Serum P^+ (mg/dL)	
Hypophosphatemia: ■ Serum P^+<3 mg/dL Clinical signs if serum P^+<1.5 mg/dL	in continuous rate infusion in calcium-free IV fluids ■ Mild hypophosphatemia → 0.01 to 0.03 mmol/kg/h ■ Severe hypophosphatemia → 0.03-0.12 mmol/kg/h If KPO is administered for phosphate supplementation, KCl supplementation is decreased accordingly Frequency of monitoring: every 8 to 12 hours
Serum Mg^{2+} (mg/dL)	
Hypomagnesemia: ■ Serum total Mg^{2+}<1.5 mg/dL ■ Ionized Mg^{2+}<1.0 mg/dL Clinical signs if serum total Mg^{2+}<1 mg/dL and/or ionized Mg^{2+}<0.4 mg/dL	in dextrose 5% in water or 0.9% sodium chloride ■ Slow replacement → 0.3-0.5 mEq/kg/day ■ Rapid replacement → 0.5-1 mEq/kg/day Frequency of monitoring: every 8 to 12 hours

Blood glucose

With the start of fluid therapy, the blood glucose (BG) concentration undergoes changes that must be monitored every hour at least in the first 24 hours of therapy. When the BG decreases to ≤250 mg/dL (14 mmol/L) or when the decrease is >50-75 mg/dL/h (>2.8-4.2 mmol/L/h) and the ketosis is still marked, a 2.5% glucose solution must be added to the IV fluid solution to maintain the BG concentration between 150 and 300 mg/dL (8.3 and 16.7 mmol/L). By implementing this strategy, it is possible to continue to administer insulin to inhibit ketogenesis, avoiding hypoglycemic episodes or osmotic shocks. A factory-calibrated flash glucose monitoring system has recently been made available for the continuous monitoring of interstitial glucose concentrations which reflect circulating BG concentrations (see chapter 21).[147]

Insulin therapy

During the treatment of DKA, the main goal of insulin therapy is not the achievement of euglycemia. Insulin is an integral part of the therapy as it inhibits lipolysis and suppresses hepatic gluconeogenesis but, above all, it allows cells to have access to glucose, present in abundant quantities in the blood, thus resolving the energy deficit and interrupting ketogenesis. The other benefits, such as the reduction of osmotic diuresis and hyperosmolality, and correction of acidosis, are a consequence of its activity. For insulin therapy to be effective in resolving the energy deficit, its administration must not be interrupted until the resolution of ketosis and acidosis. Insulin therapy should gradually reduce BG (an hourly reduction of 50-75 mg/dL/h [2.8-4.2 mmol/L/h] is ideal) until concentrations of approximately 250 mg/dL (14 mmol/L) are reached. It is subsequently advisable to maintain the BG concentration at values between 100 and 250 mg/dL (5.5 and 14 mmol/L) by lowering the doses of insulin and supplementing IV fluids with dextrose. This strategy allows the insulin to be administered continuously and safely until resolution of DKA, avoiding possible hypoglycemic episodes. In addition to hypoglycemia, other potential adverse effects of insulin therapy that should be avoided are hypokalemia and hypophosphatemia. In fact, the binding of insulin to its specific receptor determines the opening of the glucose channels and glucose can move from the extracellular to the intracellular space; this movement is accompanied by that of water, potassium and phosphorus (PO_4). Variations in serum electrolytes are unpredictable, but can be life-threatening, and represent one of the causes of therapeutic failure. The appropriate use of fluid therapy, frequent monitoring of serum electrolytes and BG, and delaying initial insulin administration are strategies to avoid the potential adverse effects of insulin therapy. It is advisable to delay insulin therapy by 2 hours after the start of fluid therapy if the kalemia is normal, but up to 4 hours if the hypokalemia persists despite potassium supplementation in the IV fluids, possibly using lower initial insulin doses (50-75%) to limit the intracellular shifts of K and PO_4. A study has demonstrated that starting insulin within 6 hours from the start of the fluid therapy was associated with a more rapid resolution of DKA without increasing the complication rate compared to starting insulin >6 hours after admission.[148]

The switch to intermediate/long-acting insulin for the long-term management of DM should only occur after resolution of the DKA. This requires that the ketosis (blood BHB <1 mmol/L or undetectable urinary AcAc using nitroprusside test strips) and the acidosis (pH >7.3 and/or bicarbonates >15) have been resolved, hydration has been restored, the electrolytes are normal or close to normal, and that the patient eats spontaneously without vomiting. In dogs with a concomitant insulin-antagonistic disease, insulin may be less effective as a result of interference with the ability to resolve the DKA and is one of the most important causes of mortality.

Given that the insulin response is subjective and difficult to predict, the insulin to be administered must have an immediate effect and a short duration of action. This allows for the rapid identification of over- and underdoses and protocol adjustments to suit patient needs. Regular insulin fulfills these requirements, and its efficacy has been demonstrated in various protocols involving IM/SC and IV use. Continuous rate IV infusion has always been considered to be the gold standard, guaranteeing the faster onset of a hypoglycemic effect, greater predictability of the glycemic trend, and the possibility of promptly modifying the insulin dosage to adapt it to the patient's response. Otherwise, IM and SC administration cause a more unpredictable uptake and a more variable time-action profile. This is because regular insulin is a solution of zinc-insulin hexamers that requires dissociation following IM or SC injection, resulting in delayed absorption, especially in dehydrated patients with compromised tissue perfusion. To overcome the limitations of regular insulin, rapid-acting insulin analogs (lispro, aspart, and glulisine) have been developed in recent decades, the structure of which differs from the original molecule by one or two amino acids. This structural feature prevents hexamerization at the IM/SC injection site and speeds up absorption, ensuring a rapid onset and a short duration of action.[149] In humans with mild-to-moderate DKA, intermittent SC injections of insulin analogs are as effective as the IV constant rate infusion of regular insulin.[150]

Low-dose intravenous constant rate infusion

The dose of regular insulin, 2.2 U/kg,[151] should be added to 48 ml of 0.9% saline. Since insulin binds to plastic, the solution obtained should remain in the infusion syringe and line for approximately 30 minutes. The entire 48 mL should then be discarded, and a fresh insulin solution prepared and administered with an infusion pump via a line separate from that used for fluid resuscitation. The initial dose should be 2 mL/h; adjustments to the infusion rate should be based on the BG concentrations (**Fig. 38.21**). Dextrose should be added to the IV fluids (generally a 2.5% solution) once the BG is reduced to ≤250 mg/dL (14 mmol/L). The protocol should be continued until the resolution of the DKA.

The effectiveness and safety of an IV lispro insulin constant rate infusion (CRI), and of IV aspart insulin CRI in dogs were compared to IV CRIs of regular insulin. All the protocols were equally efficacious and safe.[152-154]

Intramuscular and subcutaneous protocols

Regular insulin can be given at a loading dose of 0.1-0.2 U/kg IM followed by 0.1 U/kg IM every 1-2 hours[155] (**Fig. 38.21**). The insulin dose should be reduced by 25-50% in the first hours of treatment if hypokalemia is a concern. When the BG concentration approaches 250 mg/dL (14 mmol/L), insulin can be administered at a dose of 0.1-0.3 U/kg IM q4-6h hours if the patient is still dehydrated or SC q6-8h once hydration status is adequate. A 2.5-5% dextrose solution should be administered to maintain the BG concentration between 150 and 300 mg/dL (8.3-16.7 mmol/L) until the DKA resolves.

One study has investigated the use of IM/SC lispro insulin in dogs. The dogs received IM lispro insulin at an initial dose of 0.25 U/kg. When a decrease in BG of at least 10% during the following hour was not reached, the insulin dose was administered hourly; otherwise, the insulin dose was administered q3h. When the BG reached 250 mg/dL (14 mmol/L), the insulin dose was decreased to 0.125 U/kg IM or SC (based on hydration status) q3h, and enough dextrose was added to the IV fluids to arrive at a 2.5% solution. The median time to resolution of the ketosis was significantly shorter in those dogs treated as above as compared to those dogs treated with an IV CRI of regular insulin. There were no changes in the frequency or severity of adverse events.[156]

Prognosis

In recent decades, there has been a reduction in mortality of DKA from 25-35% to <10%.[152,154,156] This was possible thanks to a greater knowledge of the pathophysiological mechanisms of DKA and the strategies of dealing with them. For this purpose, constant patient supervision and frequent monitoring of the most critical parameters (BG, K^+, PO_4, Na^+, acid-base status, hydration, and tissue perfusion) are essential to be able to promptly identify those that require attention and adapt the treatment to manage such complications (e.g., hypokalemia or hypoglycemia). Any underlying disease should be identified and treated, especially those causing insulin resistance (e.g., pancreatitis, hormonal disorders, sepsis, acute kidney injury, congestive heart failure) as they represent the major cause of death, together with the client's financial constraints.

Therapy and prognosis for hyperosmolar hyperglycemic state

An HHS can be responsible for acute kidney failure leading to death. Treating HHS necessitates slowly restoring dehydration deficits (24-48h) and correcting serious hyperglycemia to avoid the occurrence of iatrogenic cerebral edema. Despite the presence of hyperosmolarity, the fluid used initially should be isotonic 0.9% saline. Serum K^+ and PO_4 concentrations must be closely monitored, and supplementation carried out according to kidney function and urine output. Beginning supplementation with 20 mEq/L of KCl is recommended. Insulin therapy for HHS should be postponed until plasma volume is restored. The BG concentration should not be reduced by more than 50 mg/dL/h (2.8 mmol/L/h) to avoid the risk of cerebral edema. The insulin protocols are identical to those for DKA. However, the beginning insulin dosage should be decreased by 50% to avoid a rapid reduction in extracellular fluid osmolality. When the BG is <250 mg/dL (14 mmol/L), administering 2.5-5% dextrose IV fluids is recommended. The prognosis of HHS is guarded to poor.[157,158]

KEY POINTS

Pathogenesis, clinical manifestations, and diagnosis

Lucy Davison

- Diabetes mellitus (DM) in dogs can be caused by a wide range of mechanisms, usually leading to beta-cell death and insulin deficiency.
- Breed predispositions suggest a genetic component to diabetes risk.
- Diagnosis is based on documentation of persistent hyperglycemia, elevation in glycated blood proteins, and clinical signs.
- Clinically, canine DM is characterized by hyperglycemia in middle-aged adult dogs, accompanied by polyuria, polydipsia, and weight loss.
- Presentation can be complicated by the presence of other conditions contributing to insulin resistance (IR), such as hyperadrenocorticism, pancreatitis, or diestrus.
- If not recognized and managed promptly, death can result from diabetic ketoacidosis.

Insulin therapy and other treatment options

Chen Gilor, Linda Fleeman

- No insulin formulation should be considered "best" by default. Rather, the choice of insulin formulation should be tailored to the specific clinical situation. Various goal-oriented treatment strategies should be considered, with pros and cons to each.
- Ideally, insulin therapy in most diabetic dogs should mimic a "basal-bolus" pattern. The "intermediate-acting" insulin formulations might provide a better approximation of "bolus" insulin secretion in many dogs than the rapid-acting formulations that are typically used for this purpose in diabetic people.
- "Basal" insulin requirements are relatively constant throughout the day. Therefore, for an insulin formulation to be effective and safe as a "basal" insulin, its action should be roughly the same every hour of the day. Currently, two formulations meet this standard in dogs: insulin glargine U300 and insulin degludec.
- Most diabetic dogs can be well-managed by using basal insulin alone. "Basal" insulin formulations should not be used in dogs unless the dose can be titrated with continuous glucose monitoring. This protocol allows for very rapid dose escalation, achieving reasonable clinical control in 1-2 weeks.
- Currently available insulin suspensions (NPH, NPH/regular mixes, lente, and PZI), insulin glargine U100, and detemir are generally used as "intermediate-acting" formulations administered twice daily.
- Compared to the traditional vial/syringe combination, insulin dosing pens improve the quality of life of the caregiver, improve adherence, and allow better dosing accuracy and precision.

Dietary management of diabetes in dogs

Linda Fleeman, Charlotte Bjørnvad

- Tailored diet recommendations should be made for diabetic dogs, taking into account the dog's age, appetite, food preferences, body composition, activity level, insulin treatment strategy, and concomitant conditions.
- Diet change does not need to routinely be recommended at the start of diabetes treatment. Instead, clinicians and owners are encouraged to first focus on insulin treatment and the dietary requirements of any other health condition.
- It is recommended to avoid hasty transitions and ensure diet palatability.
- Consistency in daily feeding routines is desirable, and includes consistent feeding times, diet composition and amount in relation to insulin injections.
- There will be possible benefit from limiting starch-containing ingredients in the diet of diabetic dogs. However, this will necessitate that more energy is derived from either protein or fat, which may not be beneficial in every case.
- Weight loss should be an integrated part of diabetes management in overweight/obese dogs.
- The postprandial "bolus" insulin secretion phase in dogs usually peaks within 30 minutes and can remain increased for 6-9 hours.
- Factors that affect "bolus" insulin requirement include diet composition, total food intake, and insulin resistance states such as Cushing's syndrome.
- Postprandial hyperglycemia occurs when there is insufficient insulin action to match "bolus" insulin requirement. This is common in insulin-treated diabetic dogs, but is typically not associated with noticeable clinical signs if peak glucose is <350 mg/dL (<19 mmol/L).

- Once the owner is accustomed to insulin administration and reasonably good control of clinical signs of diabetes is achieved, the clinical impact of postprandial hyperglycemia, if present, may then be assessed and managed.
- Potential strategies to manage excessive postprandial hyperglycemia include diet change, change to the daily feeding routine, and change to insulin therapy.

Monitoring a diabetic patient

Francesca Del Baldo

- Regular monitoring of a diabetic dog is vital to successfully achieving good control of the disease.
- The clinical signs are the most important initial parameters to assess control of glycemia. However, they are subjective and their reliability depends largely on the observational skills of the owner.
- Next to the evaluation of the clinical signs, to properly adjust the insulin therapy, clinicians should consider using more objective monitoring tools such as applying a continuous glucose monitoring system (preferred option) or generating a blood glucose curve (BGC).
- Nowadays, the use of FreeStyle Libre®, a flash glucose monitoring system, has replaced the use of blood glucose curves for monitoring most diabetic patients. It allows detailed identification of the glycemic excursions occurring throughout the day as well as the assessment of glucose variability on consecutive days, enabling the clinician to make a more informed decision regarding the insulin dose.

The unstable diabetic

Diego Miceli

- Diabetic instability could be defined as a state of "uncontrollable" DM characterized by persistent difficulties in glycemic control or treatment goals achievement. This state is potentially reversible and is associated with multiple patient, owner, and management factors.
- The causes of instability can be categorized into two groups: management-related and IR-related. These causes may entail consistent day-to-day glycemic fluctuations or dramatic increases in insulin requirements.
- Problems related to owner education and case management are common and can be evaluated during the anamnesis. It is recommended that every detail related to insulin handling/storage, injection technique, treatment regimen, monitoring, and compliance be thoroughly evaluated. Before proceeding with more complex investigations, management factors should be ruled out.
- IR is characterized by varying degrees of interference of insulin action on target cells. Several comorbidities, physiological states with hormonal antagonism (e.g., diestrus and pregnancy), and diabetogenic drugs could promote diverse IR states. Specific treatment strategies should target the cause of IR, in addition to appropriately adjusting insulin therapy.
- Hypercortisolism and progesterone-induced hypersomatotropism are probably the most common causes of IR in diabetic dogs and are often associated with extremely high insulin requirements.
- Identifying the cause of diabetic instability in dogs can be challenging, expensive, and time-consuming, and it requires good communication between clinicians and owners.
- The key strategies for successfully managing unstable diabetes are avoiding management problems, treating the cause of IR, optimizing monitoring, and employing an appropriate insulin therapy strategy for each case.

Long-term complications and prognosis

Álan G. Pöppl

- DM is a complex condition with several long-term complications that can impact the quality of life and survival of diabetic dogs.
- Increased oxidative stress and advanced glycation end-product formation are key in the process.
- The long-term complications are avoidable somehow, according to the ability to control glycemia and avoid glycemic variability.
- Most of the dramatic chronic diabetic complications observed in humans are not observed in dogs, probably because of their shortened life expectancy compared to humans.
- However, many of the ophthalmic, neurological, gastrointestinal, and kidney problems observed in people can also harm diabetic dogs.
- In this way, properly identifying these issues is a key factor in promoting a better quality of life and also should represent a discussion topic with the owners of diabetic dogs.

References

1. Mattin M, O'Neill DG, Church D, McGreevy PD, Thomson PC, Brodbelt DC. An epidemiological study of diabetes mellitus in dogs attending first opinion practice in the UK. *Vet Rec* 174:349-349, 2014.
2. Heeley AM, O'Neill DG, Davison LJ, Church DB, Corless EK, Brodbelt DC. Diabetes mellitus in dogs attending UK primary-care practices: frequency, risk factors, and survival. *Canine Med Genetics* 7:1-19, 2020.
3. Yoon S, Fleeman LM, Wilson BJ, Mansfield CS, McGreevy P. Epidemiological study of dogs with diabetes mellitus attending primary care veterinary clinics in Australia. *Vet Rec* 187, 2020.
4. Gilor C, Niessen SJM, Furrow E, Dibartola SP. What's in a name? Classification of diabetes mellitus in veterinary medicine and why it matters. *J Vet Intern Med* 30:927-940, 2016.
5. O'Kell AL, Davison LJ. Etiology and pathophysiology of diabetes mellitus in dogs. *Vet Clin North Am Small Anim Pract* 53(3):493-510, 2023.
6. Gal A, Odunayo A. Diabetes ketoacidosis and hyperosmolar hyperglycemic syndrome in companion animals. *Vet Clin North Am Small Anim Pract* 53:531-550, 2023.
7. Niessen SJ, Bjornvad C, Church DB, Davison L, Esteban-Saltiveri D, Fleeman LM, Forcada Y, Fracassi F, Gilor C, Hanson J. Agreeing Language in Veterinary Endocrinology (ALIVE): Diabetes mellitus – a modified Delphi-method-based system to create consensus disease definitions. *Vet J* 289:105910, 2022.
8. Davison L, Herrtage M, Catchpole B. Study of 253 dogs in the United Kingdom with diabetes mellitus. *Vet Rec* 156:467-471, 2005.
9. Kramer JW, Nottingham S, Robinette J, Lenz G, Sylvester S, Dessouky MI. Inherited, early onset, insulin-requiring diabetes mellitus of Keeshond dogs. *Diabetes* 29:558-565, 1980.
10. Alvarez MS, Herrería-Bustillo V, Utset AF, Martínez J. Juvenile diabetes mellitus and concurrent exocrine pancreatic insufficiency in a Labrador Retriever: long-term management. *Journal Am Anim Hosp Assoc* 51:419-423, 2015.
11. Dale MV. Canine juvenile diabetes. *Vet Rec* 159:608-608, 2006.
12. Denyer AL, Catchpole B, Davison LJ. Genetics of canine diabetes mellitus part 1: Phenotypes of disease. *Vet J* 270:105611, 2021.
13. Denyer AL, Catchpole B, Davison LJ. Genetics of canine diabetes mellitus part 2: Current understanding and future directions. *Vet J* 270:105612, 2021.
14. Gepts W, Toussaint D. Spontaneous diabetes in dogs and cats. *Diabetologia* 3:249-265, 1967.
15. Shields EJ, Lam CJ, Cox AR, Rankin MM, Van Winkle TJ, Hess RS, Kushner JA. Extreme beta-cell deficiency in pancreata of dogs with canine diabetes. *PloS One* 10:e0129809-e0129809, 2015.
16. Alejandro R, Feldman EC, Shienvold FL, Mintz DH. Advances in canine diabetes mellitus research: etiopathology and results of islet transplantation. *J Am Vet Med Assoc* 193:1050-1055, 1988.
17. Davison L. Diabetes mellitus and pancreatitis–cause or effect? *J Small Anim Pract* 56:50-59, 2015.
18. Cridge H, Lim SY, Algul H, Steiner JM. New insights into the etiology, risk factors, and pathogenesis of pancreatitis in dogs: Potential impacts on clinical practice. *J Vet Intern Med* 36:847-864, 2022.
19. Watson PJ, Herrtage ME. Use of glucagon stimulation tests to assess beta-cell function in dogs with chronic pancreatitis. *J Nutr* 134:2081S-2083S, 2004.
20. Catchpole B, Ristic JM, Fleeman LM, Davison LJ. Canine diabetes mellitus: can old dogs teach us new tricks? *Diabetologia* 48:1948-1956, 2005.
21. Davison L, Weenink S, Christie MR, Herrtage M, Catchpole B. Autoantibodies to GAD65 and IA-2 in canine diabetes mellitus. *Vet Immunol Immunopathol* 126:83-90, 2008.
22. Davison LJ, Herrtage ME, Catchpole B. Autoantibodies to recombinant canine proinsulin in canine diabetic patients. *Res Vet Sci* 91:58-63, 2011.
23. Heeley AM, Brodbelt DC, O'Neill DG, Church DB, Davison LJ. Assessment of glucocorticoid and antibiotic exposure as risk factors for diabetes mellitus in selected dog breeds attending UK primary-care clinics. *Vet Rec* 192:e2785, 2023.
24. Eigenmann JE, Eigenmann RY, Rijnberk A, Van der Gaag I, Zapf J, Froesch ER. Progesterone-controlled growth hormone overproduction and naturally occurring canine diabetes and acromegaly. *Acta Endocrinol* 104:167-176, 1983.
25. Fleeman L, Barrett R. Cushing's syndrome and other causes of insulin resistance in dogs. *Vet Clin North Am Small Anim Pract* 53:711-730, 2023.
26. Fall T, Johansson Kreuger S, Juberget Å, Bergström A, Hedhammar Å. Gestational diabetes mellitus in 13 dogs. *J Vet Intern Med* 22:1296-1300, 2008.
27. Verkest KR, Fleeman LM, Rand JS, Morton JM. Evaluation of beta-cell sensitivity to glucose and first-phase insulin secretion in obese dogs. *Am J Vet Res* 72:357-366, 2011.
28. Kuzi S, Mazaki-Tovi M, Ahmad WA, Ovadia Y, Aroch I. Clinical utility of serum fructosamine in long-term monitoring of diabetes mellitus in dogs. *Vet Rec* 192:e2236, 2023.
29. Neumann S. Reference interval of hemoglobin A1c and influence of hematological parameters on its serum concentration in dogs. *Vet Med Int* 2020:7150901-7150901, 2020.
30. Xenoulis PG, Steiner JM. Canine hyperlipidaemia. *J Small Anim Pract* 56:595-605, 2015.
31. Gilor C, Fleeman LM. One hundred years of insulin: Is it time for smart? *J Small Anim Pract* 63(9):645-660, 2022.
32. Whitley NT, Drobatz KJ, Panciera DL. Insulin overdose in dogs and cats: 28 cases (1986-1993). *J Am Vet Med Assoc* 211(3):326-330, 1997.
33. Mott J, Gilor C. Glucose counterregulation: clinical consequences of impaired sympathetic responses in diabetic dogs and cats. *Vet Clin North Am Small Anim Pract* 53(3):551-564, 2023.
34. Gilor C, Pires J, Greathouse R, et al. Loss of sympathetic innervation to islets of Langerhans in canine diabetes and pancreatitis is not associated with insulitis. *Sci Rep* 10(1):19187, 2020.
35. Gilor C, Duesberg C, Elliott DA, et al. Co-impairment of autonomic and glucagon responses to insulin-induced hypoglycemia in dogs with naturally-occurring insulin-dependent diabetes mellitus. *Am J Physiol Endocrinol Metab* 319(6):E1074-1083, 2020.
36. Hill RC, Burrows CF, Bauer JE, Ellison GW, Finke MD, Jones GL. Texturized vegetable protein containing indigestible soy carbohydrate affects blood insulin concentrations in dogs fed high fat diets. *J Nutrition* 136(7 Suppl):2024s-2027s, 2006.
37. Carciofi AC, Takakura FS, de-Oliveira LD, et al. Effects of six carbohydrate sources on dog diet digestibility and post-prandial glucose and insulin response. *J Anim Physiol Anim Nutr (Berl)* 92(3):326-336, 2008.
38. Elliott KF, Rand JS, Fleeman LM, et al. A diet lower in digestible carbohydrate results in lower postprandial glucose concentrations compared with a traditional canine diabetes diet and an adult maintenance diet in healthy dogs. *Res Vet Sci* 93(1):288-295, 2012.
39. Fleeman L, Gilor C. Insulin therapy in small animals, part 3: dogs. *Vet Clin North Am Small Anim Pract* 53(3):645-656, 2023.
40. Tardo AM, Fleeman LM, Fracassi F, Berg A, Guarino AL, Gilor C. A dose titration protocol for once daily insulin glargine 300 U/mL for the treatment of canine diabetes mellitus. *J Vet Intern Med* 38:1-9, 2024
41. Miller M, Pires J, Crakes K, Greathouse R, Quach N, Gilor C. Day-to-day variability of porcine lente, insulin glargine 300U/mL and insulin degludec in diabetic dogs. *J Vet Intern Med* 35(5):2131-2139, 2021.
42. Oda H, Mori A, Ishii S, Shono S, Onozawa E, Sako T. Time-action profiles of insulin degludec in healthy dogs and its effects on glycemic control in diabetic dogs. *J Vet Med Sci* 80(11):1720-1723, 2018.
43. Fink H, Herbert C, Gilor C. Pharmacodynamics and pharmacokinetics of insulin detemir and insulin glargine 300 U/mL in healthy dogs. *Dom Animal Endocrinol* 64:17-30, 2018.
44. Gilor C, Fracassi F, Berg A, Guarino A, Tardo A, Fleeman LM. Once-daily insulin glargine 300 U/mL for the treatment of canine diabetes mellitus (Abstract). *J Vet Intern Med* 36(6), 2022.
45. Mori A, Sako T, Lee P, et al. Comparison of time-action profiles of insulin glargine and NPH insulin in normal and diabetic dogs. *Vet Res Comm* 32(7):563-573, 2008.
46. Palm CA, Boston RC, Refsal KR, Hess RS. An investigation of the action of neutral protamine Hagedorn human analogue insulin in dogs with naturally occurring diabetes mellitus. *J Vet Intern Med* 23(1):50-55, 2009.

47. Graham PA, Nash AS, McKellar QA. Pharmacokinetics of a porcine insulin zinc suspension in diabetic dogs. *J Small Anim Pract* 38:434-438, 1997.
48. Fleeman LM, Rand JS, Morton JM. Pharmacokinetics and pharmacodynamics of porcine insulin zinc suspension in eight diabetic dogs. *Vet Rec* 164:232-237, 2009.
49. Clark M, Thomaseth K, Heit M, Hoenig M. Pharmacokinetics and pharmacodynamics of protamine zinc recombinant human insulin in healthy dogs. *J Vet Pharmacol Ther* 35(4):342-350, 2012.
50. Sako T, Mori A, Lee P, et al. Time-action profiles of insulin detemir in normal and diabetic dogs. *Res Vet Sci* 90(3):396-403, 2011.
51. Ward CR, Christiansen K, Li J, Bryson WL, Jerrentrup KA, Kroh C. Field efficacy and safety of protamine zinc recombinant human insulin in 276 dogs with diabetes mellitus. *Dom Anim Endocrinol* 75:106575, 2020.
52. Maggiore AD, Nelson RW, Dennis J, Johnson E, Kass PH. Efficacy of protamine zinc recombinant human insulin for controlling hyperglycemia in dogs with diabetes mellitus. *J Vet Intern Med* 26(1):109-115, 2012.
53. Miki Y, Mori A, Hayakawa N, et al. Evaluation of serum and urine 1,5-anhydro-D-glucitol and myo-inositol concentrations in healthy dogs. *J Vet Med Sci* 73(9):1117-1126, 2011.
54. Munroe WE, Laxton D, Fallin EA, et al. Efficacy and safety of a purified porcine insulin zinc suspension for managing diabetes mellitus in dogs. *J Vet Intern Med* 19(5):675-682, 2005.
55. Fracassi F, Corradini S, Hafner M, Boretti FS, Sieber-Ruckstuhl NS, Reusch CE. Detemir insulin for the treatment of diabetes mellitus in dogs. *J Am Vet Med Assoc* 247(1):73-78, 2015.
56. Niessen SJ, Powney S, Guitian J, et al. Evaluation of a quality-of-life tool for dogs with diabetes mellitus. *J Vet Intern Med* 26(4):953-961, 2012.
57. Niessen SJM, Hazuchova K, Powney SL, et al. The Big Pet Diabetes Survey: perceived frequency and triggers for euthanasia. *Vet Sci* 4(2):E27, 2017.
58. Fall T, Hamlin HH, Hedhammar A, Kampe O, Egenvall A. Diabetes mellitus in a population of 180,000 insured dogs: incidence, survival, and breed distribution. *J Vet Intern Med* 21(6):1209-1216, 2007.
59. Del Baldo F, Colajanni L, Corradini S, et al. Owner preference for insulin delivery device and glycaemic control in diabetic dogs. *J Small Anim Pract* 64(4):255-264, 2023.
60. Malerba E, Fracassi F, Del Baldo F, Golinelli S, Ceccherini M, Barbarossa A. The accuracy and precision of insulin administration using human and veterinary pen-injectors and syringes for administration of insulin. *J Vet Intern Med* 35(3):1255-1264, 2021.
61. Casella SJ, Mongilio MK, Plotnick LP, Hesterberg MP, Long CA. Accuracy and precision of low-dose insulin administration. *Pediatrics* 91(6):1155-1157, 1993.
62. Mitchell VD, Porter K, Beatty SJ. Administration technique and storage of disposable insulin pens reported by patients with diabetes. *Diabetes Educ* 38(5):651-658, 2012. doi:10.1177/0145721712450921
63. European Society of Veterinary Endocrinology. Project ALIVE: Euopean Society of Veterinary Endocrinology, https://www.esve.org/alive/search.aspx, accessed December 16, 2023.
64. Fleeman LM, Rand JS, Markwell PJ. Lack of advantage of high-fibre, moderate-carbohydrate diets in dogs with stabilised diabetes. *J Small Anim Pract* 50:604-614, 2009.
65. André A, Leriche I, Chaix G, et al. Recovery of insulin sensitivity and optimal body composition after rapid weight loss in obese dogs fed a high-protein medium-carbohydrate diet. *J Anim Physiol Anim Nutr (Berl)* 101 Suppl 1:21-30, 2017.
66. Teshima E, Brunetto MA, Teixeira FA, et al. Influence of type of starch and feeding management on glycaemic control in diabetic dogs. *J Anim Physiol Anim Nutr (Berl)* 105:1192-1202, 2021.
67. Graham PA, Maskell IE, Rawlings JM, et al. Influence of a high fibre diet on glycaemic control and quality of life in dogs with diabetes mellitus. *J Small Anim Pract* 43:67-73, 2002.
68. Behrend E, Holford A, Lathan P, et al. 2018 AAHA Diabetes Management Guidelines for Dogs and Cats. *J Am Anim Hosp Assoc* 54(1):1-21, 2018. doi:10.5326/JAAHA-MS-6822.
69. Casella M, Wess G, Reusch CE. Measurement of capillary blood glucose concentrations by pet owners: a new tool in the management of diabetes mellitus. *J Am Anim Hosp Assoc* 38: 239-245, 2002. doi:10.5326/0380239.
70. Casella M, Wess G, Hässig M, et al. Home monitoring of blood glucose concentration by owners of diabetic dogs. *J Small Anim Pract* 44:298-305, 2003. doi:10.1111/j.1748-5827.2003.tb00158.x.
71. Del Baldo F, Canton C, Testa S, et al. Comparison between a flash glucose monitoring system and a portable blood glucose meter for monitoring dogs with diabetes mellitus. *J Vet Intern Med* 34(6):2296-2305, 2020. doi:10.1111/jvim.15930.
72. Fleeman LM, Rand JS. Evaluation of day-to-day variability of serial blood glucose concentration curves in diabetic dogs. *J Am Vet Med Assoc* 3:317-321, 2003. doi:10.2460/javma.2003.222.317.
73. Fracassi F, Linari G, Del Baldo F, et al. Comparison of lente insulin and NPH insulin therapy for the treatment of newly diagnosed diabetic dogs: a randomised study. *Vet Rec* 183(8):262, 2018. doi:10.1136/vr.104818.
74. Monroe WE, Laxton D, Fallin EA, et al. Efficacy and safety of a purified porcine insulin zinc suspension for managing diabetes mellitus in dogs. *J Vet Intern Med* 19(5):675-682, 2005. doi:10.1892/0891 6640(2005)19[675:easoap]2.0.co;2.
75. Fracassi F, Boretti FS, Sieber-Ruckstuhl NS, et al. Use of insulin glargine in dogs with diabetes mellitus. *Vet Rec* 170(2):52, 2012. doi:10.1136/vr.100070.
76. Hess RS, Drobatz KJ. Glargine insulin for treatment of naturally occurring diabetes mellitus in dogs. *J Am Vet Med Assoc* 243(8):1154-1161, 2013. doi:10.2460/javma.243.8.1154.
77. Mori H, Okada Y, Kurozumi A, et al. Factors influencing inter-day glycemic variability in diabetic outpatients receiving insulin therapy. *J Diabetes Invest* 8:69-74, 2017. doi:10.1111/jdi.12551.
78. Suh S, Kim JH. Glycemic variability: how do we measure it why is it important? *Diabetes Metab J* 39:273-382, 2015. doi:10.4093/dmj.2015.39.4.273.
79. Dicembrini I, Cosentino C, Monami M, et al. Effects of real-time continuous glucose monitoring in type 1 diabetes: a meta-analysis of randomized controlled trials. *Acta Diabetologica* 58(4):401-410, 2021. doi:10.1007/s00592-020-01589-3.
80. Shea EK, Hess RS. Assessment of postprandial hyperglycemia and circadian fluctuation of glucose concentrations in diabetic dogs using a flash glucose monitoring system. *J Vet Intern Med* 35(2):843-52, 2021. doi:10.1111/jvim.16046.
81. Re M, Del Baldo F, Tardo AM, et al. Monitoring of diabetes mellitus using the flash glucose monitoring system: the owners' point of view. *Vet Sci* 10(3):203, 2023. doi: 10.3390/vetsci10030203.
82. Reusch CE, Haberer B. Evaluation of fructosamine in dogs and cats with hypo- or hyperproteinaemia, azotaemia, hyperlipidaemia and hyperbilirubinaemia. *Vet Rec* 148(12):370-376, 2001. doi:10.1136/vr.148.12.370.
83. Reusch CE, Gerber B, Boretti FS. Serum fructosamine concentrations in dogs with hypothyroidism. *Vet Res Comm* 26(7):531-536, 2002. doi:10.1023/a:1020287430949.
84. Zeugswetter F, Kleiter M, Wolfesberger B, et al. Elevated fructosamine concentrations caused by IgA paraproteinemia in two dogs. *J Vet Sci* 11(4):359-361, 2010. doi: 10.4142/jvs.2010.11.4.359.
85. Nelson RW. Canine diabetes mellitus. In Feldman EC, Nelson RW, Reusch CE, Scott-Moncrieff JC, Behren EN (editors). Canine and Feline Endocrinology 4th edition. St Louis, Elsevier Saunders, 2015, pp. 213-53.
86. Del Baldo F, Magna L, Dondi F, et al. Comparison of serum fructosamine and glycated hemoglobin values for assessment ofglycemic control in dogs with diabetes mellitus. *Am J Vet Res* 81(3):233-242, 2020. doi:10.2460/ajvr.81.3.233.
87. Zeugswetter FK, Beer R, Schwendenwein I. Evaluation of fructosamine concentration as an index marker for glycaemic control in diabetic dogs. *Vet Rec* 190(2):e244, 2022. doi: 10.1002/vetr.244.
88. Norris O, Schermerhorn T. Relationship between HbA1c, fructosamine and clinical assessment of glycemic control in dogs. *PLoS One* 17(2):e0264275, 2022. doi: 10.1371/journal.pone.0264275.
89. Loste A, Marca MC. Fructosamine and glycated hemoglobin in the assessment of glycaemic control in dogs. *Vet Res* 32(1):55-62, 2001. doi:10.1051/vetres:2001109.
90. Wood PA, Smith JE. Elevation rate of glycosylated hemoglobins in dogs after induction of experimental diabetes mellitus. *Metabolism* 31(9):906-909, 1982. doi:10.1016/0026-0495(82)90180-9.

91. Hasegawa S, Sako T, Takemura N, et al. Glycated hemoglobin fractions in normal and diabetic dogs measured by high performance liquid chromatography. *J Vet Med Sci* 53(1):65-68, 1991. doi:10.1292/jvms.53.65.
92. Elliott DA, Nelson RW, Feldman EC, et al. Glycosylated hemoglobin concentration for assessment of glycemic control in diabetic cats. *J Vet Intern Med* 11(3):161-165, 1997. doi:10.1111/j.1939-1676.1997.tb00084.x.
93. Mahaffey EA, Cornelius LM. Evaluation of a commercial kit for measurement of glycosylated hemoglobin in canine blood. *Vet Clin Pathol* 10(1):21-24, 1981. doi:10.1111/j.1939-165x.1981.tb00799.x.
94. Marca MC, Loste A. Glycosylated haemoglobin assay of canine blood samples. *J Small Anim Pract* 41(5):189-192, 2000. doi:10.1111/j.1748-5827.2000.tb03192.x.
95. Goemans AF, Spence SJ, Ramsey IK. Validation and determination of a reference interval for canine HbA1c using an immunoturbidimetric assay. *Vet Clin Pathol* 46(2):227-237, 2017. doi:10.1111/vcp.12477.
96. Davison LJ, Podd SL, Ristic JM, et al. Evaluation of two point-of-care analysers for measurement of fructosamine or haemoglobin A1c in dogs. *J Small Anim Pract* 43(12):526-532, 2002. doi:10.1111/j.1748-5827.2002.tb00025.x.
97. Catchpole B, Mountford S, Barabas S, et al. Evaluation of a disposable device for the measurement of haemoglobin A1c in dogs. *Vet Rec* 162(2):47-49, 2008. doi:10.1136/vr.162.2.47.
98. Oikonomidis IL, Tsouloufi TK, Soubasis N, et al. Validation, reference intervals and overlap performance of a new commercially available automated capillary electrophoresis assay for the determination of the major fraction of glycated haemoglobin (HbA1c) in dogs. *Vet J* 234:48-54, 2018. doi:10.1016/j.tvjl.2018.02.005.
99. Welsh KJ, Kirkman MS, Sacks DB. Role of glycated proteins in the diagnosis and management of diabetes: research gaps and future directions. *Diabetes Care* 39(8):1299-1306, 2016. doi:10.2337/dc15-2727.
100. Haberer B, Reusch CE. Glycated haemoglobin in various pathological conditions: investigations based on a new, fully automated method. *J Small Anim Pract* 39(11):510-517, 1998. doi:10.1111/j.1748-5827.1998.tb03696.x
101. American Diabetes Association. Standards of medical care for patients with diabetes mellitus. *Diabetes Care* 26 Suppl 1:S33-50, 2003. doi:10.2337/diacare.26.2007.s33.
102. Del Baldo F, Fracassi F. Continuous glucose monitoring in dogs and cats. Application of new technology to an old problem. *Vet Clin Nort Am Small Anim Pract* 53,591-613, 2023. doi:10.1016/j.cvsm.2023.01.008.
103. Fleeman L, Gilor C. Insulin therapy in small animals, part 1: general principles. *Vet Clin North Am Small Anim Pract* 53,615-633, 2023. doi:10.1016/j.cvsm.2023.02.002.
104. Fleeman L, Gilor C. Insulin therapy in small animals, part 3: dogs. *Vet Clin North Am Small Anim Pract* 53:645-656, 2023. doi:10.1016/j.cvsm.2023.02.003.
105. Hess RS. Insulin resistance in dogs. *Vet Clin North Am Small Anim Pract* 40,309-316, 2010. DOI:10.1016/j.cvsm.2009.12.001.
106. Miceli DD, Pignataro OP, Castillo VA. Concurrent hyperadrenocorticism and diabetes mellitus in dogs. *Res Vet Sci* 115:425-431, 2017. doi:10.1016/j.rvsc.2017.07.026.
107. Fukuta H, Mori A, Urumuhan N, et al. Characterization and comparison of insulin resistance induced by Cushing syndrome or diestrus against healthy control dogs as determined by euglycemic-hyperinsulinemic glucose clamp profile glucose infusion rate using an artificial pancreas apparatus. *J Vet Med Sci* 74(11):1527-1530, 2012. DOI: 10.1292/jvms.12-0041.
108. Peterson ME, Nesbitt GH, Schaer M. Diagnosis and management of concurrent diabetes mellitus and hyperadrenocorticism in thirty dogs. *J Am Vet Med Assoc* 178(1):66-69, 1981.
109. McLauchlan G, Knottenbelt C, Augusto M, et al. Retrospective evaluation of the effect of trilostane on insulin requirement and fructosamine concentration in eight diabetic dogs with hyperadrenocorticism. *J Small Anim Pract* 51(12):642-648, 2010. doi:10.1111/j.1748-5827.2010.01005.x.
110. Pérez-López L, Mendoza P, Melián C. Effects of concurrent canine Cushing's syndrome and diabetes mellitus on insulin requirements, trilostane dose, and survival time. *Res Vet Sci* 161:62-68, 2023. doi:10.1016/j.rvsc.2023.06.003.
111. Hofer-Inteeworn N, Panciera DL, Monroe WE, et al. Effect of hypothyroidism on insulin sensitivity and glucose tolerance in dogs. *Am J Vet Res* 73(4):529-538, 2012. doi:10.2460/ajvr.73.4.529.
112. Diaz-Espiñeira MM, Mol JA, Rijnberk A, et al. Adenohypophyseal function in dogs with primary hypothyroidism and nonthyroidal illness. *J Vet Intern Med* 23(1):100-107, 2009. doi:10.1111/j.1939-1676.2008.0240.x.
113. Mazaki-Tovi M, Feuermann Y, Segev G, et al. Increased serum leptin and insulin concentrations in canine hypothyroidism. *Vet J* 183(1):109-114, 2010. doi:10.1016/j.tvjl.2008.08.017.
114. Panciera DL. Hypothyroidism in dogs: 66 cases (1987-1992). *J Am Vet Med Assoc* 204:761-767, 1994.
115. Dixon RM, Reid SW, Mooney CT. Epidemiological, clinical, haematological and biochemical characteristics of canine hypothyroidism. *Vet Rec* 145(17):481-487, 1999. doi:10.1136/vr.145.17.481.
116. Blois SL, Dickie E, Kruth SA, et al. Multiple endocrine diseases in dogs: 35 cases (1996-2009). *J Am Vet Med Assoc* 238:1616, 2011. doi:10.2460/javma.238.12.1616.
117. Pöppl AG, Carvalho GLC, Vivian ITF, et al. Canine diabetes mellitus risk factors: a matched case-control study. *Res Vet Sci* 114:469-473, 2017. doi:10.1016/j.rvsc.2017.08.003.
118. Durocher LL, Hinchcliff KW, DiBartola SP, et al. Acid-base and hormonal abnormalities in dogs with naturally occurring diabetes mellitus. *J Am Vet Med Assoc* 232:1310-1320, 2008. doi:10.2460/javma.232.9.1310.
119. Pöppl AG, Mottin TS, González FH. Diabetes mellitus remission after resolution of inflammatory and progesterone-related conditions in bitches. *Res Vet Sci* 94(3):471-473, 2013. doi:10.1016/j.rvsc.2012.10.008.
120. Hannon AM, Thompson CJ, Sherlock M. Diabetes in patients with acromegaly. *Curr Diab Rep* 17:8, 2017. doi:10.1007/s11892-017-0838-7.
121. Fall T, Hedhammar A, Wallberg A, et al. Diabetes mellitus in elkhounds is associated with diestrus and pregnancy. *J Vet Intern Med* 24:1322-1328, 2010. doi:10.1111/j.1939-1676.2010.0630.x
122. Bhatti SFM, Duchateau L, Okkens AC, et al. Treatment of growth hormone excess in dogs with the progesterone receptor antagonist aglepristone. *Theriogenology* 66,797-803, 2006. doi:10.1016/j.theriogenology.2006.01.052.
123. Feldman EC, Nelson RW, Reusch C (editors). Canine and Feline Endocrinology 4th edition. St. Louis, Saunders, 2015.
124. Gal A, Burchel RK. Diabetes mellitus and the kidneys. *Vet Clin North Am Small Anim Pract* 53:565-580, 2023.
125. Cantero F, Ortillés A, Teresa Peña M, et al. Prevalence of ocular findings and their association with glycemia in dogs with diabetes mellitus: A 10-year clinical study (2009-2019). *Open Vet J* 13(5):620-628, 2023.
126. Beam S, Correa MT, Davidson MG. A retrospective cohort study on the development of cataracts in dogs with diabetes mellitus: 200 cases. *Vet Ophthalmol* 2:169-172, 1999.
127. Plummer CE, Specht A, Gelatt KN. Ocular manifestation of endocrine disease. *Compendium* 733-743, 2007.
128. Kador PF, Webb TR, Bras ID, Ketring K, Wyman M. Topical Kinostat™ ameliorates the clinical development and progression of cataracts in dogs with diabetes mellitus. *Vet Ophthalmol* 13(6):363-368, 2010.
129. Williams DL. Effect of oral alpha lipoic acid in preventing the genesis of canine diabetic cataract: A preliminary study. *Vet Sci* 4(18):1-6, 2017.
130. Bagley LH, Lavach JD. Comparison of postoperative phacoemulsification results in dogs with and without diabetes mellitus: 153 cases (1991-1992). *J Am Vet Med Assoc* 205(8):1165-1169, 1994.
131. Anoop S, Philip LM, Ramankutty S, et al. Ocular manifestations of endocrine disorders in small animals. *J Indian Vet Assoc* 18(2):7-19, 2020.
132. Sebastian MJ, Khan SKA, Pappachan JM, et al. Diabetes and cognitive function: An evidence-based current perspective. *World J Diabetes* 14(2): 92-109, 2023.

133. Dewey CD, Davies ES, Xie H, Wakshlag JJ. Canine cognitive dysfunction: pathophysiology, diagnosis, and treatment. *Vet Clin North Am Small Anim Pract* 49(3):477-499, 2019.
134. Verrotti A, Prezioso G, Scattoni R, et al. Autonomic neuropathy in diabetes mellitus. *Front Endocrinol* 5:205(1-7), 2014.
135. Acierno MJ, Brown S, Coleman AE, et al. ACVIM consensus statement: guidelines for the identification, evaluation, and management of systemic hypertension in dogs and cats. *J Vet Intern Med* 32(6):1803-1822, 2018.
136. Novellas R, Gopegui RR, Espada Y. Determination of renalvascular resistance in dogs with diabetes mellitus and hyperadrenocorticism. *Vet Rec* 163:592-596, 2008.
137. Brands MW, Manhiani MM. Sodium-retaining effect of insulin in diabetes. *Am J Physiol-Regul Integrative Comp Physiol* 303:R1101–R1109, 2012.
138. Herring IP, Panciera DL, Werre SR. Longitudinal prevalence of hypertension, proteinuria, and retinopathy in dogs with spontaneous diabetes mellitus. *J Vet Intern Med* 28:488-495, 2014.
139. Soares FAC, Machado L, Carvalho GLC, et al. Cardiac troponin I, fructosamine, and cardiovascular parameters in dogs with diabetes mellitus. *Austral J Vet Sci* 50:129-133, 2018.
140. Crakes KR, Pires J, Quach N, et al. Fenofibrate promotes PPARα-targeted recovery of the intestinal epithelial barrier at the host-microbe interface in dogs with diabetes mellitus. *Sci Rep* 11:13454, 2021.
141. Lombardo F, Bombaci B, Alibrandi A, et al. The impact of insulin-induced lipodystrophy on glycemic variability in pediatric patients with type 1 diabetes. *Children* 9:1087, 2022.
142. Pöppl AG, Meyrer B, Costa E, et al. Analytical accuracy of the owner's perception of exposition to risk factors for canine diabetes mellitus, and survival after its diagnosis in southern Brazil. *Acta Scientiae Veterinariae* 41:1116, 2013.
143. Tardo AM, Del Baldo F, Dondi F, et al. Survival estimates and outcome predictors in dogs with newly diagnosed diabetes mellitus treated in a veterinary teaching hospital. *Vet Rec* 185(22):692, 2019.
144. French EK, Donihi AC, Korytkowski MT. Diabetic ketoacidosis and hyperosmolar hyperglycemic syndrome: review of acute decompensated diabetes in adult patients. *BMJ* 365:1114, 2019.
145. Miles JM, Haymond MW, Nissen SL, et al. Effects of free fatty acid availability, glucagon excess, and insulin deficiency on ketone body production in postabsorptive man. *J Clin Invest* 71:1554-1561, 1983.
146. Li PK, Lee JT, MacGillivray MH, et al. Direct, fixed-time kinetic assays for beta-hydroxybutyrate and acetoacetate with a centrifugal analyzer or a computer-backed spectrophotometer. *Clin Chem* 26:1713-1717, 1980.
147. Rebrin K, Steil GM, van Antwerp WP, et al. Subcutaneous glucose predicts plasma glucose independent of insulin: implications for continuous monitoring. *Am J Physiol* 277:E561-E571, 1999.
148. DiFazio J, Fletcher DJ. Retrospective comparison of early- versus late-insulin therapy regarding effect on time to resolution of diabetic ketosis and ketoacidosis in dogs and cats: 60 cases (2003-2013). *J Vet Emerg Crit Care* 26:108-115, 2016.
149. Home PD. The pharmacokinetics and pharmacodynamics of rapid-acting insulin analogues and their clinical consequences. *Diabetes Obes Metab* 14:780-788, 2012.
150. Ersoz HO, Ukinc K, Kose M, et al. Subcutaneous lispro and intravenous regular insulin treatments are equally effective and safe for the treatment of mild and moderate diabetic ketoacidosis in adult patients. *Int J Clin Pract* 60:429-433, 2006.
151. Umpierrez GE, Latif K, Stoever J, et al. Efficacy of subcutaneous insulin lispro versus continuous intravenous regular insulin for the treatment of patients with diabetic ketoacidosis. *Am J Med* 117:291-296, 2004.
152. Sears KW, Drobatz KJ, Hess RS. Use of lispro insulin for treatment of diabetic ketoacidosis in dogs. *J Vet Emerg Crit Care* 22:211-218, 2012.
153. Malerba E, Mazzarino M, Del Baldo F, et al. Use of lispro insulin for treatment of diabetic ketoacidosis in cats. *J Fel Med Surg* 21:115-123, 2019.
154. Walsh ES, Drobatz KJ, Hess RS. Use of intravenous insulin aspart for treatment of naturally occurring diabetic ketoacidosis in dogs. *J Vet Emerg Crit Care* 26:101-107, 2016.
155. Nelson RW. Diabetic ketoacidosis. In Feldman EC, Nelson RW, Reusch CE (editors). Canine and Feline Endocrinology 4th edition. St. Louis, Elsevier, 2015, pp. 315-347.
156. Malerba E, Alessandrini F, Grossi G, et al. Efficacy and safety of intramuscular insulin lispro vs. continuous intravenous regular insulin for the treatment of dogs with diabetic ketoacidosis. *Front Vet Sci* 7:559008, 2020.
157. Koenig A, Drobatz KJ, Beale AB, King LG. Hyperglycemic, hyperosmolar syndrome in feline diabetics: 17 cases (1995-2001). *J Vet Emerg Crit Care* 14:30-40, 2004.
158. Trotman TK, Drobatz KJ, Hess RS. Retrospective evaluation of hyperosmolar hyperglycemia in 66 dogs (1993-2008). *J Vet Emerg Crit Care* 23:557-564, 2013.
159. Phillips SM, Han XX, Green HJ, Bonen A. Increments in skeletal muscle GLUT-1 and GLUT-4 after endurance training in humans. *Am J Physiol* 270(3 Pt 1):E456-462, 1996.
160. Nishida Y, Higaki Y, Tokuyama K, et al. Effect of mild exercise training on glucose effectiveness in healthy men. *Diabetes Care* 24:1008-1013, 2001.

CHAPTER 39

Insulinoma

Johan P. Schoeman
BVSc, MMedVet,
PhD, DSAM, DECVIM,
FRCVS

Insulinoma is an insulin-secreting tumor of pancreatic beta-cells that results in excessive insulin secretion and clinical signs of hypoglycemia. Canine insulinoma was first described in the dog in 1935.[30] A rapidly expanding body of knowledge has resulted in the description of approximately 600 canine cases since then (of which 260 in the past 4 years).

Pathogenesis and clinical manifestations

Insulin-secreting pancreatic beta-cells comprise approximately 70% of cells in the islets of Langerhans, which, in turn, only comprise approximately 1-2% of pancreatic volume. Most canine insulinomas are malignant. About 80% of insulinomas are solitary, located in one pancreatic limb rather than in the body of the pancreas. Occasionally, no discrete nodule is seen during gross pancreatic examination, in which case histology is required to identify the tumor.

The rate of detected metastatic lesions in dogs from different studies ranges from 45% to 64%. It is higher in studies based on necropsy versus studies using samples obtained surgically. Clinical staging of pancreatic tumors is defined in Table 39.1. Most dogs with insulinoma have stage II or III disease, and the most common sites of metastases are regional lymph nodes and the liver. Metastatic disease has an unlimited distribution.[18] Although the etiology of insulinoma is not known, local growth hormone (GH) production, which is not associated with increased plasma GH concentrations, has been paracrine or autocrine mechanisms.[25]

Neoplastic proliferation of pancreatic beta cells causes autonomous and excessive insulin secretion with resultant episodes of hypoglycemia.

Glucose enters pancreatic beta-cells and causes the closure of ATP-sensitive K^+ channels. Closure of these channels causes a build-up of K^+ ions inside the cell and the opening of voltage-sensitive Ca^{2+} channels. The resultant increased cytoplasmic Ca^{2+} leads to insulin exocytosis into the extracellular environment and, ultimately, the blood in equimolar amounts to C-peptide.

In healthy animals, insulin secretion is completely inhibited when blood glucose is <80 mg/dL (<4.4 mmol/L). However, insulin secretion from neoplastic beta-cells is independent of blood glucose concentration and persists despite low blood glucose concentrations. As a result, one of the biochemical hallmarks of insulinoma is high or normal blood insulin concentrations despite low blood glucose concentrations. The most important compensatory mechanisms for hypoglycemia are inhibition of insulin secretion and stimulation of counter-regulatory hormone secretion. The four counter-regulatory hormones secreted in response to hypoglycemia are glucagon, catecholamines, growth hormone (GH), and glucocorticoids. Of these, glucagon and catecholamines are the predominant drivers of the short-term responses to low blood glucose concentrations.

TABLE 39.1 Clinical staging of insulinoma.

Stage of disease	Primary tumor	Regional lymph node	Distant metastases
Stage 1	T_1 (Insulinoma present in pancreas)	N_0 (Negative nodes)	M_0 (no metastasis)
Stage II	T_1 (Insulinoma present in pancreas)	N_1 (Positive nodes)	M_0 (no metastasis)
Stage III	T_1 (Insulinoma present in pancreas)	N_0/N_1 (Neg. or pos. nodes)	M_1 (metastasis)

Signalment

The mean age of dogs with insulinoma is 9 years, ranging from 3 to 15 years. Although any breed of dog may develop insulinoma, it has been reported mostly in medium- to large-breed dogs. Such breeds reported to be at increased risk include Boxers, German Shepherd dogs, Golden Retrievers, Labrador Retrievers, Irish Setters, Standard Poodles, Collies, Springer Spaniels, and also some smaller breeds like Fox Terriers, West Highland White Terriers and Jack Russel Terriers.[6,9,27] There is no apparent sex predisposition for the disease.

Clinical signs

Glucose is the single most important source of energy for the brain. Brain function is dependent on a continuous glucose supply because both carbohydrate storage and the brain's ability to utilize other fuels are limited. Clinical signs are thus usually due to the effect of episodes of hypoglycemia on the central nervous system (neuroglycopenia) or to hypoglycemia-induced release of catecholamines. Clinical signs attributable to neuroglycopenia include mental dullness, disorientation, weakness, proprioceptive ataxia, visual disturbances, collapse, and focal or generalized seizures (Video 39.1). Sometimes, the signs might resemble those of paroxysmal dyskinesia.[27] Clinical signs related to excess catecholamine release and stimulation of the sympathetic nervous system include hunger, nervousness, and tremors.

The severity of clinical signs is partly correlated to the blood glucose nadir. Severe hypoglycemia may ultimately result in coma and death. However, clinical signs may also be related to the duration and the rate at which hypoglycemia develops because gradual decreases in blood glucose concentration are less likely to stimulate catecholamine secretion. Insulin secretion and clinical signs are typically episodic, and the secretion of counter-regulatory hormones tends to increase blood glucose concentration, transiently resolving the neuroglycopenic signs. Feeding can also alleviate clinical signs if blood glucose concentrations are increased. In contrast, feeding may also exacerbate clinical signs by stimulating further insulin secretion. Moreover, fasting, exercise, or excitement worsen clinical signs by decreasing blood glucose concentration or increasing sympathetic stimulation. The clinical signs of canine insulinoma are summarized in Table 39.2. Although most dogs have more than one of these clinical signs, some dogs have none. Some cases may gain weight because of the anabolic effects of insulin. Postictal changes may be apparent if a seizure occurred quite recently. A peripheral polyneuropathy characterized by posterior paresis or tetraparesis and decreased or absent appendicular reflexes has been described in dogs with insulinoma.[27] The etiology of this insulinoma-associated peripheral neuropathy has not been firmly established, yet it is most likely a paraneoplastic immune-mediated disorder.[35]

TABLE 39.2 Reported clinical signs in descending order of prevalence in 441 dogs from several studies.[5,8,14,16,18,27,29,32,33]

Clinical sign	Number of dogs (%)
Generalized seizures	183/441(41)
Generalized weakness	169/441 (38)
Collapse	132/441 (30)
Shaking/trembling/muscle twitching	79/441 (18)
Ataxia	81/441 (18)
Disorientation/behavioral changes	51/441 (12)
Hind limb weakness	43/441 (10)
Exercise intolerance	30/441 (7)
Polyphagia	20/441 (5)
Polyuria and polydipsia	20/441 (5)
Stupor/lethargy	17/441 (4)
Focal seizures	15/441(3.4)
Diarrhea	8/441 (2)
Obesity or weight gain	6/441 (1.4)
Blindness	6/441 (1.4)
Anorexia	6/441 (1.4)
Vomiting	6/441 (1.4)
Dyskinesia	3/441 (0.7)
Head tilt	2/441 (0.5)
Nervousness	2/441 (0.5)

Diagnostic procedures

Differential diagnoses

The causes of hypoglycemia may be broadly separated into those caused by decreased glucose production, those associated with excessive glucose utilization, or a combination thereof, although the exact mechanism is unknown in some cases. In elderly dogs, common differentials include hepatic insufficiency, sepsis, and nonpancreatic neoplasia-producing insulin-like growth factors (hepatocellular carcinoma, leiomyosarcoma, metastatic mammary carcinoma, and lymphoma). In middle-aged dogs, hypoadrenocorticism should be considered[31] and nesidioblastosis (hyperplasia of non-neoplastic beta-cells),[22] whilst juvenile hypoglycemia, glycogen storage diseases, portosystemic shunts, parvovirus infection, and babesiosis must be considered in young dogs. Importantly, always check for spuriously low glucose values due to a delay in processing samples or uncalibrated handheld devices. For further details regarding the differential diagnosis of hypoglycemia in dogs, see chapter 11.

Video 39.1

Video footage of a dog presenting with collapse and obtundation (mental dullness) secondary to hypoglycemia. Intravenous dextrose is administered, followed by a rapid recovery of the clinical signs.

Clinicopathological findings

Clinical suspicion of insulinoma begins with the documentation of an appropriate history and clinical signs, hypoglycemia (blood glucose concentration less than approximately 60 mg/dL [3.3 mmol/L]), and concurrent normo- or hyperinsulinemia (serum insulin concentrations within or above reference interval) (see Table 39.3 for interpretation). A pancreatic mass may be identified with imaging studies and this strengthens the suspicion for insulinoma. The diagnosis of insulinoma is ultimately confirmed with histologic examination and immunohistochemical staining of a pancreatic mass. Histopathology is usually characterized by monomorphic epitheloid cells with large amounts of fine granular basophilic cytoplasm. Often, fine connective tissue septae subdivide the cells into small chords or lobules in a characteristic neuroendocrine pattern. Immunohistochemical staining with chromogranin A is used to identify

TABLE 39.3 The clinical interpretation and suggested actions when detecting hypoglycemia in combination with variable insulin concentrations in a patient.

Glucose concentration	Insulin concentration	Interpretation and further action
<60 mg/dL (3.3 mmol/L)	Insulin above reference interval	Insulinoma
<60 mg/dL (3.3 mmol/L)	Insulin at high end of reference interval	Insulinoma
<60 mg/dL (3.3 mmol/L)	Insulin at lower end of reference interval	Equivocal; repeat insulin concentration another day; consider measuring fructosamine
<60 mg/dL (3.3 mmol/L)	Insulin undetectable	Unlikely to be insulinoma

the neuroendocrine nature of insulinoma. In addition, tumor proliferation assessed by Ki67 immunostaining is related to progression and survival. Complete blood count (CBC), serum biochemistry, and urinalysis are usually unremarkable, aside from the hypoglycemia observed in most patients. Mild hypokalemia and increased alkaline phosphatase and/or alanine aminotransferase activities have been documented.[12] Although hypoglycemia is observed on randomly obtained blood samples from the vast majority of dogs with insulinoma, especially if repeated, some patients are euglycemic at the time of presentation.[16,17] When a dog suspected of insulinoma is euglycemic, it should be fasted and closely monitored for hypoglycemia while blood glucose concentrations are measured every 30 to 60 minutes. Point-of-care analyzers are usually adequate for this purpose. In most, but not all, dogs with insulinoma, hypoglycemia (blood glucose <60 mg/dL [3.3 mmol/L]) develops within 12 hours of the previous meal.

Endocrine testing

When hypoglycemia is documented, serum for the measurement of insulin concentration should be submitted from the same sample. As mentioned above, a limited number of dogs with insulinoma do not exhibit hypoglycemia, even with repeated measurements or after a prolonged fast of 48-72 hours.[16] Low fructosamine has been used to strengthen the clinical suspicion of insulinoma in such dogs.[17] Moreover, glycosylated hemoglobin A1c concentration has been low in some, but not all, dogs with insulinoma.[7] Repetition of serum insulin measurements at a reputable laboratory may also aid in the diagnosis.

Other tests have been described for diagnosing insulinoma in euglycemic dogs with equivocal serum insulin concentrations. Of these, insulin-to-glucose and glucose-to-insulin ratios are not recommended because of their low sensitivity, and the amended insulin-to-glucose ratio is not recommended because of its low specificity.

Diagnostic imaging

Radiography and ultrasonography

Most dogs with insulinoma have unremarkable abdominal and thoracic radiographs because most insulinomas are quite small (<4 cm) and isoechoic on ultrasonographic examination when compared with surrounding pancreatic parenchyma. Metastases most commonly occur in the liver and regional pancreatic lymph nodes. Abdominal ultrasonography may be helpful in supporting the clinical suspicion of a pancreatic mass (Fig. 39.1) and metastases with a reported sensitivity of around 50-75%.[15] Nonetheless, a negative ultrasonographic examination does not rule either out. Conversely, pancreatic nodules are not specific for insulinoma and may represent changes due to chronic pancreatitis, adenomas, adenocarcinomas, endocrine-active tumors of other cell types (gastrinoma, somatostatinoma), abscesses, and cysts. Recently, contrast-enhanced ultrasound was successfully employed in discriminating insulinoma from pancreatic carcinoma.[19,36]

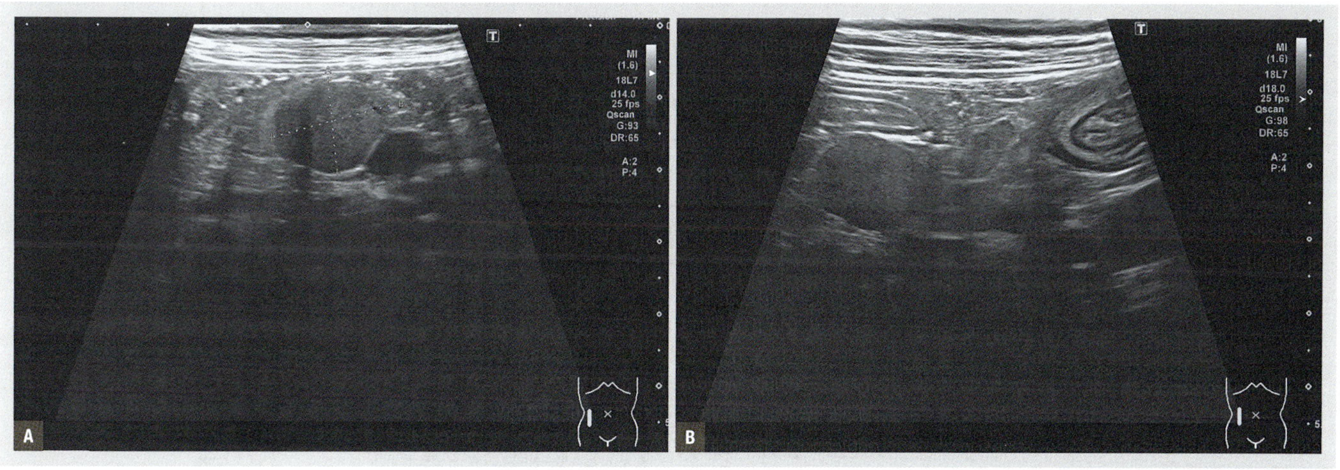

FIG. 39.1 Ultrasonographic image of a discreet mass with heterogenous, mainly hyperechoic echogenicity (approximately 13 × 17 mm) detected in the pancreas of a dog that presented with hypoglycemia. Concurrent insulin concentrations were 87 mU/L (RR: 5-10). Courtesy of Dr. Rowena Watson, Johannesburg Specialist Veterinary Centre.

Advanced diagnostic imaging

High-quality, dual-phase, thin-section multidetector computed tomography (CT) of the pancreas is effective in identifying a pancreatic mass in most affected humans.[34] The use of CT has been reported in a sizeable number of dogs with insulinoma. Contrast-enhanced CT proved more sensitive than ultrasound at detecting insulinomas,[3] and the over-riding majority of cases demonstrated hyperattenuation of the pancreatic and metastatic masses during the arterial phase of the study[6] (Fig. 39.2). Overall arterial phase sensitivity was 94% for detecting insulinomas; nevertheless, noncontrast CT examinations still have some merit, because a high proportion of lesions deformed the shape of the pancreas, rendering them visible on precontrast views.[6] A small case series documented the magnetic resonance imaging appearance of canine insulinomas as displaying a high-intensity signal on T2-weighted images and isointensity on T1-weighted images.[38] Positron emission computed tomography CT (PET-CT) with a glucose analog has also been attempted, but the inconsistent and unpredictable tumoral avidity of canine insulinomas limits the value of PET-CT for staging.[38]

Treatment

Acute treatment

During an acute hypoglycemic crisis, 50% dextrose should be given as a slow IV bolus of 1 ml/kg, diluted to a 1:4 solution in 0.9% sodium chloride). The bolus should be followed with a continuous rate infusion (CRI) of 2.5-5% dextrose. The lowest amount of glucose deemed necessary must be administered because glucose stimulates insulin secretion. This may cause rebound hypoglycemia and a subsequent vicious cycle, which may be difficult to break. In this regard, it must be emphasized that the use of dextrose should be reserved exclusively for severe clinical hypoglycemia. If hypoglycemia is not associated with clinical signs, dextrose should not be used.

Dextrose administration should be discontinued when clinical signs resolve, even if mild hypoglycemia persists. In most dogs, neuroglycopenia will resolve with the administration of dextrose, even without complete resolution of the hypoglycemia. However, some animals fail to respond clinically to dextrose administration alone. In such situations, dexamethasone or prednisolone may be considered.

Glucagon administration may also be helpful because glucagon increases blood glucose concentration by promoting glycogenolysis and gluconeogenesis. While doses vary, a CRI of glucagon of 5-10 ng/kg/min, with or without concurrent 10% dextrose, should increase glucose concentrations and resolve clinical signs. However, like glucose, glucagon also increases insulin secretion, and rebound insulin secretion is always possible but appears to be uncommon when more conservative doses are used.[12]

Some cases may be refractory to dextrose, glucocorticoids and glucagon, and this may be due to persistently high insulin secretion and/or glycogen depletion because of chronic hyperinsulinism. Additionally, prolonged and profound hypoglycemia may result in a series of changes that culminate in cerebral edema and, ultimately, irreversible brain damage. Continued neurological signs, despite normalization of blood glucose concentration, are suggestive of brain damage. If this is considered possible, ancillary treatment for seizures and cerebral edema, such as diazepam, propofol, or pentobarbital, may be implemented, but the prognosis is ultimately poor.

Chronic treatment

Chronic treatment can be divided into medical treatment aimed at the relief of clinical hypoglycemia, surgical treatment, and/or tumor-targeted therapy.

Treatment aimed at relieving clinical hypoglycemia

The main modes of relieving hypoglycemia include dietary modification and treatment with prednisone and/or diazoxide. In addition, synthetic somatostatins can be used, but not as a first choice. Small, frequent meals (every 4 to 6 hours) of a diet high in proteins, fats, and complex

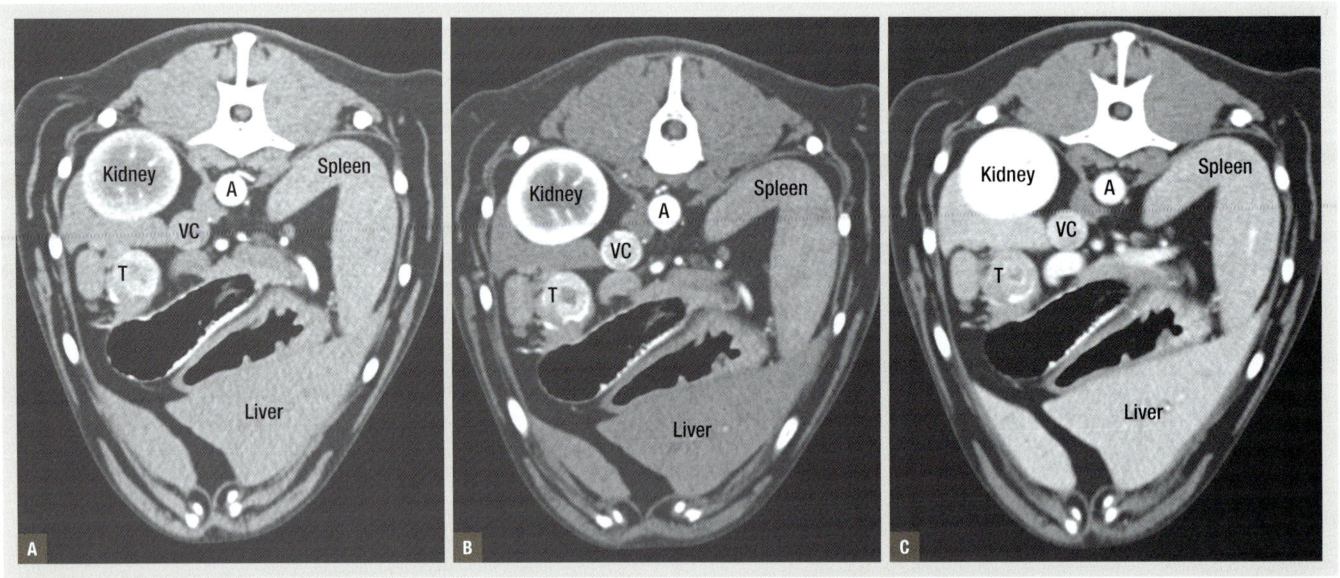

FIG. 39.2 Contrast-enhanced CT image demonstrating a hyperattenuating pancreatic mass during the arterial phase (A), early venous phase (B), and late venous phase (C), subsequently identified as an insulinoma on histopathology. A: aorta, VC: vena cava, T: pancreatic mass. Courtesy of Dr. SA van Nimwegen, Faculty of Veterinary Medicine, Utrecht University.

carbohydrates are recommended. Simple sugars (present in soft, moist dog foods) should be avoided.

Prednisolone, the least expensive and most commonly used drug, increases blood glucose concentration by increasing gluconeogenesis and glucose 6-phosphatase activity while decreasing blood glucose uptake into tissue and stimulating glucagon secretion. Prednisolone is given at an initial oral dose of about 0.2 mg/kg/day, increasing to 0.5 mg/kg/day as needed. Doses can be gradually increased as needed, usually until the drug is no longer perceived to be decreasing seizure episodes or in cases where intolerable signs of iatrogenic hypercortisolism (PU/PD) develop. Corticosteroids at higher doses of 1-2 mg/kg/day may also resolve polyneuropathy in some cases.[35]

Diazoxide is a benzothiadiazine derivative whose main action is to inhibit the closure of pancreatic beta-cell ATP-dependent K^+ channels, preventing beta-cell depolarization and inhibiting the subsequent opening of voltage-dependent Ca^{2+} channels. The resultant decreased Ca^{2+} influx causes decreased exocytosis of insulin-containing secretory vesicles. Diazoxide also increases blood glucose concentration by increasing glycogenolysis and gluconeogenesis and inhibiting tissue uptake of glucose.[1] About 70% of dogs respond to diazoxide doses of 10-40 mg/kg/day PO divided bid or tid. As is the case with prednisone, begin with the lowest dose of diazoxide and gradually increase the dose if required. Side effects in dogs are uncommon and include ptyalism, vomiting, and anorexia.

Octreotide is a long-acting synthetic somatostatin analog whose primary mode of action is the inhibition of insulin secretion through its binding affinity to any of five somatostatin receptor subtypes present in insulin-secreting tumors. Dogs show a variable response to octreotide, likely because octreotide variably inhibits glucagon and GH secretion.[26] If the suppression of glucagon and GH secretion is of greater magnitude and duration compared to the suppression of insulin secretion, octreotide may worsen hypoglycemia. While some canine insulinomas may lack somatostatin receptors, 12 dogs with insulinoma treated with a single octreotide dose of 50 µg/dog SC (median weight 23 kg) had decreases in plasma insulin concentration, yet concentrations of glucagon, GH, and ACTH were not changed.[24] These findings warrant studies on long-acting octreotide therapy in dogs with insulinoma. No adverse side effects were reported with the use of octreotide. Side effects in people include mild pain at the injection site (which is lessened if the preparation is warmed before administration), nausea, vomiting, abdominal pain, constipation, or steatorrhea.

Surgical treatment

The long-term treatment of choice for insulinoma is surgical resection of both the tumor and any obvious metastases. Lately, partial pancreatectomy through an advanced lateral approach has been performed laparoscopically in four clinical cases[13] (Video 39.2). Most tumors are readily discernible or palpable by the surgeon, depending on the surgical technique used (Fig. 39.3). Two dogs have reportedly undergone successful resection of tumor thrombi that had extended into their pancreaticoduodenal veins.[11] In addition, one dog had a prolonged disease-free interval after primary tumor resection despite the presence of metastatic lesions.[28] Surgical

Video 39.2

Video footage of the intraoperative view of the same insulinoma as in Fig. 39.3. Courtesy of Dr. SA van Nimwegen, Faculty of Veterinary Medicine, Utrecht University.

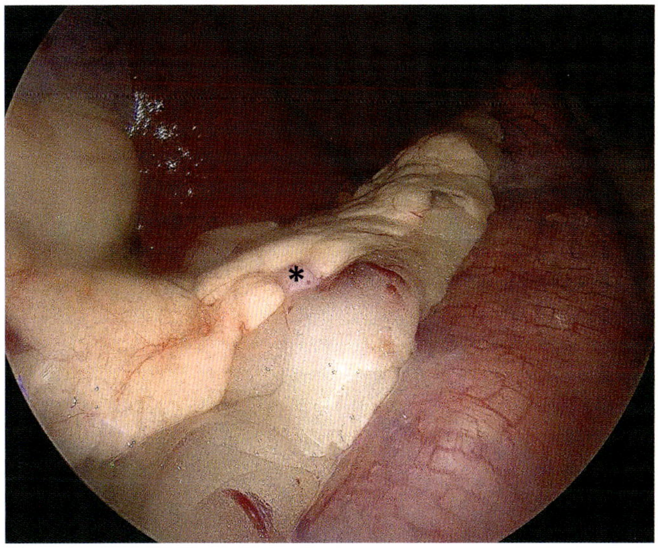

FIG. 39.3 Laparoscopic intraoperative view of an insulinoma (asterix) in the right pancreatic lobe. Courtesy of Dr SA van Nimwegen, Faculty of Veterinary Medicine, Utrecht University.

exploration and biopsy of a pancreatic mass can confirm a diagnosis and may help in estimating survival time. When postoperative hyperglycemia develops, it is usually transient and resolves once the normal beta-cells, which have been suppressed by autonomous insulin secretion from neoplastic cells, regain function. About 10-20 % of dogs with insulinoma develop diabetes mellitus after tumor removal and require exogenous insulin for an unpredictable length of time.[8] Other postoperative complications include pancreatitis, diabetic ketoacidosis, delayed wound healing, cardiac arrhythmias or arrest, hemorrhage, sepsis, and leukopenia.

Tumor-targeted therapy

Toceranib phosphate, a veterinary targeted multi-receptor tyrosine kinase inhibitor that has shown benefit in a range of solid-type tumors in dogs, has recently been evaluated in the treatment of canine insulinoma.[2,10,29] The latter study included 30 dogs, of which 21 underwent partial pancreatectomy prior to toceranib, and nine did not. Various drugs were used together or prior to the scenario, such as doxorubicin, streptozotocin, and vinorelbine. All six dogs that received prednisolone were started with toceranib when persistence or recurrence of hypoglycemia was observed, and 23 dogs that received toceranib were concurrently administered prednisolone at a median dose of 0.5 mg/kg PO once daily. The median oral starting dose of tocenarib was 2.7 mg/kg (range 2-3.3 mg/kg). Most dogs were given this dose on a Monday, Wednesday, and Friday regimen and 67% of dogs with measurable disease experienced either complete remission (CR), partial response (PR), or stable disease (SD) for a minimum of 10 weeks. All aforementioned dogs with CR, PR, or SD were reported to have normoglycemia at each assessment. Their overall median survival time was 656 days. Larger dogs were at increased risk for disease progression, and the most common adverse events were mild gastrointestinal toxicities. Clinical disease progression was defined as a return of clinical signs associated with neuroglycopenia or the development of novel metastases, metastatic progression, and/or local progressive disease according to the canine response evaluation criteria for solid tumors (cRECIST) applied based upon repeated abdominal ultrasound, CT and/or thoracic radiographs when available.[20] It was concluded that toceranib afforded these patients clinical benefits whilst causing minimal adverse events, which included mainly transient gastrointestinal signs. Further adverse events included anemia, neutropenia, and increased liver enzymes, amongst others.

Streptozocin, a nitrosourea antibiotic, selectively destroys beta-cells in pancreatic or metastatic locations. The drug is nephrotoxic in dogs, but diuresis with saline decreases drug contact time with renal tubular epithelial cells and may reduce the risk of nephrotoxicity. In one study, 17 dogs, most of whom had surgery with incomplete resection of gross lesions, were treated with 0.9% sodium chloride (18 mL/kg/h IV) for 3 hours prior to, 2 hours during, and for 2 hours following streptozocin infusion. Streptozocin (500 mg/m^2) was given every 3 weeks for five treatments. Side effects included vomiting, diabetes mellitus, transient hypoglycemia and seizures, transient hyperglycemia, transient increase in alanine aminotransferase activity, azotemia, mild thrombocytopenia, or mild neutropenia. Moreover, 30% of dogs died during treatment, while the median duration of normoglycemia in streptozocin-treated dogs was modest (163-196 days). This is not significantly different from the duration of normoglycemia in dogs that have been treated medically.[18,21]

In sum, the adverse event profile of streptozotocin is much less tolerable than that of toceranib. Therefore, the drug should only be used by experienced personnel, and further studies are necessary before streptozocin therapy can be recommended with confidence.

Prognosis

The median survival time of dogs that underwent partial pancreatectomy, reported in different older studies, was 12 to 14 months with a range of 0 days to 5 years. However, a smaller, more recent study had a median survival time of 26 months,[23] whilst the two latest studies (which had a combined total of 165 dogs) both demonstrated almost identical median survival times after surgery of approximately 20 months.[5,27] It is postulated that earlier recognition and perhaps more radical surgery and better postoperative care account for this improved survival. Moreover, dogs with clinical stage I disease have a significantly longer disease-free interval, whilst those with persistent postoperative hypoglycemia have a poorer prognosis.[5,8]

It was also demonstrated that tumor size and mitotic rate, as depicted by the Ki67 index (a proliferation marker), act as significant prognostic markers in canine insulinoma.[4]

KEY POINTS

- Insulinoma is an insulin-secreting tumor of pancreatic beta-cells that results in excessive insulin secretion and clinical signs ofhypoglycemia.
- Clinical signs are due to hypoglycemia-induced release of catecholamines or due to the effect of hypoglycemia on the central nervous system (neuroglycopenia) and include seizures, weakness, ataxia, collapse, disorientation, and behavior changes, amongst others.
- Low blood glucose 60 mg/dL (<3.3 mmol/L) and concurrent normo- or hyperinsulinemia (serum insulin concentrations within or above reference interval) in combination with the identification of a pancreatic mass through either ultrasonography or computed tomography, are diagnostic. However, many cases do not demonstrate all of these classic findings.
- Acute hypoglycemia should be treated with intravenous dextrose and, in certain cases, together with dexamethasone and/or glucagon constant rate infusion.
- The long-term treatment of choice for insulinoma is surgical resection of both the tumor and any obvious metastases.
- Toceranib phosphate has shown promise as adjuvant therapy and can be attempted as primary treatment in inoperable cases, but prospective randomized trials are required before it can be confidently recommended.

References

1. Alemzadeh R, Holshouser S. Effect of diazoxide on brain capillary insulin receptor binding and food intake in hyperphagic obese Zucker rats. *Endocrinology* 140(7):3197-3202, 1999.
2. Alonso-Miguel, D, Garcia-San Jose P, et al. Evaluation of palliative therapy, alone or in combination with toceranib phosphate, in dogs diagnosed with metastatic or recurrent beta-cell neoplasia. *New Zealand Vet J* 69:234-239, 2021.
3. Buishand FO, Kik M, Kirpensteijn J. Evaluation of clinicopathological criteria and the Ki67 index as prognostic indicators in canine insulinoma. *Vet J* 185(1):62-67, 2010.
4. Buishand, FO, Grosso, FRV, et al. Utility of contrast-enhanced computed tomography in the evaluation of canine insulinoma location. *Vet Quart* 38:53-62, 2018.
5. Cleland NT, et al. Outcome after surgical management of canine insulinoma in 49 cases. *Vet Comp Oncol* 19(3):428-441, 2021.
6. Coss P, Gilman O, Warren-Smith C, Major AC. The appearance of canine insulinoma on dual-phase computed tomographic angiography. *J Small Anim Pract* 62(7):540-546, 2021.
7. Davison, L. J., Podd, S. L., Ristic, J. M., Herrtage, M. E., Parnham, A., & Catchpole, B. Evaluation of two point-of-care analysers for measurement of fructosamine or haemoglobin A1c in dogs. *J Small Anim Pract* 43(12):526-532, 2002.
8. Del Busto I, German A, et al. Incidence of postoperative complications and outcome of 48 dogs undergoing surgical management of insulinoma. *J Vet Intern Med* 34:1135-1143, 2020.
9. Dunn J, Bostock D, Herrtage M, Jackson K, Walker M. Insulin-secreting tumours of the canine pancreas: clinical and pathological features of 11 cases. *J Small Anim Pract* 34(7):325-331,1993.
10. Flesner BK, Fletcher JM, Smithee T, Boudreaux B. Long-term survival and glycemic control with toceranib phosphate and prednisolone for a metastatic canine insulinoma. *J Am Anim Hosp Assoc* 55(1):e55105, 2019.
11. Hambrook LE, Kudnig ST. Tumor thrombus formation in two dogs with insulinomas. *J Am Vet Med Assoc* 241(8):1065-1069, 2012.
12. Harris ME, Weatherton L, Bloch CP. Glucagon therapy in canines with insulinoma: A retrospective descriptive study of 11 dogs. *Can Vet J* 61:737-742, 2020.
13. Keulen JNP, van Nimwegen SA. Laparoscopic partial pancreatectomy through an advanced lateral approach as treatment for insulinoma in dogs: a case series. *Front Vet Sci* 10:1278218, 2023.
14. Kruth SA, Feldman EC, Kennedy PC. Insulin-secreting islet cell tumors: establishing a diagnosis and the clinical course for 25 dogs. *J Am Vet Med Assoc* 181(1):54-58, 1982.
15. Lamb CR, Simpson KW, Boswood A, Matthewman LA. Ultrasonography of pancreatic neoplasia in the dog: a retrospective review of 16 cases. *Vet Rec* 137(3):65-68, 1995.
16. Leifer CE, Peterson ME, Matus RE. Insulin-secreting tumor: diagnosis, medical and surgical management in 55 dogs. *J Am Vet Med Assoc* 188:60-64, 1986.
17. Mellanby RJ, Herrtage ME. Insulinoma in a normoglycaemic dog with low serum fructosamine. *J Small Anim Pract* 43(11):506-508, 2002.
18. Moore AS, Nelson RW, Henry CJ, et al. Streptozocin for treatment of pancreatic islet cell tumors in dogs: 17 cases (1989-1999). *J Am Vet Med Assoc* 221(6): 811-818, 2002.
19. Nakamura K, Lim SY, Ochiai K, et al. Contrast-enhanced ultrasonographic findings in three dogs with pancreatic insulinoma. *Vet Radiol Ultrasound* 56(1):55-62, 2015.
20. Nguyen SM, Tham DH, et al. Response evaluation criteria for solid tumors in dogs (v1.0): a Veterinary Cooperative Oncology Group (VCOG) consensus statement. *Vet Comp Oncol* 13:176-183, 2013.
21. Northrup N, Rassnick K, Gieger T, et al. Prospective evaluation of biweekly streptozotocin in 19 dogs with insulinoma. *J Vet Intern Med* 27(3):483-490, 2013.
22. Polansky BJ, et al. Resolution of hyperinsulinemic hypoglycemia following partial pancreatectomy in a dog with nesidioblastosis. *J Am Vet Med Assoc* 253:893-896, 2018.
23. Polton GA, White RN, Brearley MJ, et al. Improved survival in a retrospective cohort of 28 dogs with insulinoma. *J Small Anim Pract* 48(3):151-156, 2007.
24. Robben JH, van den Brom WE, Mol JA, et al. Effect of octreotide on plasma concentrations of glucose, insulin, glucagon, growth hormone, and cortisol in healthy dogs and dogs with insulinoma. *Res Vet Sci* 80(1):25-32, 2006.
25. Robben JH, Van Garderen E, Mol JA, et al. Locally produced growth hormone in canine insulinomas. *Mol Cell Endocrinol* 197(1-2):187-195, 2002.
26. Robben JH, Visser-Wisselaar HA, Rutteman GR, et al. In vitro and in vivo detection of functional somatostatin receptors in canine insulinomas. *J Nuclear Med* 38(7):1036, 1997.
27. Ryan D, Pérez-Accino J, et al. Clinical findings, neurological manifestations and survival of dogs with insulinoma: 116 cases (2009-2020). *J Small Anim Pract* 62(7):531-539, 2021.
28. Rychel J, Worley DR, Hardy CS, et al. Prolonged survival in an aged Labrador retriever with a metastatic insulinoma. *J Am Anim Hosp Assoc* 49(3):224-229, 2013.
29. Sheppard Olivares S, et al. Toceranib phosphate in the management of canine insulinomas: A retrospective multicentre study of 30 cases (2009-2019). *Vet Rec Open* 9(1):e27, 2022.
30. Slye M, Wells H. Tumor of islet tissue with hyperinsulinism in a dog. *Archived Pathol* 19:537, 1935.
31. Syme HM, Scott-Moncrieff JC. Chronic hypoglycaemia in a hunting dog due to secondary hypoadrenocorticism. *J Small Anim Pract* 39(7):348-351, 1998.
32. Tobin RL, Nelson RW, Lucroy MD, Wooldridge JD, Feldman EC. Outcome of surgical versus medical treatment of dogs with beta cell neoplasia: 39 cases (1990-1997). *J Am Vet Med Assoc* 215(2):226-230, 1999.
33. Trifonidou MA, Kirpensteijn J, Robben JH. A retrospective evaluation of 51 dogs with insulinoma. *Vet Quart* 20(Suppl 1):S114-115, 1998.
34. Tucker ON, Crotty PL, Conlon KC. The management of insulinoma. *British J Surg* 93(3):264-275, 2006.
35. Van Ham L, et al. Treatment of a dog with an insulinoma-related peripheral polyneuropathy with corticosteroids. *Vet Rec* 141:98-100, 1997.
36. Vanderperren K, et al. Description of the use of contrast-enhanced ultrasonography in four dogs with pancreatic tumours. *J Small Anim Pract* 55(3):164-169, 2014.
37. Walczak R, et al. Canine insulinomas appear hyperintense on MRI T2-weighted images and isointense on T1-weighted images. *Vet Radiol Ultrasound* 60:330-337, 2019.
38. Walczak R, et al. Fluorine-18 fluorodeoxyglucose positron emission tomography-computed tomography for staging of canine insulinoma: 3 cases (2019-2020). *J Small Anim Pract* 63:227-233, 2022.

Index

B

C

D

E

F

G

H

I